Health Politics and Policy

4th edition

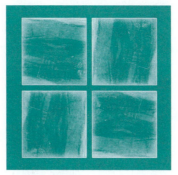

James A. Morone, Theodor J. Litman, and Leonard S. Robins

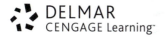

DELMAR
CENGAGE Learning™

Australia • Brazil • Japan • Korea • Mexico • Singapore • Spain • United Kingdom • United States

DELMAR
CENGAGE Learning

Health Politics and Policy
Fourth Edition
James A. Morone, Theodor
J. Litman, and Leonard S. Robins

Director of Learning Solutions:
Matthew Kane

Acquisitions Editor:
Kalen Conerly

Product Manager:
Natalie Pashoukos

Editorial Assistant:
Meaghan O'Brien

Marketing Director:
Jennifer McAvey

Marketing Manager:
Michele McTighe

Marketing Coordinator:
Chelsey Iaquinta

Production Director:
Carolyn Miller

Content Project Manager:
Thomas Heffernan

Senior Art Director:
Jack Pendleton

Technology Product Manager:
Mary Colleen Liburdi

Technology Project Manager:
Erin Zeggert

Windows is a registered trademark of the Microsoft Corporation used herein under license. Macintosh and Power Macintosh are registered trademarks of Apple Computer, Inc. Used herein under license.

© 2008 Delmar, a part of Cengage Learning. All Rights Reserved.

Library of Congress Control Number: 2007940816

ISBN-13: 978-1-4180-1428-5

ISBN-10: 1-4180-1428-1

Delmar Cengage Learning
5 Maxwell Drive
Clifton Park, NY 12065-2919
USA

Cengage Learning products are represented in Canada by Nelson Education, Ltd.

For your lifelong learning solutions, visit **delmar.cengage.com**

Visit our corporate website at **www.cengage.com**

Notice to the Reader
Publisher does not warrant or guarantee any of the products described herein or perform any independent analysis in connection with any of the product information contained herein. Publisher does not assume, and expressly disclaims, any obligation to obtain and include information other than that provided to it by the manufacturer. The reader is expressly warned to consider and adopt all safety precautions that might be indicated by the activities described herein and to avoid all potential hazards. By following the instructions contained herein, the reader willingly assumes all risks in connection with such instructions. The publisher makes no representations or warranties of any kind, including but not limited to, the warranties of fitness for particular purpose or merchantability, nor are any such representations implied with respect to the material set forth herein, and the publisher takes no responsibility with respect to such material. The publisher shall not be liable for any special, consequential, or exemplary damages resulting, in whole or part, from the readers' use of, or reliance upon, this material.

Printed in the United States of America
1 2 3 4 5 6 7 11 10 09 08 07

TABLE OF CONTENTS

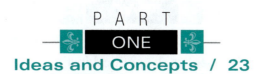

but unexpected truth: You can't have one without the other. The key question for every health care system is how to balance the two.

We usually think of public health care as scientific and secular. But there is a powerful moral component running through the ways we talk and think about public health. Here's how moral ideas shape our health policies. The chapter ends with two illustrations of moral politics in action: Obesity and School Health Care Centers.

This section adds an important point to our consideration of ideas and concepts: All health politics are not alike. There are four different types to keep in mind. Lawrence Brown explains what they are.

P A R T
TWO

Political Institutions   /   71

Part II describes the political institutions that make health care policy.

Congress has been both friend and foe of health policy. What it enacts, what it ignores, and what it defeats all tell us a great deal about America's unique legislative process.

Americans both cheer and fear strong presidents—as a result, the office has broad powers and deep constraints. Whether or not they win the laws they propose, all presidents leaves behind an important legacy: the way we think and talk about health policy.

American health law continues has been shaped by three models, each dominant in a particular historical period: the authority of the medical profession, the egalitarian social contract, and market competition.

P A R T

━━ THREE ━━

The Health Policy Process: Interest groups,
Stakeholders, and Public opinion / 201

Part III analyzes the private players. These are societal forces that interact
with government to shape our health care policies. The first two articles
provide the long historical view. Then the familiar heroes and villains.

P A R T

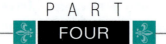

FOUR

Outcomes: Programs, Policies, and Problems / 309

Now, we put it all together. Here's how ideas (from Part I), the public institutions (Part II), and private interests (Part III) come together. Here are
the problems they face, and the programs they have made.

P A R T

FIVE

The United States in International Perspective / 415

Part V helps us understand our own system by contrasting it to it to others. Studying other nations teaches us about ourselves—by informing us
what is common among all nations and what is unique in the choices
we have made.

Dedication

To Our Mentors:
Theodore Marmor, Arnold M. Rose, and Robert T. Holt

Many students encounter a teacher who inspires them and changes their life. The three editors dedicate this book to the teachers who most inspired us.

First, Ted Marmor. If there's a mentor to an entire field, it's Theodore R. Marmor. Almost every author in this volume has been inspired by him. He guided many of us to our first jobs or book contracts. Ted got Jim Morone interested in health politics, directed his Ph.D., and mentored him through his career. More important, Marmor teaches us all by example: Ted's brilliant mind is always—always—focused by his passionate commitment to building a better society.

Arnold M. Rose was a celebrated sociologist, author of some fifteen books and over a hundred articles. Len Robins took a class with Professor Rose at the University of Minnesota and ended up becoming friends with the teaching assistant, Theodor Litman. Rose inspired both Litman and Robins. Arnold Rose died in his 40s, but lives on through the students he inspired—and this book that you hold your hands.

Robert T. Holt was Len Robins undergraduate and graduate advisor. A political scientist who specialized in comparative politics, Robins calls him one of the brightest and wisest people he's ever met—a true polymath. Professor Holt talked Len out of going to law school and got him a graduate fellowship to the University of Michigan. Like so many great teachers, he literally changed Len's life.

Contributors

Patricia M. Alt, Ph.D.
Professor
Department of Health Science
Towson University
Towson, Maryland

Robert Blendon, Sc.D.
Professor of Health Policy and Political Analysis
John F. Kennedy School of Government
Harvard University
Cambridge, Massachusetts

David Blumenthal, M.D.
Samuel O. Their Professor of Medicine and
   Professor of Health Policy
Harvard Medical School
and
Physician
Massachusetts General Hospital
Boston, Massachusetts

William P. Brandon, Ph.D., MPH
Metrolina Medical Foundation Distinguished
   Professor of Health Policy
Department of Political Science
University of North Carolina Charlotte
Charlotte, North Carolina

Mollyann Brodie
Vice President and Director of Public Opinion
   and Media Research
Henry J. Kaiser Family Foundation
Menlo Park, California

Lawrence Brown, B.A., Ph.D.
Professor of Health Policy and Management
School of Health Policy and Management
Columbia University
New York, New York

Daniel C. Ehlke
Doctoral candidate
Department of Political Science
Brown University
Providence, Rhode Island

Robert G. Evans, O.C., Ph.D., FRSC
Killam Professor (Economics)
University of British Columbia
and
Institute Fellow
Canadian Institute for Advanced Research
Vancouver, British Columbia
Canada

James W. Fossett
Associate Professor
Rockefeller College of Public Affairs and Policy
University at Albany, State University
    of New York
Albany, New York

Richard Freeman, Ph.D.
Senior Lecturer
School of Social and Political Studies
University of Edinburgh
George Square, Edinburgh
United Kingdom

Colleen M. Grogan, Ph.D.
Associate Professor
School of Social Service Administration
The University of Chicago
Chicago, Illinois

Jacob S. Hacker, Ph.D.
Professor of Political Science
Institution for Social and Policy Studies
Yale University
New Haven, Connecticut

Rogan Kersh, Ph.D.
Associate Dean and Associate Professor for
    Academic Affairs
NYU Wagner School
New York, New York

Elizabeth Kilbreth, Ph.D.
Associate Research Professor
Edmund Muskie School of Public Affairs
University of Southern Maine
Portland, Maine

Howard M. Leichter, Ph.D.
Professor and Chair, Department of
    Political Science
Linfield College
Department of Political Science
McMinnville, Oregon

Donald W. Light, Ph.D.
Professor of Comparative Health Care Systems
University of Medicine & Dentistry of New Jersey
Fellow at the Netherlands Institute for
    Advanced Study
Camden, New Jersey

Theodore R. Marmor
Professor Emeritus, Public Policy &
    Management
School of Management
Yale University
New Haven, Connecticut

Cathie Jo Martin
Professor
Department of Political Science
Boston University
Boston, Massachusetts

Jonathon Oberlander
Associate Professor of Social Medicine
University of North Carolina
Chapel Hill, North Carolina

Kieke Okma
Adjunct Associate Professor
Robert Wagner School
New York University
New York, New York

Mark Peterson
Professor of Public Policy and Political Science
UCLA School of Public Affairs
Los Angeles, California

Tom Rice, Ph.D.
Professor
Department of Health Services
UCLA School of Public Health
Los Angles, California

Rand E. Rosenblatt, J.D.
Professor of Law
Rutgers University School of Law–Camden
Camden, New Jersey

Patricia Siplon
Professor of Political Science
St. Michael's College
Colchester, Vermont

Deborah Stone, Ph.D.
Research Professor of Government
Dartmouth College
Hanover, New Hampshire

Frank J. Thompson, Ph.D.
Professor
Rockefeller College of Public Affairs and Policy
University at Albany, State University
    of New York
Albany, New York

Kelly Tzoumis
Associate Professor and Director of Public
    Policy Studies
DePaul University
Chicago, Illinois

Joseph White, Ph.D.
Luxenberg Family Professor of Public Policy
Chair, Department of Political Science
Director, Center for Policy Studies
Case Western Reserve University
Cleveland, Ohio

Preface

James A. Morone

Reverend James—a slight, handsome, black man— sat and read in the cramped study of his small Dallas church. One passage from the New Testament leapt out at him: Jesus hugged the leper. With a start, Reverend James realized he had been wrong to banish people with AIDS from the congregation. He had said that disease was God's punishment for immorality—but if Jesus hugged the leper, thought James, then he must be telling us to hug our own afflicted neighbors. He picked up the phone and called Leroy, a young man with AIDS, and invited him to come back to church.

The following Sunday Reverend James read the bible passage about the leper and told his congregation that a person with AIDS stood among them. The men and women stirred—it was the 1980s and people were not sure exactly how one contracted AIDS. At the time there was no effective treatment— diagnosis meant death. Reverend James ploughed ahead: "I want you to hug a stranger near you, he said, and as you do, imagine that you're giving comfort to a person with AIDS." The congregation broke into embraces. When they had finished, Reverend James saw tears streaming down Leroy's cheeks. That simple act of kindness "meant more than the world to me," he later said. Then James looked at the large, cheerful

woman standing next to him. Knowing he could count on her, James had asked her to stand by Leroy's side. Tears were streaming down her cheeks too. "Thank you," she told the minister after the service, "thank you for putting your faith in me."

The simple hug on an ordinary Sunday fired up this poor, black, Dallas congregation. They crowded around Reverend James after the service and asked what more they could do to minister to the AIDS community. They began to meet and brainstorm about ways they could help. Eventually, the congregation became famous for helping people with AIDS.

Health care begins with the spirit of that Dallas congregation. Health care is about providing help and comfort. After one especially contentious policy debate, I heard a medical student ask the Vice President of the American Medical Association a loaded question. "If you had it all to do over again, would you still go into this profession, troubled as it is?" "Oh yes," replied the physician. "When I look in the mirror in the morning, I see someone who takes care of people, who helps them stay healthy." Under all the sophisticated analyses of the health care system runs that simple thought: Health care providers minister to their fellow human beings.

But, of course, health care quickly gets a whole lot more complicated.

My friend and former student, Gary B., is head of psychiatry in the emergency room of a large hospital in New York City. On a busy summer night he sees our society's most disheartening cases—feral children worn down by the streets, homeless adults with endless troubles, battered people, and even predators. What makes Gary really furious, however, is the way his hands are tied when he treats the patients in his emergency room.

"Constantly after I see people who have tried to kill themselves," he says. "First, I stabilize them. Then I determine whether they are at high risk to try again. Then I check their insurance." Gary can usually tell if someone is going to attempt suicide again. If they are—and they have good health insurance—he can do a lot for them: He hospitalizes them, prescribes drugs, organizes a treatment regimen, and, if possible, talks to their family and friends. But if they have no health insurance (or if they have inadequate coverage and the insurance company refuses to pay for these services), he simply patches them up and sends them back out on the street. He knows—knows for a fact—that many will be back and that some will be beyond help when they return.

Every health provider knows this story. They know what their patients need—prescription drugs, therapy, specialist care—but can not find a way to pay for it. Again and again, health providers describe this as their biggest frustration. They believe they know what the patient needs but someone else decides if the patient is actually going to get it.

If the first story suggests the inspiring side of medicine, this second reminds us how frustrating our health care system has gotten. To many observers, it seems crazy—why, they ask, can't we just treat people who need treatment? More and more health decisions lie, not in the providers', hands, but in a great bureaucracy.

And that brings us to one last story.

Professor Robert Kane went to a large hospital in Ontario, Canada and asked a simple question. "Could I meet the staff members involved in sending out bills for hospital services?" He was introduced to four pleasant people. Since the provincial government pays most health care costs in Canada, the billing procedures are not very complicated.

Kane then went to a comparable hospital across the river in Detroit, Michigan and asked the same question. The hospital administrator laughed and handed him a list of roughly 125 people. They had a large administrative suite—practically a whole wing—to themselves. The hospital needed people to bill Blue Cross, Prudential, Cigna, and scores of private insurance companies. Other administrators in the Detroit hospital specialized in billing Medicare, Medicaid, and other government programs. When my former student, Dr. Gary, wants to treat his patients, the case quickly winds up in an administrative wing like this one. The hospital has to make ends meet. All these administrators send out bills to payers who are trying to cut their own costs in order to offer lower premiums and generate more business. Thousands of people in our hospitals, insurance companies, and government agencies negotiate with one another over who will pay how much for which patients.

Many reformers leap at Dr. Kane's study. All those bureaucrats tie the providers' hands and run up enormous costs. If Canada does not need them, why do we? If we streamline our own system, reason the reformers, we could spend more of our health care dollars on actually treating people. Others point out that all those administrative jobs are just that—jobs. Cutting back on administration would mean cutting back on health care jobs. And the really hard part comes when we start discussing just how we might want to change the system. All changes help some and harm others. Consequently, all change—all health care—involves plenty of politics. And that's what this book is all about.

POLITICS AND POLICY

If you're going to enter the health care world—as a provider, administrator, or patient—you need to know how we make decisions about your world. Some people think of politics as a dirty business. But when you stop and think about it, politics is really nothing more than how we as a society, make decisions that affect us all. And politics—our joint decisions—touch every aspect of health care.

Health politics range from the impulse to minister to others to the more complicated interaction in the emergency room and on to the thousands of decisions made by thousands of people in hospitals, clinics, government agencies, insurance companies, business corporations, and even at home at the kitchen table. All these people are guided by the rules we make as a society. Health politics and policy is about those guiding rules—how we make them, what they look like, how they might be changed.

In the pages that follow, you'll learn a great deal about health care politics and policy. But the details all add up to something more important. You'll come to understand just how politics works in the United States and how we make decisions for our society and its health system. Those decisions touch every aspect of health and health care.

PURPOSE OF THIS TEXT

You'll notice that each chapter is written by a different person. For this edition, 20 entirely new chapters have been written—it's a whole new book. In every case, we've invited the top national and international experts to write about the area that they know best. They're not just repeating what others have written. They are summarizing their own lifetime of research and experience.

The authors are not just academics. Many are active in the politics of health care. They testify before Congress, advise presidents, and participate on panels sponsored by scientific groups. For them, this is more than a job—it is a passion. They're in this business because they want to improve the American health care system. Of course, they don't all agree on what we ought to do. You will encounter plenty of different perspectives in the pages of this book. But, in a way, all of our authors are like the enthusiastic congregation following Reverend James: They're committed to making a difference.

And so can you. The American political system invites participation. You can read this book as way of learning all about health politics and policy—you'll understand what our system looks like and how and why it looks that way. Or, you can read it as way of understanding how we make political decisions. Or, you can take it a step further and use it as a primer for getting involved in the system yourself. Together with the authors of all the chapters, I invite you to read our book, reflect on where you stand, and get involved in our great national debate on health politics and policy.

ORGANIZATION

A brief word about how we organized this book. The *Introduction* gives you an overview of the subject—this is your roadmap to health politics and policy. We think *Part I* is unique: we focus on the ideas and concepts that shape health care politics and policy—after all, ideas change the world. *Part II* gets to the political nitty gritty: the government institutions that make health policy—Congress, presidents, courts, states, and so on. *Part III* turns to the private interests and groups that play an important part in framing out decisions—for example, business corporations, doctors, lobbyists and public opinion. Then, in *Part IV*, we put it all together. Here's how ideas (from *Part I*), the government institutions (*Part II*), and private interests (*Part III*) come together. We describe the problems they all face and the programs they have made. Finally, *Part V* helps us understand our own health care system by contrasting it to it to others. In some ways, the United States is unique, in other ways we look a lot like other nations. *Part V* is designed to give you a perspective on American health politics and policy.

NEW TO THIS EDITION

At the end of each Part in the text, you will find a short essay—labeled *Consider This…*—that offers an additional, brief discussion of an important topic. Each one has a special angle: It might be a personal essay, a concrete case, an additional idea, or a top 20 list.

We have also included study questions at the end of each chapter. The questions are a fun way to review the material. Some simply point to the most important features of the chapter. Others are designed to get you thinking about where you stand on the relevant issues – clarifying your own view is the first step toward plunging into the fascinating world of health politics and policy.

ACKNOWLEDGMENTS

Finally, a big thanks to the team at Delmar Cengage Learning: Natalie Pashoukos, Kalen Conerly, Maureen Rosener, Meaghan O'Brien, Thomas Heffernan, and Laurie Traver. Additional thanks to Tim Rodes. Thanks, also, to Daniel Ehlke who wrote the study questions, the teacher's manual, the PowerPoint presentation, and helped keep the entire book on track. Finally, we are grateful for editorial assistance from Si-Han Hai and Miriam Straus.

Reviewers

Amelia Broussard, Ph.D., RN, MPH
Associate Professor of Health Care Management
College of Professional Studies
Clayton State University
Morrow, Georgia

Bruce Busbee, MPH
Instructor/Professor of Health Services Management
Webster University–Columbia Metro
Columbia, South Carolina

Dena Fisher
Assistant Commissioner
Westchester County Department of Health
New Rochelle, New York

William Hayes, Ph.D.
Adjunct Faculty
Ohio State University
Columbus, Ohio
and
President
Health Policy Institute of Ohio
Columbus, Ohio

Louise Kaplan, Ph.D., ARNP
Assistant Professor
Washington State University
Vancouver, Washington

Donna Malvey, Ph.D., MHSA
Assistant Professor
Health Services Administration Program
University of Central Florida - Cocoa Campus
Cocoa, Florida

Cynthia Massie Mara, Ph.D.
Associate Professor of Health Care Administration and Policy
Pennsylvania State University
Harrisburg, Pennsylvania

Sara Rosenbaum, J.D.
Professor and Chair,
Department of Health Policy
George Washington University
Washington, DC

INTRODUCTION

Health Politics and Policy

James A. Morone

People who live in my small town of Lempster, New Hampshire make a ritual of taking their trash to the dump every Sunday afternoon. For years, a man named Darrell managed the dump. Darrell was a mess—an unshaven, sometimes scowling, tortured-looking guy who often had beer on his breath. A couple of years ago, Darrell quit his post. A few weeks later, I ran into him at the country store. He was a different man—shaved, clear eyed, cheerful. Darrell explained that he had gotten a job with the state highway. Though he was now making a good salary, he was most enthusiastic about the new health insurance his family now enjoyed— he had gotten all his cavities filled and was wearing prescription eyeglasses. For the first time in his adult life, Darrell did not have a toothache. And he could see clearly.

Welcome to the fascinating, complicated, sometimes painful world of American health politics and policy. Wealthy people fly from all over the world for treatments at the great medical centers in Houston, Boston, and New York. Nine out of ten Americans tell survey researchers that they are satisfied with the care they received at their last doctor's visit. And yet, there are 47 million people in Darrell's shoes—no health insurance, spotty health care, plenty of aches. In fact, compared to other

countries, we are not very healthy at all. The United States ranks 31st—31st!—in life expectancy at birth for men—slipping behind nations like Croatia and the sultanate of Brunei.[1]

Does the USA have outstanding health care, quite possibly the best in the world? Yes! Is American health care a mess, many would say a disgrace? Yes, again! This book explores how we got here and what we can do about it.

If you are new to health policy, you're in for a lot of surprises. Let's start out with one of the most basic. Who pays for our health care? Everyone knows the old cliché: for better or worse, the United States is the only wealthy nation without national health insurance. That's true. Does it mean that most Americans pay for health care through private insurance? No.

POLITICS IS EVERYWHERE

The biggest health care payer in the United States is the government, which pays for 44% of all American health care spending. The government spending mostly comes from two programs: Medicare (mainly for people over 65) pays 19% of our total health care bill, Medicaid (a rapidly changing program originally for low income people) pays 18%, and all other federal, state, and local programs add another 7%.

Traditionally, working people get their health insurance through employers; private insurance accounts for 36% of our health spending—that's right, the government has a larger share of the spending pie than the insurance companies. (You can see the entire pie in Figure I-1.) But even private health insurance is not a completely private matter. Congress uses tax breaks to induce employers to offer health insurance to employees—there are no taxes on the money employers pay for their worker's health insurance (in contrast, if the employer paid the same amount directly to employees so that they could buy their own health insurance, the tax breaks would not apply). The tax subsidy tops $100 billion a year in foregone revenues. Why do we put so much public money into private health insurance? Back in the 1940s and 1950s, many policy makers saw employee health insurance as a way to spread health care benefits without relying on government health insurance. So they offered business the incentive. And once you offer a tax break, it is difficult to take it away. In 2007, President George W. Bush proposed changing the system, but the proposal was rebuffed my members of both parties. Challenging a $100 billion tax break is never popular.

There is another loaded category on our spending table. Sixteen percent of payments are labeled 'out of pocket'—patients paying directly for their care. This was Darrell's category before he got the good job. Half of all personal bankruptcies are lurking here. Even families with health insurance can be ruined by the co-payments that come with a serious illness. Listen carefully to news reports about labor strikes; the fight often turns, not on salary but on an employer's effort to reduce health expenditure by getting employees to pay more of the cost. Some observers (mainly liberals) decry the growing out-of-pocket costs; they believe that

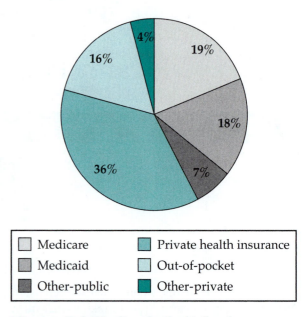

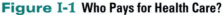

Figure I-1 **Who Pays for Health Care?**

putting this financial burden on individuals and families means that sick people won't get care and that serious illnesses will ruin families. They call on government to take up the slack. Others (mainly conservative economists) say we're finally getting a proper market in health care; consumers can best judge for themselves whether they wish to spend their money on more health care or on other goods and services. Let people chose, they say, between saving for health care or a bigger house or a more expensive college. The conservatives call on government to recast both public and private insurance in order to foster such market conditions. Many would start by repealing that tax break for employer health insurance. Some (like President George W. Bush) would shift the tax break to individuals, others would try and legislate a limit on a family's total health bill (say 10% of their income), and still others would leave the entire business to market forces.

You can already see the bottom line: politics runs into every nook and cranny of American health care. Any health care question you can think of—Who pays? Whose teeth hurt? Where will they build this hospital? What happens after a terrorist attack? Will your parents end up in a nursing home? Is there a right to life? How about a right to die?—ends up being a political question.

What is politics? It's simply how we make decisions for the whole society. Decisions that we enforce with rules, laws, and money. If you go to a hospital, a doctor, a pharmacy, an aroma therapist, or a simple walk in the woods, your experience is going to be shaped by thousands of political choices—made in your town, your state, and in Washington DC. Political decisions are different than individual economic calculations or family decisions. And here's the key: *there is a distinct logic to political decisions*. That is the point of this book. The different chapters add up. You'll learn a great deal about different political institutions (like Congress or the courts), policy choices (why do we have employer based health insurance?) the political process (public opinion, lobbyists) or specific policy programs (like Medicare and Medicaid). As you read from chapter to chapter, you'll learn something more subtle: how to understand the political world. You'll learn the logic that built and runs our health care system—and the logic by which it can be reformed.

THE STAGES OF THE POLITICAL PROCESS

Let's begin with a road map. Every public policy passes through a series of stages—running from first inspiration (the classic light bulb goes off) to the routine administration (bureaucrats shuffle papers). Each stage has its own distinctive tone, tactics, and standard procedures. Television coverage is invaluable at some points in the process and not at others. Savvy policy analysts always know just where their project stands in the process. But they have to be alert—the stage can change in a flash.

1. Setting the Agenda

A sensible engineer would expect political leaders to see problems coming and then search for efficient solutions. Lose that thought, politics does not work that way. At any moment, there are a huge number of problems that *could* grab national attention and become an issue. A handful of those problems beat out the competition and rise to the political surface; the media then run stories on the problem, people discuss it, constituents demand action. We say the problem (or issue) has become part of our political agenda.

For example, in the final three months of 1999, the national media ran fewer than a dozen stories about obesity. It was not a political issue. Then, in 2001, the Surgeon General issued an alarming report about an obesity epidemic. Over 65% of Americans were overweight, 31% clinically obese, and the health consequences—in illness and premature death—were high and growing. Suddenly obesity was all over the news. By the final quarter of 2002, the stack of media stories topped 1,200—a thousand-fold increase. People were obese in 1999. But this Surgeon General's report—like the Surgeon General's report on tobacco 25 years earlier—set off a great national debate. It put obesity on the agenda. Fat had gotten into politics.[2]

What else was rising up the national agenda around the same time? Public health and bioterrorism (thanks to the anthrax scare that followed 9/11); rising prescription drug costs (which both parties seized on as a campaign issue); social security reform (a favorite with the George W. Bush administration); and the question of whether the federal government should fund stem cell research (a hot-button issue for activists in both parties).

Now think of some of the other problems that failed to make it onto the agenda: Seven million Americans were at high risk of homelessness. Life expectancy in poor neighborhoods was terrible—that's why our health data lag behind every other wealthy nation. Soaring nursing home costs were also squeezing American elders (right along with prescription drug costs). And most independent actuaries were warning that Medicare's long-term financing looked a lot shakier than Social Security's. These alternative issues—which could (and many people thought should) have replaced some of the issues on the national agenda—sat in the background, wallflowers in our great political dance.

Problems don't rise to the agenda on their own. The battle of ideas produces political winners. Political campaigns are all about agenda formation. Elected officials use their office to put things on the agenda. Events regularly thrust items forward. The media grab one issue and ignore another. Agenda formation is more art than science. But one thing is certain: Your favorite policy is not going anywhere until it makes it onto the agenda.

And never forget the other side, the important issues that fail to get a hearing. Reformers sometimes lament the way powerful lobbies raise money, peddle influence, and defeat reforms. But that's nothing. Really deep power involves avoiding the battles altogether by keeping matters off the political agenda in the first place. Or, to put it another way, the nation's political agenda marks the limits or our political imagination and will.

2. Policy Formulation

Once a problem hits the agenda, policy makers devise solutions. Every problem has countless potential answers: We can educate, subsidize, tax, regulate, or ignore; we can rely on individuals, on markets, on local government, on states, or on Washington DC.

Take the range of answers to obesity. We could exhort people to exercise. Educate them in food nutrition. Improve nutrition labeling to guide better choices. Design tax incentives to join health clubs. Give entrepreneurs incentives to start health clubs. Redesign school lunch programs. Remove soda machines from schools (or fill them with juices and water). Tax fatty foods. Tax sugary foods. Ban fast food advertising on children's television programs. Sue fast food chains.

Every one of these alternatives has been tried somewhere in the world. But only a couple have gotten much traction in the United States. No state

is going to put a big tax on candy bars or ban television advertisements for sugary cereal. But limiting soda in schools, improving food labels, and educating consumers has gotten a great deal of political play; and people are suing fast food restaurants.

Here's a strange twist to the politics of policy formulation: The solution to the problem often precedes the problem itself. Many individuals and groups have a "pet" program they're anxious to try. The familiar trick is to wait for the agenda to offer up a likely problem and then announce that you have the perfect solution. That's why the exact same "solutions" keep coming up as an answer to different problems. For example, many health specialists think health maintenance organizations (HMOs) are a good idea. Originally, their champions saw HMOs as a way to ensure continuity of care—a full range of health services under one roof. Then the health care cost crisis hit. The solution? HMOs! Since patients paid one flat fee at the beginning of the year regardless of how much care they consumed, supporters touted HMOs as a cost control device. When the number of uninsured people rose onto the agenda, some policy analysts had a handy solution: HMOs! Worried about the quality of medicine? You guessed it, HMOs again. When a president gravely announces a dramatic new policy—President Lyndon Johnson's War on Poverty or President George W. Bush's War on Terror—mischievous political scientists like to go back and expose the many items that had been proposed (sometimes many times) long before the grave new crisis. The changing political agenda simply gave proponents of an old idea a fresh opportunity to come running in from the political sidelines with their bold "new" plans.

3. Policy Adoption

The next stage brings us to an actual decision. This may occur in many different places: Congress, the state legislature, the courts, a presidential executive order. For health policy, most big decisions eventually require action from Congress or the state legislature.

Environmental programs, on the other hand, place more emphasis on court battles and executive orders. And foreign policy shifts that balance still further toward the executive branch.

Every institution has its own process for making these decisions. The US Congress, for example, is famous for its multiple checks and balances. When the British House of Commons considers a health program, it forms a standing committee chaired by the Minister of Health, who is also a member of Parliament. In contrast, when the Clinton administration sent its national health insurance proposal to Congress, 31 different committees and subcommittees tried to claim some sliver of jurisdiction over the plan. Seven actually won a place in the process. Each felt free to substitute its own proposal for the one the president had submitted. And, in contrast to most parliamentary systems, our Constitution bars members of Congress from holding posts in the bureaucracy. As you'll see in Chapter 4, some leaders have become famous for negotiating the American legislative process; many others spend their careers ensnared in the checks built into our system.

This is the high-profile stage. If it is an important issue, the media focus on the speeches, tactics, and vote count. National Public Radio and C-Span record the debate. Demonstrations, letter writing campaigns, and highly public lobbying are all part of the process. The president or the governor will often weigh in and try to whip up public support for or against the proposed legislation. Important court cases get similar treatment.

4. Implementation

When programs pass, all that attention suddenly vanishes. The television cameras click off, the demonstrators put down their signs and go home. As the policy moves into the shadows, some of the most important work begins. Public officials in the executive branch (for health programs, often the Department of Health and Human Services) write the rules that determine how the program will actually run.

Implementation can become extremely complicated. After all, legislation can be controversial, contradictory, or just plain unrealistic. Legislators who disagree might decide to avoid conflict by passing the hot political potatoes on to the bureaucrats.

Implementation decisions seem very technical. Experts negotiate reimbursement formulae and talk in acronyms. But they are just as important as the decisions made in the limelight. Let's look at a few examples:

In 1965, Congress passed Medicare over the furious opposition of the American Medical Association. While the program was being debated (stage 3), the doctors blasted the proposal calling it "socialism," "communism," and "bureaucracy run amok." Once Medicare had passed, however, medical leaders dropped the harsh talk, rolled up their sleeves, and negotiated some extraordinary provisions. Medicare officials agreed to pay providers their "reasonable costs"—basically, anything the providers charged. In order to avoid the stigma of "government bureaucracy run amok," the implementers avoided any direct fiscal control over doctors or hospitals. Instead, private insurance companies would process the payments (a marvelous, risk-free bit of business for them). Hospitals could choose their own insurance companies (or "intermediaries"), guaranteeing that the companies would not aggressively dispute charges or squeeze costs. The predictable result: Medicare proved a financial bonanza for medical providers. Health care costs spiked. And the political agenda had a new issue, though it would be almost 20 years before the federal government (under the Reagan administration) managed to rethink the way Medicare paid health care providers. All these effects were a direct result of implementation decisions.

The implementers can even appear to override portions of the legislation. For example, in 1946, Congress passed the Hospital Construction Act (known as Hill-Burton). Over the next 35 years, Hill-Burton funded a third of all hospital construction in the United States. As a concession to the liberals, Congress required hospitals that won federal funds to provide "a reasonable volume of . . . services to persons unable to pay." Now the implementers had a decision: How to define "reasonable"? They solved that problem by simply ignoring the provision. Twenty-five years later a poverty group sued a hospital for failing to provide the required charity care. The court ruled against the group by noting that regulations had never been written for the provision. In effect, the implementing officials had put aside a section of the legislation.[3]

The Civil Rights Act of 1964 offers another dramatic example. The law forbids discrimination on the basis of race, sex, creed, or national origin. While implementation focused on racial discrimination, the provisions for sexual discrimination were originally ignored. One Congresswoman went so far as to remind the implementing federal officials that they had to "uphold the entire law, not just the parts of it that they are interested in."[4]

The entire process gets even more complex for the many programs that involve both the federal government and the states (like Medicaid). Federal legislation and federal implementation have to be matched by legislation in 50 state laws followed by 50 sets of implementing regulations.

5. Administration

Next, the dull, day-to-day process of running the program. Now there are no major political debates or big headlines (unless someone really screws up). The process becomes even more dry and technical. Participants must be ready to argue statistical models, assumptions, and formulae. This is a system for policy experts; it cannot easily be entered into by politicians, physicians, or the public.

The results are still political. There are winners, losers, and consequences. A faceless official may decide that a medical procedure will (or will not) be covered by a government program—with enormous implications for both patients and hospitals. But the entire process is bound by arcane, bureaucratic rules.

How do you enter into this world? By hiring experts. Lawyers, lobbyists and trade associations routinely negotiate with bureaucratic officials over technical rules—often with major financial implications. Congress will rarely question a bureaucratic rule. However, elected officials routinely request exceptions for constituents who get tangled in the red tape. In fact, some members of Congress become famous for helping individual citizens cut through the rules and regulations, and bureaucratic officials—with an eye on next year's budget—generally comply with these special requests.[5]

6. Consequences

Once a government program goes into effect, the politics change. Every program creates new alliances and interests. After Medicare passed in 1965, for example, the association of retired people, AARP, became a powerful political force. Notice how it worked: The *Medicare program made the powerful interest group lobby—not the other way round.* The policy changed the politics.

Take another example. When Medicaid started paying hospitals and physicians, it altered the provider's political interests and thrust them into entirely new coalitions. Now, when a state decides to cut back on, say, chiropractic services for the poor, the state chiropractic association will be right in there fighting along with the advocates for the poor. The program itself changed the politics: Health care providers, who had been fighting fiercely against government intervention in their profession, now switched sides and began fighting to maintain (and even expand) "their" government program.

Consider a very different example. Many public health advocates decry the war on drugs for "incarcerating addiction." However, the policy is very difficult to change. Why? Most people would simply chalk it up to public opinion, but that's just the tip of the political iceberg. The war on drugs funds an enormous number of jobs in both public and private sectors (from police departments to prison corporations). That does not mean, of course, that we cannot change our policy toward illegal drugs. However, because so many people, organizations, and companies are invested in the status quo, changing the policy would take enormous political energy.

Evaluation?

People who teach policy analysis like to end their description of the policy cycle with another stage, *policy evaluation*. They dream that once a program is up and running, Congress will scrutinize policy evaluations to see if the program is working properly. But you can probably already see how this works in the real world—the policy changes the politics. Groups who benefit from the policy will lobby for it; they will fund their own evaluations, which tell legislators that the program is wonderful. And elected representatives don't go around analyzing which evaluation has the most robust methodology—on the contrary, they are more likely to ask what their constituents think. As you'll see in Chapter 1, cost benefit analysis is a fundamentally ambiguous tool, steeped in political considerations. Evaluations of existing programs become one political vehicle in which allies and opponents carry on the debate.

Self Interest!

The whole question of evaluating policy raises a deeper institutional issue: The American political system does not have any neutral arbiter standing above politics. The United States never developed a skilled civil service comparable to the ones in Germany, France, Britain, or Japan. Perhaps this is because until the 20th century, positions were distributed on the basis of political loyalty. A lingering image of corruption and incompetence (quite unjustly) haunts the American bureaucracy. Consequently, public servants suffer from relatively low prestige and poor resources.

The reluctance to nourish competent public administration causes plenty of trouble in health policy. Negotiating with a well-organized, well-financed, and highly skilled professional requires competence and resources. There are plenty of energetic and talented individuals in our public service. However, they are chronically underfunded, understaffed, and underappreciated. And when government officials falter, the typical reflex is to curse all government rather than try to construct a more effective one.

Without a respected government, a prestigious civil service, or a politically independent judiciary, unabashed self-interest becomes the driving political force. Interest groups constantly press for an advantage even if it means denying the most unambiguous scientific findings. There is no shame in this. On the contrary, the single most famous American political analysis, James Madison's *Federalist #10*, argues that the best way to deal with selfish interest groups which violate the public interest is not to try to limit self interest (as classical political theory had always supposed), but rather to introduce *more* selfish interest groups into the political fray. Many different groups scrambling for their own narrow advantage will offset one another—"ambition will counteract ambition."[6]

Does that mean there is no room for idealism? Absolutely not. What it means is that advocates for any position have to mobilize and persuade. Think of the political system as a great buzzing argument. No position is "obviously" right or wrong. Everything is open for negotiation in a furious marketplace for ideas and influence.

Courts

Finally, some policy analysts overlook the enormous influence of the judiciary. The courts intervene at every stage of the political process. For starters, the courts often set the agenda. Just think about what happens when the court rules in favor of a gay person who wishes to be a beneficiary on her partner's health insurance: suddenly, the entire issue of gay beneficiaries is on the agenda. So, perhaps, are civil unions, gay politics, and the rules governing health insurance benefits. American politics turns its focus to the new item, courtesy of the courts. When the other branches of government duck an issue, reformers often turn to the courts to get the debate going.

The court should also be seen as a major policy decision maker. In fact, when Congress bogs down into stalemate, the courts are thrust into that policy-making role. The tobacco wars of the 1990s offer a good example. The politics of tobacco did not produce major legislation in Congress. However, the attorneys general of 31 states came together, filed suits, and began negotiating an extraordinary settlement with the tobacco companies that eventually became the framework for national tobacco policy. Once the obesity problem hit, litigants followed the same route and pushed the courts into the center of the controversy.[7]

The courts also play a major role in implementation and administration. Threatening litigation (and following up with a suit) is a standard part of the implementation process. And it is one of the few ways to overturn administrative decisions. As you'll see in Chapter 8, when New York City began violating national rules by cutting Medicaid recipients from the rolls, a steady stream of lawsuits proved the most effective (in fact, the only) vehicle for pushing New York's Medicaid program back into compliance with Medicaid's national rules and regulations.

A high-ranking official in the Department of Health and Human Services once told me: "If there's any stage of the process where you don't see the courts, you're just not looking very carefully."

ISSUES

Every chapter introduces new ideas. But there are some constant themes running through American health politics and policy. Let's take a quick look at our three hardiest perennials.

Costs

There is one drumbeat in American health policy: costs, costs, costs. And no wonder. Health care costs keep rising faster than the rest of the economy. Almost every year health care spending takes a larger bite of the gross domestic product (GDP).

Table I-1 tells the story. Look at how health care spending rose in the US—8.4% of the gross domestic product in 1975, 12.6% in 1990, 13.9% in 2001, and 16% by 2005. One health specialist, Uwe Reinhardt, has started speculating about "when we'll have it all—every penny in America spent on health care." His joke has a sharp point: the rise seems constant and inexorable.

And the United States stands alone: While every nation feels the cost pressure—from things like aging, new technology, and rising expectations—no other country has seen the same kind inflation in health costs. Industrial nations spend, on average, 8.5% of their gross domestic product on health care. The next biggest spenders are Germany and Switzerland—and they're both spending about 25% *less* on health care relative to the rest of their economy.

Rising costs create serious problems. Companies who provide health benefits complain because every year the same benefits cost them more. Federal and state government face the same squeeze every year: they can raise taxes, cut benefits, or let the deficit grow. And, of course, individuals face a higher health bill every year. That means the door is always open to any policy entrepreneur with a plan to tame the inflation without cutting back benefits. Taming the cost rise is always on the agenda—and explains a lot of health politics and policy over the past 30 years.

Of course, one person's crisis is another person's opportunity. Every dollar we spend on health care is a dollar earned by a health care provider.

Table I-1 Health Care Expenditures as Percentage of GNP

	1960	1975	1990	1993	1998	2001	2005
Canada	5.4	7.2	9.2	9.9	9.1	9.7	10.4
United States	5.2	8.4	12.6	13.3	13.0	13.9	16.0
Japan	3.0	5.6	6.1	6.6	7.1	8.0	7.0
UK	3.9	5.5	6.0	6.9	6.9	7.6	8.3
Germany	4.8	8.1	8.7	10.0	10.6	10.7	10.7

SOURCE: OECD Health Data, 2004, 2007.

Rising costs looks different to drug companies, hospital administrators, and physicians than to taxpayers, employers, and patients. Even so, the providers are not all cheering. That's because the payers, struggling to control their own costs, are constantly meddling with health care. American providers get the highest reimbursement in the world but, as you'll see, they pay a high price in intrusive regulations. Governments, corporations, and managed care companies constantly intervene in the practice of medicine.

Why do costs keep going up? Once upon a time, the conventional wisdom suggested a triangle of three health care values: high quality, low costs, and broad access to care. You can improve any two, said policy analysts, at the expense of the third: High quality and broad access raises costs. Lower the costs and either quality or access must suffer. Very few scholars believe in that triangle any more. Instead, many observers point to the sheer administrative cost of running a system with many different payers each setting prices, collecting premiums, and bargaining over prices. One physician, Robert Kane, illustrated the problem with a simple study. He went to a hospital in Ontario (Canada) and asked to see the people responsible for sending out the bills; the hospital administrator introduced him to four people. Then Dr. Kane went to a comparable size hospital in Minneapolis; the billing department occupies an entire wing and employs over 100 staff members. That's the difference between getting payment from one source (the Province of Ontario) and tracking down, literally, hundreds of payers (Medicare, Blue Cross, Cigna, Prudential), then matching each with the co-payments they have built into their different policies (See Table I-2). Some analysts believe that running the American system accounts for 15 to 25% of our total health care costs. Forget higher quality or better access, they conclude, the high costs we are paying comes from the large bureaucracy which runs our system of multiple health care insurers (public and private) each operating with its own rules and procedures.

You'll encounter plenty of other explanations for our rising health care costs in the pages that follow:

TABLE I-2 Percentage of National Health Expenditures Spent on Administration and Insurance, 2003

France	1.9
Japan	2.1
Canada	2.6
United Kingdom	3.3
Germany	5.6
United States	7.3

DATA: OECD Health Data 2004.

SOURCE: Commonwealth Fund National Score Card on US Health Care performance, 2006.

Extraordinary medical technology, rising consumer expectations, the high costs of malpractice, or, simply, higher prices than other countries pay. But you can begin with the simple, raw data: All societies feel the upward pressure but none have costs that are anywhere near as high as ours. Some argue that that's not necessarily bad. But rising costs is the white noise—the constant pressure—of American health policy.

Access

Another number keeps going up: Americans without health insurance. The figure has gone from 34 million in 1990 to 40 million in 2000 and 47 million in 2007. Roughly 30 million more Americans have inadequate insurance. The problem brings us right back to Darrell, the fellow at the Lempster dump. Half the people without insurance in 2003 reported putting off needed care. The Institute of Medicine estimates that at least 18,000 Americans a year die prematurely because they don't have health insurance; other researchers suggest that mortality rates could be reduced by as much as 15% if the uninsured had gained "continuous health care coverage."[8]

Gaps in health care insurance are just the tip of the American inequality problem. Comparative studies constantly report the same gloomy story.

In one study of the 13 most developed economies, the United States ranked last or near to last on almost every indicator: Infant mortality (last), low birth weight (last), years of potential life lost (last), and male life expectancy at age 1 (12th out of 13), age 15 (12th), and age 40 (9th). The average American boy can expect to live 3.5 years less than the average Japanese boy—though the Japanese child is much more likely to grow up smoking cigarettes.[9]

The dismal data mask vast differences across our population. A male born in some sections of Washington DC has a life expectancy 40 years lower than a woman born in rural Minnesota.[10] Policy analysts disagree about why: Does the problem stem from a lack of insurance for basic care? The larger problems of poverty? The more complicated dynamics of American inequality? Some combination of all three? The effort to pinpoint the causes goes on. But at a minimum we can conclude that the great American differences in wealth equate to great differences in health.

The dilemma of inequity runs through the chapters that follow. Keep the underlying problem in mind as you move from chapter to chapter. The issue often slips off the political agenda, but the trouble is acute enough that it keeps coming back. Many of us who study health care believe that addressing our health care inequities is a major imperative of a good and just society.

Quality

Another controversial matter is the question of health care quality. Many people believe that the United States serves as the world's engine for technological and medical advances. The health care for well-insured Americans with steady access to health care is, in this view, outstanding. Indeed, the vast majority of Americans report being very satisfied with their one care. Policy proposals to address the problems of high cost and spotty access often set off fears for the quality of our medical care.

Even on this ground, however, there is controversy. In 1973, Dr. John Wennberg set off an entire research tradition with a striking discovery. Physicians in different communities performed the same clinical procedures at very different rates. Local areas appeared to have their own "practice styles" or "surgical signature." Crucially, these differences could not be linked to any difference in medical outcomes. In perhaps the most famous study, Wennberg and his associates found much higher hospitalization rates (for two procedures) in Boston than in New Haven. "Boston residents incurred about $300 million more hospital expenditures [in 1982 dollars] and 795 hospital beds then they would have if the use rates of New Haven applied." Variation in medical practice, concluded Wennberg (and a long procession of followers), reflected uncertainty about appropriate treatment. Medical practice was more an artifact of local professional culture than of medical science.[11]

The rub came, of course, when researchers began to attach cost differences to the variations in practice. For years, health analysts had been delivering a painful message. Successful cost control would mean painful choices—rationing medical treatment, forgoing desirable treatments, living within tough budgets. Suddenly, policy analysts thought they saw a more palatable alternative: Find the unnecessary services and wring them out of the system. Induce the physicians to practice more efficient medicine. Better yet, use data from systematic studies—like the New Haven and Boston comparison—to guide medical providers to greater efficiency.[12]

The social scientists' dream proved illusory. Specifying the single best medical practice turned out to be extraordinarily complicated—patients differ, situations differ, technologies improve, and medicine develops new procedures before the old ones can be systematically analyzed. And, as many practitioners insist, there's always that irreducible, immeasurable touch of healing art along with the medical science.

But the studies had an enormous impact. In a system where powerful actors were almost desperate to control their costs, the studies legitimated intrusive controls over the practice of medicine. Debunking the doctor's scientific authority permitted insurance companies or government officials to deny payment for care they deemed "unnecessary."

What followed was, in effect, a long power struggle over the practice of medicine. Medical providers assert their professional expertise; payers respond by trying to control what providers do—by oversight or incentives or fiat.

Again, there is a national difference. In other nations where the government was stronger relative to the doctors (like Canada or Britain), national health insurance plans simply gave providers—whether doctors or hospitals—a budget and told them to use their professional judgment and live within it. The providers have, so far at least, been more successful than their American counterparts in fending off lay intrusion into medical practice.

At its best, American health care is extraordinary, perhaps the best in the world. But the physicians' offices, medical laboratories, and hospital rooms can also be read as the site for a great struggle over the practice of medicine. This battle, too, runs implicit through many of our health policy debates—and through the chapters of this book.

In Sum

The chapters that follow explore the nooks and crannies of the American health care enterprise—the presidency, the environment, aging, federalism, morality, the imperatives of social justice, cost benefit analysis, public opinion, and reflections on a mother dying of cancer as she shops for care. But through it all—sometimes on the surface, often just below—run the same three themes: the cost of health care, inequalities in health and care, and the great debates over medical quality and who should oversee it.

HISTORY

All politics are steeped in history. Each event shapes future possibilities. New programs create new political alignments—winners, losers, beneficiaries, bureaucracies, constituents, enemies, and fodder for the political agenda. Even small changes can have enormous political implications down the line.

Social scientists call this historical weight "path dependence."

The chapters that follow rest firmly on our history. As you'll see, some events have had an enormous influence. Sometimes big changes come in with trumpets blaring—everyone knew that it was a Big Event when Congress passed Medicare (in 1965) or defeated the Clinton administration's health reform (1993–4). Sometimes tiny, technical changes carry hidden and unintended effects—no one noticed a pension reform bill (now dubbed ERISA), but we'll see that it made a big difference.

Here's an overview of the most important health policy events that you'll encounter in this book. Some are mentioned often. Others only come up occasionally but form an important part of the background of the analysis.

1912: The Great Divide

An eminent professor at Harvard pointed to 1912 as a plausible estimate for the great dividing line in medical care when, "for the first time in human history, a random patient with a random disease consulting a doctor chosen at random stood better than a 50–50 chance of benefiting from the encounter." The spread of two 19th century innovations—antisepsis and anesthesia—helped make American medicine safer and less painful.[13]

1912–1919: National Health Insurance (I)

That same year, former president Theodore Roosevelt left the Republican party and ran for the presidency as the Progressive (or Bull Moose) Party candidate. For the first time, a presidential candidate promoted national health insurance as part of his campaign.

In 1915, a private group of reformers, the American Association for Labor Legislation (or AALL) drafted a model national health insurance bill and introduced it in 14 states. Ironically, it was especially effective at galvanizing opponents. Local medical societies ferociously denounced the effort as "socialist," "Germanic," and "un-American"—tags that became especially effective when the United States entered World War I in 1917. Physicians denounced and defeated medical leaders who had supported the legislation and turned the American Medical Association (or AMA) into a fierce enemy of government-sponsored (or compulsory) health insurance. The doctors were joined by the private health insurance industry, especially Prudential and Metropolitan; though the companies had not yet gotten into the health insurance business, they feared the implications of government-sponsored insurance. The battle came to a head in two states. In California, opponents clobbered a referendum on health reform (358,324 to 133,858). In New York, the health insurance proposal, supported by Democratic governor Al Smith, passed the Senate before dying in a House committee.

The battle left an important legacy: A powerful, self confident coalition, led by the American Medical Association, was primed to fight any whisper of national health insurance. Health reformers, on the other hand, took away the rueful lesson that proposing government insurance meant stirring up a hornet's nest.[14]

1921–1929: The Origins of Private Health Insurance

Metropolitan began selling individual health insurance in 1921, and Prudential began in 1925. A year later, Metropolitan drifted toward employee health benefits when it signed a contract with General Motors to cover 180,000 workers for disability insurance. Blue Cross—an untaxed, non-profit, hospital-based insurance plan—first began to organize in 1929 and spread during the Great Depression of the 1930s, when hospitals needed a way to guarantee payments. The American way—paying for health care through private, employment-based insurance—had begun to stir.

1935: The Social Security Act

The Social Security Act is the single most important piece of domestic legislation passed in the 20th century. It included *Old Age Insurance*, which is now known simply as Social Security and comprises the largest item in the federal budget, and *Aid to Dependent Children* (later *Aid to Families of Dependent Children* or AFDC), which was soon dubbed "welfare." Social Security became a popular and successful program; AFDC, in contrast, grew extremely unpopular and controversial before being replaced in 1996. The two programs would soon stand out from the many American social programs and offer starkly contrasting models for designing public health care benefits.

The Committee on Economic Security that drafted the Social Security Act formed a subcommittee to study health insurance. As soon as word of the subcommittee spread, "the telegraphic protests poured in upon the President." Chastened by what the committee's chair called "vilification and misrepresentation" (and mindful of what had happened back in 1919), the Roosevelt administration submitted social security legislation with just one reference to health insurance—a tepid, largely symbolic, call for further study. "That little line was responsible for so many letters to the members of Congress," recalled one administration member, "that the entire Social Security program seemed endangered." The Ways and Means Committee in the House of Representatives calmed the storm when they unanimously struck any mention of health care from the Social Security Act.[15]

National Health Insurance (II)

After his election to a fourth term in 1944, President Franklin D. Roosevelt asked a trusted advisor to prepare a report on national health insurance. When the war was over, he reportedly planned to tangle with the American Medical Association and try to win the reform. In April 1945, FDR died, and shortly thereafter President Harry Truman received the Rosenman report on health care. In November 1945, Truman made a special address to Congress recommending comprehensive national health insurance.

Truman was passionate about national health insurance. He wrote letters to constituents who had

had trouble getting care, promising them that relief was on the way, and he replied fiercely to critics, accusing them of living "in a horse and buggy era" and being opposed to "modern thinking."

Once again, however, the national health insurance proposal galvanized opponents more than supporters. Senator Robert Taft, the ranking Republican, announced that his party would not participate in socialism, and walked out of Congressional hearings. The legislation went nowhere. In the backlash, Truman's Democrats lost both houses of Congress (losing 54 seats in the House and 11 in the Senate).

Truman never abandoned his campaign for health insurance. In 1948, he ran a long shot reelection campaign—roasting the "do nothing" Republican Congress—and became the patron saint of dark horse candidates by surprising the experts and winning. The Democrats also won majorities in both houses of Congress, and national health insurance was back on the national agenda. A fierce political conflict followed. The American Medical Association denounced "the final irrevocable step to socialism," taxed every member $25, built a "war chest," and launched one of the first great public relations campaigns aimed against a single bill. The physicians found plenty of allies in the private and public sectors. Again, Senator Robert Taft denounced the plan as "the Moscow party line," torn "straight out of the Soviet Constitution." Again, the proposal (known as Murray, Wagner, Dingell, after its chief Congressional sponsors) never made it out of committee.

Many observers focus on the interest group's pyrotechnics; the AMA's effort to bury national health insurance is famous. But beneath the fury lay a simple political reality. National health insurance never had enough support to get through Congress, and President Truman was clumsy at working with legislators.

1946: The Hospital Construction Act (Hill-Burton)

The hospital industry offered an alternative that could be won without political fireworks. Rather than directly finance medical services, the government could build up American medicine by funding hospital construction—a health care strategy known, for some reason, as "the Argentina Model." Relieved politicians cheered the plan. Hill-Burton formed a prototype of postwar health policy: The federal government financed the infrastructure—the hospitals, laboratories, and research—without touching the practice or financing of medicine. The government simply distributed funds and left all the decisions to the medical industry.

Hill-Burton was an immediate hit. In less than two years, the Public Health Service provided funds for 347 construction projects in 42 states. Over the next 35 years, the program distributed $3.7 billion in federal funds, drew $9 billion more in state and local matching funds, and contributed to almost a third of all hospital construction projects in the nation.

1946–1957: The Rise of Employee Health Insurance

During World War II, corporations had faced stiff taxes on "excess profits." Employer contributions to health and pension funds counted as a business expense and were not taxed at all; companies began to set up health plans, urged on by the resurgent union movement. After the war, employer health plans boomed. In 1946, company plans insured a million workers; by 1957, they insured twelve million workers and 20 million dependents.[16] As you can see in Table 10-3, before the war few Americans (less than 1 in 10) had private health insurance; by the mid-1950s most people (60% and rising) had it. President Dwight Eisenhower cemented the trend in 1954 when he asked Congress to explicitly exempt employee health benefits from taxation. The American health insurance alternative was in place. As Jacob Hacker explains in Chapter 9, the rise of employee plans fundamentally changed the American health debate. Many workers and their families now had good health insurance. Why should they support a government alternative?

1965: Medicare and Medicaid

Liberals whittled down Truman's ambitious health plan, in a vain effort to win support, from comprehensive national health insurance to national health insurance for the elderly to a hospital plan for the elderly. After all, older Americans still had trouble getting health insurance—and they needed the care most. Here was a major gap in the employer system.

Despite liberal backpedaling, the debate never changed. The AMA and its allies tirelessly evoked the twin specters of socialist tyranny and bureaucratic incompetence.

The debate quickened when Democrats captured the Senate in 1958 and rose to a peak after President John Kennedy's election in 1960. To get a feel for the exaggerated tone of the debate, consider AMA *Operation Hometown*. The AMA sent every physician's spouse a recording with which to persuade friends and neighbors to write Congress and oppose Medicare. The final words of the exhortation crystallized the antigovernment imagery of the day:

> Write those letters now; call your friends and tell them to write them. If you don't this program, I promise you, will pass just as surely as the sun will come up tomorrow. And behind it will come other federal programs that will invade every area of freedom as we have known it in this country. Until one day we will awake to find that we have socialism. And if you don't do this, and I don't do it, one of these days you and I are going to spend our sunset years telling our children and our children's children what it was like in America when men were free.

The familiar voice behind the 1962 recording was a conservative actor named Ronald Reagan.[17]

The irony is that the rhetorical fireworks did not matter. Not in the 1940s during the Truman effort, not now. Conservative politicians—Northern Republicans and Southern Democrats—opposed the idea regardless of the American Medical Association or Ronald Reagan or public information campaigns.

Throughout the Truman, Eisenhower, and Kennedy administrations, at least one branch of government rejected the proposals. During the Kennedy years, conservative Democrats (mainly from the Southern states) blocked the proposals by bottling them up in Congressional committees. Then, in the national shock following President Kennedy's assassination, the 1964 election yielded the largest Democratic majority in 30 years. The new liberal majority stacked the Congressional committees, broke the stalemate, and prepared to pass Medicare.

Facing defeat, the American Medical Association put aside its antigovernment rhetoric and proposed an alternative. Rather than a social security–style program directed at all elders (which would grow big and popular), the AMA suggested a welfare program that could target poor people and be administered by the states (which, they reasoned, would be more like welfare and remain small and less popular). Congressman Wilbur Mills (Democrat, Arkansas), the powerful chairman of the House Ways and Means committee, had almost single-handedly stopped Medicare in the past. Now he shocked everyone by refusing to choose between the two alternatives and passing both: Medicare for the elderly and the AMA plan for eligible indigents, now titled Medicaid. The two bills became Articles 18 (Medicare) and 19 (Medicaid) of the Social Security Act.[18] Taken together, they form the most important piece of legislation in the history of American health care. They fundamentally changed our health care politics. The federal government was soon the largest payer for health care services in the nation. Eventually, this piper would soon start to call the tune.

But not for a while. Most laws begin by promising the moon. In contrast, Medicare began by promising not to change anything: "Nothing in this title shall be construed to authorize any supervision or control over the practice of medicine." The next five passages all embellish this theme, forbidding state control over medical personnel, or compensation, or organization, or administration. As I suggested above, the implementation of the program followed the spirit of the legislation and organized an extremely generous way of paying providers.

Health care prices had been growing steadily for the past decade. In the past 11 years, health care had risen from 4.4% of the gross domestic product to 5.9%. In the five years following the implementation of Medicare, it covered almost the same ground in half the time—leaping to 7.3% of GDP by 1970. And now the government was paying for it, so that rising health care costs meant either raising taxes or growing deficits. The great new health care issue came onto the political agenda: cost crisis.

1970s: Cost Control through Regulation and Planning

A scattershot of small programs first tried to address the rising costs. One effort brought together local notables for Comprehensive Health Planning (1967). Another turned to physicians and asked them to monitor colleagues who were running up excessive costs (Physician Standard Review Organizations, 1972). The American Hospital Association called for providers to do the job themselves through a Voluntary Effort (1978), and in one astonishingly ambitious program, Congress launched 205 local health planning agencies run by consumers and empowered to issue (or deny) certificates of need for every capital expenditure in the area (the Health Planning and Resources Development Act of 1975).

These many, little programs—providers might have felt sometimes like they were being stoned with popcorn—did not have much effect on costs, but they began a great shift in political power within the medical field. Decades of deferring to medical providers started coming to an end. All of a sudden hospital administrators, with the prestigious head of radiology in tow, had to go before a citizen council and request permission to buy a CAT scanner.[19]

1970s: Cost Control through Market Competition

An entirely different idea also became popular in the 1970s: Perhaps market competition could tame the beast. Guided by economic thinking, policy entrepreneurs spent the next 30 years devising and revising ways to bring market discipline to bear on health care without violating basic values (even the improvident cannot be left to die without care).

As you'll see in the following chapters, market proponents took all kinds of strategies. Let's briefly look at two of the classics.

HMOs

One early effort imagined competing health plans (like HMOs). Employers would give employees vouchers; states could do the same with Medicaid recipients. The providers, organized into HMOs or other forms of service delivery, would then compete by quality, amenity, and price. In one version, an inexpensive plan (that cost less than the voucher) would leave the extra money in your pocket; on the other hand, if you wanted a fancier plan, you'd have to pay more than the voucher set aside. In theory, providers would compete to offer the best care at the lowest cost while consumers would shop for high quality, low cost providers.

Proponents lobbied hard for HMO legislation. However, skeptics loaded the bill down with so many conditions and requirements that what finally emerged from the political process stymied HMOs as much as it fostered them. Still, the HMO legislation stands as the emblem of the long quest to bring market discipline to health care. Originally, proponents dedicated themselves to achieving market discipline without sacrificing ideals such as broad access and a rough equity.[20]

The RAND Experiment

Economic theorists also came up with a simpler market model. Insurance was the culprit, they reasoned, because it made health care seem free and that led people to consume too much of it. If people paid more, they'd seek less. In the late 1970s and 1980s, the RAND Corporation conducted a famous health insurance experiment in six communities—reputedly, the most expensive social experiment in history. Volunteers were randomly assigned to insurance plans that ranged from no cost sharing to high cost sharing. Sure enough, people who did not have to pay anything sought out more health care services. But their actual health, which was carefully monitored, proved no better than those who did not get the additional care.

The experiment inevitably drew fire: Critics refused to believe that health care was really discretionary—who goes to the hospital if they don't have to? Critics combed the data for flaws; they pointed out that the volunteers assigned to cost sharing plans dropped out of the experiment and returned to their old insurance plans at much higher rates (*16 times* higher)—perhaps, wondered the skeptics, these were the sickest people in the experiment? Despite the criticism (the debate goes on to the present day), many economists had their answer to the cost problem: Make consumers pay more for their health care and their own pocket books will impose discipline. The RAND experiment became a landmark among health care specialists.

The Great Debate

For two decades, health care politics broke into rival camps: One argued that every other nation seemed to have squared the circle of cost control and universal access; the other that markets were the American way. The first camp insisted that the only proven method—discovered by every country but ours—was right there for the taking: national health insurance. People chasing markets were indulging in the same wistful social engineering that had gotten the high-minded reformers into trouble in the past (recall the war on poverty). After all, no state or nation had successfully employed markets to manage cost and promote access in health care. It was just another high-flying impractical theory much loved by conservatives.

Market advocates responded with hoots about just who was being naïve. National health insurance was never going to happen in the United States, they said. Markets often needed oversight and adjustment, but they worked in almost every other industry and they could be made to work in this one.

For a time, each side thought it had a concept that could work, if only it could be pushed past the politics and put into place. As the stalemate continued, however, disillusionment spread. Perhaps both sides had fatal flaws. American health care never seemed to get closer to either a universal entitlement or a proper market. With time, market thinking itself would evolve and became, more bluntly, a case of every person (or payer) for themselves and devil take the hindmost.

1983: Prospective Payment Systems (PPS)

When Ronald Reagan swept into office in 1980, his administration promised competition and deregulation. It quickly chopped down the meek regulatory efforts left over from the 1970s. But the administration's most important health care contribution came in a completely unexpected realm: reimbursing hospitals. Hospitals used to charge patients the same way hotels charged guests—a basic rate for the (hospital) bed and additional charges for services. The more days a patient stayed in the hospital and the more procedures the hospital performed, the higher the bill. In 1983, Medicare administrators came up with a dramatically different way to think about paying providers: Pay by the illness, not by what providers did.

New Jersey had already begun experimenting with a new payment method which combined most hospital procedures into 363 categories known as diagnostic related groups (or DRGs)—for example, a birth without complications or an infection of the inner ear. Researchers set a price for each category (or diagnosis). Obviously, more complicated cases in a particular category would cost more than the pre-set price; but, in theory, they would be offset by simpler cases that cost less than the price. Since the price was fixed in advance, regardless of what a hospital actually did, hospitals would come out ahead if they provided fewer days and services. And they would lose (financially) if they provided more.

Do you see the revolution in thinking? Traditionally, the more a hospital did for a patient, the more it got paid. Suddenly, the less it did to a patient—the fewer days in the hospital, the fewer tests, the fewer procedures—the higher its revenue. The physician who ordered an extra test or prescribed expensive meds suddenly became a liability. Needless to say, medical staffs were infuriated. Hospital administrators who knew nothing about medicine were suddenly badgering them about ordering too many services or hospitalizing patients for too many days.

The idea of paying a pre-set price—DRGs were simply one example—is known as *prospective payment* (or PPS). It changed the financial incentives in the hospital. It also changed the power relations. Administrators assumed more authority relative to physicians. The Reagan administration—really, the Medicare administrators in collaboration with the administrators in the New Jersey Department of Health—were using financial incentives to change the practice of medicine. As any social scientist would predict, changes did indeed follow. For example, the average length of a hospital stay rapidly started going down.

Payer Competition

Prospective payment set off another earthquake in the health care business. Rather than trying to cut the costs for the entire system, Medicare had focused only on its own costs. A savvy hospital manager might make up the lost income by raising prices for patients insured by, say, Prudential or Cigna (this is known as *cost shifting*). The payers found themselves in a race. If Prudential could lower its costs more effectively than Cigna, it could charge lower premiums and win more business. A new competition developed: not among providers seeking health consumers but among payers seeking to lower their own costs, lower their premiums, and enroll new groups into their health plans.

There were lots of strategies for trying to pay hospitals less than a rival plan. You could, for example, negotiate hard for a better rate. Or monitor the care more closely. But social critics began to worry that there was a simpler way to win this contest: Enroll

healthier people who will require less expensive health care. Even a freshman actuary could tell you how to do that. Sign up young, healthy, well-educated, well-off people and avoid poor, old, or chronically ill people. The insurance industry confronted an odd incentive: seek the healthy, shun the sick.

As you'll see in Chapter 1, a new view of health insurance emerged. The classic perspective had placed everyone into a big insurance pool. You never knew when you might get sick, so the lucky who stayed healthy subsidized the unlucky who fell ill. Now a new thought insinuated itself: My family is young and healthy, we're a lot less likely to get sick than someone who is poor or old or has a dangerous job. Why should we subsidize them?

The competition among payers did not reduce costs; on the contrary, costs continued to rise. So did the number of people without health insurance. Individuals unaffiliated with a large employment group found health insurance increasingly difficult to get—the insurance company actuaries fingered them as the most likely to run up health care costs.

Managed Care

With their new payment scheme, Medicare officials had stopped deferring to professional authority. Doctors, drawing on their expertise, could insist that this or that patient needed more care, but Medicare would not pay for it. Payers (mainly insurance companies and government programs) took the next step and began thinking about directing medical practice. Remember the study that found "surgical signatures," or different practice patterns in different cities? Health services researchers reasoned that careful studies would reveal the most effective treatments. They could study thousands of cases and then, drawing on their data, guide health care providers toward better practice—higher quality at lower prices. Many health services researchers began to disparage the intuition, on-the-job experience, and internalized norms of the individual health care practitioner. A good technician sitting at a computer could draw on a much wider range of experience and, so went the theory, guide the nurses and doctors to better medical decisions than those individuals could make relying on their own limited experience.

The logic produced managed care: health care guided by a manager who would impose statistical order on the therapeutic chaos. The managers and their trusty computers would keep track of patient Jones as she moved through the medical system. When a provider proposed a procedure, the manager would have all the most recent studies at her fingertips and could help guide the provider away from ineffective or inefficient regimens and toward more effective, economical, state-of-the-art treatment.

1993–4: The Clinton Health Care Reform Plan

Costs continued to rise. Large employers complained about the rising burden of covering employees. The number of people without health insurance grew. Hospitals that faced too many uninsured patients sank into debt. Many states tried to take action but, despite great promise, none managed to fully launch and sustain a viable universal program (Howard Leichter explains why in Chapter 7).

In this setting, Bill Clinton ran for president in 1992 and promised national health insurance. The old liberal dream had appeared during the Truman administration (1945, 1949), the Nixon administration (1973, when the Democrats, focused on impeaching Nixon, shortsightedly spiked the idea), and the Carter administration (1979–80). Now, with Democrats in control of Washington, the Clinton administration tried again. What followed was one of the decisive battles of recent political history. Almost every chapter refers to it—and for good reason.

The Clinton plan would take existing programs (employer health care, Medicare, Medicaid), add insurance for those who did not have it, and place them all under a federally designed, regionally run, managed care system. Beneath the policy details, Democrats were making a political bet: Like Social

Security (in 1935) and Medicare (in 1965), this would become a popular program that changed the political environment and rebuilt the Democratic party base around a celebrated new entitlement.

Republicans responded with the tried-and-true way. If you go back and read the outcry that greeted each national health insurance, you'll find similar language, modified slightly to reflect the times. The Clinton proposal ran right into variations of the traditional themes: bureaucracy run amok, bloated (naïve, arrogant) government, the end of decent American medicine, and the return of socialism just three years after Eastern Europeans had broken through the Berlin Wall and buried Communism. Many Republican constituencies—notably, small business—genuinely feared the proposal. Beneath the clash, however, Republicans made precisely the same political calculation as the Democrats. Winning the reform would burnish the Clinton administration's reputation and rouse the Democratic party base; on the other hand, killing the reform would embarrass Clinton, disgruntle Democrats, and help inspire Republican voters.

The Republicans won the battle. More important, they won the post-contest spin. After the defeat, the Clinton administration dropped the idea of national health insurance and stopped defending its own plan. The Republican interpretation went unchallenged: the plan had been a bloated, maladroit, overreaching mess. The next election—only three months later—brought the largest Republican victory of the 20th century: The GOP took the Senate, the House of Representatives, both houses of the state legislature in 11 *new* states, and won 15 *new* governors, giving the party control of the executive office in 32 states (that last figure for governors covers elections between 1993 and 1996). Some of the top leaders of the Democratic party, like Governor Mario Cuomo (New York) and Governor Ann Richards (Texas), lost to political neophytes such as George Pataki and George W. Bush.

American politics changed. The minority party for most of the past 60 years had leapt into the majority on both the national and state levels. Six years later it would consolidate its control by taking the presidency and, for six years (until the midterm election of 2006) controlling American politics. One great question for health policy analysts—you'll see it often in the chapters that follow—is simple to ask but difficult to answer: What difference did the Republican revolution make for health care political and policy? On the one hand you'll see ways in which the Republican majority had a very different view of health care programs (see Chapter 15 for a powerful statement of this perspective); on the other hand, you'll learn (in Chapter 5) that every modern Republican president—Eisenhower, Nixon, Ford, Reagan, the first president Bush, and the second president Bush—proposed a significant expansion of government health care benefits. There was no hiding from health care programs.

Managed Care: Revolution and Backlash

In the short run, something funny happened to health policy. The Clinton plan would have relied heavily on managed care (organized into something more grandiose known as "managed competition"). Well, the managed care revolution took off without the revolutionaries. Individual payers all seized on the managed care idea to try and control their own costs. Hospitals and other health care institutions, expecting Clinton's national health insurance to pass, also geared up for the change. A failed proposal helped transform the health care system—or perhaps simply sped up reforms that were already under way. In either case, the dead plan prompted sweeping changes.

Managed care offered a marvelous ideal: Health services research would produce the data that would guide health care providers. You may have already noticed that in the real world of health policy, most ideas do not work out exactly as expected. In this case, the data that would guide effective health care practice never materialized. The studies never managed to keep pace with the progress of medicine itself.

That did not stop the payers. They took control and insisted on authorizing expensive medical procedures. No approval meant no payment. However, without the promised data to back up decisions, the managed care decisions often seemed arbitrary. Providers felt they knew what the patients needed. They complained bitterly that managed care had become nothing more than a very blunt cost control device. It was, they said, nothing but a hammer with which payers pounded down costs.

For a short time the hammer seemed to work. The relentless escalation in health care costs abated. Health care costs had stood at 13.3% of GDP in 1993 when Clinton launched his plan; five years later, with managed care widely in use, costs had slipped to 13.0% (of a booming GDP). This was one of the only periods in the past half century when health care costs stopped their inexorable conquest of the American dollar.

However, health care providers and patients did not bear the squeeze quietly. Providers routinely told patients that they needed a procedure that their insurers refused to authorize. Patients and their families screamed. Over 1,000 pieces of proposed legislation sprouted across all 50 states. In Congress, Democrats read the names of people who had allegedly died at the hands of managed care. Popular books and movies—*The Rainmaker*, *John Q*—framed dramas around what you might call managed care murders. Evil insurance company executives or cash-register hospital administrators left people to die from treatable (but expensive) maladies. Patients complained to their political representatives, their insurers, and their employers' benefits offices (which select insurers for the company). Before long the managed care regime began to loosen. Some insurers began marketing promises that they would never deny treatments.

By 2000, costs began to leap up—rapidly making up for the brief restraint of the mid-1990s. Managed care's advocates grumbled that the strategy had been working; Americans were just not willing to face the needed constraints. Skeptics surmised that all that cost control had merely masked the inevitable inflation. Even while costs were low in the mid-1990s, one insurance executive told me that the insurers were like swimmers holding their breath underwater; once the other guys quit and leave the market, he predicted, the winners would raise health care premiums big time to make up for the lean years. Sure enough, the 2000s saw soaring insurance premiums and rapidly rising health care costs.

Where We Stand

All the old troubles remain: Americans still face escalating health care costs. Employers grow increasingly weary of their rising premiums and try to shift more of the costs to their workers. Governments struggle with their own costs. The number of uninsured people grows. But as Pogo, the comic strip character and sometime philosopher once remarked, "the future just ain't what it used to be." That's because all the surefire solutions—competition, managed care, national health insurance—appear to have lost their luster. The agenda is wide open for anyone with a new idea.

And yet the health care glass remains more than half full. Medicine continues to find almost-miraculous cures. Treatments grow simpler, less complicated, and less painful.

Most of us know people—grandparents, parents, and friends—who live normal lives with conditions that would have killed them a generation (or even a decade) ago.

Health care politics and policy is an emotional ride: On the one hand, the triumph of healing, caring, and progress. On the other hand, frustration at our own social and economic limits—the burden of high prices, the sad reality of inequity and social injustice.

Finally, the wise policy analyst understands that there is no final solution, no program that will simply solve our health care dilemmas once and for all. Payers want to pay less; health providers want to do more and better; citizens and patients want both. Every policy carries unanticipated consequences. Every innovation reveals new problems. Each program generates winners, losers, and new issues for

the political agenda. Every move in politics and policy prompts a counter move. The health care debates always go on.

A FINAL WORD

There is an old political saw: If you want to enjoy either sausages or laws, don't look too closely at how they are made. Americans love to disparage the political process—how many times have you heard people say "its all politics"? But stop and think for a minute. Politics is how we decide—as a community, as a nation—what really matters to us. Yes, we want efficient programs. But we also want to give ourselves lots of say in the process—and the more input people have, the more complicated and drawn out that process is going to be. Democracy is messy.

The chapters that follow engage almost every feature of health care politics and policy. They explain how things happen. But there is common thread: The American system invites people to get involved. In fact, it only works well with broad and enthusiastic participation. Think, as you read the chapters, about where you stand—and where you might make your voice heard.

It is not "only politics." It is our health care. And our democracy—with ugly warts and high flying ideals. Naturally, I hope that this book teaches you a great deal about health politics and policy. But I have a deeper wish. I hope we also inspire you to get involved. That's the only way Americans will ever make progress against the many problems you are about to encounter.

STUDY QUESTIONS

1. What are the stages through which each item of public policy passes?
2. Imagine that you are political activist working hard to win a program. How would your

strategies change with each stage of the
policy process?

3. Your statistics professor tells you that good
public policy requires robust cost/benefits
analyses so that legislators will know what to
do next. Give her a little lecture about how
policies change politics.

4. How does health policy suffer from the
relative lack of prestige accorded to the
American governmental bureaucracy?

5. How much of an impact has the judiciary
had on health policymaking in America?

6. What are some of the common explanations
for America's rising health care costs?

7. What is 'path dependence'? How can it be
related to health policy?

8. Why has managed care failed to keep health
care costs down over the long term?

NOTES

1. See Morone and Jacobs, 2005.
2. For details on obesity, see Kersh and Morone,
2005.
3. For a description of this case, see Rand
Rosenblatt, 1978; and Chapter 6.
4. The civil rights case is described in detail in
Morone, 2003, quoted at 441.
5. For a classic description of the process, see
Arnold, 1980.
6. James Madison, *Federalist #10*; quotation
from *Federalist #51*.
7. See Kersh and Morone, 2005.
8. Kaiser Family Foundation, *Kaiser Commission
on Medicaid and the Uninsured,* "The Uninsured and Their Access to Health Care," November 2004. Accessed (January 18, 2006) at:
http://www.kff.org/uninsured/upload/The-
Uninsured-and-Their-Access-to-Health-Care-
November-2004-Fact-Sheet.pdf.
9. See the data and arguments by Ichuro Kawachi
(p 20) and James Morone and Lawrence Jacobs
(p 5) in Morone and Jacobs, 2005.
10. Morone and Jacobs, 5; *USA Today*.

11. John Wennberg, 1202-4.
12. John Wennberg, 1202-4.
13. Harris, 1966, 5; Marmor, 2000, 3.
14. See Quadagno, 2005, 18-21; Starr, 1981,
243–54.
15. See Morone, 1998, 257–8.
16. Quadagno, 50-2 (employee plans).
17. Morone, 1998, 262.
18. As you'll see in Chapter 15, there were actually
three bills that came together—a three layer
cake. Medicare Part A (which pays for hospital
care), Medicare Part B (doctors), and Medicaid
(described in Chapter 16) were originally competing bills that Wilbur Mills pressed together
into one huge package.
19. For a description, see Morone, 1998, Chapter 7.
20. On HMOs, see Lawrence Brown, 1982.

REFERENCES

Arnold, Douglas. 1980. *Congress and the Bureaucracy:
A Theory of Influence.* New Haven: Yale University
Press.

Brown, Lawrence. 1982. *HMOs as Federal Policy.*
Washington DC: Brookings Press.

Kawachi, Ichuro. 2005. "Why the US is Not Number 1
in Health Care." James Morone and Lawrence
Jacobs, eds. *Healthy, Wealthy and Fair: Health
Care and the Good Society.* New York: Oxford
University Press.

Kersh, Rogan, and James Morone. 2005. "Obesity,
Courts, and the New Politics of Public Health,"
Journal of Health Politics, Policy and Law 30 (5):
839-68.

John Jay, Alexander Hamilton, James Madison. 1788.
The Federalist Papers.

Marmor, Theodor, and Jan Marmor. 2000. *The Politics
of Medicare.* New York: Aldine.

Morone, James, and Lawrence Jacobs. 2005. *Healthy,
Wealthy and Fair: Health Care and the Good Society.*
New York: Oxford University Press.

—— 2003. *Hellfire Nation: The Politics of Sin in
American History.* New Haven: Yale University
Press.

—— 1998. *The Democratic Wish: Popular Participation
and the Limits of American Government.* New Haven:
Yale University Press

Rosenblatt, Rand. 1977. Health Care Reform and
    Administrative Law: A Structural Approach. *Yale
    Law Journal* 88 (2): 243-336.
Starr, Paul. 1982. *The Social Transformation of American
    Medicine*. New York: Basic Books.
Quadagno, Jill. 1995. *One Nation Uninsured: Why the
    US Has No Health Insurance*. New York: Oxford
    University Press.

Wennberg, John. 1990. "Sounding Board: Outcomes
    Research, Cost Containment and the Fear of Health
    Care Rationing," *New England Journal of Medicine*
    323 (17): 102–4.

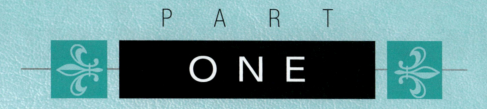

Ideas
and
Concepts

CHAPTER 1

Values in Health Policy: Understanding Fairness and Efficiency

Deborah Stone

Deborah Stone introduces us to the two most important values in health care. We can't have all we want of both fairness and efficiency, so we have to think about tradeoffs between them. In the process we learn a more fundamental lesson: how to think about values in health policy.

Two powerful ideals—fairness and efficiency—tower over health policy. These ideas unite us around lofty goals, only to divide us the minute we get down to details. That's not only because there is an inherent tension between fairness and efficiency, but also because each has multiple meanings. Different interpretations of fairness and efficiency define different kinds of community. They draw different boundaries, gather different memberships and offer different levels of inclusiveness. In the shadow of these grand ideals lurk many dilemmas for those who would use them as yardsticks for policy evaluation.

EFFICIENCY

Let's start with efficiency, for though it is less inspiring than fairness, it is the more deceptively simple of the two, and more often taken for granted as an incontrovertible value in health policy.

Efficiency is another word for a bargain. It is getting the most for the least, or, in slightly more economic terms, producing the most output for a given input. All policy reformers promise to give the country a bargain. Every person with a program to peddle promises that this program will save more than it costs. Efficiency is one of those motherhood values that everybody is *for,* so long as no one spells out exactly what it means—but it papers over a lot of conflicts.

The idea behind efficiency is engagingly simple: First, we measure the costs and benefits of any program, proposal, or procedure. Then, with measurements in hand, we can compare them and choose the course of action with the highest ratio of benefits to costs.

There are lots of problems with this vision, but the most basic is the core assumption that efficiency is an empirically measurable fact. I want to suggest, instead, that efficiency is a concept that must have and come from a point of view. Efficiency can be judged only with reference to a vantage point, and vantage points are particular, not universal. With multiple vantage points come multiple efficiencies. Efficiency is not the one best way to do things for society as a whole (as Pareto would have it). Efficiencies, like politicians, are tied to constituencies. Let me illustrate with five examples.

The Waiting Room

A doctor's waiting room is set up to be efficient. With long training and very expensive expertise, a doctor is a valuable resource. A doctor can't know in advance how much time each patient will need, so to use the resource most efficiently, the receptionist schedules patients so that there are always several waiting in the waiting room. The doctor never has an unused minute. The patients kill a lot of time. You know the drill—how much time have *you* killed in doctors' waiting rooms in your life? (I venture to say it is more time than you have bought yourself by reducing your cholesterol.)

The waiting room game is efficient only if we regard it from the doctor's point of view. The doctor, as a resource, is being used to the max. His or her time is never wasted. Now look at it from the patients' point of view. Some of their time is always wasted. In order to say that the waiting room system produces the most medical care for the least amount of time, we have to ignore all the patients' wasted time. Or we have to value patients' time much less than the doctor's time. Or both.

The point is simple. One person's efficiency is another person's waste. Even if we think that organizing medical care so that patients wait for doctors is the most efficient use of medical resources for society as a whole, we still buy societal efficiency at the cost of lots of wasted time for lots of people. Somebody is hurt. The doctor's waiting room is a good metaphor for the core notion of efficiency itself—every gain and every loss belongs to somebody.

The Million-Dollar Catheter Lab

Under the headline "Doctors Say They Can Save Lives and Still Save Money," the *New York Times* ran an article touting the Geisinger Foundation in Minnesota as the wave of the future. The Geisinger Foundation had figured out how to increase efficiency in medical care. Among its tricks was a grand version of the waiting room game. The health plan avoided "duplication of costly equipment" by doing all cardiac catheterizations at one hospital. "This does mean," the *New York Times* allowed, "that some patients have to travel up to 100 miles for major procedures that in a less efficient system might be available at a community hospital."[1]

It might be more efficient to have only one cardiac catheterization lab for the entire community served by the Geisinger Foundation, but we shouldn't leap to that conclusion before we tally up all the costs of centralization. First, there are the costs of patients' time; then the time of their spouses, friends, or whomever accompanies the patients; then the travel and lodging costs for all the people who have to travel so far from home. There are the emotional costs of making this procedure into an even bigger deal than it already it is by embedding it in a trip away from home. There may be still more costs associated with leaving home—paying someone else to mind the kids, for example, or the burden to yet another relative who comes into the home to mind the kids. One can imagine an infinite chain of disturbance: John needs a cardiac catheterization, his wife Janice goes with him, her sister Janeen takes time off from work to mind their kids, Janeen's husband Arthur eats out because Janeen's not there to cook, Janeen's colleagues work harder to fill in for her, and some of Janeen's work doesn't get done, with attendant costs to her employer.

A full efficiency calculus has to take into account all these points of view—the points of view of all the people who are affected by the remote location of catheterization labs. Tracing out such chains of consequences is rather like doing genealogy: We can decide to go only so far as our great-grandparents, but drawing those limits is an arbitrary decision.

This represents what I call the boundary problem in efficiency measurement. How do we know where to draw the boundaries in including the ramifications and costs of any way of organizing medical care? There are no natural or correct or obvious boundaries, because people live embedded in social networks, just as they are born into unbounded genealogical trees.

The Paycheck

Every paycheck is an expenditure to a hospital and a livelihood to an employee, and therein lies a tale. Whether that paycheck goes on the output side or the input side of an efficiency ratio depends on who is doing the accounting.

We could adopt the point of view of the hospital CEO, and say we are trying to measure efficiency from the point of view of the hospital. How much input does it take to produce our output? To the CEO, the paycheck is input, and she or he wants to write as few paychecks as possible and keep each one of them as low as possible.

But the hospital is also a community institution and a major local employer. To the governor, the mayor, and even the neighbors, the hospital's role is not only to make sick people well but also to provide economic stability to the neighborhood. From the point of view of the local community, each hospital payroll check is output many times over. It means a livelihood to a hospital employee and her family. Because employees will spend most of their paychecks, each check means revenue to local businesses and, in turn, paychecks to those businesses' employees.

Robert Reich, the former secretary of labor, has made a career on the idea that economies produce not only goods and services, but jobs. Reich has taught us that while labor counts as "inputs" to production in classic market models, employment is also an economic output. Societies whose economies produce more employment for their members are usually better off than those whose economies produce less.

Thus, President Bill Clinton was only half right when he said in his first inaugural address that we can't fix our economy without doing something about health care costs. The half he didn't mention is that our health care system is the strongest part of our economy in terms of jobs. Between 1988 and 1992, in the run-up to the Clinton presidency, jobs in health care grew 43%, while jobs elsewhere in the private sector inched up a paltry 1%.[2] Thanks largely to a graying population, jobs in the health sector are projected to increase almost twice as fast as jobs in all industries—27% compared with 14%—over the next several years.[3] There's a nasty double bind here. Health care expenditures are eating up our GNP and raising the cost of American goods, but every health care expenditure is income to someone employed in the health sector, or to someone employed by someone who makes things for the health care sector. We can't get a handle on health care costs unless we are willing to put a lot of people out of work.

There's another wrinkle to the paycheck story. Jobs, on balance, probably contribute to people's health: Paychecks feed families. Jobs give people pride, satisfaction, something to do. For the lucky employees of large businesses, jobs provide health insurance and access to medical care. To be sure, not all jobs provide decent wages, stress-free work, or even safe and healthy work, much less health insurance. But to the extent that jobs do provide these things, reducing the input side of health production by reducing paychecks doesn't necessarily increase the ratio of output (health) to input (dollars).

Only from the vantage point of someone whose vision stops at the hospital walls does cutting staff increase efficiency. From a wider community vantage point, such as the mayor's, the efficiency calculus is much different. To extend the analogy, insofar as health analysts look only at the efficiency of health providers, they neglect all the important ways health activities are *outputs* to the communities in which providers provide.

The Leaky Bladder

To talk about producing health care most efficiently requires us to think that health care production can be analyzed like widget production. The most important difference is that medicine works not by people doing something to inert objects, but by people interacting in a relationship. Trust and warmth in the relationship contribute to better diagnosis and more effective therapy. Without getting sentimental about old fashioned doctoring, it is probably fair to say that time and talk are the two great healers. When time and talk are treated as inputs in a production process, to be measured and minimized, medical care will suffer.

Economists traditionally measure productivity in manufacturing as output per labor hour. In the service sector, this definition becomes something like "number of people processed per labor hour," since handling people is what service industries do. Thus, hospital productivity is measured in patient days. Extra personnel, such as more nurses or ombudspersons, no doubt add to patients' comfort and sense of well-being, and maybe even to their health; but they lower productivity statistics because now there are more workers spread over the same number of patients.

If we adopt the point of view of the consumers, patients, and families instead of the CEOs, productivity looks very different. In choosing a hospital or a nursing home for a relative, you would look for a *high* staff-to-patient ratio. The very qualities that make hospitals and other human services more attractive to consumers—more useful and helpful to them—make them less productive in efficiency statistics.

What happens when we use economic notions of efficiency to re-shape health services and drive down costs? Consider New York's effort to reduce its spending for home care during the 1990s. New York has the most extensive and generous Medicaid home care program. In 1991, 63 cents of every Medicaid dollar spent nationally on home care were spent in New York.[4] The state department of social services decided to apply Scientific Taylorism to home care. The department devised a system of defining precise client needs—such as feeding, toileting, and bathing—and designated an amount of time necessary for each task. The goal was to pay home care workers only for the time necessary to do these instrumental tasks and to cut out the unproductive or "dead time." The dead time is the time a home care worker spends chatting with the client—schmoozing, joking, just being together in a human relationship. Under the new system, an elderly woman whose chief problem is incontinence would no longer be eligible for a full-time live-in attendant. Her allotment of care would be ten-and-a-half hours per week. That was apparently the time it took to service someone without bladder control. The department thought of paying for her care in the same way an auto mechanic would figure out how much time it takes service a car with a leaky gas tank. The pursuit of instrumental efficiency reduced this woman to a leaky container that needed mopping up.[5]

In health care, it is hard to tell what efficiency is because we don't know what "output" is in the first place. We use some crude population measures, such as infant mortality and life expectancy, but these are not good measures of a health system's output since they are influenced by lots of factors besides medical care. Researchers in the field of outcomes research have come up with a host of indicators about specific treatments, such as survival rates for cardiac bypass operations or recurrence rates for urinary tract infections. Others have developed "report cards" to measure organizational performance on such indicators as consumer satisfaction, delivery of preventive care, and administrative efficiency.

Most of what the health system produces is not so easily definable and measurable—things such as better functioning, lowered risk of future disease, reduced pain, education about caring for oneself, and, let us not forget, reassurance, hope, and a sense of well-being. Health researchers are going to be hard-put to provide consumers with this kind of outcome data.

Pain control, peace of mind, dignity, hope, and other important features of medical care are notoriously hard to measure. And when the only incentive is to score well on the measures, that which is measurable drives out the unmeasurable. Suppose, for example, that all the outcome studies found that waiting a month or two to investigate a mildly suspicious breast lump had no discernible impact on survival rates among women whose lumps turn out to be malignant. Health plans might save money—without sacrificing longevity—by reducing their capacity for ultrasounds and biopsies and making women (and their anxious families) wait a few months for diagnoses. The outcome data on those plans would look just fine to regulators and consumers. The price would look good, too. Yet the human costs and benefits—private terror versus peace of mind—would not be measured, much less factored into the efficiency calculus.

These are some of the traps that await the health care efficiency experts. Without carefully specifying *whose* costs count, what kinds of costs we want to control, and what kinds of output we want from the medical system, we end up simply shifting the burden and producing all kinds of perverse results.

The Cost-Ineffective TB Program[6]

Paul Farmer, doctor, anthropologist, and international medical activist, was troubled by the large number of cases of drug-resistant tuberculosis in Haiti and Peru. When he and his colleague Dr. Jim Yong Kim tried to interest the World Health Organization in funding public health campaigns against MDR-TB (multi-drug-resistant tuberculosis, as the disease is nicknamed), they learned that WHO had deemed treating the disease in developing countries as not cost-effective. Indeed, it did cost about $15,000 per person to treat a patient with MDR-TB. Treating the simpler forms of TB that do respond to standard antibiotics was much cheaper. And so, in the deadly jargon of policy analysis, WHO had declared in one of its manuals: "In settings of resource constraint [read: poor countries], it is necessary for rational resource allocation to prioritise TB treatment categories according to the

cost-effectiveness of treatment of each category."[7] In other words, doctors like Farmer and Kim were supposed to ignore patients with MDR-TB because they could cure more people by putting all their resources into treating those with ordinary TB.

With WHO's seal-of-disapproval for treating MDR-TB in developing countries, it was nearly impossible for Farmer and Kim to raise money to support their programs. They were so committed to treating the disease, though, that they went ahead treating a small number of patients, begging and borrowing the money and drugs to do it. (At one point, they were "found out" by Brigham and Women's Hospital; they had taken $92,000 worth of drugs from its pharmacy to Haiti and Peru. But they never intended to steal; they had a philanthropist in their corner who wrote a check to the hospital, with a note saying he thought the hospital "ought to be more generous toward the poor.") They were determined to prove that at least the disease was curable. And they were incensed by the way that cost-effectiveness analysis, as they saw it, "rationalized an irrational status quo: MDR treatment was cost-effective in a place like New York, but not in a place like Peru."

Farmer and Kim had been buying some drugs to treat MDR-TB in different places. They noticed that one of the drugs, manufactured by Eli Lilly, cost $29.90 per vial at the Brigham and Women's Hospital in Boston, $21.00 a vial in Peru, and only $8.80 per vial in Paris. When their Paris supplier suddenly refused to sell them any more drugs, a light bulb went on: The price of drugs is set by the pharmaceutical manufacturers, and they set radically different prices for different markets. If that were true—and it still is—then the "cost" of treating MDR-TB wasn't a given. The "cost" in cost-effectiveness analysis was an artifact of the drug manufacturer's pricing policies.

Dr. Kim, Dr. Farmer, and their allies browbeat, jawboned, and negotiated. They persuaded some manufacturers to lower their prices for the MDR-TB drugs, and persuaded one of them, Eli Lilly, which had a patent on one of the most effective drugs, to donate large amounts of its drug. Suddenly, the cost of curing a case of drug-resistant TB plummeted from $15,000 a year to $1,500 a year, and cure rates were very high.

But it wasn't enough to get one or two companies to lower prices for a small amount of drugs. Farmer and Kim set about trying to change the market for MDR-TB drugs, to change the entire system of supply and demand. They knew they needed to get someone to manufacture large quantities of these drugs for less money. They joined forces with other non-profit organizations to stimulate smaller drug manufacturers to make generic versions of MDR-TB drugs. In order to convince generic manufacturers to develop and produce the drugs, they had to show that there was a market for them, meaning that a lot of TB projects would use (and buy) them. They masterminded a plan to get MDR-TB drugs listed on WHO's official list of "essential drugs," a list that in itself symbolically signaled a market demand. If a drug were on WHO's essential list, then firms should manufacture it regardless.

Farmer and Kim's public health coup turns cost-effectiveness analysis inside out. Cost-effectiveness and cost-benefit analyses depend on knowing the cost of whatever outcome you are trying to produce. You've got to plug *some* price into your equation. But if cost is simply a matter of what a supplier charges, then it, in turn, depends on the power relationships between buyers and sellers. When the World Health Organization evaluated the cost-effectiveness of treating MDR-TB in developing countries, it took the price of drugs as a given— something fixed, inherent, and unchangeable. Implicitly, then, WHO also took as a given the political economy of pharmaceuticals—the dominant market position of large American pharmaceutical companies, the monopoly pricing permitted by American patent protection, the power of manufacturers to dictate prices, and WHO's power to dictate what diseases public health programs would treat, and therefore which drugs they would purchase.

If instead, we regard the cost of inputs as themselves outputs of a political-economic system, then they are not objective measures, and the cost-benefit analysis that derives from them is no more objective.

Prices and cost-effectiveness judgments are captives of the political status quo, and cost-effectiveness analysis is a recipe for preserving the current distribution of resources.

FAIRNESS

Elsewhere in the world, medical insurance is called "sickness insurance" and it covers sick people. In the United States, we have "health insurance," and as befits its name, insurers strive to weed out sick people and cover only the healthy. This is about as perverse a system as one can imagine, and one that poses an extraordinary puzzle: Why and how does a country's political system produce a health-policy sub-system whose result is absolutely antithetical to its public purpose? The result can only be explained as a long history of political conflict between world-views about fairness and equity. This conflict is vividly illustrated—quite literally, illustrated with photographs—in the advertising campaigns of health insurance and other interest groups.

In the late 1980s, the trade associations of the health and life insurance industry sponsored an advertising campaign to persuade the public that "paying for someone else's risks" is a bad idea. In one of these ads, a photo of a worker in a hard hat and tool belt straddling the girders of a steel tower was captioned "If you don't take risks, why should you pay for someone else's?" Another ad showed a young man and woman playing basketball one-on-one, and asked "Why should men and women pay different rates for their health and life insurance?" The choral refrain at the bottom of each ad in the series went "The lower your risk, the lower your premium," and the small print explained the relevant facts. For example,

> Women under 55 normally incur more health care expenses than men of the same age, so they pay more for individual health insurance than men. After age 55, women

generally have lower claims costs, so they normally pay less for individual health insurance than men of the same age.

That's why insurers have to group people with similar risks when they calculate premiums. If they didn't, people with low risks would end up subsidizing people with high risks. And that wouldn't be fair.

In 1991, with Bill Clinton running on a platform of universal access to health care, The Prudential Insurance Company ran a very different sort of ad campaign. In the *New York Times, Wall Street Journal,* and many news weeklies, readers saw a photo of a chest X-ray with a large white mass in the lower right quadrant. Though most readers couldn't interpret the X-ray, the caption explained its significance: "Because he works for a small company, the prognosis isn't good for his fellow workers either." The small-print text went on to explain how one employee's serious illness might cause a small company to be charged "excessively high premiums" come renewal time, and how the company might even be forced to drop its health insurance coverage. Prudential, readers were assured, didn't consider this situation fair, and so it was backing legislation to "regulate the guidelines and rating practices of insurers." Offering a rather different interpretation of fairness from the one in the trade association series a few years back, Prudential opined: "After all, a small company shouldn't be forced to drop its health plan because an employee was sick enough to need it."

These advertisements have many layers of meaning. On the surface, the issue is how commercial insurers ought to price their health insurance policies. Just below the surface lurks the struggle over health insurance reform proposals in the states and Congress. But the underlying question is whether medical care should be distributed as a right of citizenship or as a market commodity. If, as "the lower-your-risk-the-lower-your-premium" series commends, we charge people as closely as possible for the medical care they need and consume, then we are treating medical care like other consumer goods

distributed through the market. If, like Prudential, we are unwilling to throw sick people and their fellow employees out of the insurance lifeboat, if we think that perhaps the healthy should help pay for the care of others, then medical care becomes more like things we distribute as a basic right, such as education. These advertisements symbolize two very different logics of insurance: the actuarial fairness principle and the solidarity principle.

At a still deeper level, these advertisements offer competing visions of community. They suggest how Americans should think about what ties them together, and to whom they have ties. In one view, no one else should feel an obligation to pay for the medical care of those who get injured while doing constructive work for society. Similarly, women of childbearing age are exhorted daily to assure the health of their babies, even those not yet conceived; yet no one else should finance their extra medical care, least of all the men with whom they are creating the next generation. Alternatively, says the Prudential ad, we should not abandon those who are sick or attached to people who are sick; sick and healthy, we are all one community.

Many things go into the making of community. Communities share a common culture and a way of perpetuating it. They establish processes for governance, conflict resolution, and self-defense. But above all, the people in a community help each other. Mutual aid among a group of people who see themselves as sharing common interests is the essence of community. A willingness to help each other is the glue that holds people together as a society, whether a simple peasant community, an urban neighborhood, or a modern welfare state. What distinguishes the mutual aid in the modern welfare state from that in peasant societies is largely a matter of scale: the number of people encompassed in the mutual aid network, the complexity of the rules that govern how we aid one another, and the variety of goods and services that we provide.

All mutual aid systems are based on a communal agreement—why, when, and to whom should people give up something of their own and offer help? This is not to say there is no conflict over redistribution in a community; on the contrary, the agreements are constantly under challenge, the communal boundaries are always being re-drawn. But there is also a core of stable expectations about when people can expect help from one another.

In most societies, sickness is widely accepted as a condition that should trigger mutual aid; the American polity, however, has had a weak and wavering commitment to that principle. The politics of medical insurance can only be understood as a struggle over the meaning of sickness and whether it is a condition that should automatically generate mutual assistance. This is more than a cultural conflict, however—more than a fight over meanings. The private insurance industry, the first line of defense in the U.S. system of mutual aid for sickness, is organized around a principle profoundly antithetical to the idea of mutual aid. Indeed, the growth and survival of the industry depends on its ability to finance health care by charging the sick and convincing the public that "each person should pay for his own risk."

Actuarial fairness—each person paying for his or her own risk—is more than an idea about distributive justice. It is a method of organizing mutual aid by fragmenting communities into ever smaller, more homogeneous groups. It is a method that leads ultimately to the destruction of mutual aid. This fragmentation must be accomplished by fostering in people a sense of their differences rather than their commonalities; it emphasizes responsibility for self rather than interdependence within a community. Moreover, insurance necessarily operates on the logic of actuarial fairness when it, in turn, is organized as a competitive market.

Both social and commercial health insurance are mechanisms for pooling savings and redistributing funds from healthy premium-payers to sick ones. However, they operate by two fundamentally different logics—the solidarity principle and actuarial fairness.

The Solidarity Principle

Social insurance operates by the logic of *solidarity*. Its purpose is to guarantee that certain agreed-upon individual needs will be paid for by a community or group. This is the logic of mutual aid societies and fraternal associations, as well as government social insurance programs. Having decided in advance that some need is deserving of social aid, a society undertakes to guarantee that the need is met for all its members. The argument for financing medical care via social insurance rests on the prior assumption that medical care should be distributed according to medical need.

If medical care were financed like most market goods, by charging people for exactly the goods and services they consume, medical care would only be partially distributed according to need. Those who are sick and need care would come forward to purchase it, but only those who could afford it would actually receive care. In addition, some who are not sick but who have plenty of resources might try to purchase care as well. People who could not afford to buy care would not receive any, regardless of their need for it.

Social insurance unties the two essential connections of the market, the link between the amount one pays for care and the amount one consumes, and the link between the amount of care one buys and one's ability to pay. Under a social insurance scheme, individuals are entitled to receive whatever care they need, and the amounts they pay to finance the scheme are totally unrelated to the amount or cost of care they actually use. (Of course, to the extent there are coinsurance and deductibles in a social insurance scheme, the amount a person pays is slightly related to the amount one consumes.)

Of course, even social insurance doesn't guarantee that medical care is distributed exactly according to medical need. Need, after all, is a rather elusive concept, all the more so in medicine. Unlike most consumer goods, the value of medical care depends on its being customized. Whether someone can benefit from a particular medical procedure doesn't hinge on personal "tastes and preferences," as classical economic theory would have it, but rather on a correct match between a medical procedure and the person's pathology. The degree to which social insurance results in allocation of care according to need is mediated by the professional skill of medical personnel in matching procedures to pathologies. Many other factors influence the distribution of care as well, such as local professional norms about the appropriate use of procedures, the supply of medical facilities and personnel and equipment, and ownership of diagnostic and therapeutic facilities, such as imaging centers and dialysis clinics.[8] All of these factors mean that even under a system of pure social insurance, medical care will not be perfectly distributed according to medical need. But the *ideal* of the solidarity principle is that we should strive to distribute medical care according to medical need, and to limit the influence of one's ability to pay.

The solidarity principle doesn't require that medical care be distributed equally in the sense that everyone gets the same amount. Social insurance is not a fixed-shares arrangement, where each contributing member gets an equal slice of the pie. When people "pool their risks" and their savings in social insurance, they are taking their chances that they may never become sick or need expensive care, and that most of their contributions will go to help the members who do incur a need for expensive care. As in any lottery, they pay into the pot, regardless of whether they ultimately get to draw out of it.

In fact, only some members of a risk pool will get sick enough to need care. Since only those who get seriously sick will receive a payout, the others necessarily pay to help them. Thus, redistribution from the healthy to the sick is built into insurance. Payouts are made on the basis of need (or loss incurred), not on the basis of contributions to the scheme. Health policy analysts and corporate benefits managers frequently discover with great alarm that a small portion of insured people accounts for a huge proportion of claims expenditures, as though this skewing means that something is amiss. But subsidy from the vast majority of insured people to a small minority is precisely what is supposed to happen in insurance. Such skewing is what people agree to when they join a social insurance risk-pool. They accept it because they don't know, when they join, whether they will be on the giving end or

the receiving end, and they want to protect themselves in case they are part of the unlucky minority. They accept it, too, because they believe that sickness is one of those contingencies when society should rally around the individual.

Actuarial Fairness

Commercial insurers—that is, private firms selling insurance as a profit-making venture—operate on a deep contradiction. They provide for pooling of risks and mutual aid among policyholders, much as social insurance does; yet they select their policyholders, group them, and price their policies according to market logic. When they speak of equity, commercial insurers espouse the principle of actuarial fairness: Premium rates should be differentiated so that "each insured [person] will pay in accordance with the quality of his risk."[9] By quality of risk, insurers mean the likelihood a person will incur whatever loss he or she is insured against. In life insurance, they are principally interested in factors that might affect life expectancy; in health insurance, they are interested in factors that affect or predict a person's use of medical care. These include one's occupation, hobbies (since some are very dangerous), family medical history, personal medical history, and any medical information such as family history or a genetic marker that predicts disease, even if the disease hasn't yet occurred.

Insurers assert that actuarial fairness requires them to seek the most complete risk information on applicants. An insurer has the "responsibility to treat all its policy holders fairly by establishing premiums at a level consistent with risk represented by each individual policyholder."[10] To accomplish this task, insurers must have the "right . . . to create classifications to recognize the many differences which exist among individuals." People who have diseases or serious risks to their health are in a sense getting a more valuable insurance policy than those with lesser risks, so they ought to pay more for the extra value. Or, to see the matter another way, if insurers did not identify people with higher risks, separate them from the general pool of policyholders, and charge them more, insurers would be causing a "forced subsidy from the healthy to the less healthy."[11] "An applicant presenting a low risk of loss to the insurer should not be required to subsidize another applicant who presents a higher degree of risk."[12]

Here is the crux of the conflict: The very redistribution from the healthy to the sick that is the essential purpose of medical insurance under the solidarity principle is anathema to commercial insurers under the actuarial principle. Tellingly, insurers virtually never use the word "subsidy" without a pejorative modifier such as "coerced," "forced," or "unfair." Although all insurance entails a subsidy from the lucky to the unlucky (whether luck concerns car accidents, diseases, or fires), commercial insurers eschew subsidy from one "class" of policyholders to another. "Class," in insurance jargon, means risk class, or a group of people with similar probabilities of becoming sick (or perhaps more accurately, with similar probabilities of generating costs to the insurer). To commercial insurers, subsidy is not what they pursue, but the *unwanted result* of their failure to segregate people into homogeneous risk classes.

If the actuarial fairness principle could be perfectly implemented, if we had perfect predictive information and precise rating, each person would pay for himself. This, of course, would be the antithesis of insurance. In fact, in a world of perfect predictive information, there would be no need and no market demand for insurance, because no one would stand to gain by "beating the odds." Since each insurance policy would be priced according to the medical care actually consumed by each policyholder, people would do better to pay for their care directly and avoid paying for the administrative expenses and profits of insurance companies. And since the price of insurance would be the same as the price of needed medical care, those who couldn't afford to pay for their own care couldn't afford to pay for insurance either. Insurers rarely acknowledge that actuarial fairness undermines the solidarity principle of insurance—the very reason to have insurance— but the ultimate conclusion of the logic of actuarial fairness is clear. In the words of Robert Goldstone,

vice president and medical director of Pacific Mutual Life Company,

> In theory, every individual should have a different rate, based on a multivariate analysis of every possible health condition and risk factor that can be evaluated.[13]

Actuarial Fairness and the Politics of Exclusion

To put the matter simply, the U.S got a "health insurance" system instead of a "sickness insurance" system because our government fostered privatization of the social welfare function from the beginning. Because government allowed the private sector to provide the first line of defense against illness, and because the private sector operated on the logic of actuarial fairness, the door was open for a politics of exclusion.

The first battles over insurance company underwriting practices concerned race, specifically the use of race as an underwriting criterion in life insurance. As early as the 1880s, several states tried to prohibit life insurance companies from charging higher rates to blacks than whites.[14] Insurers found it quite easy to avoid public interference with their "scientific principles." In 1900, Frederick Hoffman, then chief statistician of The Prudential Company, wrote that many states had passed laws "compelling Industrial [life insurance] companies to accept Negro risks at the same rates as those charged the white population. Fortunately," he boasted, "the companies cannot be compelled to solicit this class of risks, and very little business of this class is now written by Industrial companies, practically none by the Prudential."[15]

In the ensuing century, there have been more battles between the public and private sectors over race and other social groupings. In the late 1960s and 1970s, the property insurance field was plagued by the issue of "redlining"; the racial composition of a neighborhood became an explicit factor in determining the availability of mortgages and property insurance. Also in the 1970s, activists challenged the use of gender as a factor the price of life and disability insurance, as well as automobile insurance. Disease-based interest groups (notably Tay-Sachs Disease, Sickle Cell Anemia, and DES mothers and daughters) challenged the use of "their disease" as a criterion in underwriting life and health insurance, and succeeded in winning protections in several states. In the late 1980s, the dominant underwriting issue was life and health insurers' use of sexual orientation as a proxy for AIDS risk and then HIV tests.

For the most part, insurers have been able to block restrictions on their underwriting criteria, either by defeating bills and regulations or by inserting narrow language to permit the use of criteria that are "actuarially sound." What risk classification and segregation insurers cannot accomplish through direct medical underwriting, they can often accomplish through targeted marketing or pricing. Prudential's early strategy of simply not soliciting Negro business was the prototype. Today we see HMOs and other managed care plans featuring their maternity and fitness club benefits when they market plans to employee groups; they market to the young and healthy. Some health plans quietly avoid contracting with physicians in minority neighborhoods, another way of making their insurance inaccessible to populations against whom they cannot discriminate outright.

And finally, commercial insurers by-and-large have been able to capture public regulators. Most state insurance departments and commissions are controlled by men who come from commercial insurance and will return to lucrative jobs there. They share the insurers' worldview in which equity is actuarial fairness. In the 1980s, when the battle over HIV testing by health and life insurers was largely perceived as a struggle about the inclusion of gays in the insurance lifeboat, a state commissioner told the Office of Technology Assessment (emphasis added):

"We encourage insurers to test where appropriate because we don't want insurance companies to issue policies to people who are sick, likely to be sick, or likely to die."[16]

When public regulators see their job as protecting private health insurers from covering sick people, we get a system of "health insurance" instead of "sickness insurance."

It is not going to be easy to eradicate the actuarial fairness principle from the American insurance system. We have had nearly a century of industry promoting the "each person should pay for himself" principle as the ideal of fairness. The public servants who are responsible for regulating insurance generally believe in this principle as both a matter of fairness and a matter of financial necessity. Actuarial fairness makes sense as a business strategy in competitive insurance markets. With this combination of elements, it will be extraordinarily difficult to prevent insurers from engaging in implicit and explicit underwriting within any foreseeable system based on market competition among insurers.

Efficiency and fairness are fine aspirations for public programs, but no one should be lulled into thinking they are neutral criteria for judging the virtues of health care systems or reform proposals. They are more like empty packages, craftily gift-wrapped with glitter and bows, tempting us to imagine their contents. Political actors, stakeholders in the complex world of health insurance, conduct much of their politics by offering visions of what might be in these boxes under different political and economic scenarios. When the boxes are finally opened, some people will be showered with useful and lucrative gifts; others will go away empty-handed.

STUDY QUESTIONS

1. What are some examples that demonstrate that efficiency is a subjective concept?
2. What are some of the costs pertaining to centralization of (medical) procedures?
3. How does the 'boundary problem' arise in the measurement of efficiency?

4. How can rising health care costs be seen as a positive development? Whose perspective would this require one to adopt?

5. Why is it difficult to identify (much less measure) health 'outputs'?

6. Why is it important to treat health input costs as products of a particular politico-economic configuration, rather than absolute?

7. What are the actuarial fairness and solidarity principles? What is their relevance to the finance of health care?

8. Develop an opinion: Which principle—actuarial fairness or solidarity—orms a superior basis for insuring health care? Why? Note the strengths and weaknesses of each principle.

9. Why are there limitations on the extent to which health care can be matched to patient need, even under a system governed by the principles of mutual aid?

10. In what sense do commercial insurers act in ways that, taken to their logical conclusion, would render insurance superfluous?

11. How has the issue of insuring populations become racially charged?

NOTES

1. Erik Eckholm, 1991, A1.
2. Robert Pear, 1993, A1.
3. US Department of Labor, Bureau of Labor Statistics, Bulletin 2601, "The 2006–07 Career Guide To Industries, Table 3 (www.bls.gov/oco/cg/print/cgs035.htm, visited Jan. 15, 2006).
4. Bennett, 1992, p A1.
5. This story is from the *New York Times* article, *ibid*.
6. I take the details of this story from Kidder, 2003. All quotations in this section are from this book unless otherwise noted.
7. World Health Organization, *Treatment of Tuberculosis: Guidelines for National Programmes*. 2nd ed. Geneva, 1997, quoted in Kidder, 2003, p 141.

8. Hillman, B.J., et al., 1990, 1604–8
9. Bailey, H.T., T.M. Hutchinson, and G.R. Narber, 1976.
10. Clifford, K., and R. Iuculano, 1987.
11. Clifford, K., and R. Iuculano, *ibid*.
12. Hoffman, J.N., and E.Z. Kincaid. 1986–7. "AIDS: The Challenge to Life and Health Insurers' Freedom of Contract." *Drake Law Review* 35: 709–71.
13. Goldstone, R., 1992.
14. James, Marquis, 1947.
15. Hoffman, F.L., 1900.
16. Statement made at a meeting (February 17, 1987) of the Advisory Panel to the Office of Technology Assessment for its study, *Medical Testing and Health Insurance* (US Congress, 1988). I was a member of this panel.

REFERENCES

Bailey, H.T., T.M. Hutchinson, and G.R. Narber. 1976. The Regulatory Challenge to Life Insurance Classification. *Drake Law Review* 25: 779–827.

Bennett, James. 1992. "Home Care in New York, A Model Plan, Awaits Cuts," *New York Times* November 20. p A1.

Clifford, K., and R. Iuculano. 1987. "AIDS and Insurance: The Rationale for AIDS-related Testing," *Harvard Law Review* 100: 1806–24.

Eckholm, Erik. 1991. "Doctors Say They Can Save Lives and Still Save Money." *New York Times* March 18. p A1.

Goldstone, R. 1992. "Substandard, Not Inferior." *Best's Review* 92 (March): 24–8, 90.

Hillman, B. J., et al. 1990. "Frequency and Costs of Diagnostic Imaging in Office Practice—A comparison of Referring and Radiologist-Referring Physicians. *New England Journal of Medicine* 323: 1604–8.

Hoffman, F.L. 1900. History of The Prudential Insurance Company of America (Industrial Insurance) 1875–1900. Prudential Press.

Hoffman, J.N., and E.Z. Kincaid. 1986–7. "AIDS: The Challenge to Life and Health Insurers' Freedom of Contract." *Drake Law Review* 35: 709–71.

Kidder, Tracy. 2003. Mountains Beyond Mountains: The Quest of Dr. Paul Farmer, A Man Who Would Cure the World. New York: Random House.

James, Marquis. 1947. The Metropolitan Life: A Study in Business Growth. New York: Viking Press.

Pear, Robert. 1993. "Health-Care Cots Up Sharply Again, Posing New Threat," *New York Times* January 5. p A1.

US Department of Labor, Bureau of Labor Statistics. Bulletin 2601, "The 2006–07 Career Guide To Industries, "Table 3 (www.bls.gov/oco/cg/print/cgs035.htm, visited January 15, 2006).

US Congress. 1988. Advisory Panel to the Office of Technology Assessment for its study, *Medical Testing Health Insurance*.

CHAPTER 2

Markets and Politics

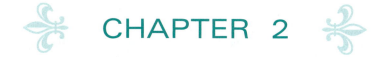

In this chapter, Thomas Rice explains how economists think about the two most important concepts in health care economics—markets and government.

MARKETS

Since the publication by Adam Smith of *Wealth of Nations* in 1776, economists have been enamored with markets. This is understandable. Smith and subsequent analysts demonstrated that markets can, through an "invisible hand," make the self-interested actions of disparate individuals result in—at least by some definitions—an "optimal" allocation of society's resources.

The logic of markets is now well understood. People "demand" the things that they want most, ensuring that they purchase the market basket of goods and services that maximizes their "utilities" given their limited budgets. Suppliers produce only those things that are demanded by consumers, and in doing so must use inputs as efficiently as possible so as to price their products low enough to attract buyers. Thus, people are able to buy the things they desire, and these things are

produced using the least costly set of inputs. Furthermore, the profit motive encourages firms and would-be firms to be innovative in developing new products and techniques to meet future consumer demands.

Economists have shown that if certain assumptions are met, then a market economy will result in a state called "Pareto optimality," named after Italian economist Vilfredo Pareto. Under Pareto optimality, it is impossible to make someone better off without making someone else worse off. This might seem to be an odd criterion for optimality, but upon reflection it is logical. If an economy were not in Pareto optimality, then it would be possible to make someone better off without harming another person. But if that were the case, then things hardly would be optimal. Rather, changes could be instituted to help those who might benefit without resulting in any harm to others. Only when no such changes are any longer possible would the economy be in a Pareto optimal state.

Aside from its reliance on certain assumptions, it is critical to understand Pareto optimality does not address issues of equity or the desirability of the distribution of income that results from the workings of a competitive economy. Thus, a market outcome in which one person has nearly all of the output, and another has almost none, could still be consistent with Pareto optimality. In fact, this can easily occur if the former person begins with the vast majority of initial wealth or input. Amartya Sen makes this point graphically:

> An economy can be [Pareto] optimal . . . even when some people are rolling in luxury and others are near starvation as long as the starvers cannot be made better off without cutting into the pleasures of the rich. If preventing the burning of Rome would have made Emperor Nero feel worse off, then letting him burn Rome would have been Pareto-optimal. In short, a society or an economy can be Pareto-optimal and still be perfectly disgusting.[1]

Although it might seem desirable to transfer wealth from the rich person to the poor person, doing so cannot be viewed as improving the economy from a Pareto optimality standpoint because the change will involve making the rich person worse off.

In summary, under a market-based economic model, competition is designed to enhance efficiency; it does not necessarily improve equity. In thinking about the impact of markets on health care, we will need to consider both the applicability of the model's assumptions as well as any concerns we have about the resulting distribution of wealth.

ASSUMPTIONS UNDERLYING THE SUCCESSFUL OPERATION OF MARKETS

There is no single agreed-upon list of assumptions about which the competitive economic model is based. A simple, abbreviated list emphasizing the

implications for health policy would include the following key requirements:[2]

- Individuals are rational; they know what goods and services are likely to make them best off; and they can effectively use available information to achieve this best-off position given their wealth.

- Individuals' tastes for goods and services are predetermined and cannot be unduly influenced by physicians or other providers.

- The distribution of wealth is approved of by society, and furthermore, individuals care only about their own resources and not those of others.

What happens if these conditions are not met (as, I will argue, is the case in health care)? One policy alternative to markets is government intervention in the marketplace. Government can try to correct imperfections through direct regulation or control, or alternatively, institute policies to counteract some of the potentially undesirable consequences of market competition. To make this more concrete, suppose that direct-to-consumer advertising results in patients demanding prescription medications from their physicians that are both medically inappropriate and cost-increasing—resulting is poorer health and higher costs. A way to address this problem might be to further regulate the content and extent of such advertising (as was the case in the past). A different strategy would be for government to engage in its own advertising campaign to counteract what it believes to be misleading messages from industry. Sometimes both strategies are employed. In the case of cigarette smoking, government has banned or severely limited various types of advertising, and concurrently, created its own advertisements aimed at convincing smokers to quit and at others not to start.

The alternative to government action is for government to do nothing. Even if markets do a poor job in some areas, government might perform even worse. There are several possible reasons for this. Government officials may lack the expertise of those in the private sector. Moreover, they may be beholden to special interests, particularly those that contribute materially to these officials' power or wealth. And even in the absence of such undue influence, government is often inefficient because it does not face competition for the services it provides.[3]

Over the years many economists have weighted in over this issue. Henry Sidgwick (1887) once stated that, "It does not follow that whenever laissez-faire falls short government interference is expedient; since the inevitable drawbacks of the latter may, in any particular case, be worse than the shortcomings of private enterprise."[4] More than 100 years later, Mark Pauly expresses a similar view when noting that "a government staffed by angels could undoubtedly do a better job than markets run by humans"[5] he is less sure when humans run the government. Charles Wolf (1993) adds, "The actual choice is among imperfect markets, imperfect governments, and various combinations of the two. The cardinal economic choice concerns the degree to which markets or governments—each with their respective flaws—should determine the allocation, use, and distribution of resources in the economy."[6] We will return to the issue of how markets and government can work together to improve the health care.

MARKETS IN HEALTH CARE: ARE THE ASSUMPTIONS MET?

This section briefly reviews evidence drawn from health care systems about the three assumptions underlying markets, discussed earlier.

- Assumption No. 1: Individuals are rational; they know what goods and services are likely to make them best off; and they can effectively use available information to achieve this best-off position (given their wealth).

In most areas, health included, individuals tend to act fairly rationally and know what is best for themselves, at least as evaluated by conventional norms. There are obvious exceptions. People ride motorcycles without helmets. Some desperate people in developing countries sell their own organs, a practice that reduces rather increases their economic status.[7] Others kill themselves when an objective observer might have viewed the person's circumstances as remediable. In general, though, government does not interfere too much with markets to deal with these issues; rather, it lets people make good or bad decisions for themselves.

A more troubling issue is people's ability to successfully use information about health-related issues. This involves both care and coverage decisions. They face at least two types of problems. One relates to the concept of the "counterfactual." Counterfactual questions are those that are hypothetical in that they concern what would have happened if history had been different. Questions such as these can never be answered with certainty. Some examples in health: "Would the problem have gone away if I had left it untreated?" "What would have happened if I had sought the care of a specialist instead of a primary care physician?" And "Would the result have been different if I had seen a different primary care physician than the one I sought?"

In this regard, Burton Weisbrod has written that,

For ordinary goods, the buyer has little difficulty in evaluating the counterfactual—that is, what the situation will be if the good is not obtained. Not so for the bulk of health care . . . Because the human physiological system is itself an adaptive system, it is likely to correct itself and deal effectively with an ailment, even without any medical care services. Thus, a consumer of such services who gets better after the purchase does not know whether the improvement was because of, or even in spite of, the "care" that was received. Or if no health care services are purchased and the individual's problem becomes worse, he is generally not in a strong position to determine whether the results would have been different, and better, if he had purchased certain health care. And the consumer, not being a medical expert, may learn little from experience or from friends' experience . . . because of the difficulty of determining whether the counterfactual to a particular type of health care today is the same as it was the previous time the consumer, or a friend, had "similar" symptoms. The noteworthy point is not simply that it is difficult for the consumer to judge quality before the purchase . . . but that it is difficult even after the purchase.[8]

Decisions about whether to obtain care, what to obtain, and from whom to obtain it present extraordinary challenges to the consumer because markets are ill equipped to assist in answering counterfactual questions. But consumers also face a second set of challenges involving which health plan, hospital, or physician generalists and specialists to choose.

We focus here on choosing a health plan. There are many types of health plans available in the United States, including health maintenance organizations (HMOs), point-of-service plans (POSs), preferred provider organizations (PPOs), traditional or indemnity plans, and new-fangled "consumer-driven" health plans. Usually HMOs, POSs, and sometimes PPOs are referred to as examples of "managed care" while indemnity and consumer-driven plans are not. If consumers are going to choose the plan type that is best for their own preferences and circumstances, it behooves them to understand managed care—not just general issues but very particular ones, such as whether they can seek care directly from specialists and even what financial incentives their doctors and hospital face.

When surveyed, however, most consumers do not understand even rudimentary issues, such as the difference between fee-for-service medicine and managed care plans.[9] Consumers are particularly bad at understanding certain key features of their own health plans. One US survey, for example, found that whereas 62% of plan members believed that plans

had to approve specialty referrals, in reality approval was needed just 28% of the time.[10]

An area in which consumers need to be particularly skilled at using information is "report cards" on their health plans. People often obtain these report cards from their employer, and then are supposed to choose a health plan by weighing such factors as quality, convenience, flexibility, and costs. Currently, there is no one standard report card format.

Good report cards should be easy to understand. Some items, such as satisfaction ratings, are comprehensible to most people, but other elements are more problematic. It is not clear, for example, that consumers know how to make effective use of information on utilization rates for alternative services, or that they understand the relative importance of survival rates from high-incidence (i.e., heart disease) versus low-incidence (i.e., kidney failure) diseases. As a result, more recent iterations of report cards tend to be somewhat simpler than previous versions, presenting a limited number of items and often rating health plans by showing, say, between one and five stars for each measure of quality. Even then, consumers often do not know how to interpret the information being presented.[11]

Some of the early work on consumer response to health plan report cards was discouraging: not only did people not understand the report cards, but their availability did not seem to draw people to better-rated health plans.[12] There is some evidence that things may be beginning to change, however. One recent study that examined employees of General Motors found that although there is no evidence that people gravitated to health plans that receive high report card scores, there is evidence that they avoid plans with low scores. One limitation with the study, however, is the difficulty of determining whether the report cards themselves, or alternatively, other attributes of the health plans that receive low scores, cause people to move away from such plans.[13]

Challenges remain if we are to rely on the market to develop and disseminate report cards. Marc Rodwin notes a number of problems with the report cards in use today. One problem is that they ignore key aspects concerning how health plans operate such as the stringency of utilization review and the financial incentives that providers face. Another is that many of the tasks previously performed by health plans have now devolved to capitated physician groups, whose performance is only occasionally available from report cards. A third is that report cards—in order to simplify—tend to be aggregated and not focused on performance for particular medical conditions. It is the management of chronic conditions, however, that are perhaps the most important barometer of the success of a health plan since most serious illnesses are chronic ones and because they are responsible for the large majority of health care costs.[14]

- Assumption No. 2: Individuals' tastes for goods and services are predetermined and cannot be unduly influenced by physicians or other providers.

Economists often have a peculiar view of the genesis of human preferences or tastes. They are believed to be endemic to the individual—that is, something that is not influenced by the environment in which a person exists. (This may seem odd in light of the way in which advertising tends to work.) In economic theory, according to Lester Thurow, individual tastes and preferences "simply exist—fully developed and immutable."[15] This is what Kenneth Boulding has referred to as the "Immaculate Conception of the Indifference Curve," because "tastes are simply given, and . . . we cannot inquire into the process by which they are formed."[16]

How else could one account for the following statement by Nobel Prize winners George Stigler and Gary Becker, who write that, "[T]astes neither change capriciously nor differ importantly between people. . . . [O]ne does not argue over tastes for the same reason that one does not argue over the Rocky Mountains—both are there, will be there next year, too, and are the same for all men."[17] (Becker has also written that, "preferences are assumed not to change substantially over time, nor to be very different

between wealthy and poor persons, or even between persons in different societies and cultures."[18])

One natural application of this theory of the sovereignty of consumer preferences is the firm belief that physicians cannot "induce" demand among their patients, convincing them to receive services they would not want had they the same medical expertise as the physician. Perhaps no topic in health policy has generated more disagreements among economists, as well as between economists and other disciplines.

The existence of physician-induced demand would be at odds with a health care marketplace that is operating competitively. Two examples will help clarify why this is the case. Economists would normally expect that an increase in physician supply would lower prices, but that is not necessarily the case if physicians induce demand. Furthermore, we would also expect physicians to supply fewer services if they are paid less per service, but again, this would not necessarily be true if demand inducement were present.

Unfortunately, whether demand inducement exists and is an important element of the health care marketplace is terribly difficult, if not impossible, to demonstrate—there are many reasons for this,[19] but the most important is simple: to know for certain if physicians are inducing demand, we would have to know what patients would demand if they knew as much about medicine as the physician—but testing that appears to be nearly impossible.[20]

The types of policies a society might develop regarding physician supply and payment depend crucially on beliefs about the importance of demand inducement. If the amount of patient demand induced by physicians is negligible, then policy makers may wish to encourage the training of more physicians and payment on a fee-for-service basis. In contrast, if demand inducement is commonplace, then physician supply should perhaps be controlled, and physicians paid in a way whereby they do not have an incentive to provide more services (e.g., salary or capitation). A similar argument can be made about the appropriateness of public policies aimed at regulating the diffusion of medical technologies.

- <u>Assumption No. 3:</u> The distribution of wealth is approved of by society, and furthermore, individuals care only about their own resources and not those of others.

Markets are not designed to solve problems of income distribution. Rather, the outcome of the competitive process will be a distribution of income that is highly correlated with how many resources an individual brought into the process in the first place. Clearly then, if there is dissatisfaction with income distribution, government needs to intervene.

Where disagreements arise is *how* to intervene. If one believes Assumption No. 1 ("Individuals know their own interests"), then cash subsidies are the best method because individuals would know the best use of additional monies. If there is some doubt about the assumption, then it might make more sense to provide poorer people with additional wealth through services—e.g., health care, housing—than cash. An equally important reason to provide services is that wealthier people are much more likely to willingly pay taxes or voluntarily contribute to charities if they know that their contributions will be used in the way they intend. As David Collard notes, "any reader who believes himself to be entirely non-paternalistic in his concern is asked to perform the following mental experiment. I notice that my neighbour is badly fed and badly clothed so I give him some money which he then spends on beer and tobacco. Do I feel entirely happy about this or do I somehow feel that my intentions have been thwarted?"[21]

A final assumption is somewhat more abstract, but gets at some of the key differences between markets and regulations. It is the assumption that individuals care only about their absolute wealth rather than how it compares to others. This goes by the technical economic term of "externalities of consumption." If there are positive externalities of consumption, then person B is happier if person A has more wealth. If there are negative externalities, person B would be less happy, probably due to envy. A casual observation of human nature is that

people often exhibit positive externalities toward those who have little, and negative externalities toward those with more than them—consistent with the quotation by H.L. Mencken, who reputedly defined "wealth" as "any income that is at least one hundred dollars more a year than the income of one's wife's sister's husband."[22]

This seemingly abstract issue becomes real when one considers a new scarce medical technology that is only available to the very rich. Is society made better off by allowing them to purchase it? The concept of Pareto optimality would give an unambiguous "yes"—allow someone to be made better off so long as no one is made worse off? But if people care about how they compare to others, then providing something to a wealthy person that a poor person cannot afford could indeed make the latter psychologically worse off. Thus, allowing the former to purchase it has ambiguous implications for overall social welfare.[23]

A similar and perhaps less abstract example of a positive externality of consumption is altruism—your consumption of a good, like medical care, might not only you better off, but me better off as well. Since markets underproduce positive externalities of consumption, one would expect that external channels would be necessary to produce the "right" amount. as discussed in the following section.

REGULATION IN HEALTH CARE

An alternative to allowing markets to operate unencumbered is to regulate them. There are various theories regarding the motivation for regulation. The traditional viewpoint is sometimes called the "public interest" model, which hypothesizes that regulations are instituted to help the public. An opposite viewpoint—sometimes called the "economic theory of regulation" (and not terribly dissimilar to "public choice" theory in political science) is that regulations are instituted to serve special interest groups.[24] For example, it has been claimed that the American Medical Association and affiliated organizations used their political power to keep HMOs out of the medical marketplace during the middle of the 20th century—not as a way of preserving quality but rather to further increase physicians' incomes.[25] Undoubtedly, there is an element of truth in both theories of regulation: some do appear to serve the public interest and some don't. And some classic political theories suggest a "life cycle" of regulatory agencies—governments create regulatory agencies with good public-interest intentions (often after a tragedy or a crisis), but, over time, the regulators slowly fall under the political influence of the most interested groups or parties (who continue to lobby the agency long after the general public has stopped paying attention).[26]

"Regulation" is a rather vague term, however, encompassing many different strategies, some of which intervene in market activity far more than others. Stepping back for a moment, consider the various ways that government can intervene in a market. One can come up with any number of continuums of government involvement. One useful set, developed by Philip Musgrove, lists five types, ordered from the least to most intrusive: (1) provide information; (2) regulate, e.g., set rules for private providers; (3) mandate, e.g., stipulate that private entities act in a certain manner, such as requiring employers to provide health insurance coverage; (4) finance with public monies; and (5) have government provide services directly.[27]

It is perhaps noteworthy that "regulation" appears on this list as the second-least intrusive. To see why this is the case, consider the case of health insurance. Private markets can indeed provide coverage, but they are imperfect because they will strive to avoid the most costly individuals who, if they had to pay their expected costs (plus a "loading fee"), would not be able to afford coverage. If, as is the case in most countries, policy makers find this unacceptable, there is a continuum of approaches. One would be to regulate the market—for example,

require that insurance be "community rated" so that everyone is charged the same premium, and that there be "open enrollment" so people are not excluded from coverage because of their health status. This essentially permits a hidden network of cross subsidies to develop—when everyone pays the same price the good risks (healthy, young, and affluent) subsidize the poor risks (ill, old, and poor). This is what Deborah Stone called the *solidarity culture* in Chapter 1. A more intensive way for government to become involved would be to directly finance the insurance, because in doing so, it will undoubtedly set very stringent rules (e.g., coverage requirements, fee controls, or global budgets). The most intrusive involvement, of course, would be to replace the private insurance market with government-provided coverage.

Up till now the discussion has implied that regulation is solely carried out by government, but that is not necessarily the case. To give just two of many possible examples, health plans exercise regulation when they require physicians to obtain permission before hospitalizing a patient, or require a patient to obtain a referral from a "gatekeeper" primary care doctor before consulting a specialist.

There is an important distinction between "microregulation" and "macroregulation."[28] Microregulation implies direct observation and, potentially, control over the organization and/or individuals being regulated, whereas macroregulation is more indirect: setting the ground rules and stepping back, letting the organization and/or individuals choose how to respond. Other developed countries rely on macroregulation much more than the United States, using such tools as regional global budgets, where private entities (hospitals, nursing homes) must act under strict financial limits (say an annual budget) but do not face much direct oversight. The United States relies much more on microregulation that is carried out privately. Examples include utilization management techniques such as pre-certification requirements for hospital stays, monitoring physicians' utilization patterns, and the like. Many Americans are surprised to learn that while foreign physicians face more stringent fiscal constraints (from macroregulations), they enjoy considerably more professional autonomy over medicine itself than their American counterparts (who face a wide array of intrusive microregulations).

POLICY CHOICES

Economists often distinguish between two broad sets of policy levels: those aimed at the demand side of the market, and those targeting the supply side.[29] In general, those espousing market solutions tend to favor demand-side policies, while those who believe in greater government regulatory action tend to favor the side.

Demand-side policies seek to improve the workings of the price mechanism. To illustrate, economists often cite inefficiencies in the health care system due to overinsurance, which, it is claimed, cause people to consume services that they don't value very much. This theory, originally applied to health care markets by Mark Pauly, postulates that society incurs a "welfare loss," estimated by some to be on the order of 10% to 30% of total health care costs in the United States.[30]

The idea behind welfare loss is as follows. Economic theory postulates that people will purchase goods so long as the utility they confer to a person exceeds the price. Insurance brings down the price of services—sometimes to zero—meaning that people will find it advantageous to use services even if they convey very little utility. In such instances, the social costs of producing the services may far exceed the utility a person derives from its consumption.[31] If one compares the costs and benefits, it is argued that the former exceeds the latter, leading to a welfare loss on part of society.

Patient cost-sharing is one way to reduce the welfare loss of overinsurance. If people have to pay more for services, then they will, it is theorized, demand only those services that convey higher utility. Indeed, cost-sharing requirements are rising rapidly in the United States as a way of trying to quell the increased demand for services—although this is also a simple way to shift costs from larger payers (employers, governments) to the consumers themselves. For example, in the two-year period between 2001 and 2003, average annual deductibles for in-network services in PPOs rose by 60%.[32]

A related strategy called "consumer-driven health care is spreading rapidly."[33] The basic idea is to have the consumer bear the economic consequences of the insurance and utilization choices they make. Consumer-driven health plans often provide a choice of coverage and relatively large deductibles. They are often touted as an alternative to managed care because, rather than having an HMO say "no" to patients, these plans provide financial incentives for people to say "no" to themselves. Their success will depend on many factors. Most crucial are challenging issues surrounding favorable selection (i.e., healthier people joining them, leaving sicker individuals in the risk pools of other plans, which could potentially cause their premiums to spin out of control) and consumers' ability to make informed choices about whether to seek services in the face of large deductibles.

A final issue about demand-side strategies concerns equity. Robert Evans and colleagues eloquently state the issue:

> [P]eople pay taxes in rough proportion to their incomes, and use health care in rough proportion to their health status or need for care. The relationships are not exact, but in general sicker people use more health care, and richer people pay more taxes. It follows that when health care is paid for from taxes, people with higher incomes pay a larger share of the total cost; when it is paid for by the users, sick people pay a larger share . . . Whether one is a gainer or loser, then, depends upon where one is located in the distribution of both income . . . and health . . . In general, a shift to more user fee financing redistributes net income . . . from lower to higher income people, and from sicker to healthier people. The wealthy and healthy gain, the poor and sick lose.[34]

The alternative to demand-side policies are those focused on the supply side. As Joseph White explains in Chapter 19, most developed countries rely far more on supply-side policies. These include global budgets, control of the diffusion of medical technologies, limits on the number of hospital beds and physicians, hospital and physician payment incentives, practice guidelines, and utilization review.

Supply-side methods have two main advantages over those aimed at the demand side. First, with respect to efficiency, informational problems often make demand-side policies less effective. As noted above, consumers often do not respond to information about health plan quality by choosing more cost-effective plans. Second, unlike demand-side policies such as increased patient cost-sharing, those aimed at suppliers are not, by nature, regressive. In short, proponents of these policies claim that they are more effective at controlling costs and more equitable across the population.

Supply-side approaches do have their problems, however. Several of the methods just noted, especially limits on technologies and hospital beds and funding, may result in long waits for services. Conversely, reliance on price—the key market mechanism—tends to result in shorter waits because services are rationed on ability to pay. It is difficult to generalize much more than this, however, because waiting times vary a great deal between countries, and each has its own way of grappling with the problem.

MARKETS AND REGULATION IN HEALTH CARE SYSTEMS

Beyond the broad statement that the United States tends to rely more on markets in health care and other countries, more on regulation, few generalizations are possible. This isn't surprising. Every nation mixes markets and regulation. As James Morone describes in the Introduction, more than half of all health care spending in the United States is by government; and private providers (if not private financing) play a dominant role in most developed countries.

It should be apparent by now that markets and governments are not all-or-nothing propositions. Rather, they need to be used in conjunction with each other. Private markets help assure that government is not too inefficient or too beholden to special interest groups; government helps ensure that insurers do not select only the healthiest people, that providers are available to the general public, and that people can afford access to care (to name just a few things). The real issue is the balance between the two.

Can we say unambiguously what this balance should be? Unfortunately, the answer is no. There are at least four reasons why countries may want to approach these issues differently:

- Different countries want different things from their health systems. Some may want to emphasize access, others cost control; some opt for efficiency over equity, and others the opposite. Moreover, historical and cultural factors are critical determinants of how different countries health services systems have developed, making it risky to suggest that any one country's system be replicated by others.

- It is probably impossible to come up with an agreed-upon set of weights among the different outcomes. How does one weigh, for example, the short waits (a characteristic of the market-based US system) against the equity of health system financing (a characteristic of the government-controlled British system)? Selecting between such clashing values is the heart and soul of politics. When it comes to these basic trade-offs, the often heard plea—"can't we get beyond politics?"—is a sure sign of political naïveté.

- It is also hard to characterize the countries according to the reliance of each on markets versus regulation. Germany offers a good example. Although there is little explicit government involvement in health care financing (which is largely left up to the insurers, which are called "sickness funds"), there is a great deal of government oversight and direction, particularly on the supply side. Further complicating matters is that health systems change, sometimes fairly rapidly. Both Great Britain and the Netherlands, for example, went from fairly non-market-like systems to ones relying much more on competition; then both nations stepped back from the market somewhat.

- Although cross-national measures of access and costs are reasonably good, little is known about the quality of care provided in different countries.

Ultimately, we should see markets and regulation as tools that can be combined in very different ways. Each choice involves complicated trade offs between different values such as equality, efficiency, freedom, solidarity, fairness, and the acquisition of wealth. Economists perform a vital function by developing empirical comparisons of the performance of countries that rely on alternative mixes of markets and regulation. But, in the end, basic health system choices involve more than evidence and computation. They require nations to make judgments about their own ideals.

STUDY QUESTIONS

1. What is Pareto optimality? How can the concept be applied to health care?
2. What are the three key assumptions underlying markets, according to Rice? Where does the health care 'market' fail to meet these criteria?
3. What are some ways government (and other actors) can affect the demand side in health care? How can it impact, or regulate, the supply side?
4. Can health plan report cards be improved, to allow for a more informed health care 'consumer'?
5. What ways can the U.S. be seen to microregulate health care? What are some alternatives to microregulation?

6. What is the theory behind consumer-driven health plans? How can they keep health care costs down?
7. At the very end of the article, the author mentions six values that a health care system can chose to emphasize. What are they?
8. Develop your own view: Which values in the preceding answer do you think are most important?

NOTES

1. Sen, A.K. 1970. *Collective Choice and Social Welfare*. San Francisco: Holden-Day, p 22.
2. For a fuller discussion—including fifteen assumptions—see T. Rice, 2003. *The Economics of Health Reconsidered*. Chicago: Health Administration Press, p 6.
3. For further discussion of "government failure," see: Wolf, C., Jr. 1979. "A Theory of Nonmarket Failure: Framework for Implementation Analysis." *Journal of Law and Economics* 22 (1): 107–39; and Wolf, C., Jr. 1993. *Markets or Governments: Choosing Between Imperfect Alternatives*. Cambridge, MA: MIT Press.
4. Sidgwick, H. 1887. *Principles of Political Economy*. London: MacMillan, p 414.
5. Pauly, M.V. 1997. "Who Was That Straw Man Anyway? A Comment on Evans and Rice." *Journal of Health Politics, Policy and Law* 22 (2): 467–73 (quotation on p 470).
6. Wolfe, 1993 (endnote 3), p 7.
7. Goyal, M., R.L. Mehta, L.J. Schneiderman, and A.R. Sehgal. 2002. "Economics and Health Consequences of Selling a Kidney in India." *Journal of the American Medical Association* 288 (13): 1589–93.
8. Weisbrod, B.A. 1978. "Comment on Paper by Mark Pauly." In: *Competition in the Health Care Sector: Past, Present, and Future*, edited by W. Greenberg, pp 49–56. Washington DC: Bureau of Economics, Federal Trade Commission, p 52.

9. Isaacs, S.L. 1996. "Consumers' Information Needs: Results of a National Survey." *Health Affairs* 15 (4): 31–41.

10. Cunningham, P.J., C. Denk, and M. Sinclair. 2001. "Do Consumers Know How Their Health Plan Works?" *Health Affairs* 20 (2): 159–66.

11. Hibbard, J.H., and J.J. Jewett. 1997. "Will Quality Report Cards Help Consumers?" *Health Affairs* 16 (3): 218–28.

12. Hibbard, J.H., and J.J. Jewett. 1996. "What Type of Quality Information Do Consumers Want in a Health Care Report Card?" *Medical Care Research and Review* 53 (1): 28–47; and Chernew, M., and D.P. Scanlon. 1998. "Health Plan Report Cards and Insurance Choice." *Inquiry* 35: 9–22.

13. Scanlon, D.P., M. Chernew, C. McLaughlin, and G. Solon. 2002. "The Impact of Health Plan Report Cards on Managed Care Enrollment." *Journal of Health Economics* 21: 19–41.

14. Rodwin, M.A. 2001. "Consumer Voice and Representation in Managed Healthcare." *Journal of Health Law* 34 (2): 233–76.

15. Thurow, L.C. 1983. *Dangerous Currents: The State of Economics*. New York: Random House, p 219.

16. Boulding, K.E. 1969. "Economics as a Moral Science." *American Economic Review* 59 (1): 1–12. Quotation on p 2.

17. Stigler, G.J., and G.S. Becker. 1977. "*De Gustibus Non Est Disputandum.*" *American Economic Review* 67 (2): 76–90.

18. Becker, G.S. 1979. "Economic Analysis and Human Behavior." In *Sociological Economics*, ed. by L. Levy-Garboua. Beverly Hills, CA: Sage Publications, p 9.

19. For a more complete listing and discussion see Rice (2003), Chapter 3.

20. Mooney, G. 1994. *Key Issues in Health Economics*. New York: Harvester Wheatsheaf.

21. Collard, D. 1978. *Altruism and Economy: A Study in Non-Selfish Economics*. Oxford: Martin Robertson & Co., p 122.

22. This quotation was obtained from: Frank, R.H. 1985. *Choosing the Right Pond: Human Behavior and the Quest for Status*. New York: Oxford University Press, p 5.

23. For further discussion of this and other examples, see: Reinhardt, U.E. 1992. "Reflections on the Meaning of Efficiency: Can Efficiency Be Separated from Equity?" *Yale Law & Policy Review* 10: 302–15.

24. For one of the earliest and most readable essays on the economic theory of regulation, see: Stigler, G.J. 1971. "The Theory of Economic Regulation." *Bell Journal of Economics and Management Science* 2: 3–21.

25. Kessel, R.A. 1958. Price Discrimination in Medicine. *Journal of Law and Economics* 1(1): 20–53.

26. Downs, A. 1993. *Inside Bureaucracy*. Long Grove, IL: Waveland Press.

27. Musgrove, P. 1996. *Public and Private Roles in Health: Theory and Financing Patterns*. Discussion paper no. 339. Washington DC: The World Bank.

28. For a discussion of this distinction, see Rice, T., "Macro Versus Micro Regulation," in *Regulating Managed Care: Theory, Practice, and Future Options*, ed. S.H. Altman, U.E. Reinhardt, and D Shactman (San Francisco: Jossey Bass, 1999).

29. A good discussion of one aspect of supply vs. demand-side policies, involving cost-sharing, is in: Ellis, R.P., and T.G. McGuire. 1993. "Supply-Side and Demand-Side Cost Sharing in Health Care." *Journal of Economic Perspectives* 7 (4): 135–51.

30. Pauly, M.V. 1968. "The Economics of Moral Hazard: Comment." *American Economic Review* 58 (4): 531–7.

31. Feldman, R., and B. Dowd. 1991. "A New Estimate of the Welfare Loss of Excess Health Insurance." *American Economic Review* 81 (1): 297–301.

32. For a critique of this theory, see Rice (endnote 2) or: Rice, T. 1992. "An Alternative Framework for Evaluating Welfare Losses in the Health

Care Market." *Journal of Health Economics* 11 (1): 88–92.

33. Gabel, J., G. Claxton, E. Holve, J. Pickreign, H. Whitmore, K. Dhont, S. Hawkins, and D. Rowland. 2003. "Health Benefits in 2003: Premiums Reach Thirteen-Year High as Employers Adopt Now Forms of Cost Sharing." *Health Affairs* 22 (5): 117–26.

34. For more information on these plans, see: Gabel, J.R., A.T. Lo Sasso, and T. Rice. 2002. "Consumer-Choice Plans: Are They More than Talk Now? *Health Affairs,* November: W395–W407.

REFERENCES

Culyer, A.J. 1989. "The Normative Economics of Health Care Finance and Provision." *Oxford Review of Economic Policy* 5 (1): 34–58.

Ellis, R.P., and T.G. McGuire. 1993. "Supply-Side and Demand-Side Cost Sharing in Health Care." *Journal of Economic Perspectives* 7 (4): 135–51.

Enthoven, A. 1978. "Consumer Choice Health Plan." *The New England Journal of Medicine* 298 (12): 650–8.

Enthoven, A. 1978. "Consumer Choice Health Plan." *The New England Journal of Medicine* 298 (13): 709–20.

Evans, R.G. 1984. *Strained Mercy.* Toronto, Ontario: Butterworth.

Frank, R.H. 1985. *Choosing the Right Pond: Human Behavior and the Quest for Status.* New York: Oxford University Press.

Frank R.H. 1999. *Luxury Fever.* New York: Free Press.

Friedman, M. 1962. "Occupational Licensure," in *Capitalism and Freedom.* Chicago: University of Chicago Press: 137–60.

Hausman, D.M., and M.S. McPherson. 1993. "Taking Ethics Seriously: Economics and Contemporary Moral Philosophy." *Journal of Economic Literature* 31 (2): 671–731.

Hibbard, J.H. 1997. "Will Quality Report Cards Help Consumers?" *Health Affairs* 16 (5): 218–28.

Kuttner, R. 1997. *Everything for Sale: The Virtue and Limits of Markets.* New York: Alfred A. Knopf.

Labelle, R., G. Stoddart, and T. Rice. 1994. "A Re-Examination of the Meaning and Importance of

Supplier-Induced Demand." *Journal of Health Economics* 13 (3): 347–68.

Lohr, K.N., et al. 1986. "Effect of Cost Sharing on Use of Medically Effective and Less Effective Care." *Medical Care* 24 (Supplement): S31–S38.

Mooney, G. 1994. *Key Issues in Health Economics.* New York: Harvester Wheatsheaf.

Musgrove, P. 1996. *Public and Private Roles in Health: Theory and Financing Patterns.* Discussion paper no. 339. Washington DC: The World Bank.

Newhouse, J.P., et al. 1993. *Free for All? Lessons from the RAND Health Insurance Experiment.* Cambridge, MA: Harvard University Press.

Pauly, M.V. 1968. "The Economics of Moral Hazard: Comment." *American Economic Review* 58 (4): 531–7.

Preker, A.S., A. Harding, and P. Travis. 2000. "'Make or Buy' Decisions in the Production of Health Care Goods and Services: New Insights from Institutional Economics and Organizational Theory." *Bulletin of the World Health Organization* 78 (6): 779–90.

Reinhardt, U.E. 1992. "Reflections on the Meaning of Efficiency: Can Efficiency Be Separated from Equity?" *Yale Law & Policy Review* 10: 302–15.

Rice, T. 2003. *The Economics of Health Reconsidered.* Chicago: Health Administration Press.

Saltman, R.B., and J. Figueras. 1998. "Analyzing the Evidence on European Health Care Reforms." *Health Affairs* 17 (2): 85–108.

Sen, A.K. 1987. *On Ethics and Economics.* Oxford: Basil Blackwell.

Sen, A.K. 1992. *Inequality Revisited.* Cambridge, MA: Harvard University Press.

Stigler, G.J. 1971. "The Theory of Economic Regulation." *Bell Journal of Economics and Management Science* 2: 3–21.

Thaler, R.H. 1992. *The Winner's Curse: Paradoxes and Anomalies of Economic Life.* New York: The Free Press, Macmillan and Co.

Thurow, L.C. 1983. *Dangerous Currents: The State of Economics.* New York: Random House.

Wagstaff, A., and E. van Doorslaer. 2000. "Income Inequality and Health: What Does the Literature Tell Us?" *Annual Review of Public Health* 21: 543–67.

Wolf, C., Jr. 1993. *Markets or Governments: Choosing Between Imperfect Alternatives.* Cambridge, MA: MIT Press.

CHAPTER 3

Morals and Health Policy

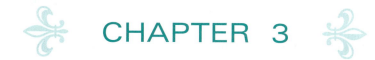

James A. Morone

We usually think of public health care as scientific and secular. But morality deeply shapes the way Americans talk and think about public health. This chapter explains how.

American health care policy is different from health policy in other nations.[1] Of course, the United States has no national health insurance but that simply reflects a deeper contrast in the ways we Americans think about politics and health care. European health policy analysts regularly invoke a "solidarity culture"—a staunch belief in sharing resources, a concern for what might be called "the people's health." European political cultures and institutions often reflect this collective ideal.[2]

What most observers first notice about the American process is the unabashed pursuit of self-interest. In our dynamic (some would say raucous) system, stakeholders and interest groups jockey for advantage on every issue. One wily 19th century politician put it famously after double-crossing a rival: "politics is not a branch of the Sunday school business."[3] This process poses a challenge for health specialists: Groups pushing their own interests will stand up and oppose even the most unambiguous scientific findings.

Political scientists usually view health policy through the lens of interest group politics. Stakeholders and politicians pursue their preferences. They negotiate with one another, cajole neutral parties, and mobilize their own supporters. The entire political system lurches along, operating its celebrated checks, balancing public programs with private markets, blunting radical changes, and producing incremental adjustments to the status quo. From this perspective, health science constantly wrestles with self-interested politics. Even robust findings are only as good as the policy coalition that assembles around them.

However, interest group politics are only the most obvious story. Two other traditions run through American policies. First, Americans also share a more intermittent legacy of collective cooperation (that grows especially vivid during a crisis). Millions of Americans volunteer their time and energy to enrich their communities or help their neighbors; national service programs (like VISTA or AmeriCorps) tap the same civic energy; even obscure government programs often invite public commentary and direct citizen participation. Public health advocates, in particular, often try to get beyond self interest competition and appeal to shared interests and values. Deborah Stone describes the logic of this solidarity in Chapter 1.

Morality offers Americans still another political framework. As foreign observers often point out, the United States remains the industrial world's foremost Puritan nation. The Puritan colonists bequeathed America a tendency to turn political differences into moral disputes. The debates that gust up around our social programs often go directly to the moral worth of the beneficiaries—are they deserving? Such questions put vivid and contested moral images—of virtue and vice, good and evil, us and them—at the heart of American politics.

This chapter examines the way social scientists normally think about our health policies and contrasts it with the moral framework. As we'll see, moral framing helps define American politics and shapes the way we think and talk about health politics and policy. Where does morality politics spring from? How does it work? And how, exactly, does it affect issues?

TRADITIONAL MODELS OF AMERICAN POLITICS

We begin with the more familiar models of American politics—individualism and community.

Individualism

Why are Americans so committed to individualism (or what political theorists call "classical liberalism")? One of our great national myths offers a popular answer: The first colonists sailed away from old world tyranny and settled a vast unpopulated land—the place almost thrust freedom on them. American settlers did not have to push aside kings or nobles to get ahead. Instead, as

Tocqueville famously put it, "Americans were born equal instead of becoming so."[4] Men (and maybe women, the myth gets a bit shaky here) faced extraordinary opportunities. The land and its riches awaited—all it took was a little capital and a lot of work. The irresistible result would be the nation's celebrated individualism, a deep faith in free economic markets (some foreign observers think its almost a cult), and a corresponding belief in limited government.

The US Constitution organized this ideology into the nation's political rules. An elaborate system of checks and balances limited national power. But it also offered political participants many different venues in which to pursue their interests. In the past, political systems had tried to suppress self-interest; the American founders opened the door to it. The answer to the problem of faction (or interests), wrote James Madison in *Federalist #10*, is to inject an "even greater variety" into the political process. Today, political scientists sometimes lament the "hyper-pluralism" of a system crowded with clashing interests, lobbyists, and lawyers.

The result is that almost no political arena stands above the scramble. There are very few non-partisan agencies; there is no prestigious civil service trusted by all sides; and even the judiciary has become just another political branch of government.[5]

The ferocity of this scramble for advantage poses a particular dilemma for health care policy. After all, medical science seeks objective answers to questions about health and health care. It documents, for example, the dangers of smoking, obesity, stress, unsafe sex practices or delayed medical care. The same pattern constantly appears: The surgeon general, the Institute of Medicine, or the Centers for Disease Control might issues a health warning based on solid science. However, any effort to follow up and actually do anything promptly triggers the politics of self-interest. Our political culture does not penalize such a reaction—in politics, self-interest is just as legitimate as medical science.

The result appears to pose a conflict between medicine and politics. No matter how robust the scientific findings, interested groups mobilize and often delay or derail action. The politics of individualism offers health-minded reformers unambiguous advice: use your scientific findings to organize your own supporters. In the political arena, your science is only as strong as your political coalition.

Community

During the 1980s, critics began growing uneasy about unabashed self-interest and untrammeled markets. What happens to the common good when every one pushes only for number one? Back to early America trooped the social theorists. There they discovered an entirely different American political tradition, one grounded in a robust collective life. In contrast to the legends of rugged individualism, historians documented rich networks of communal assistance. If a barn burned down, the townsfolk got together and helped their neighbor raise another. If iron pots were expensive, families shared them with the neighbors—early American household inventories often list one half or one third of a pot or a skillet.[6]

The communal story sparks enthusiasm across the political spectrum. Here, say proponents, lies firm ground on which to imagine a renewed civic culture. Americans are not just celebrants of self but partners in a shared public life, not just individualists but communitarians. Conservatives saw an opportunity to restore traditional American values; progressives stressed our obligations to one another, our shared communal fate.

The legacy of community recalls an often-overlooked public health legacy. After all, American cities have a long history of funding clinics and fighting infectious diseases. A communal heritage—if it can somehow be tapped—opens the prospect of putting self-interest in a larger, civic-minded context.[7]

Franklin D. Roosevelt introduced the idea of social security in 1932 with the classic communal appeal for public health. "The causes of poverty . . . are beyond the control of any individual." Well, so much for the individualistic version of American politics. What was the alternative? "Community effort."

When a modern civilization faces a disease epidemic, said Roosevelt, "it takes care of the victims after they are stricken." But it also roots out the source of the contagion. Roosevelt proposed an entire social program built on the public health model. He would put aside "jungle law of economic competition" for "brotherly" cooperation.[8]

Of course, President Roosevelt introduced his program in response to the Great Depression. The communal alternative has always been more fragile and intermittent, displacing individualism largely during crisis and extraordinary circumstances. Moreover, political theorists warn us against romanticizing the American communal tradition. After all, that tradition also animates a more painful historical legacy—the urge to reject entire groups based on race, gender, ethnicity, or religion. The Ku Klux Klan, lynching, anti-immigrant riots, militia groups, and a long, harsh line of nativist organizations reflect the dark side of community.[9]

Still, the communal vision offers a potential rejoinder to the politics of self-interest. Communitarians were critical of the Clinton administration's health reform effort, for example, because officials tried to sell it by promising one group after another that the plan was in their self-interest. The moral of that story, warned White House advisor Paul Starr, is that with "so many people on board . . . our boat may sink from its own weight." The communitarian perspective would have appealed bluntly to the common good, to the notion that we all share values as citizens of the same nation.[10]

Could such a collective appeal work? Under what circumstances? What conditions stir America's communal legacy? And what about the ugly urge to reject some Americans? We can find some of the answers to these questions in another tradition, American morality politics.

MORALITY POLITICS

Americans take religion and morality more seriously than the citizens in most other industrial

countries. Ninety-five percent of all Americans believe in God—a distinct contrast to Sweden (52%),
France (62%), or Britain (76%). While other industrial nations grow secular over time, the United
States keeps experiencing religious revivals. That social fact has deep consequences for American politics. In a nation marked by moral and religious
fervor, partisans often take their faith into politics.[11]
Moral fervor drove—drives—an extraordinary
range of political movements—civil rights, temperance, tobacco, anti-abortion, and many others.
Moral judgment seeps into all kinds of political
issues in both dramatic and subtle ways.

Moral politics comes with its own founding
story. "It seems to me," wrote Alexis de Tocqueville,
"that I can see the entire destiny of America contained in the first Puritan who came ashore."[12]
Those first settlers arrived in the New World facing
the essential communal question: "Who are we?"
Who were they? The Puritans concocted an extraordinary answer: They were the community of
Saints. Leadership, in both state and church, went
to men who could prove that they were pre-
ordained for salvation. The saints could vote, hold
office, and enjoy full church membership. (The
methodology for proving salvation was complicated, but wealth and health were taken as pretty
reliable indicators.) People who were morally
uncertain—those who had not demonstrated
salvation—were expected to follow the proven
saints; they went to church, for example, but did not
hold office, vote, or become full church members.
And the damned were driven out—witches were
hung, Native Americans slaughtered and heretics
sent packing (mainly to Rhode Island, "the *latrina*
of New England" for all its noxious heresies). In
short, moral standing defined leaders, allocated
privileges (like voting), defined communities and
identified the dangerous "other."

The Puritan idea burst out of New England and
spread across America (thanks to the purest Puritans, the Baptists). The essential Puritan trope still
persists and flourishes: Moral virtue continues to
define the community and still distinguishes "us"
from "them." Moral images specify privilege or
punishment, inclusion or exclusion, deserving poor
or dangerous other. These images of potential
beneficiaries—often shifting, constantly contested—
lie under every American social policy. "We" get
assistance; "they" face social controls.

The individualist model of American politics, described above, emphasizes a sharp line between private realm and public sphere. Constitutional rights
bar any public authority from meddling with people's private lives. "However strange it may seem,"
wrote John Locke in 1689, "the lawgiver hath nothing to do with moral virtues and vices." In this view,
citizens draw on their private desires and values and
then charge into the public, the political, realm to
advance their goals. In the patois of economics,
every agent maximizes her own utilities. In contrast,
moral politics refuses to honor the private–public
distinction. Moral politics explicitly enters the private sphere. Individual virtue—character—affects
the public good. The citizen's private behavior, ruled
right out of politics in traditional models, now becomes crucial. Some group's private behavior (real
or imagined) seems to threaten the community.

The Puritans bequeathed America two distinct
moral visions, two answers to that political bottom
line—whom should we blame for our troubles? I
call the two answers, the Puritan and the Social
Gospel.

Puritans

The Puritan approach focuses on dangerous sinners
lurking in our society. Fears of "them" tilt our political
debates and destroy the communal urge by eroding
our sense of common values. The policy problem
turns, instead, to protecting us from them.

The personal transgressions—the sins—that ostensibly endanger the nation are most often public
health sins. For example, the most sustained moral
campaign in American history targeted substance
abuse. Temperance crusaders organized in the early
19th century, won their first statewide prohibition
in 1851, managed national prohibition by 1920,
and now inspire a formidable drug war (that draws
heavily on Prohibition era jurisprudence).[13]

Sexual threats pose another political perennial. The American Medical Association launched its first great political campaign against abortion—a common practice in the mid-nineteenth century (when there was about one abortion for every six live births). Physicians consolidated their own role as social leaders and healers by turning abortion into a crime. Abortions, they argued, were subverting the good community by undermining the white, middle class birth rate while the foreign immigrants multiplied and threatened to swamp American blood.[14]

Similarly, sexually transmitted diseases bred in the urban ghettos and spread into middle class families. After all, reported the *American Journal of Public Health*, "many . . . white . . . boys are going to sow their wild oats." In the South, the syphilis rate among African Americans became a familiar justification for Jim Crow apartheid. A similar argument reappeared during the first wave of AIDS hysteria; frightened Americans dreamed up all sorts of ways to keep homosexuals from slipping "their" disease into the mainstream population.[15]

In each case the same general pattern recurs. Some dangerous personal behavior—drinking, drugs, sexual practices, teen pregnancy, birth control, abortion, the list goes on—threatens the community. The questionable behavior becomes associated with some group. Moral politics triggers vibrant stereotypes: Irish drink, Italian immigrants have too many babies, Muslims are terrorists, and black people commit almost every possible sin. Political leaders warn that America faces terrible decline if we don't find a way to rein in the dangerous people and their bad behavior. Standard solutions run to pledges ("just say 'no'" to alcohol, drugs, and sex before marriage), prohibitions, restrictions, regulations, more prisons, and tougher laws.

Of course all societies impose controls. The political key lies in the emphasis on personal discipline, in the balance between restrictive policies and social welfare benefits. I experienced a vivid illustration of the difference during a debate about the Clinton health reform proposal in 1994.

I was debating a Republican senator who opposed the Clinton plan. We were before a young,

liberal audience that was giving the Republican a very chilly hearing. Then, toward the end of the debate, he abruptly turned to face me. The body language said, "Okay, let's quit kidding around." And here's what followed: "Look, professor, you can't expect the hard-working people of suburban Cook County to go into the same health care alliance [a kind of insurance pool] as the crackheads in the city of Chicago." When I turned to face the audience, all set to brush aside this fatuous dichotomy, I saw a room of suddenly sobered liberals. "Yes," they were thinking, "that is a terrible problem." "Hey," I yelped, "those uninsured people in the city of Chicago are college students and hard-working nurses and taxi drivers doing double shifts and single moms holding down two jobs . . ." No dice. In fact, it only got worse. Crackheads and single moms. Our imagined community, struggling together to fix a troubled health care system, had vanished in an instant. Now, it was a hard-working us against a drug-abusing, sexually promiscuous them. Forget about extending health care coverage—what "those people" need is moral discipline. The politics of social policy always turns on the mental images we create of the beneficiaries.

The Social Gospel

An alternative moral tradition once offered a sharp alternative to blaming individuals. I call it the social gospel (borrowing the name from a group of reformers at the end of the 19th century). Social gospel thinking shifts the focus from individual sinners to an unjust system. The neo-puritans blame individual misbehavior for society's troubles; the social gospel approach blames society—or socioeconomic pressures—for individual troubles. The causal arrow runs in precisely the opposite direction: the economic system, race prejudice, underprivilege, or social stress put pressures on people. If those people behave badly (by using illegal drugs, for example) it is largely because social and economic forces have pushed them into a tough corner. The social gospel solution appears in countless variations but they converge on the same familiar points: fix the system and give every American a fair chance to prosper; don't blame those who fall by the wayside; we all share a common duty to help the disadvantaged.

Thinkers in the late 19th and early 20th century first systematically articulated a version of the social gospel. Reformers like Jane Addams began challenging the dominant Victorian paradigm: poverty caused drunkenness, they said, as much as the other way around. Low salaries and harsh factory conditions—deprivation, not depravity—pushed women into prostitution. This way of thinking came to power with the Roosevelt administration in 1933.[16] Roosevelt constantly articulated the social gospel and his administration hammered out policies that reflected the approach. The social gospel, like the Puritan perspective, turns on images of health and disease. However, while the neo Puritans tend to fear contagions, the social gospel seizes on community health as a public policy model.

Roosevelt first introduced the idea of social security while campaigning for president in October 1932. Roosevelt began by declaring that because it was a Sunday, he would not be "talking politics" but "preaching a sermon." True to his word, the candidate packed his address with religious quotations and allusions. As I noted above, he used a public health analogy to draw a picture of the good society, one that protected the weak and the disadvantaged.[17]

Roosevelt brought these generalities down to political earth with sad stories about good people. An 89 year old neighbor had died while milking a cow—after a blizzard no less; now, it was our collective responsibility to help his "83 year old kid sister" who was languishing in an insane asylum because she had nowhere else to go. Roosevelt was off and running down a roster of needy innocents who needed help: hungry children in public schools, injured workers, sick men and women, crippled children, the unemployed, and many more. Each example came with the same political spin: poor people are virtuous neighbors who have fallen on hard times. Roosevelt was consciously displacing the past icons of depravity—undisciplined

black men or lazy immigrants lounging about the saloons.[18]

That last example, drinking, carried plenty of baggage for these were the last days of Prohibition. In the New Dealer's hands, excess drinking turned from sin to illness; dry pledges and national prohibition gave way to treatment and education. The fault line between neo-Puritans and social gospel would run right through the next half century: vice versus illness, crime versus public health, sin versus social responsibility. The social gospel view reached its high tide during the southern civil rights movement and the Lyndon Johnson administration's Great Society. "Should we double our wealth and conquer the stars," declared Johnson in his most beautiful speech, "and still be unequal to this issue [of racial inequality] then we will have failed as a people and as a nation. For with a country as with a person. What is a man profited, if he shall gain the whole world, and lose his own soul?"[19]

The Ronald Reagan administration eventually buried the whole approach. Reagan scoffed at the idea of collective responsibility. Instead, he turned personal responsibility—"just say no!"—into a formidable policy mantra. Today, the old social gospel idea that crime or drug abuse might stem from "underprivilege" finds almost no policy traction. Contemporary politics includes plenty of moralizing. But there is scant evidence of the old social gospel claim that we share collective responsibility for fostering social justice toward everyone.

MORAL POLITICS IN ACTION

Morality politics are protean and pervasive. They spring up in unexpected places, surprising unwary policy makers. Consider two recent cases—school based health centers and the politics of obesity.

School Based Health Clinics

Teenagers face difficult health problems—like substance abuse, reproductive health, and depression—that often land them in trouble.[20] Given the nature of these problems, perhaps it is not surprising that as a group they are slow to seek care. However, ignoring adolescent health leads to serious problems: one million unintended pregnancies a year, three million sexually transmitted diseases, more than four thousand suicides, and terrible incidents of school violence. The United States has a high adolescent and young adult death rate—1.5 deaths per thousand young males (in contrast to 0.7 in England, 0.6 in Sweden, and 0.9 in Germany).

One policy response that grew increasingly popular in the 1990s sprang from a simple intuition: put the health care where the kids are. Local hospitals, community health centers, or public health departments opened health centers directly in the schools, especially in poor neighborhoods.

Across the country, the school based health centers immediately set off a political storm as they inevitably faced issues like substance abuse and reproductive health. Cultural and religious conservatives feared that providing treatment (possibly without parental notification) would implicitly condone illegal drug use, underage drinking, and premarital sex. Conservatives countered with calls for stronger discipline, personal responsibility ("just say no"), and abstinence education. By 1997, The Personal Responsibility and Work Opportunity Act (or welfare reform) had introduced abstinence education into schools across the country.[21]

Some liberals confronted the moral issues head on. They responded that young people needed counseling on sexuality and chemical dependency. If teens were going to have sex, argued these advocates, they ought to be prepared. Dr. Jocelyn Elders set off a firestorm in her first press conference as director of the Arkansas Department of Health: "We are not going to put them on their lunch trays. But yes, we intend to distribute condoms [through] . . . school based clinics."[22]

The battle was on. However, liberals soon discovered that cultural (often Christian) conservatives had formed powerful local organizations across the nation. Those groups were focused, in particular, on school boards. In the Northeast, cultural conservatives found allies in the Catholic bishops who were chary of birth control. In the South and West they worked with the Christian Coalition. In the Pacific states they allied with anti-tax advocates. When the Christian coalition helped Mike Foster come from far behind and win the governorship in Louisiana, the organization's first demand was an end to the school health centers.

Parental notification posed another thorny issue. When the California legislature passed a bill guaranteeing privacy in school health centers, critics charged the government with undermining parental control. More than 10,000 people rallied against the bill (which conservative talk show host, Dr. Laura, turned into a highly publicized cause). Governor Gray Davis responded by vetoing the legislation.

Yet, despite ardent opposition, the clinics survived and flourished. Even the school centers in Louisiana weathered the storm and spread. How? Proponents turned moral politics into a classic interest group issue. Where opponents opposed reproductive health services or sex education, the centers backed off (usually referring their student patients to other providers). More important, advocates employed that classic political wisdom: build a constituency. As children started receiving treatment, parents, teachers, and health providers rallied around the centers, countering moral complaints with down to earth descriptions of kids getting care.

Respectable locals—parents, teachers, and health care providers—went to legislators and told heartwarming stories about their children and the school clinics. Legislators are always primed to deliver concrete benefits to "responsible" community members and the school clinics have become a prime constituent service. They combine education and health care. They do not bust the budget. They are simple to understand. They offer fine photo opportunities. And they can be doled out one school at a time. In the end, the health centers overcame the opposition and expanded—from some 150 in 1990 to more than 1,300 by 2007. But both sides of the story are important. Although, advocates defused the moral attack, the criticism powerfully shaped both the health centers and their politics. The health centers reflect the larger politics of public health. Reviewing the response to AIDS, for example, the *American Journal of Public Health* (*AJPH*) reported that Americans engaged in far more premarital sex than their British counterparts and, at the same time, condemned promiscuity at much higher rates. The colonists still stick to the old Puritan spirit, chortled *The Economist*, reporting on the *AJPH* survey, and they pay the price.[23]

American public health policies must steer carefully between sin and censure. When AIDS hit the more tolerant and abstemious Europeans quickly launched forceful public health campaigns that included leaflets, television advertisements, and needle exchanges. Across the Atlantic, Americans delayed their effort while they pondered the exact moral nuance of the message, particularly the degree of emphasis on abstinence. The American incidence of AIDS soon measured ten times higher than Britain's. Of course, many factors underlie the difference.

In the AIDS case, as with the school health centers, Americans eventually sorted out the tension between education and abstinence. But both cases illustrate how moral conflicts can profoundly shape health programs and their outcomes. Health policy makers constantly have to negotiate complicated moral politics. The school based health centers offer a fine example of how local health advocates and officials—initially surprised by the political heat—managed to address the moral concerns and solidify their program.

Obesity

In 2001, Surgeon General David Satcher issued a startling report: Over 65% of Americans were overweight and 30% clinically obese.[24] Obesity, rising at epidemic rates, threatened to overtake tobacco as the chief cause of preventable death. Americans (in fact, residents of almost every nation) suddenly found themselves bombarded by data about obesity's toll—on our lives, our health, and our budgets.

At first, the issue provoked derisive commentaries about the "menace" of "big chocolate." The critics drew on the familiar model of America as a nation of individualists who celebrate free markets and vehemently oppose big government meddling in private lives. What could be more personal than food? The critics were pointing to a genuine dilemma. How could public health advocates possibly make a political issue out of such a private matter?

One classic response lies in the moral realm. Nothing moves the political system like a threat from greedy companies who put profits before the public's welfare. Demonizing providers regularly offers reformers a way to cross into the private sphere and control, limit, or prohibit. In the early twentieth century temperance advocates gained considerable political mileage by charging breweries and saloons with pouring poison into the American workingman. Tobacco offers a more contemporary example. Public health officials spent years trying to publicize the danger but for political effect, nothing matched the revelations that the industry had consciously lied about the health effects of smoking.

The same kinds of condemnation rapidly entered the obesity debates. Public health scholars explain the startling rise in obesity by pointing to an "unhealthy food environment." For starters, portion sizes have undergone an extraordinary expansion. In his influential book, *Food Fight*, Kelly Brownell describes the growth of the all-American burger. In 1957, reports Brownell, the typical hamburger weighed in at one ounce and 210 calories. Today, that burger is up to six ounces (618 calories)—and that's before your bacon, cheese, supersized fries (another 610 calories) and double gulp (64 ounce) soft drink.[25] Entrepreneurs in the highly competitive food service business trumpet ever-larger portions— think "whopper," "Xtreme gulp," "Big Grab," and "The Beast." Each innovation ups the ante in serving sizes. Even ostensibly healthy products come loaded with hidden ingredients. Sugar (or high fructose corn syrup) is the first ingredient in Kellogg's Strawberry Nutri-Grain yogurt bars and the second in Skippy super chunk peanut butter.[26]

It only took a small step to move from these analyses to charges of corporate villainy. As the most ardent critics put it, a cynical industry targets children and reshapes their eating habits. The companies put soda machines in schools and fast food outlets in lunchrooms. The result, argues Eric Schlosser in *Fast Food Nation*, is "a lifetime of weight problems" and "emotional pain." And that is just the beginning. Fast food, continues Schlosser, has trashed the countryside, widened the social gap between rich and poor, and turned the meatpacking industry into a labor nightmare. Schlosser's descriptions of the food business are every bit as horrifying as Upton Sinclair's famous exposé, *The Jungle*. Schlosser's book became a surprise best seller and a steady stream of exposés rapidly followed.[27]

A backlash against fast food muckrakers simply shifts the blame. If some liberals demonize the industry, some conservatives blame overweight individuals. Heavy people lack will power, they make foolish food choices, they live in unhealthy ways. Obese people—like smokers, drug abusers, and heavy drinkers—have made personal choices; they should "just say no" and push away from the table. And just like those other forms of substance abuse, obesity is concentrated in poor and minority communities.

Each picture of blame—the industry versus the individual—carries different policy implications. A focus on the industry suggests requiring stricter food labels, rethinking school nutrition, restricting advertising, regulating fat content, punishing misleading claims, taxing unhealthy ingredients, and so on. Successfully demonizing "big food"—directing popular anger at the industry—may cut through the checks and balances of the political system and lead to action on these issues.

However, the politics of demonization cuts two ways. Some observers charge that food stamps and school lunches only encourage poor people—who are already fat enough—to overeat.[28] Others have suggested an insurance premium surcharge on heavy people. Once policy makers start condemning heavy people, the list of new policy solutions will quickly grow.

The larger lessons from America's long moral history suggest that demonization is always tempting, since it gets political results, but always dangerous: it fractures our communities, limits the range of health policy alternatives, and lands hardest on poor and weak populations. In the long run, public health advocates do best when they focus on policies that foster healthy lives and build good communities.

What next in obesity politics? Past efforts to regulate private behavior, such as alcohol and tobacco use, take us beyond politics and into the cultural realm: Americans dramatically reduced their drinking, their smoking, and even their tolerance for second hand smoke. When advocates detect a crisis, define a problem, and seek a solution, they are—indirectly, perhaps often unexpectedly—educating the public. The obesity wars are likely to grow, spread, and generate considerable political heat. However, if the history of drinking and smoking serve as a guide, the most important consequence may lie in the conclusions that citizens draw about their own personal lifestyles.

EPILOGUE

Moral fears and aspirations change American politics. One forgotten consequence lies in the sheer political power of moral claims. Franklin D. Roosevelt and Martin Luther King, Jr. made moral arguments as they redefined American social policy. President Ronald Reagan asserted a very different moral framework: neo-Puritan rather than social gospel. The force with which he championed his alternative, and the success he met, may be Reagan's most enduring domestic legacy.

When it comes to moral politics, every side seizes on health care. What I have called the Puritan approach focuses on threats to our public health: drinking, drug abuse, out of wedlock births, sexually transmitted diseases, and more. The fears often lead to powerful public action: to restrictions, regulations, and prohibitions.

Proponents of the social gospel reframe the problem away from sin and sinners. They see illness rather than crime, addiction rather than moral weakness. They would treat rather than punish; they look past personal behavior and focus on complex social causes. They constantly echo Franklin Roosevelt's "Sunday sermon" on social security and call for public health solutions. Puritan drug wars elicit social gospel calls for treatment, education, and harm reduction. More broadly, the social gospel pushes for social justice; it promotes collective responsibility toward every member of the community. However, today's call for social gospel programs is a weak echo of the powerful reforming tradition that dominated American politics in the 1930s and 1960s.

Still, down through American history and across a wide political spectrum today, every side uses images of health to articulate its hopes and aspirations, to voice its fears and warnings. The problems we face and the solutions we contrive ultimately revolve around our definitions of health and illness. Our health care policies rest on the pictures we construct of one another. In the end, American morality politics reminds us of the importance—the sheer cultural power—of health, health care, and health studies in forging a good society.

STUDY QUESTIONS

1. How does the American political conception of health care contrast with that prevailing across Europe?
2. In what way(s) does the politics of self-interest pose a challenge to scientists and their efforts to be objective?
3. This chapter describes three different frameworks—individualism, community and morality. Briefly describe each framework.
4. What's your view: Do you think one of these frameworks is more useful than the others? If so, say which one and explain why. Alternately, you can agree with the

author and explain how they 'all work together'?
5. What are some of the maladies and/or public health issues that have taken on moral dimensions in political discourse?
6. What are the two main forms taken by morality politics in America?
7. How, and why, did school health centers become a battleground in the politics of morality?
8. How did school health centers weather the opposition posed by morally charged interest groups?
9. How did leaders concerned about obesity overcome considerations of self-interest to place the issue on the political agenda?
10. In what way would 'neopuritans' conceptualize the obesity problem facing America?

NOTES

1. For a book-length treatment of morality politics, see James Morone, 2003. A slightly different version of this article was published in David Mechanic, et al., 2005, 13–25. Special thanks to the editors of that volume, David Mechanic, Lynn Rogut, David Colby, and James Knickman. I am grateful to the Robert Wood Johnson Foundation and the RWJ Investigators Awards Program for funding. I am also grateful to Rogan Kersh and Elizabeth Kilbreth—my collaborators in studying obesity and schools centers, respectively. Finally, thanks to John DiIulio, Steve Macedo, Gretchen Ritter, Deborah Stone, and Rick Vallely for comments.
2. Morone, 2000.
3. Morone, 1998.
4. Tocqueville, 1969, p 509; Hartz, 1955; Greenstone, 1986.
5. For the classic description, McConnell, 1966; for the update, see Kersh and Morone, 2004.
6. See Morone, 2003a, 7–8.
7. For terrific efforts to rouse the civic minded, see Putnam, 2000 and Skocpol, 2003.

8. Roosevelt gave his speech during the 1932 election campaign. Roosevelt, 1932, p 38–46.
9. See Rogers Smith, 1997.
10. Hacker, 1997, p 138.
11. Data in this paragraph comes from Morone, 2003, p 23–4. For details, data, and quotes in this section, see Morone, 2003a, Introduction. People often wonder about the Constitutional separation of church and state. In fact, that is precisely what fostered the American religious tumult. By keeping government out of the religious sphere (and refusing to privilege any one sect or faith), the Constitution facilitates a robust competition—precisely what makes the American religious culture so fluid and vital.
12. Tocqueville, 1969, p 279.
13. See Morone, 2003a, Chapters 10–11.
14. Storer, 1867; Morone, 2003a, Chapters 8.
15. Allen, 1915, 200–1; Morone, 1997.
16. Historians would not categorize Roosevelt with the social gospel thinkers. I've redefined the category (around its most salient features) and applied it more generally. For details, see Morone, 2003, Part IV.
17. Roosevelt, 1932, 38–46.
18. Roosevelt, 1932, 38–46.
19. Quoted in Morone, 2003a, 426–7.
20. This discussion of school centers comes from work I have done with Elizabeth Kilbreth. We are grateful to the Robert Wood Johnson Foundation for funding the research. For a further discussion of school based health centers, see Morone, Kilberth, and Langwell, 2001.
21. See Morone, 2003b.
22. Elders, 1996, p 242.
23. Morone, 2003a, p 481.
24. My discussion of obesity is shaped by the insights of my collaborator, Rogan Kersh. For further discussion, see Kersh and Morone, 2002a, 2002b, 2005.
25. See Bronwell and Horgen, 183.
26. Brownell and Horgen, 2003, 29–30; Nestle, 2002; Kersh and Morone, 2005.
27. Schlosser, 2001, 240–3.
28. For example, see Kaufman, 2003.

REFERERNCES

Allen, L.C. 1915. *American Journal of Public Health* 5: 194–203.

Brownell, K., and K.B. Horgen. 2003. *Food Fight.* New York: Contemporary Books.

Elders, J. 1996. *Joycelyn Elders, M.D.: From Sharecropper's Daughter to Surgeon General of the United States of America.* New York: Avon Books.

Greenstone, D. 1986. "Political Culture and American Political Development: Liberty, Union and the Liberal Bipolarity." *Studies in American Political Development* I (1): 1–49.

Hacker, J. 1997. *The Road to Nowhere: The Genesis of President Clinton's Plan for Health Security.* Princeton, NJ: Princeton University Press.

Hartz, L. 1955. *The Liberal Tradition in America.* New York: Harcourt, Brace and World.

Kaufman, L. 2003. "Welfare Wars: Are the Poor Suffering from Hunger Anymore?" *New York Times* February 23, p 4.

Kersh, R., and J.A. Morone. 2002a. "The Politics of Obesity." *Health Affairs* 20 (6): 142–53

—— 2002b. "How the Personal Becomes Political: Prohibitions, Public Health and Obesity." *Studies in American Political Development* 16 (fall): 162–75.

—— 2005. "Obesity, Courts and the New Politics of Public Health." *Journal of Health Politics, Policy and Law* 30 (5): 839–68.

McConnell, G. 1966. *Private Power and American Democracy.* New York: Knopf.

Mechanic, D., L.B. Rogut, D. Colby, and J. Knickman. 2005. *Policy Challenges in Modern Health Care.* New Brunswick: Rutgers University Press.

Morone, J.A. 2003a. *Hellfire Nation: The Politics of Sin in American History.* New Haven: Yale University Press.

—— 2003b. "American Ways of Welfare." *Perspectives on Politics.* 1 (March): 137–46.

—— 2000. "Citizens or Shoppers? Solidarity Under Siege." *Journal of Health Politics, Policy and Law* 25 (October): 959–69.

—— 1998. *The Democratic Wish: Popular Participation and the Limits of American Government,* rev. ed. New Haven: Yale University Press.

—— 1997. "Enemies of the People: The Moral Dimension to Public-Health." *Journal of Health Politics, Policy and Law* 22 (4): 993–1010.

Kilbreth, E., and K.M. Langwell. 2001. "Back to School: A Health Care Strategy for Youth." *Health Affairs* 20 (1): 122–36.

Nestle, M. 2002. *Food Politics: How the Food Industry Influences Nutrition and Health*. Berkeley: University of California Press.

Putnam, R. 2000. *Bowling Alone: The Collapse and Revival of American Community*. New York: Simon and Schuster.

Roosevelt, F. 1932. "The Philosophy of Social Justice Through Social Action." October, 2. *The Public Papers and Addresses of Franklin D. Roosevelt*. New York: Random House.

Schlosser, E. 2001. *Fast Food Nation: The Dark Side of the All-American Meal*. New York: Houghton Mifflin.

Smith, R. 1997. *Civic Ideals: Conflicting Ideals of Citizenship in the US History*. New Haven: Yale University Press.

Skocpol, T. 2003. *Diminished Democracy: From Membership to Management in American Civic Life*. Norman: University of Oklahoma Press.

Storer, H.R. 1867. *Is it I? A Book for Every Man*. Boston: Lee and Shepherd.

Tocqueville, Alexis de. 1969 [1835]. *Democracy in America*. New York: Doubleday.

Lawrence D. Brown

Consider This... sections are brief discussions of an important topic. In the first Consider This... section, Lawrence Brown adds an important, missing dimension to the discussion of key concepts and ideas—all health politics are not alike. There are four different types to keep in mind.

Health politics is not a unitary process marked by neat and tidy models. Rather the patterns of health politics vary with policy "arenas"—defined by strategies of intervention that emerged sequentially since 1945 as the federal government has constructed programs that address the demands of the public, interest groups, and (increasingly) the government itself. Students of health policy should be aware of four very different policy arenas—*subsidy, financing, reorganization,* and *regulation.* Each area evinces its own very different brand of politics.

SUBSIDY ARENA

The top health policy preoccupation in most Western nations struggling back to normalcy after World War II was to achieve and sustain universal coverage. The United States, by contrast, had deadlocked since the Progressive Era (1900–1915) over national health insurance, a circumstance itself symptomatic of intense conservative and professional opposition to federal intrusion in health affairs. On the other hand, professional, public, and political opinion concurred that rapid innovation in medical technology brought the conquest of dread diseases into view, that modern hospitals were community centers for advanced care, and that

the nation faced a shortage of physicians. Policy entrepreneurs who looked beyond the stalemate over universal coverage increasingly discerned a safe political harbor for federal interventions that enlarged the supply side of the health care system.

The subsidy strategy, by means of which the federal government funded providers (notably researchers, hospitals, and physicians) to expand their activities and to innovate, encompassed policies of formidable political appeal despite, indeed perhaps because of, America's ingrained suspicion of a governmental hand in health care. "More is better" resonated both with the general public (attuned as in no other policy field to innovations that migrated rapidly from laboratory to learned medical journals to *Reader's Digest* and the evening news). A host of special groups—academic medical centers, medical researchers, drug companies, medical suppliers, hospitals, the construction unions, businesses, and community residents—identified with hospitals, sought care in them, and looked to them for employment. Benefits were spread broadly across both general and special publics; costs were widely diffused. Here was a serviceable a wedge as can readily be imagined for the entry of federal policy into hostile political precincts. Everyone wanted more of the more that is better.

Although the expansion of the National Institutes of Health (NIH), the enactment of the Hill-Burton hospital construction program, and new programs to expand the medial workforce put the federal government squarely in the health policy game, the politics that produced these programs were surprisingly consensual and quiescent. Contrary to Poli.Sci. 101 texts (the executive leads, Congress oversees), Congress took the lead when presidents Truman and Eisenhower were slow to mount the subsidy bandwagon. Partisan and ideological conflict were notably absent. Many interest groups lined up to support these programs, hardly any opposed them. The main exception, which in effect proves the rule, is the legislative breakthrough by means of which the federal government helped to finance medical education, delayed by AMA opposition until 1963, when the association decided to concentrate all its political fire against the Medicare proposal.

From 1945–65 these subsidy programs were the heart of federal health care policy, so much so that some observers saw in them the sordid spectacle of "social pork barrels" and "iron triangles" (alliances among executive agencies, congressional committees, and interest groups so strong as virtually to preclude changes proposed by publicly interested protagonists).[1]

The arena's history, however, presents a political puzzle. How and why would a more-is-better dynamic ever slow or cease? And yet it did. While National Institutes of Health waxed, Hill-Burton hospital construction and the professional workforce subsidies waned. Even as the ink dried on David Stockman's article of 1975, which lampooned Hill-Burton as a plate of social pork, Congress was enfolding the program into new health planning legislation, ending its separate legislation existence and most of its funding.[2] In short order the federal payments to medical schools and their students came under fire. Rising health costs cannot explain the puzzle: hospitals and physicians are powerful cost drivers but so too is

medical technology. The fracturing of supportive coalitions also comes up short: to be sure Hill-Burton was beset by battles about the relative merits of new construction of hospitals versus renovation of existing (especially large urban) facilities and of investment in inpatient versus ambulatory treatment capacity; proponents of medical education quarreled over the right proportions of generalist versus specialist training. The NIH, however, sustained bitter fights over basic versus applied research, over the right organizational arrangements for the National Cancer Institute, and over its seeming indifference to prevention and health promotion.

The answer to the puzzle is that in the privileged preserve of producers and providers encased in iron triangles, ideas and analysis can pack a surprisingly potent policy punch. Policy makers came to believe (rightly or wrongly) that the ranks of hospitals and physicians had expanded into an ominous and reliably quantifiable "surplus," whereas no comparably concrete and seemingly actionable indictment came to attach to technology and medical research.

FINANCING ARENA

Subsidy programs, which in effect hypothesized that the benefits of research, technology, hospitals, and physicians would trickle down and across the population, thus creating universal access, were a distinctively American riposte to advocates of national health insurance. Critics insisted all along that this scenario was ridiculously rosy, and by the mid 1950s the fate of those outside the scope of work-based coverage—especially the aged and the unemployed poor—won national notice. In the aftermath of John F. Kennedy's assassination (in 1963) and Lyndon B. Johnson's landslide victory in the presidential election of 1964, the federal government enacted a torrent of "social" legislation, including Medicare and Medicaid, which committed the federal government to funding important and costly medical services for a sizable subset of the population.

Financing policy posed challenges of legitimacy ("role of government") very different from those the subsidizers faced. In a society where "mere" citizenship does not vindicate a right to health coverage, such programs posed a formidable question: who deserves this public benefit and who should pay for it? Because private coverage was widespread, the ideas that anyone can get sick and that security against the high costs of care is society's business never anchored universalism. Moreover, financing programs meant raising and redistributing massive sums of tax revenue—a prospect that connoted "welfare" (as in public assistance), an ideological ordeal the subsidy programs never faced.

These salient features of financing policy shaped political dynamics that differed markedly from those of the subsidy arena. Whereas subsidy politics seldom generated much partisan or ideological heat, financing politics triggered intense conflict. Interest groups in the subsidy arena were almost all pro, rarely con, but financing programs were a bitter battleground on which the AMA and other conservative groups struggled to kill Medicare over the objections of its core supporters, organized labor and the elderly. Low levels of conflict over subsidy initiatives enabled Congress to lead and steer in the absence of strong presidential leadership. Battles over a new federal financing role fragmented Congress, which put presidential leadership at a premium. Not until—and not since—Johnson did the presidential will to enact public expansions of coverage coincide with the power to do so, that is, with ideologically supportive majorities in Congress.

Reformers made a series of astute policy improvisations: linking Medicare to social security, thus averting images of "welfare"; bifurcating the program into compulsory hospital coverage and a voluntary physician counterpart; excluding costly and controverted benefits such as coverage for long-term care and prescription drugs; and agreeing to pay providers their "actual" and "customary" costs. These stratagems helped carry Medicare into law. The political barricades that had blocked a major federal role in the financing of care seemingly crumbled, as too (supposedly) did the veto power of the AMA and its allies.

In the aftermath of Medicare's enactment, national health insurance itself looked imminent. These great expectations, however, quickly yielded to a puzzle—namely four decades of intermittent "imminence" of national health insurance followed by (in John Donne's words) "perplexed discomposition" of coverage initiatives whose time, it seemed, had incontestably come. In the early 70s Richard Nixon's proposed employer mandate failed to attract sufficient support among single-payer–minded liberals to overcome conservative resistance. In 1974 rumors of an impending consensus on national health insurance ceased after the three principal power holders (Richard Nixon, Edward Kennedy, and Wilbur Mills) confirmed what Randall Bovbjerg memorably termed the "hydraulic theory" of the failure of national health insurance by immersing themselves respectively in Watergate, Chappaquiddick, and the Tidal Basin (the last with a stripper in the car). In the 1970s Jimmy Carter's quest for an efficient model of national health insurance produced no legislative action but put policy entrepreneur Alain Enthoven on the case and his managed competition proposals on the national agenda. That doctrine won pride of place in the Clinton reform plan, widely viewed as a sure thing in fall 1993, universally dismissed as a dead duck six months later.[3]

No less puzzling is the other side of the coin, notably expansion of Medicaid coverage to 13 million beneficiaries in a series of federal enactments in the Reagan and (first) Bush administrations and the creation of the State Children's Health Insurance Program (SCHIP) in 1997 when conservative Republican contractarians with America controlled both houses of Congress. The solution to this puzzle lies in the interplay between policy properties and political power. The arena's political history suggests that, contrary to lingering leftist conventional wisdom, reform struggles premised on universalism—pitched battles in which fervently mobilized reformist groups triumph over insurers, providers, and the conservative ire invariably triggered by the "t" word (tax) and the "w" word (welfare)—gain little traction. The strategies that "work," as exemplified by the Medicaid expansion and SCHIP, target delimited and clearly "legitimate" beneficiary groups (poor mothers and children), modulate the otherwise intense pluralism of financing politics by working quietly within the insulating framework of the federal budget process, and fund coverage expansions with general revenues (including tobacco tax moneys), not by fiscal stratagems that inflame opposition in the private sector. This prospect raises a tough question for liberal reformers: Is Medicare (itself a pale but far from pointless imitation of European-style national health insurance) defunct as a guide to the perplexities of universal coverage in 21st century America?

REORGANIZATION ARENA

The arrival of Medicare and Medicaid transformed the politics of US health policy. Now that Washington political leaders were intervening on both the supply and demand sides of the policy equation, they watched their budget obligation rise quickly. By 1968 "uncontrollable spending," on "entitlements" had become troublesome, health care costs containment became perforce a high priority, and policy imperatives pushed politics into new institutional patterns.

The *subsidy* and *financing* arenas, notwithstanding the sharp political differences between them, fit the preconditions of pluralist politics fairly well. Popular sensibilities (favoring greater public investment in health care infrastructure, and in time, public coverage for those left behind by the private system) were taken up by political organizations that pushed for the subsidies and engaged in fierce pulling and hauling in the financing arena). National political leaders balanced, refined, mediated, compromised, and finally shaped the interest group demands into acceptable programmatic outcomes.

Around 1970 a new "state-centered" policy-making style entered the picture. Government itself replaced interest groups as the prime mover. The earliest evidence was the politics by which federal leaders endorsed a reorganization strategy—the creation of new organizations or a new division of labor among existing ones, as a means to national policy goals. This first prominent case in point was the "discovery" of HMOs.[4] Obliged to "do something" about health costs, the Nixon administration surveyed with distaste the options on the shelf—cuts in benefits in the recently enacted Medicare and Medicaid programs, comprehensive reforms that would both expand coverage and limit payments to providers, and "public utility" regulation of the health sector. Then Paul Ellwood proposed a fresh diagnosis and prescription: The cost problem was rooted in the ill-advised conjunction of fee-for-service practice and third party payment, which in tandem produced pervasively perverse incentives; the cure was federal promotion of prepaid group practices (PGPs), which enfolded care and coverage within organizations that employed or contracted with physicians whose incomes did not rise directly with the volume of services they rendered, thus incorporating the inestimable blessing of "correct incentives." The administration embraced the HMO strategy, which neither cut nor enlarged benefits; featured competition and choice; worked through private incentives rather than public regulation; and cost the federal budget very little money.

The state-centered politics that produced the HMO Act of 1973 differed radically from those that drove the *subsidy* and *financing* arenas. The public did not clamor for HMOs. In 1970 only about two percent of the population was in such a plan and it is safe to say that few citizens knew what HMOs were. No powerful interest groups fought for them, and one formidable group—the AMA—fought the legislation tooth and nail. The innovation and the political resolve to advance it came from a new heavyweight "group" on the scene—the federal government itself, now running, in effect, a ceaseless RFP (Request For Proposal) for bright ideas that would help it manage its budget strains in a politically tolerable fashion. The nation now had two distinct models of health politics—one addressing benefits, the other costs, and the two simultaneously coexisted, competed for primacy among policy makers, and occasionally worked at confusing cross purposes.

The durable federal devotion to reorganization of the health system by means of HMOs, managed care, managed competition, and other variations on market themes presents an intriguing set of political puzzles. Why did the conservative Republican Nixon administration, well-supported by organized medicine and leery of overpromising and overreaching by government, unleash not only a blistering postmodern critique of the health system's status quo but also an HMO development initiative that asked of market forces far more than any private entrepreneur then dreamed of? Why did HMOs kindle slowly for more than a decade and then, around 1985, under the moniker of managed care, come blazing into the mainstream of medical care? How did managed care, generally sold as a market based alternative to more extensive public intervention, give birth to managed competition, an ambitious scheme to make managed care the centerpiece of universal coverage within a sophisticated, elaborated framework of government rules? Why was the Clinton administration blind to the political liabilities with which managed care and managed competition saddled its health reform proposal of 1993? How did managed care become an economic success but a political failure?[5]

These mysteries are explained by the policy properties of managed care. Simply put, managed care embodied a dialectical tension between economic and political success that admitted not (as it briefly seemed in the 1990s) a higher synthesis but rather ineradicable contradiction. HMOs were a political construction, or better put, a political reconstruction of prepaid group practice that enabled diverse partisan and ideological players to see, in this new posited organizational form, the policy virtues they preferred. Conservatives such as Nixon could find in HMOs the magic of the marketplace (competition, correct incentives); but Congress's leading liberal health specialist, Senator Edward Kennedy (DMA), embraced them as an assault on the hegemony of organized medicine, hence a political step toward national health insurance.

In Canada and most nations of Continental Europe, the combination of universal coverage and settled understandings that providers who collectively bargain over fees stand exempt from clinical micro-management makes reorganization a radical enterprise indeed. Unlike the United States, moreover, these nations know that fee-for-service can coexist with third party payment quite successfully so long as governments set firm rules of the health policy game. In the United States, which combined multiple and heterogeneous sources of coverage (uneven and nonuniversal) with a long history of professional rejection of anything resembling a collective settlement with government, reorganization was, all things considered, the path of least resistance for a national government that had become a Very Important Payer and therefore acutely cost conscious.

The porpous, amorphous character of the HMO was also, however, the source of its political vulnerability. Neither Ellwood nor Nixon imagined that an HMO development policy would mean sprinkling the nation with facsimiles of the Kaiser plans or other "true" prepaid group practices. The HMO strategy would conjoin the correct incentives at the logical core of prepaid group practices with amorphous institutional variations, including independent practice associations, and in time, preferred provider organizations, point of service plans, and what wags came to call OWAs (Other Weird Arrangements). The institutional flexibility that allowed employers and consumers to avoid the rigors of "bureaucratic medicine" was crucial to the economic success of managed care but also carried the seeds of its political destruction.

By allowing managed care to amass market share, the hybridization of its organizational forms gave purchasers and managed care executives, eager to slow health care costs, the confidence to tighten economic and administrative screws on providers and consumers. That tightening, in turn, triggered a "backlash"; media indignation at managed care abuses; consumer–provider coalitions demanding legislative and regulatory protections against heartless plans; and market adaptations by plans determined to give aggrieved parties the looser, less disciplined, albeit more costly, arrangements they sought. Political success thus changed the definition of economic success for the plans themselves: expanding their market share required them to turn away from forcing premiums down (which produced furious customers) and instead, to use an ever lighter hand on the levers of efficiency.

An uncritical infatuation with the policy logic of markets generated a politics of diffusion at odds with the enduring economic success of managed care, leaving US policy after three credulous decades with but two options for cost containment: higher consumer cost sharing or tougher public regulation of providers, payers, and perhaps purchasers.

REGULATORY ARENA

Policy analysts often postulated an "either . . . or" choice: market reorganization of the system or cost regulation by public authorities. Policy makers, however, quickly opted for "both . . . and."

A steady parade of regulatory programs came on the scene. With the Professional Standards Review Organization (PSRO) program of 1972 the federal government tried to promote peer oversight of the physician use of hospital care in Medicare and Medicaid. The commitment continued with the conversion of PSROs into Peer Review Organizations (PROs) in 1983. In 1972 Congress also gave states authority to experiment with replacing retrospective reimbursement in Medicare by prospective payment. In 1974 the feds created a state and regional health planning program and coupled to it a requirement that all states enact certificate of need programs that reviewed major capital expenditure projects proposed by hospitals. (Before the requirement of 1974 about half the states had adopted such laws; after the requirement lapsed in 1986 about 2/3 of the states retained CON.) In 1977–78 the Carter administration's plans to regulate increases in hospital spending faltered and died, but before long (1983) a prospective payment system for hospitals in Medicare sailed into federal law. In 1989 legislation introduced a fee schedule to replace "usual and customary but reasonable" charges as the basis for Medicare payment to physicians. In the Health Insurance Portability and Accountability Act of 1996 the federal government asserted new authority over the regulation of health insurance, entering preserves that had hitherto belonged to the states. Around the same time new federal constraints on managed care plans joined the regulatory crowd.

The political robustness of the regulatory arena is a puzzle that demands explanation. After all, the national regimes under which it grew honored some variant of the maxim that the era of big government was over and often voiced overt distaste for regulation. Many economists, steadily looming larger in the councils of policy analysis, dismissed regulation as a classic misadventure in unintended consequences. And the interests to be regulated sometimes fought the proposed enactments, while few countervailing groups supported more regulation.

Health care regulation has thrived in this seemingly inhospitable environment precisely because the policies in question had a flexible and improvisatory character that circumvented most of the rigidities and dysfunctions widely attributed to such classic regulatory agencies as, say, the Interstate Commerce Commission. The origins of the PSROs were no less state centered than those of the HMOs. In both cases the federal government seized on an obscure organizational species that (seemingly) permitted it to attack rising economic costs at acceptable political cost. The same relentless quest for politically tolerable variations on conceptual themes that morphed prepaid group practices into "managed care," also animated the search for feasible regulatory innovations.

Far from seeking to "acquire" regulation for their own ends (as economists have traditionally argued) physicians deplored the PSROs as "cook book medicine." Once the 200-odd PSROs were up and running—or limping—the problem was less the physicians' determination to "capture" then than their unwillingness to engage with them at all. (Likewise CON laws emerged not from the anticompetitive schemes of hospitals but from wise policy heads who had concluded that Roemer's law—"a bed built is a bed filled"—meant that the supply of hospital beds induced demand.) The PSROs, so distasteful to organized medicine, were the brainchild of conservative Republican Senator Wallace Bennett of Utah, who was impressed with a prototype of the peer review approach in his home state and conjectured that a national program along such lines might enlist physicians themselves to challenge excessive use of hospital services by their colleagues. In vivid illustration of the capacious and accommodating character of the emerging health regulatory arena, Edward Kennedy and fellow liberals were at the same time sculpting the health planning program that, they hoped, would endow the nation with a national infrastructure for allocating health care resources once national health insurance again became imminent. Kennedy's national planning program produced a network of supposedly consumer led regulatory and planning agencies (known as health systems agencies or HSAs).

The state centered pattern—programs borne of the federal government's search for solutions to its own health costs problems, often over the objections of "special interests" and without salient support among the public or organized groups—continued into the 1980s as the feds upped the policy ante from "decentralized behavioral" to "centralized budgetary" regulatory endeavors. For example, the hospital industry killed Carter's bold hospital cost containment proposal with a temporarily successful "voluntary effort" to slow the growth of costs. As soon as the Carter proposal was dead, hospitals returned to their wonted wanton ways. The Senate Republicans who had presided over demise of Carter's effort, notably Robert Dole of Kansas and Richard Schweiker of Pennsylvania who became the head of Health and Human Services in the Reagan administration), accelerated the design of a tough new system of hospital payment. The hospitals came to the proverbial bargaining table to help shape the new plan, not because they wanted change but because they knew that in winning the battle over Carter's regulatory plan they had lost the war (once their voluntary effort fizzled and costs again soared). The Reagan administration cheerfully endorsed the new venture in federal government rate setting for hospitals, ironically touting its "pro-competitive" incentives.

Regulation, moreover, has proved serviceable for pluralistic as well as state centered political purposes. After the Clinton reform plan collapsed, both the Democratic administration and the Republican-controlled Congress concurred that new federal regulatory powers in the health insurance market might redeem at least a little of the agenda—portability and accountability—that had spurred the supposed popular mandate for health reform in the first place. Nor did the growing "success" of market reform—the supplanting of fee-for-service medicine by managed care at the center of the system—dampen political taste for the regulatory alternative. If anything, it whetted that appetite as provider organizations and consumer groups coalesced to implore the State to protect them from "greedy" HMOs.

In the 1970s regulation—PSROs, HSAs, CON, rate-setting—mainly sought to constrain the excesses of programs built up in the *subsidy arena*. In the 1980s new federal rate setting schemes—PPS, RBRVS—began to trim the sails of the retrospective cost based payment encoded into Medicare in the *financing arena* which had made its bow in 1965. In the 1990s regulation picked up a few pieces of Clinton's failed plan to lead the nation into affordable universal coverage by means of a reorganization of the system and was invoked to counter abuses of the unmanaged competition that passed for (private) reform after public management of competition had been roundly rejected. Contrary to three decades of ideological pronouncements, this suspect fourth (*regulatory*) arena comes in to bat clean-up for its three predecessors.

CONCLUSION: DISPELLING THE DEMOCRATIC DISCONNECT

Federal health care politics is not one process but rather four arenas—four reasonably distinct strategies of intervention that exhibit four distinct political patterns. Academic neglect of health politics leaves the basic policy history sketched here little understood, and the political dynamics that drive it are more obscure still. The result is a gaping democratic disconnect: neither the public nor enlightened would-be shapers of its opinion are well equipped to explain and evaluate how and why, amid assurances that the era of big government is over, the role of big government has grown, and steadily continues to grow, in the steering of this nearly one-sixth of the national economy. The larger the health system grows, the stronger grow the political imperatives to control it. But the larger the system grows, the stronger grow the political obstacles hindering that control—a policy paradox that repeatedly frustrates reforms befuddled by the bewildering admixture of persistence and mutability in a status quo the political foundations and workings of which remain largely mysterious. Understanding the interplay among arenas may help dispel the democratic disconnect between policy words and political deeds.

NOTES

1. See Ginzberg, 1990; Peterson, 1994.
2. Stockman, 1975.
3. See Hacker, 1997; Skocpol, 1997.
4. See Brown, 1983.
5. See Robinson, 2001.

REFERENCES

Brown, L.D. 1983. *Politics and Health Care Organization: HMOs as Federal Policy.* Washington DC: Brookings Institution.

Ginzberg, E. 1990. *The Medical Triangle: Physicians, Politicians, and the Public* Cambridge, MA: Harvard University Press.

Hacker, J. 1997. *Road to Nowhere: The Genesis of President Clinton's Plan for Health Security.* Princeton: Princeton University Press.

Peterson, M.A. 1994. "Congress in the 1990s: From Iron Triangles to Policy Networks," in J.A. Morone and G.S. Belkin, eds., *The Politics of Health Care Reform: Lessons from the Past, Prospects for the Future.* Durham, NC: Duke University Press.

Robinson, J.A. 2001. "The End of Managed Care." *Journal of the American Medical Association* 285 (May 23/30): 2622–8.

Skocpol, T. 1997. *Boomerang: Health Care Reform and the Turn Against Government.* New York: Norton.

Stockman, D. 1975. "The Public Pork Barrel." *The Public Interest* 39 (Spring): 3–30

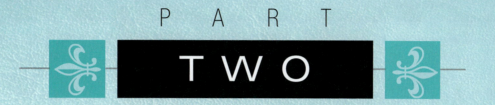

PART
TWO

Political
Institutions

CHAPTER 4

Congress

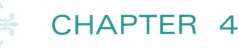

Mark A. Peterson

We cannot understand health politics and policy without understanding Congress. In this chapter, Mark Peterson explores the logic of our legislature, shows how it is unique, and explains why it matters.

Congress has been both friend and foe of health policy. What it enacts, what it ignores, and what it defeats all reveal a good deal about the legislative process in the United States and reflect the changes that, over time, remake American lawmaking.

Congress has constructed a far-reaching national health policy with enormous financial consequences. A comprehensive analysis of all federal expenditures and tax benefits in 1999 estimated that federal dollars represent 40.8% of all health care spending and 50% of expenditure on personal health care.[1] But for all of its engagement with health policy, Capitol Hill has presented an insurmountable hurdle for particular kinds of policies. Except for legislation that cuts projected spending for public programs like Medicare and Medicaid, Congress has consistently rejected proposals designed to contain health care costs, even when overall health care expenditures have increased at more than two or three times the overall rate of inflation in the economy. Congress has also refused, time

and again, all attempts to establish universal health insurance coverage. Even as every other advanced democracy achieved, each in its own way, the "international standard" of universal coverage and cost-containment mechanisms, Congress has rejected every effort in the United States.[2]

How are we to understand the American legislative process—with its emphasis on distributive policymaking, bursts of regulation, episodic focus on particular populations and constituencies, and (thus far) the blunt refusal to discipline health care spending or provide universal insurance coverage? What does one need to know about Congress to explain this mix of activism and denial, to ascertain "the logic of congressional action" and inaction in health policymaking?[3] In this chapter, I describe the core features of Congress. I consider how unusual election results as well as changes in the structure of Congress can alter the internal politics of lawmaking. With these fundamentals of the legislative branch in hand, I turn to the issue that is often of paramount interest to students of health politics and policy, offering a relatively detailed analysis of the repeated failures of comprehensive health care reform. Finally, I assess how Congress has changed. Since the last round in the health care reform debates in the early 1990s, Congressional decision-making has become more partisan and more centralized.

THE BASELINE CONGRESS

One fact about Congress stands above all others. "Among the national legislatures of major countries, Congress is the only one that still plays a powerful independent role in public policymaking. . . . Only Congress initiates legislation, makes decisions on major provisions, and says 'no' to executive proposals."[4] Consider the stark difference between the United States and the United Kingdom. Three major empirical studies reveal that Congress in the post-war period adopted, typically only in part, just 6 in 10 presidential initiatives. Some presidents faired particularly poorly—Gerald Ford and Jimmy Carter could get Capitol Hill to accept only about a third of their legislative agendas.[5] In contrast, British Prime Minister Tony Blair was in office *for more than eight years* before the parliament defeated one of his major legislative proposals.[6] Congress not only frequently exercises its authority to block or substantially alter initiatives from the executive, it often plays a critical leadership role in the formative stages of policymaking. Policy ideas "proposed" by presidents often begin as bills drafted much earlier by members of Congress.[7] Based on his detailed historical analysis of 28 major statutes enacted from 1947 to 1990, Charles O. Jones determined that the impact of the legislature was "preponderant" for a quarter of the laws, and in more than half the cases Congress shared roughly equal influence with the president.[8]

What permits Congress to be so different from other national legislatures, and therefore of such unique consequence to health policymaking? The "separation of powers" and attendant checks and balances established by the US Constitution. This system of independent legislative, executive, and judicial branches of government, each with a formal claim over some aspect of lawmaking and implementation—more accurately captured by Richard Neustadt's phrase, "separated institutions *sharing* powers"—ensures that Congress is a central player in national policymaking.[9] It also fosters decision-making complexity by injecting multiple perspectives into legislative policymaking. Both the Constitution and institutional arrangements that developed later (through law, rules, and interpretation) make enacting statutes difficult; successful legislation requires assembling a daunting series of like-minded coalitions in numerous venues—committees and subcommittees within the House and the Senate, while also garnering the support of the president (or sufficiently larger majorities in both the House and Senate to override a presidential veto). Just about everything engineered by the Constitution makes legislating difficult, such as the separate constituencies and election timetables for the president, the House, and the Senate.

Elaborating on the comparative context illustrates the point. Arend Lijpjart identified two "ideal types" of democratic, constitutional design: "*majoritarian*" and "*consensus*."[10] Majoritarian systems simplify the burdens of decisionmaking by concentrating power in the hands of the leadership of the political party that won the most recent election. They dramatically limit the opportunities for independent action by the legislature. Such systems have a prime minister as the single executive leader; the prime minister and the cabinet (together forming "the government") are generally members of parliament, thus fusing the executive and legislative authority; and the legislature has only one body with policy-making power. In addition, only two parties compete meaningfully in elections and take stances on issues that clearly differentiate the parties; in those elections a legislative district is represented by the candidate who won a plurality of the vote; lower level governments are under the authority of the national government; and the constitution is unwritten, interpreted by the parliament instead of an independent judicial branch of government. Majority party members in parliament are expected to follow the lead of their prime minister and cabinet. New Zealand's political system fits this image nearly perfectly.[11] The United Kingdom and Canada come close to this model.

Alternatively, nations that comport with "consensus" arrangements have governing systems in which taking action requires nurturing pervasive agreement among myriad policy makers located in multiple institutional settings. Everything about these systems fragments power where majoritarian systems concentrate it. As a result, consensus systems invite any interest groups with a large stakes in any policy question to work the institutional crevices of dispersed policymaking in order to shape laws more to its liking or to "veto" provisions with which it disagrees.[12] The United States possesses a number of majoritarian attributes (executive power concentrated in a single president, a two-party system, single-member legislative districts, and "first-past-the-post" plurality elections for Congress and the president); however, because of the separation of powers and the equal authority granted the two chambers of Congress, each with distinctive constituencies, along with federalism that protects the autonomy of the states (further reflected back in the Senate and tensions between the House and Senate), and a written constitution with the independent judiciary as the final interpreter, our system tilts heavily in the direction of the consensus model. In addition, the United States has few of the other social institutions—such as muscular political parties, a tradition of a strong administrative state, and a widely organized and influential labor movement—that bridge institutional divides in other countries.[13]

Knowing that Congress matters more than most national legislatures as a policy-making body, and that legislating is a complicated endeavor, does not yet tell us how and why Congress acts, or fails to act, in response to particular policy issues. For insights on these issues, we must first examine the role and orientation of legislators in the American context and the effects of specific features of Congress as an institution have on legislative decisionmaking.

The Legislator

Congress is ultimately an aggregation of its members. Its actions reflect the motivations, preferences, and choices of the individuals elected to serve as Representatives and Senators. One starting assumption is that members of Congress are "single-minded seekers of re-election."[14] That proposition may be too narrow and cynical, but even when members are primarily intent upon wielding power or pursuing the public interest through good public policy, re-election is the necessary predicate and thus an inescapable objective.[15] However, that goal creates different behavioral incentives in different systems. In many parliamentary systems, the political parties maintain close control over the slates of legislative candidates, not only determining who will run (or "stand") for election and re-election, but even what districts or constituencies they will represent. Electoral success in such settings, therefore, hinges first on satisfying the party's needs, including supporting the expressed policy positions of the party once in office.

Although there have been times in American history when the major political parties have played a significant role in candidate selection and promotion, congressional candidates and incumbents running for re-election are usually independent agents who promote their individual political interests. In some instances, party figures from local or national organizations try to entice particular individuals to seek election to Congress with promises of support but most candidates launch the race for office under their own volition. The party's nomination is determined by voters in primary elections, not the party's leadership. In 1938, incumbent conservative Southern Democrats who opposed FDR's New Deal easily won renomination and re-election despite the president's bold efforts to defeat them. In 1990, GOP leaders were embarrassed when the white supremacist David Duke ran as the Republican challenger to incumbent Democratic Senator J. Bennett Johnston in Louisiana. In the general election, various party organizations inside and outside of Congress may provide some campaign funding, media assistance, or campaign visits by their partisan luminaries, such as the president or congressional leaders, but for the most part congressional candidates assemble their own electoral teams, hire their own consultants, do their own polling, and craft their own themes attuned to their particular constituencies. As a result, both congressional campaigns and legislative decisionmaking are especially responsive to local considerations. Members of Congress must judge even national policy issues like funding Medicaid, educating health care professionals, or containing hospital costs through the lens of their constituencies. The late Thomas "Tip" O'Neill of Massachusetts, Democratic Speaker of the House from 1977 to 1987, famously endorsed the well-worn line that "all politics is local."[16]

Congressional Organization— Legislative Parties

Political parties in Congress are the most single most important *organizational* feature of the legislature. In both the House and Senate, the party that wins the majority of seats in the election chooses the leaders of the chamber who, in turn, determine which committees will be assigned bills and organize floor deliberations. Committee and subcommittee chairs come from the ranks of the majority party, and they determine the schedule of the committee's work and hire most of its professional staff. Party affiliation is also the best single predictor of how members of the House and Senate will vote on pending rules and legislation.[17] That, however, is where any apparent similarities between Congress and other national legislatures ends. In many parliamentary systems the majority party has to hang together on important votes or, in the extreme case, the government "falls" and new elections are called.

In purely "majoritarian" systems, a "government" (prime minister and cabinet) can almost always secure a legislative victory, even for the most sweeping and controversial legislation. Congress could not be more different. Since most members of Congress have their own independent constituent base, Democratic and Republican leaders often have had trouble motivating individual members to support the party's positions. House and Senate leaders of both parties understand the strong local ties. They rarely try to compel members to comply with party positions, if it would risk electoral damage, and few mavericks have been punished when they have broken ranks, even on major party priorities.[18] The effect is reflected in average "party unity scores"—the percentage of a party's members who voted with a majority of their compatriots when on a recorded roll-call vote a majority of one party countered the majority of the other party. Since 1954, for example, Democratic party unity on all such votes in the House ranged from a low of 70% in the early 1970s to a peak of 89% in 1993 (Republicans followed a similar pattern, although they acted with more sustained unity since 1993; the Senate also closely matches the House).[19]

Congressional Organization— Structural Characteristics

Any legislature has structural design features— established by the constitution, legislation, or the rules of each chamber—that largely determine which legislators can significantly affect lawmaking. Put bluntly, are institutional power and resources concentrated in the hands of the majority and its leadership or are they dispersed? With Congress, we start with the knowledge that authority is constitutionally divided between two houses with very different organizational characteristics, constituencies, electoral schedules, and incentives. But we can go further. One can imagine three possible "pure types" of organizational arrangements in each chamber. The first would be a "centralized" structure, with the majority party leadership in command of decisionmaking—agendas, organization of the committees, staff resources, legislative mark-ups, floor debates, and so on. Given the previous discussion, it should not be surprising that the most centralized form is the Westminster-style parliament found in New Zealand or the United Kingdom. When the majority party leadership wishes to act, those in opposition do not have the institutional assets needed to block the way. The second form of legislative organization would be a "decentralized" institution in which power and resources are distributed beyond the majority party's leadership. For example, considerable authority is often granted to standing committees of jurisdiction, and thus their chairs (or the members), which provide detailed review of all bills introduced in their areas of policy jurisdiction. The consequences are most pronounced when the policy preferences of a committee—the chair, the committee members, or both—differ measurably from the rest of the party members. In this setting, committees might become veto points, unwilling to report out bills that would otherwise be agreeable to the whole chamber. Powerful committees might also be able to help move an initiative forward that the majority leadership may prefer to avoid. Other members of the chamber from both parties turn to the committee of jurisdiction for substantive policy cues and know that their future legislative interests in the policy area may be well served by supporting legislation favored by the committee. The final type of legislative structure—"fragmented"—disperses power even further. In its most pronounced form, individual legislators are provided with the kind of staff resources, institutional positions, and access to the bill amending process that permits them to influence the course and substance of legislation. Working coalitions are difficult to orchestrate and maintain when so many individuals have a claim on the legislative process. Such diffused power, however, also offers multiple legislative pathways to overcome the opposition of the leadership or a single committee.

What kind of structure best describes Congress? As a complex institution, one finds attributes of all three types, but historically there have also been some clear tendencies. First, power has almost always been more "fragmented" in the Senate than in

the House. Individual senators possess more resources and larger staffs. The opportunity to filibuster during floor debates—long ago forbidden in the House—grants each senator the potential capacity to bring the institution to a halt (a powerful bargaining tool). Over the course of the 20th century, the House of Representatives cycled through all three forms of legislative organization.[20] Very early in the 20th century there was considerable centralization; the majority party leadership commanded the agenda and shaped legislative outcomes. After a revolt against the leadership (in 1910), the institution became what the congressional literature sometimes calls a "textbook Congress" (roughly 1920 to 1960). The work became decentralized. A limited number of autonomous or semi-autonomous committees run by powerful, "baron"-like chairmen—the "whales" of the legislative enterprise—dominated the agenda and often thwarted legislation desired by the leadership and the majority. Major political shifts that cumulated in the 1970s led to what is usually referred to as the "reform" Congress. Liberal Democrats in particular wanted to get around conservative committee chairs who stood in the way of progressive legislation. Lacking the wherewithal for a frontal assault on the chairs, they instead pursued new rules that ended up fragmenting power by shifting authority and resources to innumerable subcommittees and individual representatives. The 1980s witnessed the "post-reform" Congress. While power remained fragmented, leaders took more control and committees (and their chairs), now less out-of-step from the House as a whole, regained influence.[21] The mid-1990s saw a return to the highly centralized House reminiscent of the early 1900s (more on this last stage later in this chapter).

Organized Interests Present and Accounted For

Congressional policy deliberations do not, of course, occur in a vacuum, free of efforts at intervention by organized interests with stakes in the legislative outcomes. Although there is some controversy about whether or not parliamentary systems are more resistant to interest groups, there is no question that Congress is an open target for attempts at influence, both directly through lobbying and indirectly using the media and other methods to pique Congressional constituents. Mobilizing large memberships, leveraging skilled lobbying operations, fertilizing congressional access with hefty campaign contributions, and sometimes financing sophisticated public relations drives, well-endowed interest groups—especially large, commercial interests—seek to gain entry to and to shape the views of congressional powers. For much of the 20th century this meant targeting the committees.[22] Indeed, health care policy in the United States has often been characterized as the natural product of interest group politics.[23] The American Medical Association (AMA) was the paradigmatic case in point for a long period.

The rise of social movements in the 1960s and 1970s altered this picture. They gave birth to new organizations representing consumers, women, environmentalists, and others dedicated to social change and competing with the older interests for the attention of policy makers. New "patrons of political action," including foundations and wealthy individuals, emerged to help these organizations acquire the resources they needed to organize and maintain themselves by overcoming the inherent difficulty of mobilizing large, dispersed groups of individuals for collective action.[24] The new mix of organized interests could at times make it more difficult for the established interests to work as successfully with Congress. They also helped to open up the policy-making process and broaden the agenda to include popular issues like environmental protection and occupational safety.

The Legislative Consequences

Put these pieces together—the near self-selection of locally-oriented legislators who can act independently, parties in Congress generally unable and rarely willing to force the adherence and discipline of their members; legislative power often concentrated in committees (or dispersed even more widely); and

the open access of the institution to organized interests, especially those with strong constituency ties— and it is easy to ascertain what members of Congress consider to be "politically attractive" policies.[25] They create identifiable benefits that can be broadly allocated and traced back to the votes and actions of individual legislators who claim credit for their enactment. If the law entails costs, they are widely diffused, without imposing significant burdens on targeted payers. In short, they look a lot like Hill-Burton hospital construction and expansion, training of the health professions and development of their schools, and funding for biomedical research. Proposed legislation that would yield obscure benefits sometime in the relatively distant future, or whose returns are not obvious for attentive citizens, but would demand the bearing of substantial costs by powerful interests, or a bill that would explicitly redistribute the tax dollars of politically engaged constituents to the benefit of the politically withdrawn, are the most difficult to enact.

Changing circumstances, however, can modify this "baseline" dynamic of the legislative process. The rise of the environmental and consumer movements, for example, transformed the otherwise antagonistic politics of regulation by bringing competing organized interests to the legislative arena, making the costs of inaction more stark, and clarifying the benefits of pollution control for the middle class electorate.[26] Elections can bring dramatic shifts that disrupt the simple "distributive" status quo of Congress. The election of 1932 not only put FDR in the White House, but also huge new Democratic majorities in Congress that temporarily led to greater centralization of the House and a willingness to enact programs like Social Security. The election of 1964 gave Lyndon Johnson an unprecedented landslide and infused Congress with liberal Democrats who overwhelmed the House Ways and Means Committee which had been blocking Medicare.[27] In 1994, Republicans—under the leadership of Newt Gingrich—successfully nationalized the election, breaking the hold of the local imperatives in Congress. Capturing both chambers of Congress in that election, the GOP enjoyed bicameral legislative majorities for the first time in two generations, unified their ranks, centralized House decisionmaking, and passed legislation that would have privatized Medicare (only to be thwarted by President Clinton's veto), block-granted Medicaid to the states, and carved out hundreds of billions of dollars in projected spending for these programs, which would have imposed substantial costs on beneficiaries and providers.[28]

Elections need not be so dramatic to reconfigure the internal politics of Congress. After great battles lead to stalemate (and the appearance of failed legislative responsiveness to the public), the coming of the next election can incite both parties to reach agreement on lesser programs that they deem to be sufficiently distant from partisan cleavages, popular with voters, and providing benefits that incumbents can bring home to their constituents. For example, the Health Insurance Portability and Accountability Act (HIPAA) of 1996 passed with bipartisan votes in the wake of health care reform's defeat.[29] Alternatively, the continued policy and electoral success of one party in a policy area may entice the other party to poach the issue, in the hope of eviscerating the original partisan advantage. Clinton and centrist Democrats tried that with welfare reform. President George W. Bush and the Republican Congress, in turn, used every institutional advantage of their majorities and centralized control of the House to push the Medicare Prescription Drug, Improvement, and Modernization Act (MMA) of 2003.[30]

COMPREHENSIVE HEALTH CARE REFORM: A WINDOW INTO CONGRESS

The history of comprehensive health care reform reveals all of the elements of congressional policymaking presented in this chapter, from legislative barriers to the changing constellation of interest groups, from the role of partisanship to the changing institutional structure of legislative power.

We can begin by returning to the puzzle of American health care policy. All industrial nations and many poorer developing ones endow their citizens with some form of universal health insurance. The latter half of the 20th century brought the emergence of the near universal and reasonably consistent "international standard" of coverage and financing for medical services, albeit using quite different institutional arrangements across nations.[31] Even the Anglo countries with the most pronounced traditions of individual liberty and responsibility—England, Canada, and Australia—recognize the degree to which ill health has to do with genetic and experiential bad luck, and provide universal care. The United States is the one startling exception. The reason? When it comes to national proposals for comprehensive health care reform Congress has been an unrelenting graveyard. Not all the "homicides," however, were equally quick or certain.

Not Coming to Our Consensus

The lack of universal insurance coverage is not for want of popular support. At least as reflected in opinion polls, substantial public majorities consistently affirm that individuals ought to have coverage for medical services regardless of their incomes and social standing. Even in the context of the 2000 elections, which produced the first conservative, unified Republican government in nearly a half century, 64% of the public agreed that "it is the responsibility of the federal government to make sure all Americans have health care coverage." Significant majorities—in the range of 70% to 90% for the last 20 years—have found fault with the existing arrangements for financing and delivering health care and called, in some fashion, for major changes. Typically that support comes with the understanding that government would have to play an important role.[32]

Though universal health care had strong advocates by the 1910s, it was not until 1939, when New York Senator Robert Wagner introduced a relatively modest, state-based health care reform bill, that something resembling national health insurance formally entered the congressional arena. That set the ball rolling. In 1943 Wagner was joined by Senator James Murray (Democrat from Montana) and Representative John Dingell (D. Michigan) to introduce the first bill to develop a national, comprehensive, universal health insurance program, this one tied to Social Security (Dingell's son replaced his father in 1955 and has re-introduced the national health insurance bill in every Congress since). In the fall of 1945, shortly after he assumed the presidency, Harry Truman became the first sitting president to propose a national, compulsory health insurance plan. He granted it a prominent place on his legislative agenda throughout the late 1940s. Some 30 years later, politicians like Democratic Senator Ted Kennedy and Republican President Richard Nixon returned national health insurance to the political agenda. By early 1974, President Nixon offered an expansive Comprehensive Health Insurance Program (CHIP), designed to use employer mandates and public coverage for the working poor and unemployed to yield universal coverage. Nixon's plan, along with the competing Democratic plans, was the first health care reform proposal to engender serious congressional attention. President Jimmy Carter proposed universal coverage in 1979 to be provided by competing private health care plans financed by both employers and government. Although President Ronald Reagan avoided the issue, President George H.W. Bush offered modest legislative overtures to expand insurance coverage, a defensive posture stimulated by rapidly escalating calls for comprehensive health care reform and the introduction of major proposals by both Democratic and Republican leaders in the House and Senate. Finally, Bill Clinton went even further, campaigning in 1992 with health care reform and universal coverage as a centerpiece of his platform. He made his Health Security Act a lead issue on his subsequent presidential agenda.

Despite all of this attention to the issue at multiple times in the previous century, and notwithstanding the hundreds of plans formed and bills introduced, some offered by presidents and a few given the full weight of their administrations, *not a single health care reform initiative has ever come to a vote on the floor of either chamber of the US Congress*. They have all been deflected by wanton congressional inaction. The first health care reform floor *debate*, held in the Senate, did not even ensue until the 103rd Congress and the presentation of Clinton's plan. How is it possible that Congress has proven so incapable of, or so unwilling to, join the international standard of universal coverage? Sven Steinmo and Jon Watts, students of cross-national politics and social policymaking, have a simple answer: "It's the Institutions, Stupid!"[33] First written before the failure of Clinton's health care reform effort, their article, subtitled "Why Comprehensive National Health Insurance Always Fails in America," argues that the design of our governing arrangements, especially Congress and its relationship with other institutions as described earlier, have made and will always make it impossible to enact such sweeping reform.

To end the story here, though, would be premature. However profound the differences noted earlier between the governing structures of the United States and the other industrial nations, American institutional arrangements and health care politics have actually varied considerably over time. They have dramatically altered the prospects of reform from one period to the next. There have been times when Congress could have enacted universal coverage, and perhaps almost did. The consistency of the policy outcome in the United States has obscured the substantial variability of the legislative policy process. Steinmo and Watts have simply drawn too bright a line. We have to ask ourselves what real opportunities for policy innovation in Congress have emerged in the past, what policy makers did with those opportunities, and exactly why health care reform met repeatedly with congressional inaction on each of those occasions.

Barriers to Coalition Building in Congress

My earlier discussion of shifts from the congressional baseline noted that new opportunities emerge in the legislative setting when a changed context boosts the potential for pulling together winning coalitions. Let us return to three dimensions important for defining the congressional setting at any given time. I will call them "party" (the percentage of seats held by the political party that generally favors the policy change), "cohesion" (the level of unity or agreement among the members of that party), and "structural coherence" (the degree to which the legislature's decision-making authority is concentrated rather than dispersed, and thus can be coordinated by the majority party).

When examining an issue like health care reform, we would like to know what proportion of a legislative chamber's membership has a predisposition to support a general course of action, such as assuring universal coverage. That information is not available, especially over an extended number of years. On many issues, though, including health care reform, a reasonable surrogate is the relative stature of the political party most likely to endorse such a policy innovation. Although many Republicans in Congress have worked earnestly for health care reforms (the late Senator John Chafee of Rhode Island comes to mind), the most ardent advocates of universal coverage have consistently been Democrats. And they have been a fairly numerous bunch. Between 1933 and 1994 (during which the most important health care reform debates transpired), Democrats held majorities in the House of Representatives for all but four years (1947–48 and 1953–54) and in the Senate for all but 10 years (1947–48, 1953–54, and 1981–86). Sometimes those majorities were stunning in their size. During FDR's Second New Deal, Lyndon Johnson's Great Society, and Jimmy Carter's first two years, Democrats controlled 77%, 68%, and 67% of the House, respectively, and roughly the same proportions of the Senate. When in the majority since 1932, Democrats have held on average of approximately six in ten House and Senate seats. These are healthy margins and with majority control the Democrats have held the House Speakership, leadership positions, considerable leverage over the floor agenda, the chairs of all committees and subcommittees, as well as the bulk of the staff and other legislative

resources. Universal coverage should have had a leg up in Congress.

However, the second dimension of relevance to coalition building, cohesion, draws attention to how limited the utility of party majorities can be, especially in the American context. Continue with political party as a proxy for the potential coalition base. A deeply divided party, even if nominally in the majority, will not be able to deliver reliable votes for significant policy initiatives like health care reform. Recall that for both Democrats and Republicans unity has never been universal and dipped quite low in the 1970s.

The evidence from 1955 to 1994, during which Democrats enjoyed continuous control of the House of Representatives, illustrates the potential problem of achieving what might be called a *reliable* majority (one that would be of sufficient size *and* unity to produce an expected majority vote in favor of policy approaches presented on the floor). If one multiplies the number of seats controlled by the Democrats (the starting base in the calculation) by the average percentage of Democrats who voted with their party on party unity votes (a measure of how likely it was at that time for individual Democratic members to vote with their party), in only 18 out of the 40 years does the result produce a slim reliable majority. Most of the time, therefore, having a majority of seats did not translate into mustering a majority of votes on contentious issues.

Of those 18 years, only five had a Democratic president (thus a chief executive who would have endorsed Democratic health care reform efforts): Kennedy's third year, the 89th Congress during Johnson's Great Society, and President Bill Clinton's first two years. As we will see in Chapter 5, President Lyndon Johnson led the passage of Medicare and Medicaid when the combined size and unity of the Democratic majority in the House was at its postwar zenith, but did not feel he had to votes to offer a more expansive health reform agenda. The situation in the Senate made successful action even less likely. Because of the filibuster, which allows any individual senator or small group of senators to block floor action by conducting endless debate, legislation can be thwarted unless a supermajority of sixty votes is available to cut off debate (known as enforcing "cloture"). Even during LBJ's heyday in the 89th Congress, the combined Democratic seats and unity nudged a slim majority in the Senate, well short of the sustained effective coalition that would be needed in the face of serious opposition on the floor. In short, if enactment of universal coverage depended on the Democratic Party in Congress alone, there have been precious few windows of real opportunity (neither Truman nor Carter launched their initiatives during an opportune period).

The challenge to health care reformers becomes even more complicated—and daunting—when we introduce the third dimension of coalition building: the structural coherence of the legislature itself. Consider the features associated with centralization, decentralization, and fragmentation that I noted earlier. Using extensive empirical measures of the institutional attributes of specific relevance to legislating in the realm of health care reform, I have developed indices to represent the presence of factors associated with centralization, decentralization, and fragmentation in the House of Representatives and Senate from 1909 to 2000.[34] The House of Truman's day, for example, ranked low in centralization and fragmentation, but high on the second dimension, decentralization—that is, the committee chairs wielded significant power. In Truman's time, the committees that had jurisdiction over health care reform legislation were more conservative than the House as a whole, and their chairs opposed the president's national health insurance plan. Veto they could and veto they did.

Fast forward to Carter's administration and one discovers a fundamentally changed legislative institution. The Democratic majority in the House was much larger, but also much more divided within itself. The power of the committee chairs (decentralization) had been supplanted by widespread fragmentation. Every committee was required to have subcommittees of jurisdiction with their own staff resources and agenda control, and every subcommittee throughout the chamber was chaired by a different member of the House Democratic majority.

Rank-and-file members also had more staff and increased influence (the House came to look a lot more like the Senate, which has always been a more fragmented institution).[35] The Carter years (and Nixon's just before) did not offer an opportune context for putting together a coalition on an issue as significant, complicated, and threatening to so many stakeholders as health care reform and universal coverage.

The Congresses during the time when Bill Clinton ran for president and took office, however, showed more promising signs.[36] Many features of fragmentation remained. However, the committees of jurisdiction—all with chairs supportive of reform and members more liberal than the House as a whole—had regained some of their influence (the decentralization index was higher) and there were more rules that enhanced the influence of the Speaker of the House to coordinate the legislative process. There were still plenty of institutional barriers, but the 103rd Congress at the start of the Clinton administration combined the attributes—Democratic majority, unity, and institutional coherence—that gave health care reform–minded coalition-builders a better organizational chance than they had had in any previous round of national health insurance debates.

Congress in the Web of Interests

For much of the 20th century, the politics of health care reform seemed to be a paradigmatic example of the power of organized interests with strong stakes in the status quo. The American Medical Association (AMA) in particular possessed all of the instruments of interest group influence, including an enormous membership residing in every legislative district, unity of purpose, the authority to speak for its membership, unrivaled expertise on the issues, and vast organizational and financial resources to lobby legislators and support candidates for office. Under its leadership, physicians, hospitals, insurers, and employers are thought to have channeled their way into the open congressional arena, striving effectively to preserve their own interests, and fend off health care reform and universal coverage.[37] For a long time, that imagery was consistent with the observable patterns of policymaking on issues both small and large.[38] When FDR contemplated health care coverage next to Social Security and Truman proposed national health insurance, the American Medical Association led a powerful antireform alliance that included medicine, insurance, and business. It dominated the interest group scene and out-influenced what we might term the stake challengers, mainly labor unions who endorsed national health insurance. For the most part, in the decentralized Congress of that era, this antireform alliance found ready partners among the chairs and members of the committees of jurisdiction. As presidents for the first time were moving universal coverage to their programmatic agendas, reform did not stand a chance in Congress. Anticipating the result, Roosevelt pulled back from even launching an initiative, and Truman's proposal could garner no more than a single, brief committee hearing.[39]

By the time that Richard Nixon and Jimmy Carter were engaged in their own health care reform efforts, the interest group world had begun to change. Their administrations came in the wake of the social movements of the 1960s and 1970s. Many of new "citizen" organizations would eventually join with organized labor in challenging the health care "industry" and promoting universal coverage.[40] However, the antireform alliance remained unified in its opposition to such large-scale government intervention. Although the reform debates of the 1970s remained largely "inside-the-beltway" contests, reformers faced significant challenges due to the idiosyncratic features of presidential politics at the time (e.g., the ramifications of Nixon's Watergate scandal), the general divisions among congressional Democrats, and the chaotic setting of the increasingly fragmented House and Senate. However, Congress did more than hold brief perfunctory committee hearings—considerable committee attention was devoted to the issue. One possible path to compromise on health care reform even emerged

that possibly could have been passed.[41] More on that story in a moment.

Between Jimmy Carter's return home to Plains, Georgia, in 1981 and Bill Clinton's bus trip from Jefferson's Monticello to his inauguration in 1993, a metamorphosis took place in the community of organized interests focused on health care reform. More than a decade of sharply rising health care costs, partial cost control programs (introduced by government and business), huge disparities in coverage provided by large and small employers, and increased medical specialization splintered the old antireform alliance. The divisions emerged both across and within the domains of medicine, insurance, and business. In the meantime, more citizen groups arrived on the scene; most were sympathetic to universal coverage but some, such as the Christian Coalition, reflected a conservative countermobilization against greater government taxation and economic regulation.[42] Ironically, the two leading antagonists in the health care reform wars of the past—the American Medical Association and organized labor—had both diminished considerably in strength. Instead of including nearly all practicing physicians, as in the past, the AMA's membership slipped to just four in ten doctors by the early 1990s. Labor's ranks had declined from representing better than a third of the labor force at its 1950s zenith to just under 15 percent.[43] By the late 1980s, these "peak associations" that once spoke for whole sectors of the economy had become "just another interest group" or "just one more PAC."[44] The AMA, for all intents and purposes, dropped entirely from the relevant set of organized interests on health care reform. Labor remained a player, but became weakened on this issue by its diminished base and its commitment to employer-based insurance.[45]

On both sides of the reform debate new organizational leaders would emerge. The National Federation of Independent Business (NFIB), the hard-right point organization for small business; the Health Insurance Association of America (HIAA), the trade association for commercial insurers; and the Pharmaceutical Research and Manufacturing Association (PhRMA), representing the drug companies, took up the charge against government reform. On the other side, the AARP, Families USA, and Citizen Action—all either relatively recently founded or newly revitalized groups—provided much of the organizational wherewithal and grassroots mobilization for the proreform forces.[46] The early 1990s offered an opportunity for each side of the health care reform debate. Which interest group coalition would coalesce most effectively, succeed in the court of public opinion, and demonstrate efficacious use of the legislative levers of influence? The gates to the congressional graveyard were unlocked, but would they open?

Presidents in the Legislative Arena

The legislative dictum of the modern era is that the president proposes and Congress disposes. Like most maxims, this one is too simplistic. Even with the post-war enlargement of the presidency's aura in all matters of policy, foreign and domestic, Congress continues to be the source of much legislative energy and policy innovation.[47] Nonetheless, it would be difficult to envision the enactment of a reform as expansive as universal health care coverage without the collaboration, indeed the leadership, of the chief executive.[48] The only times that health care reform has been seriously on the agenda, regardless of the trends in the ranks of the uninsured or the costs of the health care system, has been when presidents have initiated formal proposals. That is not to say that their involvement has always been purely voluntary. Both Richard Nixon, with his comprehensive plan, tentatively carried forward by Gerald Ford and George H.W. Bush, with his more incremental approach, were responding to the Democrats' potential advantage on this issue. Many presidents, of course, have also used their influence to thwart reform impulses by simply ignoring the issue. Still, if one wants to assess those moments when something substantive about reform was in the air, one has to look to the actions of particular presidents.

Three possible strategies have been available for presidents interested in health care reform: combat,

collaboration, and co-optation. And all three have been tried. Perhaps befitting his personality, and clearly linked to the context in which he served, Harry Truman chose combat. His plan for compulsory national health insurance, publicly financed and linked to Social Security, was favorably received by the public but ran entirely counter to the constellation of organized interests and the preferences of members of Congress who dominated health care legislation, especially (but not only) during the Republican Congress of 1947–48. This was no effort to engage the stakeholder interests or skeptics in Congress. He sought to "give 'em hell," to attack the "do nothing Republican Congress," and to mobilize public opinion (although far too casually to be effective). No matter what he might have tried, however, an institutional analysis reveals that no strategy was available that could break the lock against health care reform. Defeat was ensured by the partnership of the antireform alliance's policy monopoly with the relevant committee chairs and members in Congress who were antagonistic to major government intervention in health care financing.

A second strategy is collaboration. To a large extent, that was the theme of the 1970s. Both Nixon and Carter sought to build universal coverage on the existing system of employer-sponsored insurance, filling in the gaps with a publicly financed program. Private insurers would not be put out of business, and employers (along with labor) would continue to have a primary in offering coverage. By collaborating with both stakeholders and opposition members of Congress, each president envisioned a grand compromise.

A collaborative, bipartisan process might have won reform. In August 1974, Congress came very close to enacting universal coverage predicated on employer mandates and some public financing. A compromise appeared to be in motion among President Richard Nixon (later Gerald Ford), Senator Ted Kennedy (who had earlier advocated full public funding), Senator Russell Long (the fairly conservative Democratic chair of the Senate Finance Committee), and Wilbur Mills (the chair of the House Ways and Means Committee who was always seeking ways to control the agenda on his terms). Losing some Southern Democrats but picking up a few Republicans, as well as holding onto all of the liberal Democrats on the Committee, Mills came within a vote or two of reporting out a bill that would have given universal coverage some momentum.[49] One can only speculate whether such a bill sent to the floor on a deeply split vote by the Committee on Ways and Means would have survived in the full House and then the Senate. Several Democrats, for example, were anticipating huge Democratic gains in the fall elections following Nixon's resignation. Many were further convinced that 1976 would bring the election of a Democratic president committed to more expansive health care reform. They might have thwarted Mills's efforts in exchange for a better package in the future.[50] In any case, two clear results stand out from the efforts of the mid-1970s. First, congressional committees (including Senate Finance) actually marked-up legislation for the first time, suggesting that some version of reform emerged into the realm of the possible. But, second, universal coverage died again—never making it out of committee, never coming to the floor of either chamber.

The Clinton period is the most beguiling of all. In the early 1990s, the problems in the health care system were more pronounced than ever. Health care costs escalated rapidly. For the first time the United States had become an unmistakable outlier, spending far more than any other nation on health care per capita and as a percent of the gross domestic product. In addition, commencing around the mid-1980s, the percentage of people with health insurance coverage started to shrink, reversing decades of broadening employer-based insurance and the enormous coverage gains achieved by Medicare and Medicaid. In another first, the AMA was hardly relevant as a health care power any longer, and to the extent it was involved in the debate, it had even endorsed universal coverage. The interest group politics of health care reform were up for grabs. As I noted earlier, too, Clinton could work with a Congress in which the size of the Democratic majorities and the general unity within them offered an

unusual window of opportunity. The institutional character of the House, at least, afforded coalition-building advantages not found in previous periods. Taken together, by 1993 almost all the participants in health care reform politics and policymaking, even stakeholders who were vehemently opposed to the idea, had concluded that some version of reform would soon be enacted.[51]

Four obvious risks remained, however. President Clinton was pursuing a popular idea—health care reform—but with no particular electoral mandate generated by his feeble plurality win of just 43% in the 1992 presidential election. Both the House and Senate still yielded opportunities for many members to delay or thwart legislative action, if they chose to do so, and significant divisions remained—even among Democrats—about the best way to solve the nation's health care problems. The Republicans in Congress had, in opposition, become just as unified in their ranks as had the Democrats. Finally, all other advanced democracies had enacted and implemented their systems for universal coverage *before* the stakes in the status quo arrangements had grown so enormous for providers of all kinds, private insurers, and employers.[52]

Both during the presidential campaign and once in office, Clinton chose a health care reform strategy of co-optation. The more combative approaches taken by Democrats in the past had led to defeat. Their proposals for publicly-financed programs fed Republican rhetoric about Democrats as the "tax-and-spend" party. Several initially collaborative bipartisan efforts had also come up short, losing the support of both conservatives and liberals.[53] Clinton's approach, reflected in the "managed competition under a budget" rubric of the Health Security Act, was to co-opt the left and right simultaneously, and along the way capture the voters, interest groups, and centrist members of Congress. Liberals would be energized by his commitment to universal coverage, achieved through a combination of employer mandates and an expanded public program that replaced Medicaid for the poor and unemployed; the cost-control discipline ensured by imposing a budget on health care expenditures backed up by insurance premium caps; and the standardization of basic coverage for people regardless of their socio-economic standing. Conservatives would resonate with the "private," market-oriented features of the initiative—the primary use of private insurance carriers, the role of competition among insurance plans to discipline costs, empowering consumers with choices between insurance products, and the movement of Medicaid beneficiaries into private insurance.[54] Other provisions and subsidies would mitigate concerns about the employer mandate's impact on small businesses. With the left and right joined, reasoned the program's architects, health providers, major business groups, insurance carriers, and other moderate stakeholders would all enlist in the coalition.

To avoid the pitfalls of previous bipartisan efforts, however, the *process* toward enacting legislation would follow the pattern Charles Jones describes as "co-partisanship."[55] Clinton and the Democrats would initially craft their version of health care reform, the Republicans would pursue their own. Then—each plan falling somewhere in the general domain of managed competition among private health insurance plans—a final compromise could be struck that was more expensive and regulatory than Republicans favored and launched more slowly, with greater variability in insurance arrangements than Democrats preferred.

That was the projection. In the end, however, Congress was once again the graveyard of reform. Despite full engagement by several House and Senate committees, intense on-going negotiations over alternatives and possible compromises, and even formal debate in the Senate chamber, universal coverage died once again without a single vote being taken on the floor of either the House or Senate. The full story, of course, is nuanced and complicated, the subject of numerous books, including my own.[56]

For our purposes here, let me highlight a few issues of particular relevance to Congress. To start, bicameralism became a major barrier. Because the Senate was more institutionally fragmented and more conservative than the House, the White House and Democratic leaders in Congress expected to pass legislation in the House first. That success would create the impetus needed to leverage favorable action in the Senate. But this strategy was stymied by the political damage of Clinton's budget and economic program, enacted a year earlier in the summer of 1993. That initiative had originally included a tax on energy consumption, calibrated using British thermal units (BTUs), a standard measure of energy. House Democrats—blasted by Republicans for raising taxes—stuck with the president in support of this controversial, strange sounding provision because he twisted arms, scrounged votes, and promised not to drop the BTU tax in the Senate. However, energy producers are more effectively represented in the Senate. To get the Senate's agreement on the economic program Clinton ultimately felt compelled to sacrifice the energy tax (Vice President Al Gore had to cast a tie-breaking final vote on the package). House members, who had taken an unpopular position on a provision that was dropped in the Senate declared they would not be "BTUed" again. They insisted that the Senate move first on health care reform, which had equally controversial elements. Action in the Senate, however, was much harder to achieve—again, it operates under more fragmented rules that permit minorities to block action by, among other things, threatening filibusters. After intense and lengthy efforts, the Senate Finance Committee was not able to report out an acceptable compromise.

Passage of health care reform in either the Senate or the House was stymied by an intense, highly mobilized opposition that brought together most Republicans, including much of their leadership, with the "No-Name Coalition," the new antireform alliance that emerged under the leadership of small business (operating through the NFIB), the private insurance carriers (HIAA), and the pharmaceutical companies (PhRMA). Clinton's method of drafting the Health Security Act, and the Byzantine substantive policy requirements of achieving universal coverage and cost control using disparate private institutions, also gave the opponents of health care reform the ammunition they needed to defeat the proposed legislation.

Because of the complexities involved in designing a fresh health care reform, and the emergence of divisive issues like the budget fight, ratification of the North American Free Trade Agreement (NAFTA, which split organized labor from the Clinton administration), and unexpected foreign policy set-backs, it took much longer to develop the president's initiative than expected. Clinton announced the plan in a major speech to the public from a joint session of Congress in September 1993, but the actual proposal was not available to Congress until the start of 1994. That gave the opposition time to find allies, marshal resources, develop a strategy, and hone a message. The Health Security Act itself, an intricate plan articulated in 1,342 pages of legislative language, provided keys to that message. Clinton's opponents unrelentingly declared the president's plan a "government takeover of health care," a bureaucrat's dream for government intervention into every nook and cranny of one's relationship with doctors, hospitals, and insurers. In short, opponents offered new variations on the trusty old arguments against universal health care. In the meantime, liberal groups, and liberal members of Congress—disgruntled by unrelated issues or unhappy with the compromises in the plan—often refused to sign on.[57]

The co-optation strategy failed on both the left and the right. Mike Lux, the White House liaison to health care groups, wrote in a May 3, 1993, confidential memorandum to Hilary Clinton, who was leading the president's health care reform effort, "I'm beginning to grow a little concerned that in our health care decisionmaking, we may end up with a reform package that excites no one except our opposition—in other words, we could end up with a bill that generates intense opposition from several powerful special interests, but only lukewarm support from the people we've counted on to be our base."[58] In a survey I conducted of health care interest groups ($N = 120$) after the end of the reform debate, the results are exactly as Lux predicted. Among groups that held positions and had resources that made them likely allies of Republican opponents to reform, almost 60 percent actively fought to defeat the Health Security Act. Among

those organized interests that should have been targeted by Democrats and been fully mobilized advocates of reform, only about one quarter endorsed the president's plan. Another quarter favored it but did not formally lend their endorsement. Fully one half of these groups remained neutral. They liked some features of the plan but opposed others, thus preventing them from becoming active members of a coalition favorable to reform. These interest group results, I believe, closely parallel the reactions of both the public and members of Congress.[59]

Had Clinton chosen an alternative legislative strategy, would the outcome have been different? Congress may have been the graveyard, but did the president commit involuntary manslaughter? One answer is that Clinton, pursuing another strategy, could hardly have done worse. Given what appeared to be new reform coalition-building opportunities in Congress in 1993–94, it is striking that more was not accomplished. It is impossible to know whether another approach might have shifted the result all the way from one that never saw floor action in either house of Congress to enactment by both chambers. Two crucial lessons, however, can be gleaned from the recent and past congressional experiences with health care reform. First, even under the best of circumstances (albeit in relative, not absolute, terms), accomplishing major health policy change is hard in the American system. Not surprisingly, in a 2004 survey of the legislative staff in the personal offices of representatives and senators, fully nine out of ten said that it is "very true" or "somewhat true" that "significant policy change (is/was) extremely difficult" in the House and Senate.[60] Second, for those wishing to pursue significant health policy innovation, it is essential both to identify accurately the prevailing characteristics of the overall legislative setting and to match the policy approach and the political strategy supporting it to those contextual parameters. Although there were no floor votes in either the 1970s or 1990s, the legislative machinations had progressed sufficiently far that it is possible that had reform proponents made more astute connections between policy and the politics of the time, significant reforms might have survived the legislative gauntlet.

HEALTH POLITICS AND POLICY IN A PARTISAN CONGRESS

Those concerned about either the distributive tendencies of what I call the baseline Congress or the legislative barriers to major health policy innovation may harbor a longing for Westminster-style parliamentary government. Reform advocates in Canada eventually overcame past failures and finally witnessed the enactment of universal coverage, unlike their US counterparts, precisely because of their parliamentary institutions.[61] Such a constitutional change in the United States—the value of which would be highly debatable on other grounds—is about the least likely political proposition that one could imagine. Is there a more plausible substitute and what would be its consequences?

For many decades political scientists have called for a system of "responsible party government."[62] Each of the political parties would present clear and distinctive policy platforms to the electorate and, following elections, the institutions of government splintered by the constitutional separation of powers would be joined under the umbrella of unified party government (the same party would control the presidency, House, and Senate). Presumably such an arrangement would create enhanced incentives for legislators to focus on national concerns and perspectives, as well as provide additional political "glue" to bind legislative coalitions led by the president. For a long time such a conception of American government also seemed farfetched. After 1954, the government was more frequently divided than unified. Both parties were internally split ideologically, hardly projecting clear and distinctive policy images to the electorate. In the 93rd Congress (1973–74), for example, based on roll-call votes there was considerable overlap between Democrats

and Republicans. Perhaps a third of the House was lodged at the center and could have comfortably resided in either party (in addition, many Democrats were, in fact, conservative, while a number of Republicans voted like liberals).[63]

In the last decade, however, the profile changed. Largely as a result of Republican "conservatives replacing more moderate Republicans outside of the southern states and [Republican] conservatives replacing moderate and conservative Democrats in the South," the congressional parties in both the House and Senate have become both more ideologically coherent within their respective ranks and increasingly separated from one another. The ideological distance between the parties in the legislature is the largest in about a century and the most substantial since the current party system emerged in the midst of the Great Depression in the 1930s.[64] By the 107th Congress (in 2001–02), the "center" had all but disappeared. Fewer than 3% of the House members inhabited the middle, and under 4% were encompassed by the entire ideological range in roll-call voting in which both Republicans and Democrats could be found (in contrast to more than *three quarters* of the House in 1973–74).[65] Throw in unified party government—such as what Republicans have achieved for the most part since the 2000 elections—and the opportunities for effective legislative action would seem to be particularly pronounced.

At first blush, there is some evidence to suggest this result has occurred. The most significant may be in the realm of health care policy: the December 2003 enactment of the Medicare Modernization Act, arguably the most expensive and expansive piece of social policy making since the establishment of Medicare itself also incorporates more conservative, private sector approaches to social policy than any previous law. President Bush and his Republican allies in Congress succeeded with this program, designed almost entirely in their terms over Democratic objections, only because of unified party government, solidarity within Republican ranks, and the capacity of the House Republican leadership to exploit its command of the rules and procedures to reverse a fifteen-vote defeat at the close of the normal fifteen minute voting period (in an unprecedented move, the Speaker held open voting period for nearly three hours to orchestrate some successful arm-twisting).

Experience reveals, however, that highly partisan legislative politics do not sit well within the separation of powers framework. Not only may it fail to surmount the dispersion of policy-making authority in the American system, its interaction with a system based on multiple competing institutions can exacerbate, rather than mitigate, problems in policymaking. On the first point, even with shared party majorities, the "bicameral hurdle" remains, because the House and Senate have "different electoral constituencies (district-based versus statewide), . . . just one-third of the Senate up for re-election every two years, . . . different forces that shape House and Senate election outcomes, . . . [and] the uneven powers afforded House and Senate party leaders."[66] When different parties control the House and Senate in an intense partisan environment, as happened briefly in 2001 and 2002 when Senator James Jeffords left the GOP to become an independent, the incentives against cross-chamber accommodations become even stronger. In addition, the president—still constitutionally separated from the legislature and with divergent perspectives and political needs—cannot command serious legislative attention, much less be successful. Consider the failure of President Bush to gain any legislative leverage on his proposal for partial Social Security privatization.

It is perhaps ironic that in the American institutional setting, ideologically focused parties in Congress can also lead to greater legislative dysfunction rather than less.[67] The distributive impulses of the House and Senate, for example, have not been mitigated. Indeed, in some respects they have grown worse, reflecting the continued self-selection, autonomy, and local orientation of individual legislators, as well as the capacity of favored interest groups to gain unchecked entrée through the majority party.[68] Members of the House now request about 35,000 "earmarked" individual spending requests for their districts, attempts to "secure federal dollars

for pork-barrel projects by covertly attaching them to huge spending bills." In 2005, about 15,000 earmarks were incorporated into enacted legislation, a jump from 4,000 about 10 years ago. The growth in earmarks has complicated efforts to rein in the deficit and reinforces bargaining over legislation based on particularistic log-rolling rather than substantive debate.[69] Of perhaps greater significance, the separation of powers—with the multiple perspectives and constituencies represented by the different branches of government and house of Congress—requires accommodation and compromise for action to be taken.[70] Moderate members of Congress, who have credibility with both parties, may be a necessary ingredient. Sarah Binder has determined empirically that

> [a]s Congress moderates ideologically, stalemate becomes less likely. Although single party control of the branches may help to break deadlock, there are clearly limits to the power of political parties to smooth the way for legislative agreement. Intense polarization seems counter-productive to fostering major policy change . . . [because] parties have an electoral, as well as a policy-based, incentive to distinguish their records and positions, and a less incentive to bargain and compromise.[71]

At the current levels of partisan polarization, such legislative impasses are likely to become even more pronounced if the parties continue to split control of the presidency and Congress (as they did after the 2006 election). Paul Quirk and Sarah Binder, who co-chaired a recent Annenberg Institutions of American Democracy commission on the status of the legislative branch, offer a particularly worrisome assessment:

> With the relative strength of the two parties quite comparable, divided control—especially with a Democratic president and a Republican Congress—is highly likely. In the most recent period of divided control, from 1995 to 2000,

President Bill Clinton and the Republican Congress fought a vicious battle over health care reform, ending in stalemate; allowed the federal government to be shut down for several days in a budget impasse; and spent a full year contesting a doomed effort to remove Clinton from office through impeachment. The next [period] of divided party control . . . could witness even more destructive conflict.[72]

Only time will tell whether heightened polarization will persist and congressional policymaking will remain so problematic under conditions of either unified or divided government. It is incumbent upon students of health politics and policy, however, to recognize the inherent tendencies of a legislature that is both embedded in a separation of powers system and is populated by individual members who play such an independent role in their own selection. Around that "baseline" of congressional behavior one must then assess, for any given period, the effects of changes in party control, size of party majorities, unity within party ranks, and organization of legislative authority and power. Legislative success will often depend on matching the contours of policy proposals to the dynamics of the prevailing congressional context.

STUDY QUESTIONS

1. How does the U.S. Congress stand out among the legislatures of the world? Why?
2. This chapter argues that our system makes legislation much more difficult to pass. Do you believe this an advantage (because it checks government power) or a disadvantage (because voters do not get what they want) in a modern democracy? Why?
3. How did the House of Representatives vary in its degree of centralization over the course of the 20th century (and beyond)?
4. How have scholars attempted to explain congressional reluctance to take on the matter of national health insurance?

5. In what ways did the interest group landscape change during the 1980s and 1990s, and what ramifications did this transformation have on the possibility of enacting health care reform?
6. What are the three main types of strategy employed by presidents in their attempts to shape health care policy in concert with Congress?
7. How did Congress help stymie the health care reform program of the mid-1990s?
8. Why has unified party control of the presidency and Congress, as well as increased intraparty unity, failed to significantly ease the way toward more significant legislative action?

NOTES

1. Cowan and Hartman, 2005, pp. 18, 24; Himmelstein and Woodhandler, 2002, p 92. On the second figure, see James Morone, Introduction.
2. White, 1995.
3. Arnold, 1992.
4. Binder and Quirk, 2005, p xix.
5. Barrett and Edwards, 2000; Peterson, 1990, p 232; Rudalevige, 2002, p 137.
6. Regan, 2005.
7. Peterson, 1990, pp 47–48.
8. Jones, 1994, Chapter 7.
9. Neustadt, 1960, p 42.
10. Lijphart, 1984.
11. The consequences for health care policymaking can be seen in Gauld, 2000, p 815.
12. Immergut, 1992; Adolino and Blake, 2001, pp 679–708.
13. Jacobs, 2005; Adolino and Blake, 2001, pp 679–708; Immergut, 1992; Longstreth et al., 1992.
14. Mayhew, 1974, p 5.
15. Arnold, 1992, pp 5–6; Fenno, 1973, Chapter 1.
16. Novak and O'Neill, 1987.
17. Cox and McCubbins, 1993.
18. Davidson, 1992; Hertzke and Peters, 1992; Jacobs and Shapiro, 2000; Mann and Ornstein,

1981; Rhode, 1991; Sinclair, 1982; Sinclair, 1983; Sinclair, 1989.

19. Malbin et al., 2002, p 173.

20. Peterson, forthcoming.

21. Shickler, 2005; Davidson, 1992; Rhode, 1991.

22. The extent to which interest groups wield influence over Congress remains a complicated and unsettled issue, the subject of an enormous body of literature. A useful overview can be found in Ainsworth, 2002.

23. Alford, 1975; Feldstein, 1977; Starr, 1983; Weissert and Weissert, 1996.

24. Olson, 1965; Walker, 1991.

25. Arnold, 1992, p 75.

26. See, for example, Bosso, 1987.

27. Marmor, 2000, especially ch. 4; Oberlander, 2000, Chapter 16.

28. Peterson, 1998, pp 197–208.

29. Peterson, 1998, pp 214–18.

30. Toner, 2006, pp A1, A17.

31. White, 1995.

32. Gallup Poll, September 2001; Jacobs and Shapiro, 1995.

33. Steinmo and Watts, 1995, pp 329–72.

34. Peterson, forthcoming. My measures include the characteristic and allocation of staff resources, legislative mark-up and hearing activities, the process of selecting committee chairs, and the availability of rules that empower leadership.

35. Davidson, 1992; Deering and Smith, 1984; Hertzke and Peters, 1992; Mann and Ornstein, 1981; Rhode, 1991; Sinclair, 1982; Sinclair, 1983; Sinclair, 1989.

36. Peterson, forthcoming.

37. Peterson, 2001, pp 1145–63.

38. Quadagno, 2005.

39. Campion, 1984; Peterson, forthcoming; Peterson, 1994, 103–47; Poen, 1979.

40. Peterson, 2004.

41. Peterson, forthcoming; Wainess, 1999, p 305–33.

42. Peterson, forthcoming; Skocpol, 1996.

43. Feder, 1993, p A22; Goldfield, 1987; Gottschalk, 2000.

44. Heinz et al., 1993; Peterson, 2001; Peterson, forthcoming; Sammon, 1992, p 1810.

45. Gottschalk, 2000.

46. Broder and Johnson, 1996; Peterson, forthcoming.

47. Jones, 1994.

48. Peterson, 1990.

49. Wainess, 1999.

50. Starr, 1983.

51. Peterson, 1992, pp 553–73; Peterson, 1998.

52. Jacobs, 1995, pp 143–57.

53. Peterson, 1998.

54. Hacker, 1997; Starr, 1994.

55. Jones, 1994.

56. See, for example: Gottschalk, 2000; Hacker, 1997; Jacobs and Shapiro, 2000; Broder and Johnson, 1996; Martin, 2000; Mayes, 2005; Peterson, forthcoming; Quadagno, 2005; Skocpol, 1996.

57. Peterson, forthcoming; Peterson, 1998.

58. Memorandum, 1993, p 1.

59. Brady and Buckley, 1995, pp 447–54; Brodie and Blendon, 1995, pp 403–10; Hacker, 1997; Jacobs and Shapiro, 2000.

60. Annenberg, 2004, question 9a.

61. Maioni, 1994, pp 5–30.

62. Schattschneider, 1942; Committee, 1950.

63. The estimate is based on using the NOMINATE scores developed by Keith T. Poole and Howard Rosenthal and the distribution of House members in the 93rd Congress, with "center" defined as in the range of –0.1 to +0.1 on the NOMINATE liberal–conservative scale (the full scale goes from –1.0 (most liberal) to 1.0 (most conservative).

64. Poole, 2005, p 8; Sundquist, 1973, Chapter 10.

65. The "entire range" is defined as the range on the Poole-Rosenthal NOMINATE liberal–conservative scale that is inclusive of the left-most voting Republican and the right-most voting Democrat.

66. Binder, 2005, p 12.

67. Fiorina, 2006.

68. Binder and Quirk, 2005, p 541. The most extreme example is the scandal surrounding lobbyist and former Republican congressional staffer Jack Abramoff, as well as the general

difficulties confronting Representative Tom DeLay, who was forced to resign from his post as Republican Majority Leader in the House. See Cochran, 2006, p 174; Cochran, 2005, pp 2636–41; Koszczuk and Ota, 2005, pp 2642–7.

69. Flake, 2006, p 27; Hulse, 2006, p 16.
70. See Peterson, forthcoming.
71. Binder, 2005, p 12–13; Binder, 2003.
72. Binder and Quirk, 2005, p 546.

REFERENCES

Adolino, J.R., and C.H. Blake. 2001. "The Enactment of National Health Insurance: A Boolean Analysis of Twenty Advanced Industrial Countries," *Journal of Health Politics, Policy and Law* 26 (August): 679–708.

Ainsworth, S.H. 2002. Analyzing Interest Groups: Group Influence on People and Policies. New York: W.W. Norton.

Alford, R.R. 1975. Health Care Politics: Ideological and Interest Group Barriers to Reform. Chicago: University of Chicago Press.

Annenberg Congress Survey (in the field August 4 to November 22, 2004; *N* = 252). Question 9a; are part of the Annenberg Institutions of American Democracy Surveys.

Arnold, R.D. 1992. *The Logic of Congressional Action.* Yale University Press.

Barrett, A., and G.C. Edwards, III. 2000. "Presidential Agenda Setting in Congress," in J.R. Bond and R. Fleischer, eds., *Polarized Politics: Congress and the President in a Partisan Era.* Washington DC: CQ Press.

Binder, S.A. 2005. "Elections and Congress's Governing Capacity," *extensions: A Journal of the Carl Albert Congressional and Studies Center* (Fall): 12–13.

—— 2003. Stalemate: Causes and Consequences of Legislative Gridlock Washington DC: Brookings Institution Press.

Binder, S.A., and P.J. Quirk. 2005. "Congress and American Democracy: Assessing Institutional Performance," in P.J. Quirk and S.A. Binder, eds., *Institutions of American Democracy: The Legislative Branch.* New York: Oxford University Press, pp 541–6.

—— 2005. "Introduction: Congress and American Democracy: Institutions and Performance," in P.J. Quirk and S.A. Binder, eds., *Institutions of American Democracy: The Legislative Branch.* New York: Oxford University Press, p xix.

Bosso C.J. 1987. *Pesticides and Politics: The Life Cycle of a Public Issue.* Pittsburgh: University of Pittsburgh Press.

Brady, D.W., and K.M. Buckley. 1995. "Health Care Reform in the 103rd Congress: A Predictable Failure," *Journal of Health Politics, Policy and Law* 20 (Summer): 447–54.

Broder, D.S., and Johnson, H. 1996. The System: The American Way of Politics at the Breaking Point. Boston: Little, Brown.

Brodie, M., and Blendon, R.J. 1995. "The Public's Contribution to Congressional Gridlock on Health Care Reform," *Journal of Health Politics, Policy and Law* 20 (Summer): 403–10.

Campion, F.D. 1984. *The A.M.A. and U.S. Health Policy Since 1940.* Chicago: Chicago Review Press.

Cochran, J. 2005. "Debacles, DeLay, and Disarray," CQ Weekly, October 3, pp 2636–41.

—— 2006. "The Influence Implosion," CQ Weekly, January 16, p 174.

Committee on Political Parties. 1950. "Towards a More Responsible Two-Party System." New York: American Political Science Association.

Cowan, C.A., and M.B. Hartman. 2005. "Financing Health Care: Business, Households, and Governments, 1987–2003," *Health Care Financing Review*/Web Exclusive 1 (July): 18, 24.

Cox, G.W., and M.D. McCubbins. 1993. *Legislative Leviathan: Party Government in the House.* Berkeley: University of California Press.

Davidson, R.H., ed. 1992. *The Postreform Congress.* New York: St. Martin's Press.

Deering, C.J., and S.S. Smith. 1984. *Committees in Congress.* Washington DC: CQ Press.

Feder, B.J. 1993. "Medical Group Battles to be Heard Over Others on Health-Care Changes," *New York Times,* June 11, p A22.

Feldstein, P.J. 1977. Health Associations and the Demand for Legislation: The Political Economy of Health. Cambridge: Ballinger Publishing.

Fenno, R.F. Jr. 1973. *Congressmen in Committees.* Boston: Little, Brown, Chapter 1.

Fiorina, M.P. 2006. "Parties as Problem Solvers," in A. Gerber and E. Patashnick, eds., *Promoting the General Welfare: American Democracy and the Political Economy of Government Performance.* Washington DC: The Brookings Institution Press.

Flake, J. 2006. "Earmarked Men," *New York Times,* February 9, p 27.

Gauld, R.D.C. 2000. "Big Bang and the Policy Prescription: Health Care Meets the Market in New Zealand," *Journal of Health Politics, Policy and Law* 25 (October): 815; White, *Competing Solutions.*

Goldfield, M. 1987. *The Decline of Organized Labor in the United States.* Chicago: University of Chicago Press.

Gottschalk, M. 2000. The Shadow Welfare State: Labor, Business, and the Politics of Health Care in the United States. Ithaca: Cornell University Press.

Hacker, J. 1997. The Road to Nowhere: The Genesis of President Clinton's Plan for Health Security. Princeton: Princeton University Press.

Heinz, J.P., E.O. Laumann, R.L. Nelson and R.H. Salisbury. 1993. *The Hollow Core: Private Interests in National Policy Making.* Cambridge: Harvard University Press.

Hertzke, A.D., and R.M. Peters, Jr., eds. 1992. *The Atomistic Congress: An Interpretation of Congressional Change.* New York: M.E. Sharpe.

Himelfarb, R. 1995. Catastrophic Politics: The Rise and Fall of the Medicare Catastrophic Coverage Act of 1988. University Park, PA: Penn State University Press.

Himmelstein, D.U., and S. Woolhandler. 2002. "Paying for National Health Insurance—And Not Getting It," *Health Affairs* 21 (July-August): 92.

Hulse, C. 2006. "Lawmakers Seeking Curbs on Special Spending Requests," *New York Times,* February 7, p 16.

Immergut, E.M. 1992. Health Politics: Interests and Institutions in Western Europe. New York: Cambridge University Press.

Jacobs, L.R. 1995. "The Politics of America's Supply State: Health Reform and Technology," *Health Affairs* 14 (Summer): 143–57.

—— 2005. "Health Disparities in the Land of Equality," in J.A. Morone and L.R. Jacobs, eds., *Health, Wealthy, and Fair: Health Care and the Good Society.* New York: Oxford University Press.

Jacobs, L.R., and R.Y. Shapiro. 1995. "Don't Blame the Public for Failed Health Care Reform," *Journal of Health Politics, Policy and Law* 20 (Summer): 416–7.

—— 2000. Politicians Don't Pander: Political Manipulation and the Loss of Democratic Responsiveness. Chicago: University of Chicago Press.

Jones, C.O. 1994. *The Presidency in a Separated System.* Washington DC: Brookings Institution Press, Chapter 7.

Koszczuk, J., and A.K. Ota. 2005. "The Slow Decline of a GOP 'Godfather,'" CQ Weekly, October 3, pp 2642–7.

Lijphart, A. 1984. Democracies: Patterns of Majoritarian and Consensus Government in Twenty-One Countries. New Haven: Yale University Press.

Longest, Jr., B.B. 2002. *Health Policymaking in the United States,* 3rd ed. Ann Arbor: Health Administration Press.

Longstreth, F., S. Steinmo, K. Thelen, eds. 1992. *Structuring Politics: Historical Institutionalism in Comparative Analysis.* New York: Cambridge University Press.

Mayhew, D.R. 1974. *Congress: The Electoral Connection.* New Haven: Yale University Press, p 5.

Maioni, A. 1994. "Nothing Succeeds Like the Right Kind of Failure: Postwar National Health Initiatives in Canada and the United States," *Journal of Health Politics, Policy and Law* 19 (Winter): 5–30.

Malbin, M.J., T.E. Mann and N.J. Ornstein. 2002. *Vital Statistics on Congress, 2001–2002.* Washington DC: AEI Press, p 173.

Mann, T.E., and N.J. Ornstein, eds. 1981. *The New Congress.* Washington DC: American Enterprise Institute.

Marmor, T.R. 2000. *The Politics of Medicare*, 2nd ed. Aldine Transaction.

Martin, C.J. 2000. Stuck in Neutral: Business and the Politics of Human Capital Investment Policy. Princeton: Princeton University Press.

Mayes, R. 2005. Universal Coverage: The Elusive Quest for National Health Insurance. Ann Arbor: University of Michigan Press.

Memorandum for Hillary Rodham Clinton, from Mike Lux, subject Positioning Ourselves on Health Care, May 3, 1993, Privileged and Confidential, p 1.

Morone, J.A., and L.R. Jacobs. 2005. *Healthy, Wealthy, and Fair: Health Care and the Good Society.* New York: Oxford University Press.

Neustadt, R.E. 1960. *Presidential Power.* New York: John Wiley & Sons, p 42.

Novak, W., and T.P. O'Neill. 1987. Man of the House: The Life and Political Memoirs of Speaker Tip O'Neill. New York: Random House.

Olson, M. 1965. *The Logic of Collective Action*. Cambridge: Harvard University Press.

Peterson, M.A. 1994. "Congress in the 1990s: From Iron Triangles to Policy Networks," in J.A. Morone and G.S. Belkin, eds., *The Politics of Health Care Reform: Lessons from the Past, Prospects for the Future*. Durham: Duke University Press, pp 103–47.

—— 1990. Legislating Together: The White House and Capitol Hill from Eisenhower to Reagan. Cambridge: Harvard University Press, p 232.

—— 1992. "Report from Congress: Momentum Toward Health Care Reform in the U.S. Senate," *Journal of Health Politics, Policy and Law* 17 (Fall): 553–73.

—— (forthcoming). "Stalemate: Opportunity, Gambles, and Miscalculations in Health Policy Innovation."

—— 1998. "The Politics of Health Care Policy: Overreaching in an Age of Polarization," in M. Weir, ed., *The Social Divide: Political Parties and the Future of Activist Government*. Washington DC and New York: Brookings Institution and Russell Sage Foundation.

—— 2001. "From Trust to Political Power: Interest Groups, Public Choice, and Health Care Markets," *Journal of Health Politics, Policy and Law* 26 (October): 1145–63.

—— 2004. "The Politics of Health: The Changing Community of Organized Interests." Paper prepared for delivery at the annual meeting of the American Political Science Association, IL, September 2–5.

—— (forthcoming). "The Three Branches of Government: Checks, Roles, and Performance," in The Annenberg Democracy Group, *Institutions of American Democracy: A Nation Divided* (tentative title). New York: Oxford University Press.

Poen, M.M. 1979. *Harry S. Truman versus the Medical Lobby*. Columbia: University of Missouri Press.

Poole, K.T. 2005. "The Decline and Rise of Party Polarization in Congress During the Twentieth Century," *extensions: A Journal of the Carl Albert Congressional and Studies Center* (Fall): 8.

Quadagno, J. 2005. One Nation Uninsured: Why the U.S. Has No National Health Insurance. New York: Oxford University Press.

Regan, T. 2005. "Blair Loses Key Terror Vote," CSMonitor.Com (*Christian Science Monitor*), posted November 10, at 11:00 a.m., http://www.csmonitor.com/2005/1110/dailyUpdate.html?s=rel.

Rhode, D.W. 1991. *Parties and Leaders in the Postreform House*. Chicago: University of Chicago Press.

Rudalevige, A. 2002. Managing the President's Program: Presidential Leadership and Legislative Policy Formulation. Princeton: Princeton University Press, p 137.

Sammon, R. 1992. "Fall of Striker Bill Spotlights Doubts about Labor Lobby," *Congressional Quarterly Weekly Report*, June 20, p 1810.

Schattschneider, E.E. 1942. *Party Government I*. New York: Farrar and Reinhart.

Shickler, E. 2005. "Institutional Development of Congress," in P.J. Quirk and S.A. Binder, *Institutions of American Democracy: The Legislative Branch*. New York: Oxford University Press.

Skocpol, T. 1996. Boomerang: Clinton's Health Security Effort and the Turn Against Government in U.S. Politics. New York: W. W. Norton.

Sinclair, B. 1982. Legislators, Leaders, and Lawmaking: The U.S. House of Representatives in the Post-Reform Era. Baltimore: Johns Hopkins University Press.

—— 1983. *Majority Leadership in the U.S. House*. Baltimore: Johns Hopkins University Press.

—— 1989. *The Transformation of the U.S. Senate*. Baltimore: Johns Hopkins University Press.

Starr, Paul. 1994. The Logic of Health Care Reform: Why and How the President's Plan Will Work. New York: Whittle.

—— 1983. The Transformation of American Medicine. New York: Basic Books.

Steinmo, S., and J. Watts. 1995. "It's the Institutions, Stupid! Why Comprehensive National Health Insurance Always Fails in America," *Journal of Health Politics, Policy and Law* 20 (Summer): 329–72.

Sundquist, J.L. 1973. Dynamics of the Party System: Alignment and Realignment of Political Parties in the United States. Washington DC: The Brookings Institution, Chapter 10.

Toner, R. 2006. "Rival Visions Led to Rocky Start for Drug Benefit," *New York Times*, February 6, pp A1, A17.

Wainess, F.J. 1999. "The Ways and Means of National Health Care Reform, 1974 and Beyond," *Journal of Health Politics, Policy and Law* 24 (April): 305–33.

Walker, J.L. Jr. 1991. Mobilizing Interest Groups in America: Patrons, Professions, and Social Movements. Ann Arbor: University of Michigan Press.

Weissert, C.S., W.G. Weissert. 1996. *Governing Health: The Politics of Health Policy*. Baltimore: John Hopkins University Press.

White, J. 1995. Competing Solutions: American Health Care Proposals and International Experience. Washington DC: Brookings Institution, pp 5–7.

CHAPTER 5

Presidents

David Blumenthal and James Morone

This chapter examines the president's role in health politics and policy. Presidents are the only nationally elected officials; big health policy changes rarely occur without their active leadership. The authors first examine the institution itself, then review the modern presidents and their health care legacies, and conclude with policy lessons from presidential history.

Presidents energize health care policy—they set the political agenda, propose solutions, and organize programs. Bold health policies almost always require presidential leadership. How do presidents play their role? The answer requires us to ask two completely different kinds of questions.

On the one hand, scholars focus on the organization, rules, roles, powers, and limits that define the presidency itself. Each president operates in a well defined setting and manages an office of some 500 employees (up from three when Franklin Roosevelt took office in 1932). On the other hand, the presidency is uniquely personal. Only 19 men held the post across the entire 20th century. Each brought strengths and weaknesses to the job, each redefined the office. For example, John Kennedy used his charisma to become the first television president; Bill Clinton ran the White House like an invigorating and chaotic Oxford seminar (as we'll see, creative chaos is a familiar Democratic syndrome); and

George W. Bush turned to a corporate business model (a common Republican aspiration).

This chapter explains the dynamics of the presidency by exploring both the institution and the individuals. Understanding where health care fits in the presidency means understanding what was unique about each president—and what they all shared in common. We begin by explaining the essential dynamics of the office, then take a closer look at the health care legacy of each modern president and, finally, conclude with generalizations—policy do's and don'ts—that seem to hold across all modern incumbents.

AMERICAN PARADOX: DEFINING THE PRESIDENCY

"We give the president more work than a man can do," wrote John Steinbeck, "more responsibility than a man should take, and more pressure than a man can bear." Thomas Jefferson (president from 1801 to 1809) called the job "a splendid misery." The crush of people seeking favors made James Garfield (1881–83) "cry out in the agony of my soul"; one dissatisfied pleader shot him—though it was his doctors who eventually killed him when they prodded the wound with unwashed hands. Grover Cleveland (elected in 1884 and again in 1892) described the presidency as "a dreadful, self-inflicted penance for the good of the country." Henry Adams sarcastically suggested that the first 15 presidents—from George Washington to Ulysses Grant—refuted Darwin's theory about evolution through survival of the fittest.[1]

The choir of complaining rings right down to the present and tells us something important about the presidency itself. The office straddles a national paradox: Americans both cheer and fear strong presidents.

The Limited President

On the one hand, Americans are wary of their own leaders. Even Alexander Hamilton—the great proponent of executive power—conceded that Americans find "a vigorous executive . . . inconsistent with the genius of republican government."[2] The Constitution is studded with limits to government power; to clinch the point, the founders announced that all powers that are not explicitly granted to federal officials are "reserved to the states" or "to the people."[3] Henry David Thoreau spoke for many Americans when he wrote, "the government that governs least governs best." President Ronald Reagan began his first inaugural address with a steelier version of the same idea: "Government is not the solution to our problem; government is the problem." Americans fear their own government and, especially, presidential power.[4]

Congress, courts, rival parties, interest groups, economic busts, and foreign crises all check the executive. When Presidents Jimmy Carter and Bill Clinton proposed national health insurance, they were each surprised by the sheer force of the resistance, especially from organized interest groups.

They were not learning anything new. Lord James Bryce visited the United States in 1888 and reported that "In ordinary times, the president may be compared to a senior or managing clerk . . . hampered at every turn by . . . Congress, which may be jealous or indifferent or hostile."[5]

The Powerful President

On the other side lies the powerful American presidency. "Energy in the executive is the leading character in the definition of good government," insisted Alexander Hamilton. At the Constitutional Convention, he had even argued that the president should be elected for life (no one else supported the idea). "A feeble executive," sniffed Hamilton in *The Federalist Papers*, is but another phrase for . . . bad government."[6] The president wears an impressive number of hats (and helmets): he is Commander in Chief (a Constitutional provision), he is responsible for a smooth economy (thanks to the Full Employment Act of 1946), he faces up to national problems, represents America to the world, embodies our cultural values, and occupies a great bully pulpit. The highly regarded presidents were forceful leaders. "Give 'em hell Harry!" shouted Truman's supporters—their man is still best remembered for doing just that.

Crises empower presidents. During the civil war, reported Lord Bryce, the American mouse turned into a lion: "Abraham Lincoln . . . wielded more authority than any Englishman has done since Oliver Cromwell" 200 years earlier.[7] In particular, the president exercises almost unchecked power over foreign crises. Some observers even detect two presidencies—a vigorous international office and a flaccid domestic one. Presidents regularly try to tap their strong side by declaring "war" on major problems—a war on poverty, a war on crime, a war on drugs, a war on inflation, a war on terror. Presidents draw on their powers more easily when they can make the war metaphor—the sense of international crisis—stick.

Still, when Presidents Lyndon Johnson (1963–69) and Richard Nixon (1969–73) pushed the boundaries of presidential power, historian Arthur Schlesinger warned that an "imperial presidency" threatened the republic; legislators forced Nixon to resign, and Congress eagerly promulgated new rules to reign in the powers of the office.[8]

So what do Americans want? A powerful president who shapes the nation's destiny? Or a robust republic that firmly checks its chief executive? American history offers a clear answer: We want both. From the very start, the presidency spanned the great American contradiction and the tension between an energetic executive and a vibrant republic only became stronger as the United States grew more powerful.

Ambiguous Powers

The presidential paradox is increased by the puzzling way the Constitution defines the office. The Constitution's *Article I* gives Congress a detailed and specific charge. In contrast, *Article II*, on the presidency, is short and dominated by an enigmatic phrase—"the executive power shall be vested in a President." What precisely is that executive power? The founders did not say. The presidency had to be defined—and still has to be defined—in actual practice. Even very basic questions have been hammered out in the political hurly burly. For example, may a president fire members of his cabinet? Andrew Jackson set off a firestorm when he first tried it (in 1833); Congress impeached Andrew Johnson for removing his Secretary of War (in 1868); but by the 20th century firing cabinet secretaries fell perfectly within a president's authority.

Each president remakes his role and bargains over the limits of his powers. Great presidents don't simply solve problems, sign laws, and launch programs. They redefine the office itself. In contrast, other presidents seem overwhelmed by events, "managing clerks" who fail to meet national problems. Jimmy Carter told Americans, in July 1979, that a crisis of confidence "at the very heart, soul and spirit of our national will . . . is threatening to destroy . . . America." Many Americans thought the crisis lay in the Oval Office. A mischievous typesetter at the *Boston*

Globe captured the national mood with a mock headline that slipped into the first edition: "More mush from the wimp."

The Individual and the Context

What makes some presidents strong and others weak? The answers fall into two categories. Some analysts focus on the individual, others on the context.

Popular writers highlight the presidents themselves. They emphasize the genius of a Franklin Roosevelt (1933–45) or a Ronald Reagan (1981–89). Both Roosevelt and Reagan adroitly worked the machinery of Washington politics. Both skillfully used the media to go directly to the people. Each articulated a new vision of politics. "These dark days will be worth all they cost us," promised Roosevelt in the trough of the Great Depression, "if they teach us that our true destiny is . . . to minister to . . . our fellow man." Ronald Reagan invoked Franklin Roosevelt even as he called the United States away from a collective ideal and back to a kind of rugged individualism. It's easy to imagine that presidential greatness lies in the vision of such men and their administrations. Outstanding individuals succeed where weaker and less skillful men fail.[9]

On the other hand, the president operates in a tangle of constraints. Different men confront problems with more or less political capital. How big was the president's electoral victory? Members of Congress tread far more deferentially if the president got more votes in their district than they did. Does the president's party control Congress? How big is the majority? Is the party united? Fractious? What is the economic situation? The international situation? The mood of the country? The strength of the opposition?

Political scientists often analyze the president's constraints through the lens of "political time"—the cycles of a party's waxing and waning influence. For example, Franklin Roosevelt rode a formidable political wave into power surrounded by energetic, like-minded men and women, and enjoyed large majorities in Congress. Political scientists, following Stephen Skowronek, say the Democrats built a new *political regime* in the 1930s. Over time regimes wear out. The excitement wanes as fresh ideas fade into old saws; coalition members begin to clash; new problems pose fresh challenges. By the time Jimmy Carter comes along, more than 40 years later, the New Deal order was springing apart at the seams. Following Carter, Ronald Reagan constructed an entirely new majority coalition drawing on new regions (the Sunbelt), new groups (the Christian right), and new ideas (less government, lower taxes). Never mind the talents of the individual, say many political scientists. There is a more important question about presidential power: Where does the president stand in the great cycle of regime evolution? Is his coalition fresh and vigorous? Or is it tired and falling apart?[10]

Analyzing the presidency always means striking the right balance. A talented president can wield great power but the political context empowers and constrains every administration. The policy analyst's job is to sort out the individual and the context, to appreciate each president's talent while locating him (and, someday, her) in political time.

THE THREE FACES OF THE PRESIDENCY

Scholars have explored every aspect of the presidency—personality, elections, rhetoric, regimes, and even presidential doodles. Health care introduces a unique set of pressures and demands. Three dimensions are especially important for understanding how presidents negotiate health politics and policy: the president as an individual, as a political operator, and as a manager of the policy process.

The Individual

Presidential studies begin with biography. Presidential personalities invariably stamp the times. The president is the only nationally elected official, the only politician who answers to all Americans. That

gives the presidents their first and, in some ways, their most formidable power: putting ideas before the nation.

Presidents pick our problems and suggest solutions. When the president identifies a problem it immediately zooms to the top of the political charts. For example, in early 1977 political scientist John Kingdon interviewed members of Congress and reported that only 18% mentioned controlling hospital costs as a priority. Later that year, President Carter introduced a hospital cost containment plan. Kingdon returned to Congress and found the members buzzing about the issue (81% brought it up). Jimmy Carter had taken hospital cost control from the pile of health care problems and placed it at the top of the political agenda.[11]

To take another famous example, in 1985, less than 1% of Americans tagged illegal drugs as "the number one problem facing the nation today." In September 1986, President and Mrs. Reagan delivered an impassioned joint address from the White House in which they declared their war on drugs. "For the sake of our children," said the First Lady, "I implore each of you to be unyielding and inflexible in your opposition to drugs." The number of Americans who identified drugs as America's number one problem quickly leapt to 54%.[12]

Of course, illegal drugs and hospital costs were both real problems, but there were plenty of other health care issues the presidents might have emphasized. Senator Ted Kennedy (D-MA) illustrated the point by blasting Carter for focusing on hospital cost containment rather than universal health insurance.

The president can only pick a few items for national attention. If he chooses too many, they will elbow each other on the airwaves and crowd out one another on the Congressional docket. Every president faces the same question: What does he care about most? Of all the issues and problems that face the nation, which two or three or four is he going to pluck out and emphasize?

There are many reasons to propose a major program—campaign promises, interest group pressure, political rivals, popular opinion, a dangerous crisis. But beneath all the political push and shove lies the ultimate question: What does the president really care about? How do they want to define their legacy? This becomes especially important for health care policy where the big issues—controlling costs, extending coverage—always raise fierce political resistance and can be numbingly complicated.

Even so, every modern president has proposed a major expansion of health care coverage. Why? For two reasons: First, some presidents care about health care. As usual, Lyndon Johnson (1963–69) put it with the most flair when he promised to fund any Medicare bill that Congress passed.

I'll go a hundred million or a billion on health or education. I don't argue about that any more than I argue with [my wife] Lady Bird about buying flour. You got to have to have flour and coffee in your house and [you got to have] education and health. I'll spend the goddamn money. I may cut back some tanks. But not on health. That's the go sign I gave them.[13]

Second, political pressures push presidents into health care. True believers come to office with a full-throated call for ambitious reform (Harry Truman, Lyndon Johnson, Bill Clinton). Others resist or agonize, Hamlet-like, for years and then squeeze out a plan (Jimmy Carter, George H.W. Bush). Health care is always difficult but plans patched together under political pressure rarely get very far.

In many policy areas, we measure the presidents by the programs they pass. In health, there is also a more subtle metric. Every president shapes the national conversation, each reframes both problems and solutions. We can ask the same question of every administration: How did they change the way Americans think and talk about health policy? What legacy did they leave?

The Political President

Great ideas may change the world, but every administration faces a more basic test: How skillfully does it operate the political machinery? Can it run the government smoothly? Meet its goals? Get things done?

The first seven modern presidents entered the White House with experience—in some cases, a lifetime of experience—in the federal service. Then, in 1976, Jimmy Carter ran for the White House with none at all. His outsider's stance fit the national mood after Watergate as well as the more enduring American distrust of government. Following Jimmy Carter's surprise election, only one president (out of four) came to power with any national government experience on his resume.

Running as an outsider—denouncing Washington business as usual and promising a fresh approach—is an effective campaign strategy. But no administration can govern from the outside. Presidents do not accomplish anything until they learn to master the political system and that means managing both Congress and the public.

Congress

As President Lyndon Johnson once put it, "there is only one way to deal with Congress and that is continuously, incessantly and without interruption."[14] Johnson himself had been the Senate majority leader and he knew the Congressional folkways better than any man alive. He tracked each of his bills through the legislative process—advising, cajoling, and arm-twisting the members of Congress. For example, when the House Ways and Means Committee voted in favor of Medicare (after blocking the legislation for years), Democratic House leaders triumphantly telephoned the President to report the good news. LBJ immediately looked ahead to the next political hurdle—insuring that the Rules Committee quickly sent the bill to the floor for a vote before opposition could develop. Johnson put it memorably:

Now remember this. Nine out of ten things I get in trouble on is because they [the bills] lay around . . . . It stinks. It's just like a dead cat on the door . . . For god sakes, don't let dead cats stand on your porch . . . . Mr. Rayburn [the legendary Speaker of the

House of Representatives] used to say: "they
stunk and they stunk and they stunk." When
you get one out of your committee, you call
that son of a bitch up before they can get
their letters written.[15]

Speed is crucial. Every day in office, said Johnson
on another occasion, "I lose part of my power. Every
day . . . I have less power left." In a landmark study,
Paul Light discovered how right Johnson had been.
Legislation submitted in the first three months of a
presidency succeeded 73% of the time; legislation
submitted just six months later (between July and
September) had a 25% success rate. The Congressional docket gets crowded, the president begins to
use up his political capital, and politicians all start
positioning themselves for the next election. By the
end of the president's first year, Washington is
already focused on the midterm election the following November. The key message for presidents who
want to reform the health care system could be
delivered the day after the election: hurry up, you're
almost out of time.[16]

Other presidents discover the same political rules
the hard way. President Jimmy Carter (1977–81) violated LBJ's dictum about continuously working
with Congress. Carter infuriated members when he
refused small courtesies like extra tickets to the inauguration (no special favors, he said); he ambushed
Congress by cutting local projects from the budget
(Washington needed to learn fiscal discipline, he insisted.). Carter might have been correct, but that did
not help his cause on Capitol Hill. "You don't have
to be a legislative genius to figure out that Pennsylvania Avenue is a two way street," complained powerful House Speaker Tip O'Neil (D-MA). Carter soon
learned, as he put it in his autobiography, that "each
legislator had to be wooed and won individually."
Carter slowly cast off his outsider's stance, learned
how to work the Washington process, and began to
enjoy more success with his proposals.

Another outsider, Bill Clinton (1993–2001),
staked his party's political fate on an ambitious
health care plan that violated the rule of speed. He
failed to submit the legislation till the last day of

the 1993 Congressional session. By the time the
legislature got to the measure, in early 1994, all
political eyes were on the midterm election later
that year. The Republicans outmaneuvered Clinton,
killed the bill, and rode the backlash to a huge
election victory.

Going to the People

Presidents often try to nudge Congress by speaking directly to the people. Going public involves an entirely
different set of skills from the insider game of maneuvering Congress. President Franklin Roosevelt was a
master of the radio and John F. Kennedy—young,
handsome, and charismatic—became America's first
television president. Today, media operations are a
major White House function and presidents who fail
to invest in them, such as George H.W. Bush, pay a
high political price. Campaigning for an issue involves
constant polling to find the best way to cast the message; big media "roll outs" involve speeches, talk
shows, newspapers, blogs, and coordinating allies
and interest groups.[17]

Going public is an alluring strategy for the only
politician elected by the entire nation. Congress cannot ignore an avalanche of phone calls and emails.
However, rousing the nation to prod Congress is a
tricky business. Opponents often undermine the
president's program by dragging out the process
and riding out the surge of public opinion. Even
savvy media campaigns wear thin. Time takes it toll
on every president's agenda.

Some presidents take an issue public simply to
get it on the agenda, to get the nation talking. For example, when President Harry Truman proposed national health insurance in 1946, Congress flatly
turned him down. Truman unexpectedly won reelection in 1948 by thumping national health insurance
and tarring the "do nothing" Congress. No matter.
Congress turned him down again. Undaunted, Truman tirelessly championed his lost cause and, by
doing so, helped turn national health insurance into
an essential liberal reform. When Lyndon Johnson
won Medicare in 1965 he flew to Independence,
Missouri and signed the bill sitting along side an
aging Harry Truman—a rare homage to the man

who had put expanding public health insurance on the national agenda.

The President as Policy Manager

The presidents are the policy makers in chief. They manage a great federal bureaucracy tasked with running the nations programs. They frame new policies to take to Congress or the put before the people.

The Executive Branch

The president's own branch—1.8 million workers strong—is both a source of power and a management problem. The president coordinates three centers of power: his own White House staff; the Executive Office of the President (EOP), which includes agencies directly under presidential control like the Office of Management and Budget and the Council of Economic Advisors; and the vast federal bureaucracy headed by the president's cabinet members. Each administration recalibrates the balance of power. Every incumbent tinkers with executive branch organization—another illustration of the American presidency as a constant work in progress.

Over time, power has gradually slipped from the cabinet agencies and toward the president's advisors—turning the executive branch ever more political. Early presidents simply relied on their cabinets to develop policy and submit it directly to Congress. President Franklin Roosevelt changed all that. Facing the Great Depression, he made his first term a whirlwind of proposals and programs. Roosevelt seemed positively exuberant about his overlapping advisors, committees, and programs—he called it all his "three ring circus." President Roosevelt left Democrats a seductive but dangerous model—the freewheeling administration long on creativity and short on discipline. Democrats have often emulated the free form Roosevelt style with advisors playing multiple and loosely defined roles. Republicans generally prefer tightly organized and carefully specified administrative lines.

Roosevelt himself learned the limits of administrative free-for-all. In 1938, he asked a distinguished committee of public management specialists to impose order. Many Democrats would travel the same route from a free wheeling staff to a tighter, more carefully managed organization.

On the Republican side, President Eisenhower (1953–61) set a modern standard. He ran his White House like the military and treated cabinet officials as his general staff. President Richard Nixon entered office (in 1969) and worried that after 35 years of Democratic dominance the bureaucracy reflected Democratic attitudes. In response, President Nixon centralized power in his own office. The Nixon administration put over 600 people on the White House staff and almost 5,000 in the EOP. Seven years later, President Reagan (1981–89) took a different tack, placed trusted allies in key positions through out the bureaucracy, then shifted power and control back to the cabinet. Reagan reduced the size and scope of the EOP by more than half (to just under 2,000 which is roughly where it remains today).[18]

The growing power and sophistication of the White House bureaucracy is a double-edged sword. In an earlier era, President Johnson could negotiate Medicare with down-home metaphors about flour and coffee. Today, a hive of EOP economists and policy specialists would be buzzing cautions in Johnson's ear. The director of the Office of Management and Budget warns of budget deficits, the head of the Council of Economic Advisors weighs in with macroeconomic cautions, and the US Trade Representative might be on hand to spell out the implications on international markets. And that's all before the pollsters and the communication directors barge into the president's office.

Over time, the president's office has grown more technical, more sophisticated, more powerful, and more overtly political. Every president must learn how to manage his own office, decide how much to delegate to the cabinet agencies, and then find a way to coordinate the entire enterprise. Every administration faces the same structural dilemma: A very small group of men and women in the oval office must find a way to control the great executive leviathan.

Finally, the executive branch is also a source of policy and power. Congressional deliberations generate publicity and debate. In contrast, administrative decisions are generally silent, almost stealthy. They often slip through with no publicity. Yet, even small technical changes can have very large impacts on health policy and health care delivery.

Framing Policies

Of course, ideas have to be hammered into policies before they can be taken to Congress or promulgated by executive agencies. Presidents generally delegate this job. They champion the big idea, carry them through the political system, and leave the program details to others.

Whom? The president is surrounded by institutions designed to hammer out policies. He can charge a cabinet agency, task his advisors, name an informal committee, or announce a formal commission. Naturally, each method has its own strength and weakness. But all presidents must negotiate twin perils as they translate general ideas into concrete policies.

First, some presidents get too deeply enmeshed in policy detail. Successful presidents almost all leave the fine print to subordinates. Franklin Roosevelt, Lyndon Johnson, and Ronald Reagan laid out the guiding philosophy. They did not delve into the minutiae of the programs they championed. On the other hand, President Carter famously dove into the details of almost every policy. Such deep involvement distracts presidents from tasks that only they can perform—like persuading Congress and the nation to buy into the policies.

A second problem comes at the other extreme. A president who is not engaged (or wise) enough to broker the policy battles within his administration. The president is surrounded by agencies with their own turf to protect, advisors with their own axes to grind, and supporters with their own interests to promote. Ultimately, a successful president learns to draw on a range of policy advisors without becoming captive to any one.

Finally, careful policy design often clashes with the imperatives of time and diminishing presidential

capital. As a result, successful presidents often enter the White House with major policy proposals in hand. This, in turn, puts a premium on the issue network—the informal group of thinkers, advisors, and policy entrepreneurs that surrounds candidates and parties. If the president's influence wanes a little every day, administrations benefit from coming to power with their plans all ready to go.

INDIVIDUAL PRESIDENTS

Health is a personal issue that reflects the men inside the office. Presidents suffer heart attacks, live with painful conditions, and lose people they love. They deal with (or duck) health issues as governors, legislators, or county commissioners long before ascending to the Oval Office. Moreover, the archives are full of moving letters from people who got tangled in the medical system and write to the president—in hope or sadness or anger. Health care troubles surround every president.

However, expanding health care coverage or controlling its costs is a tough job that tests the political mettle of even the best leaders. Some presidents make it a signature issue. Others approach the topic reluctantly—prodded by allies or nervous about a looming election.

Regardless of how they come to the issue, health reform draws on every aspect of the presidency—the personal, the political, and the policy maker. Watching the presidents take on health care offers a window on the presidency itself. And it helps explain the great arc of American health care policy by showing us how each president reshaped our programs, our institutions, our aspirations, and the ways we think about health policy.

Franklin D. Roosevelt (1933–45)

President Roosevelt came to office under extraordinary circumstances. The nation was in the pit of the great depression and almost a quarter of the work force was unemployed. More important, the men who had led America through the roaring 20s were, as one historian puts it, "exposed as nincompoops." "They know only the rules of a generation of self-seekers," charged President Roosevelt who promised to restore social values that were "more noble than mere monetary profit."[19]

Roosevelt introduced a whirlwind of programs, agencies, and chaos. His health care policy reflected the tumult. The president tapped experts and advisors for health care committees who studied the issue, devised plans, and engaged opponents. Three different rounds (1934–35, 1938–39, and 1945) produced at least the rough outline of three health care proposals. An enigmatic President Roosevelt stirred the pot, encouraged the advocates, avoided committing himself, and—in the end—always put the health care battle off for another day.

The first round began in 1934 when Roosevelt charged the Committee on Economic Security with drafting Social Security. The Committee crafted an extraordinary program that included old age pensions (what we now call Social Security), unemployment compensation, maternal benefits, and Aid to Families with Children (later dubbed welfare). It debated including health care but when physicians rebelled, Roosevelt organized a subcommittee of physicians, and put the question about including health insurance to them. The subcommittee could not agree and Roosevelt quickly backed off.

When the administration unveiled its Social Security package, in January 1935, it included only a wan promise to "study" the issue of health insurance. However, as one official put it, "that little line was responsible for so many letters to Congress that the entire Social Security bill seemed endangered." The administration dropped even the usually harmless call for further study.[20]

In October 1936, Roosevelt seemed to put the entire issue to rest by offering the profession precisely what it wanted to hear: Doctors and nurses . . . "can rest assured that the Federal Administration contemplates action only in their interest . . . . Attempts have been made in the past to put medicine into politics.

Such attempts have failed and always will fail." That should have been that. The former president of the American Medical Association (AMA) responded with an effusive thank you letter.[21]

Except the armies refused to leave the field. Eight months later, in June 1937, Democratic Senator James "Ham" Lewis (a celebrated orator known as "pink whiskers") chilled the annual meeting of the AMA by warning them that if they failed "to help the helpless" the government would "take charge of medicine and turn it into a federal institution." To spice up his address, Lewis announced that his remarks had the "direct authority" of the president (much to the surprise of the White House). *Time Magazine* covered the speech with a cover story in June 1937 titled, "Nationalized Doctors?" The battle was on again.[22]

Roosevelt's second health care round emerged that fall. The Social Security program itself now offered an institutional home for planning expansions of social programs. Health reformers gathered on a subcommittee—the name itself radiates bureaucracy—the *Technical Committee on Medical Care* established under the *Interdepartmental Committee to Coordinate Health and Welfare Activities* for the *Social Security Board*. The committee drafted a health care proposal by early 1938.

Roosevelt kept the issue simmering. He published the Committee's findings about American health—their five principles would form the backbone of American health proposals for the next decade. On the one hand, Roosevelt encouraged the reformers to hold a conference in which they could refine their proposals. On the other hand, the president—always at arms length from health reform—regretted that he could not attend as he was on a cruise. The conference fired up health reformers. Josephine Roche, Assistant Secretary of the Treasury and chair of the committee that had sponsored the conference captured the excitement when she cabled the president:

CANNOT RESIST SENDING YOU WORD AMAZING PUBLIC SUPPORT AT NATIONAL HEALTH CONFERENCE FOR

NATIONAL HEALTH PROGRAM AND WHICH IS MOUNTING DAILY . . . OUR TECHINICIANS ARE WORKING WITH ALL SPEED TO DEVELOP SPECIFIC PROPOSALS.

The reformers follow up with a detailed memo about both their health insurance plan and the politics of taking on the AMA. The AMA, in turn, called an emergency meeting of its House of Delegates and, while opposing compulsory health insurance, made some tactical concessions by supporting some aid to indigent people and the use of private health insurance.[23]

Roosevelt pondered the advantages of making health care an issue in the 1938 midterm election campaign. Again, he backed off. When he passed on the Committee's health report to Congress in January 1939, he mildly recommended it "for careful study by the Congress." Senator Robert Wagner (D-NY) sponsored the bill but without White House support it had no chance.[24]

For the second time, FDR had encouraged his advisors to study a national health care program. After committees, studies, a conference, and a formal report, Roosevelt decided not to press the issue. He remained aloof as the health insurance debate continued to sweep up partisans and passions on both sides.

There would be still another round for health reform. Beginning with his 1943 State of the Union Message, Roosevelt began calling for social insurance "from the cradle to the grave." The following year, the president began touting "an economic bill of rights" that prominently included "the right to adequate medical care and the opportunity to achieve and enjoy good health."

Still Roosevelt kept spinning a mixed message. In 1943, he told a Senate committee chair, "We can't go up against the state medical societies. We just can't do it." A year later, Roosevelt organized yet another committee, led by trusted advisor Samuel Rosenman to consider national health insurance. One member of the committee later told a reporter, that after being elected to his fourth term, Roosevelt was "clearly

looking forward to doing battle with those [AMA] fellows from Chicago."[25]

Was he? Was national health insurance going to be FDR's great post-war campaign? Or was this just another round in which the master politician prepared multiple political possibilities before choosing which to pursue? Certainly the setting had changed. His advisors were more unified. The English had impressed Roosevelt with their own national health care proposal, the Beveridge report (described in Chapter 20). But we'll never know. FDR died just before the war ended.

The Roosevelt administration illustrates the presidency as health care policy maker. The executive offices buzzed with overlapping committees and new health plans. The president formed the committees but never pursued the plans they developed. The New Deal's policy apparatus spawned an ideal and a plan. They would be Roosevelt's greatest health care legacy. The man himself would take audacious risks on a multitude of programs, both foreign and domestic. But health care was never one of them.

Harry Truman (1945–53)

Harry Truman is the Democrat's patron saint of national health insurance. Truman's status as the icon of the lost reform shines a light on what Americans admire in a president—he did not design national health insurance or come close to winning it, but no one ever fought more passionately for a reform than Truman did for health care.

This was the personal presidency in its purest form. Truman felt health care in his bones. Why? When an interviewer put the question to him, Truman pointed to his first political triumph as a county judge (or commissioner) in Missouri. An old army buddy induced the Prendergast political machine to run Harry for the post. Rather than simply dole out special favors like other machine politicians, Judge Truman raised the money (through a bond issue) for a hospital. "There were derelicts who had lost all they had, and they didn't have any ambition," explained Truman later. "We took good care of them. And then there were those who were just making a living. . . . If sickness overtook these families they were sunk. I've seen people turned away from the big hospitals in town to die, just because they did not have the money to get in. I built a hospital to take care of these people." The experience gave Truman a special affinity for health care reform.[26]

President Truman inherited national health insurance when the Rosenman committee delivered the plan they had been preparing for Roosevelt. Three months after the war ended (in November 1945), President Truman issued a special message to the Congress recommending a comprehensive health program: The five features of the plan—hospital construction, maternal and child care, medical research, health insurance, and disability insurance—revised the five planks that had had emerged from Roosevelt's 1938 conference; to enact the plan, the same senator (Robert Wagner, D-NY) co-sponsored the same bill he had introduced before (in 1943). The ideas, the Congressional sponsors, and the proposed legislation were all familiar. This time, however, the package came with the ardent support of the president.[27]

The national physicians committee responded with a dramatic emergency bulletin: "This is the beginning of the final showdown on the collectivist issue. Not one day dare be lost."[28] For all the operatic drama they injected into the issue, the AMA did not matter. Congress had no intention of passing the legislation.

Senate hearings on the national health insurance bill began on April 2nd, 1946. Senator Murray, the committee chair, asked that out of respect for the president, the legislation not be described as socialistic or communistic. Robert Taft (the ranking Republican from Ohio) interrupted. "I consider it socialism. It is to my mind, the most socialistic measure this Congress has ever had before it." He then led the Republicans out of the room. The Committee in the House of Representatives went further. The chair flatly refused to schedule hearings at all.[29]

The health debate offered an early contest between the two great arguments of the post-war debate. Truman and the Democrats argued that a rich, powerful, modern society should guarantee security for all its citizens; they would extend the New Deal welfare state to include health insurance. Compulsory health insurance, retorted Republicans and conservative Southern Democrats, was a strand of socialism. The Republicans framed their health care arguments within a larger attack: Democrats subverted America's strength before the communist danger.

In the 1946 midterm election, six months after defeating health insurance, the Republicans retook Congress after 16 years in the New Deal wilderness (picking up 13 seats in the Senate and 55 in the House). Truman did not back off. In his 1947 state of the union message, he bravely made civil rights his first priority and national health insurance his second. In 1948, he ran for reelection by attacking the "do nothing" Republican Congress for blocking health care. To everyone's surprise, Truman won reelection and the Democrats regained their congressional majorities.

National health insurance was back in play but it did not get much further on Truman's second try. "There was nothing unusual about a President being rebuffed by Congress," wrote historian David McCullough. "What was novel was a President who, when repeatedly rebuffed, refused to change his tactics."[30]

Once again Truman delivered his health care message. Once again, allies and enemies mobilized. Once again Congress defeated the plan. After this defeat, some officials began to reduce universal health insurance to health insurance for the elderly—an idea that would finally bear legislative fruit more than 15 years later.

Harry Truman remained a feisty, dogged supporter of his favorite reform. He constantly tried to set people straight on the matter. When one of his old Missouri constituents wrote a cheerful letter in April 1949, Harry cut him no slack for opposing "socialized medicine."

The main difficulty is that you start off with the wrong premise. Nobody is working for socialized medicine—all my health program calls for is an insurance plan that will enable people to receive the hospital treatment when they need it.

I can't understand the rabid approach of the American Medical Association—they have distorted and misrepresented the whole program so that it will be necessary for me to go out and tell the people just exactly what we are asking for.

I am trying to fix it so the people in the middle income bracket can live as long as the very rich and very poor.

He was no kinder to a Democratic Congressman from West Virginia who forwarded him a constituent letter about lazy free loaders: "I fear some of our Senators and Representatives . . . are still living in 1890. Perhaps like Rip Van Winkle they will come out of their slumber and find how the world has progressed."

Even after he left office, Truman wrote letter after letter chasing what now seemed a political chimera. "I had some bitter disappointments as President," admitted Truman, "but the one that has troubled me most in a personal way has been the failure to the defeat the organized opposition to the national health insurance program."

Long after the architects of the policy are forgotten, we still celebrate its political champion. Truman took the idea of national health insurance and supported it—ardently, vigorously, to the last. In doing so, he inspired reformers through the generations.

Truman illustrates how a presidential passion can echo through the years. When Lyndon Johnson and the Democrats finally won Medicare, President Johnson flew out to Independence, Missouri and signed the legislation sitting next to a delighted Harry Truman.

Dwight Eisenhower (1953–61)

After two decades of Democratic fireworks, this modest Republican lowered the political heat in the oval office. He suggested that power should be nudged back from president to Congress. He declined to propose a legislative program in his first year. One correspondent summed up the Washington view: "The

memory of Franklin Roosevelt's voracious seizure and joyous exercise of presidential power 20 years earlier contributes to a companion illusion of a man who slipped in the White House by the back door and still hasn't yet found his way to the presidential desk.[31]

However, Eisenhower fooled people. He had skillfully led the international coalition of allies through World War II. Now he governed with what one political scientist called "a hidden hand."[32] Right from the start, Eisenhower organized the White House along crisp lines of authority marked by orderly decisions taken in direct consultation with cabinet members. His administration originated the chief of staff to oversee the president's office, introduced a formal legislative liaison to Congress, and created the department of Health Education and Welfare (HEW).

The Eisenhower administration never challenged the New Deal programs or its premises. On the contrary, as historian Oscar Handlin observed at the time, Eisenhower made "the social welfare legislation of the past two decades . . . palatable to most Republicans."[33] Eisenhower tried to turn future social policy in a Republican direction by emphasizing private markets, smaller government, and restoring authority to the states.

Eisenhower had a secret affinity for health care programs, but his commitment was expressed within the narrow constraints of a firmly held and enduring belief that the federal power was a threat to the nation. His interest in health care contended throughout his presidency with his conservative principles. At times, the desire to move a health issue forward prevailed. In 1954, Oveta Culp Hobby, the first Secretary of HEW, proposed a health plan. The Bureau of the Budget resisted, not simply because of the expense but for "philosophical reasons"—opposing government in health care. Eisenhower thanked the budget director for making such a clear case, then sided with Hobby.

However, when he submitted the plan to Congress in January 1954, he emphasized the prospect of strengthening the private sector. He broke with Truman's national health insurance by pointing to the great change in American health care: "During the past decade, private and non-profit health insurance organizations have made striking progress"—in fact, the numbers of workers covered by negotiated health insurance plans had shot up from 1 to 12 million (along with 20 million dependents). The administration's plan would bolster this trend by subsidizing (or reinsuring) private health insurers who could then offer lower premiums to families.[34]

Democratic Senator James Murray pounced: "a paltry, puny, picayune proposal."[35] The AMA also opposed the bill, despite energetic efforts by the White House to turn the doctors around. The Senate rejected the Eisenhower administration's bill by a single vote. "Just plain stupid," seethed the president about the AMA, "a little group of reactionary men dead set against change."[36]

Eisenhower turned back to health care in the waning months of his administration when electoral politics thrust the issue forward. Senator John Kennedy (D-MA), already running for president, introduced a plan providing health insurance to the elderly through Social Security (and sponsored in the House by representative Clinton Anderson [D-NM]). Vice President Richard Nixon, running for president on the Republican side, needed an answer to Kennedy. Eisenhower is often characterized as reluctant—even uncaring—about health care. This was not the case. Then secretary of HEW, Arthur Fleming, recounts how Eisenhower was moved by the issue—and lived it first hand during the serious illness of his mother-in-law, who lived with him in the White House. However, his feelings about health care clashed with his conservative principles and stymied a decisive response to the need.

Eventually, Fleming and Nixon persuaded Eisenhower to introduce a Republican answer to the Kennedy-Anderson bill, *A Medicare Program for the Aged*. The program, financed by federal and state governments, would pay lower income elders so they could buy private health insurance. A program with so many moving parts—federal government, state government, private insurance companies—might cost more, admitted Eisenhower. But "I am

against compulsory medicine and that is exactly what I am against, and I don't care if that does cost the treasury a little bit more money . . . the price of freedom is not always measured just in dollars."[37]

To complicate matters, Senator Robert Kerr (D-OK), introduced a bill that offered federal grants to states for health care to the aged poor. Southern hospitals were still racially segregated and by funneling the money through state welfare programs rather than through federal Social Security (like Kennedy's bill) Kerr's plan did not threaten Jim Crow. Another Southern representative, Wilbur Mills (D-AK), proposed a similar bill in the House.

Just months before election day, the two presidential candidates—Senator John Kennedy and Vice President Richard Nixon (the vice president presides over the Senate) dueled on the Senate floor. First, the liberal Kennedy-Anderson bill came up. With Southern Democrats opposed and Nixon frenetically twisting arms, the bill failed, 51–44. The administration plan did even worse, falling 67–28. The Senate then agreed to Senator Kerr's middle ground, by a whopping margin, 91–2. The Kerr-Mills bill produced a modest program for elders.

The congressional debate offers a scorecard for the health care landscape in 1960:

- John Kennedy and the northern liberals had a campaign issue—universal health care coverage for people over 65 funded by Social Security. This was a reduced version of Truman's national health insurance.

- Kerr and Mills staked out a position for conservative Democrats: federally funded, state sponsored programs for indigent elders. Their bill looked more like welfare, controlled by the states, than Kennedy's Social Security bill that was financed and run by Washington.[38]

- The Eisenhower administration introduced a moderate Republican position that used federal and state funds to bolster private health insurance, which was rapidly expanding among working Americans. The administration would help the private markets expand into more difficult territory—the poor and the elderly. Like the liberal Democrats, the administration accepted the principle of social concern for the needy. Like the conservative Democrats, they emphasized state involvement. Every Republican administration would return to the Eisenhower combination—social concern, federal incentives, state decisionmaking, and private markets.

- Finally, notice that two senators voted against Kerr-Mills. One of them, Barry Goldwater (R-AZ) would for president in 1964. He propounded a simple principle: the federal government had no business in health care. In fact, it had no business in any business. Goldwater would get buried in 1964. But his *laissez faire* vision would revolutionize the Republican party and eventually inspire a new national majority. What is most striking is that Goldwater's perspective never gained traction in health care. No president, no matter how conservative, would subscribe to the Goldwater view that the government had no business helping Americans get access to health care.

In short, the full American health policy menu swirled through the Senate at the end of the Eisenhower era: a universal social security plan, a state based welfare program for the needy; assistance to private markets sold as the American Way; and a flat out rejection of federal government action. These four health care templates—shifting, mixing, matching, and clashing—would define the American health care debates to the present day.

John F. Kennedy (1961–63)

John Kennedy won the White House by a whisker (118,000 out of 68 million cast), lost most of his domestic agenda in Congress, and had a mixed foreign policy record. Yet, he transformed the presidency. Kennedy, radiating glamour and energy, was the first television president. After the Kennedy administration, television became the presidency's essential tool.[39]

Kennedy rejected Eisenhower's disciplined organizational chart—too stuffy, too traditional. Instead,

his administration introduced a free wheeling, unscripted, ad hoc executive style marked by aides who moved from issue to issue. Kennedy drew power from the executive branch into the White House. As he put it, "this nation needs a Chief Executive who is the vital center of action in our whole scheme of government." For the next 15 years, each president would up the ante on that aspiration.[40]

The president's style and ambition raised expectations for a powerfully constrained administration. Kennedy had squeaked into office and faced a Congress stacked against his liberal agenda since the Southern Democrats (there were 99 of them in the House) often voted with the Republicans. The administration's first congressional effort vividly illustrated the problem. The House Rules Committee, which could stop legislation from coming to a vote, had eight Democrats and four Republicans, but two of the Democrats regularly voted with the Republicans to block liberal action. To make room for his agenda, Kennedy moved to add three more Democrats to the committee. Even with Sam Rayburn, the influential Speaker of the House, pushing the measure, it scraped through, 217–212. As Arthur Schlesinger later wrote, "nothing brought the precariousness of the administration's position home more grimly than [that] first . . . battle."[41]

Kennedy had a well defined health plan (a variation of the one he had sponsored a year earlier) and declared that it would be one of his administration's first bills. Ironically, the media began referring to the proposal as *Medicare*—the name of Eisenhower's proposal.

The new Medicare would cover all social security beneficiaries over 65 with 90 days of hospital care. But this was more easily promised than achieved. The *New York Times* reflected the problem on page one: "President Kennedy outlined a broad and controversial program of Federal insurance . . . to cope with the country's needs in the field of health. The insurance plan [is] similar to plans rejected in the last session."[42]

The political problem was simple. The bill had to pass through the House Ways and Means Committee where it was five votes short. The administration responded in two ways—an outside strategy of taking the issue to the people and insider negotiations with Congress.[43]

"Presidents have tried to marshal public opinion before this for a favored . . . bill," commented the *New York Times*, "but probably never on such a scale as has Mr. Kennedy for health insurance." The new techniques were all on display in May 1962, when Kennedy addressed a Medicare rally at Madison Square Garden. The event was carried live on all three television networks. Swept up in the excitement, the president put aside his speech, spoke extemporaneously to the cheering mob—and flopped on television. Many supporters thought it was one of the president's worst speeches.[44]

The AMA poured resources into blunting the campaign. In a public relations counter coup, the Association rented out Madison Square Garden the day after Kennedy's speech. Alone in the quiet arena, the litter from the previous day's rally still scattered about, AMA president Dr. Edward Anis, spoke quietly. "I am not a cheerleader," he said. "I am a physician. Nobody—certainly not your doctors—can compete in this unfamiliar art of public persuasion, against such massive publicity, such enormous professional machinery, such unexpected money and such skillful manipulation!" The AMA won that exchange, but it could not blunt Medicare's popularity. Kennedy had introduced formidable new media techniques in his effort to win Medicare. Still, none of the rhetorical pyrotechnics changed the situation in Congress.[45]

The Kennedy administration tried to address that by lobbying members of the Ways and Means Committee and working with House leaders to place Medicare supporters on the committee as vacancies occurred. When they were still short of votes by the summer of 1962, the administration shifted to the Senate. There they attached Medicare to a welfare bill that had already passed in the house. (If the bill passed the Senate, it would go to conference committee to iron out differences between Senate version—with Medicare—and the House version—without Medicare—and then onto the floor of both Chambers for final approval.) This way, Medicare could bypass the Ways and Means Committee. On July 17, 1962, with Lyndon Johnson on the Senate floor to break an expected tie, two supporters defected and Medicare went down to defeat. An angry Kennedy went on television called it "a serious defeat for every American family" and promised to reintroduce the bill the following session.[46]

The debate heated up all over again the following year. This time, Medicare failed to clear the Ways and Means Committee by just a single vote. The administration was making slow progress in Congress. Even so, the Kennedy administration was not especially effective in lobbying Congress. A rural congressman from Tennessee explained why in 1962: "All that Mozart string music and ballet dancing down there [in the White House] . . . He's too elegant for me. I can't talk to him." The sophistication seemed fabulous to northeastern elites, but rural congressmen did not buy it.[47]

On November 22, 1963 the president was murdered in Dallas. The event defined an entire generation—as the attack on Pearl Harbor had done for an earlier age and the attack on 9/11 would a later one. Americans gathered around their television screens and watched numbly. As the president's young son saluted the caisson carrying his father's flag draped coffin, John F. Kennedy leapt from popular president to a national icon, a legend. At the very moment he was killed, Wilbur Cohen, Kennedy's effervescent health care policy leader, was meeting with Wilbur Mills in an effort to revive Medicare.

For political scientists, Kennedy's legacy lies in the way he made direct appeals to the people. Yet, even as he remade the presidency around television, Kennedy illustrated the age-old dilemma of all presidential politics: Even a very popular bill can be blocked in Congress. And not just in Congress, but by a handful of members on a key committee in Congress.

Ultimately, the Kennedy administration illustrates the power of old fashioned institutional dynamics. Few interest groups ever lobbied as long or as hard as the AMA lobbied against government health insurance. However the real political story lies in the organization of Congress: a small number of powerful legislators sitting on the Ways and Means Committee could block Medicare regardless of Kennedy or the AMA or public opinion.

Like Harry Truman, John Kennedy's major health care legacy lay in setting the political agenda. After his murder, John Kennedy's entire agenda took on a special status. Roosevelt had died in office and left his successor an ambiguous health care legacy. In contrast, John F. Kennedy left one that was clear and popular. Lyndon B. Johnson would receive that agenda and, using his extraordinary skills, would run with it like no president had run with a health agenda before or since.

Lyndon B. Johnson (1963–69)

Lyndon Johnson (LBJ) came up through the Senate ranks and understood Congress better than any modern president. Johnson took office, seized the Kennedy agenda and—invoking the fallen president—began pulling laws out of Congress. He won Kennedy's stalled tax cut in February 1964; persuaded moderate Republicans to help break an 87-day filibuster and pass the blockbuster Civil Rights Act of 1964 (in July); and launched the War on Poverty (in August).

Medicare was more complicated. The usual story goes like this: The Ways and Means Committee remained opposed until a Democratic landslide in November 1964 made Medicare inevitable. Wilbur Mills, chairman of the Ways and Means Committee, then switched sides and led the Democrats to the victory he had long denied them. Mills took the administration's Medicare proposal and, in a move that stunned Washington, linked it to two rival bills, tripling the size of the program. Taken by happy surprise, Johnson cheerfully acquiesced in Mills's coup and watched the new and improved Medicare sail through Congress.

Recently released telephone recordings paint a different picture. Johnson reintroduced Medicare less than three months after Kennedy's death. Through the spring of 1964, Johnson courted Wilbur Mills. In one of their conversations, Wilbur Mills fretted that he had to give conservative Democrats who had long opposed Medicare some cover for changing their

vote. Suppose, said Mills, he combined all the rival health insurance proposals that were floating around Congress into one great package. "If you give me that bill, I'll underwrite it," responded Johnson, who then urged Congressman Mills to go ahead and add even more. As Mills warmed up, LBJ flattered him, "it will be the biggest thing you have ever done for the country." We will come in and "applaud you," he said. Mills would get all the credit. In typical fashion, Johnson added, "I am not trying to go into details . . . I trust your judgment on that."[48]

Wilbur Mills would eventually come around, but not that spring. When it became clear that the Ways and Means Committee would not release the bill to the House, LBJ worked on the Senate. He wheedled and cajoled and managed Medicare's first win, 49–44. "I don't want to leave the impression we twisted arms or forced individuals," exulted the president, "but I'd say we did what we do on a lot of legislation." Some aides wanted Johnson to emulate Kennedy and go public to pressure the House to join the Senate. Johnson refused. He was an inside player and knew the limits of public pressure (and perhaps also the limits of his own stiff television style). Medicare never made it through the House in 1964. With a touch of Texas populism, Johnson explained how the administration would use the quest for Medicare in the November election: "We are really trying to do something for the people. We think the average mother wants peace, she wants her husband to have a job, and they're looking for somethin' to take care of 'em in their old age, and that's what we're trying to do . . . ."[49]

The 1964 election, held in the shadow of President Kennedy's murder, produced the biggest Democratic victory since 1936. House leaders promptly packed the Ways and Means Committee with liberal supporters. The Democrat's singled out Medicare's importance by labeling it HR1 and S1—the first bill in the queue on both sides of Congress.

Four months later, in the middle of a packed Ways and Means Committee meeting, Wilbur Mills made his celebrated move, bundling three competing bills into a single "three layer cake"—eventually known as Medicare Part A (hospital services), Medicare Part B (physician services), and Medicaid. "Like everyone else in the room I was stunned by Mill's strategy," averred Wilbur Cohen, the influential health advisor. "President Johnson was also surprised and amused," reported a prominent journalist. Only after the White House telephone transcripts became available did we discover that Lyndon Johnson had been in on the surprise and had pushed Mills to expand it. As LBJ had promised, all the credit fell to Wilbur Mills.[50]

Johnson swooped in every time he saw a potential roadblock. As soon as House leaders called Johnson to tell him the bill had cleared the committee, he dished out the salty advice about the Rules Committee quoted above: "For god sakes, don't let dead cats stand on your porch . . . you call that son of a bitch up [for a floor vote] before they can get their letters written."[51]

Three days after the Ways and Means Committee vote, President Johnson turned to another potential hurdle. He invited Senator Harry Byrd (D-WV), the chairman of the Committee on Finance to the White House. Byrd was a powerful Southern conservative who had always voted against Medicare. White House advisors thought he might bury the bill by postponing hearings. Johnson had also invited Medicare's congressional supporters and surprised them all by ushering them before the press. With television camera's rolling, the president smiled and ambushed Harry Byrd.

- LBJ: "I know that you will take an interest in the orderly scheduling of the matter and give it a thorough hearing."

- Byrd: [taken aback] "If I had known all this was going to happen I would have dressed more formally."

- LBJ: "Would you care to make an observation [regarding Medicare]?"

- Byrd: [shaking his head] "There is no observation I can make now, because the bill hasn't come before the Senate. Naturally I'm not familiar with it."

- LBJ: [pressing him by the elbow] "And you have nothing that you know of that would prevent

[hearings] coming about in reasonable time, not anything ahead of it in the committee?"

- Byrd: [softly] "Nothing in the committee now."

- LBJ: [leaning forward] "So . . . you will arrange for prompt hearings and thorough hearings?"

- Byrd: [barely audible] "Yes."[52]

Byrd kept his word and did not delay the bill. Presidential advisor Larry O'Brien later commented that Senator Byrd "was enough of an old pro himself to recognize a pro in action and probably admired it a little bit." The coup was, continued O'Brien, pure LBJ—none of his advisors were in on the plan.[53]

Even after all that, passage was no cakewalk. In the crucial House vote, on whether to bury Medicare back in committee, Medicare passed by just 45 votes—44 of them from newly elected members (both Democrats and Republicans). It was only after the relatively close vote that the bill enjoyed a 313–115 victory.

The Medicare victory invariably raises two questions. First, did the president matter or is the story all about the electoral constraints? Not even Lyndon Johnson could get the bill through in 1964. Perhaps any president could have won the legislation in 1965. Researchers put the question to Wilbur Mills more than 20 years later—Would John Kennedy have won the program had he been president in 1965? "No. No," responded Mills, "and that's where Johnson doesn't get the credit. He had the greatest ability of any president to get things done."[54] With time, we can see the potential hurdles more clearly: compromises in Ways and Means might have made have made the bill smaller rather than larger; the House Rules Committee might have delayed; the Senate Finance committee might have delayed further; the administration itself might have been tempted to rethink the legislation and put it off.

A familiar second question asks if Johnson could have won even more. Given the reforms flying out of Congress after the 1964 landslide, might the Democrats have won a full national health insurance plan? More than 40 years after the fact, it is easy to imagine Truman's ideal as another irresistible feature of the Great Society. But delve into the details—the caution of Wilbur Mills, the 45 vote margin in the House, the reluctance of Harry Byrd, the long negotiations on every side—and it becomes clear what an immense leap it would have been. In fact, as LBJ so often warned, delays might have lost the entire bill. Immerse yourself in the fears of the era and a full blown national health insurance seems like a great stretch—it is no surprise that none of the president's advisors suggested it.

The question itself suggests both strength and weakness in the Johnson White House. His most successful programs—Medicare, Medicaid, Civil Rights—came to him carefully crafted and ready to go. With a program already in hand, LBJ could do what he did best, negotiate the politics of passage.

The administration was not always as effective when it was planning or packaging new programs. Johnson was impatient with abstract ideas, formal policy studies, and budget analyses. "Those fools had to go to projecting it [my health program] down the road five or six years," he grumbled to Senator Ted Kennedy.[55] "You just make this thing work, I don't give a damn about the details," Johnson told the architects of the War on Poverty. "I'm not trying to go into details," he said to Wilbur Mills, about Medicare.[56]

Lyndon Johnson's executive branch was loose and chaotic. There was no Office of Management and Budget to hold everyone's feet to the numbers. There was very little formal policy analysis, few links between policy development and budgeting, until new advisors like Joseph Califano began imposing some order in late 1965. Ironically, the rise of a more robust policy analysis framework—introduced in the following years—would yield more careful policy development but inhibit decisive action on domestic problems.

For two years, Johnson acted like a supermajority leader and—together with a rare Democratic supermajority—won programs like no other modern president except Franklin Roosevelt. Medicare and Medicaid transformed American social policy. Together they would make the federal government the largest purchaser of health care services, eventually add up to second largest item in the federal budget, and comprise 37% of all health care spending.

Still, Lyndon Johnson's great reforms mark the end of the Democratic era. There was no future administration to build on the legacy. Bogged down by Vietnam, race riots, student protests, and economic trouble, Johnson declined to run another term. His successor would construct an entirely new regime in American health politics and policy.

Richard M. Nixon (1969–74)

President Nixon stands at the crossroads of American health politics. *An era of expansion*—marked by a free-wheeling debate over spreading health care benefits—turned into an *era of retrenchment* marked by concern over cost control. In this changed context, Nixon devised the first new universal health plan since Roosevelt.

Health care mattered to Nixon. He had been deeply affected by his brothers' painful, expensive, and fatal bouts with tuberculosis. Right after taking office, Nixon requested a health care study from HEW Secretary Robert Finch. Six months later, report in hand, the president told the nation "The problem is much greater than I had realized. We face a massive crisis in this area and unless action is taken . . . to meet that crisis within the next two to three years, we will have a breakdown in our medical care system."[57]

What to do? The Finch report pointed to prepaid groups or HMOs. Policy entrepreneurs had taken an old idea, prepaid group practice, and repackaged it as a way to inject market competition into the health care chaos. The administration came to see the idea of HMOs competing for enrollees as the solution to every problem. In July 1969, the administration floated the idea of HMOs for Medicaid. In March 1970, undersecretary of HEW, John Veneman, briefed the Ways and Means Committee on plans to introduce widespread use of HMOs into a proposed Medicare Part C. In February 1971, the administration unveiled a national health strategy that would push the entire population toward HMOs. "An HMO . . . cannot afford to waste resources that costs more money in the short run," explained the president. "But neither can it afford to economize in ways which hurt patients for that increases long-run expense." They would solve the age-old problem of getting high quality at low costs. Assistant Secretary of Health Lewis Butler speculated that 90% of all Americans might be in HMOs by 1980.[58]

Prepaid group health plans had been in operation for decades. They were not very well known or especially popular. Few people imagined that they were a "solution" to any policy problem—much less costs, access, coordination, and preventive care. The Nixon administration plucked the idea from a small group of policy entrepreneurs, placed it before the public and turned it into a perennial solution to American health policy woes.[59]

In the short run, however, the administration's HMOs initiative foundered in the political maelstrom. Liberals, led by Ted Kennedy, seized on the concept for their own goals. The Nixon administration found itself fighting expensive add-ons that, in its eyes, threatened to turn a cost cutter into a budget buster. The final policy result, The HMO Act of 1973, pleased almost no one and did nothing to help the fledgling HMO market.

The Nixon administration introduced another important break with Democratic proposals by rejecting a universal government health insurance program on the social security model; "there simply is no need to eliminate an entire segment of our private economy," said the president. Instead, he proposed "a partnership" between "government and our people, business and labor, the insurance industry and the health profession." Employers would continue to cover employees through private plans; government would fill in the gaps and cover the poor and old.

The Nixon plan (known by its acronym, CHIP) became part of the national debate in 1971, although it was not formally introduced until 1974. Inevitably, the CHIP proposal joined rival bills in Congress. Senator Ted Kennedy submitted a classic national health insurance package that looked like an extension of Medicare. The Nixon administration would extend the private health insurance system and fill in its gaps while Kennedy countered with a universal public program.

Time ran out on the Nixon administration. In March 1974, a grand jury indicted three of Nixon's closest aides; in June he was implicated as an unindicted coconspirator; in August, he became the only president to resign and leave office. National health insurance was lost in the storm. Liberals, expecting to win back the presidency at the next election, saw no reason to compromise with the conservative public–private "partnership" tossed up by a sinking administration. Of course, getting big health care change through Congress is never easy. Winning the reform under the looming shadow of impeachment and disgrace was, perhaps, impossible.

However, the Nixon administration left behind what may be the most ironic legacy in health care policy. It shifted the focus from a national health program to a government program that fills gaps in the private sector. Nixon's proposal—with its public–private partnership—would become the prototype for almost every subsequent effort. Nixon flew off to his disgrace leaving behind a bitter fate for liberal reformers: They would spend the rest of the century unsuccessfully chasing variations of the reform they rejected from Richard Nixon.

Jimmy Carter (1977–81)

Jimmy Carter ran for president as an outsider, untainted by Washington politics. After winning, he tried to govern that way. Rather than take up his role as the leader of a majority party that controlled every branch of government, he continued posing as an outsider.

One advisor pictured the difficult political context immediately after the election: "The Democratic Party is in serious national trouble—with a shrinking and ill-defined coalition." The solution? Vigorously "educate" incoming administration officials in Jimmy Carter's "philosophy." Most presidents lead a movement into power; this one would have to begin by instructing his own appointees. What lay at the heart of the president's philosophy? Not substance or ideology or passion. Rather, Jimmy Carter put an engineer's faith on efficiency and detail.[60]

Carter's health care policies reflected a great clash between engineering cost control on the one side and living up to political commitments on the other. In order to win organized labor's support during his long-shot campaign, Carter had tepidly endorsed national health insurance.[61] Congressional liberals soon began to call in that commitment. "Health reform is in danger of becoming the [Carter Administration's] missing promise," charged Ted Kennedy in May 1977. "The American people should not tolerate delay on national health care simply because other reforms are already lined up bumper to bumper."[62]

While Democratic liberals pushed for quick action, Democratic moderates pushed back. Ways and Means chairman, Representative Al Ullman (D-OR) snapped, "If Carter sends an NHI bill up here, it will destroy his presidency because it seems so counter to his fight on inflation . . . You tell the president that I will have to publicly call the act of submitting a proposal to Congress this year a major disaster."[63]

The Carter administration eventually spurned the liberals and proposed cost control. As Carter described it, "*The Hospital Cost Containment Act* will restrain increases in the reimbursements which hospitals receive from all sources: Medicare, Medicaid, Blue Cross, commercial insurers, and individuals."[64] The engineer in Carter, and perhaps the ascetic, saw cost control as the necessary prelude to expanding access to care. Only after the system was fixed—after the spinach was downed—would it be safe and proper to expand access, which was the inflationary dessert.

Of course, the hospital industry worked furiously against the legislation. More important, Jimmy Carter never roused the public over the issue. Members of Congress reported getting no constituent mail on the subject and the proposal died in the Senate Finance Committee.[65]

Undaunted, Carter continued to push for hospital cost containment. When Ted Kennedy developed a national health insurance plan and decided to challenge Carter for the democratic nomination, the White House responded by promising its own proposal. The clashing health plans might have turned into a battle for the soul of the Democratic party. But while Kennedy was committed to bold action, the Carter administration remained half hearted about national health insurance. In Carter's 1979 State of the Union Message, national health insurance got little more than a squeak: "This year, we will take our first steps to develop a national health plan."[66]

In 1978, despite long odds, the administration got the Hospital Cost Containment bill through the Senate. Stunned industry lobbyists descended on the House (bearing campaign contributions for members on both sides of the aisle) and, in July 1978, soundly beat back the regulatory effort. The whole cost control plan fit oddly with the spirit of the times and the president's own rhetoric. Carter called for deregulation and free markets across the economy—except for hospitals that would face a heavy dose of old fashioned regulation.

On June 6, 1978, an antigovernment wave rolled out of California with a victory for "Proposition 13" which sharply limited property taxes.[67] The great Republican tax rebellion had begun. President Carter—immersed in policy details, full of dry, good government reforms, presiding over a collapsing coalition—had no answer for the hot, antitax, antigovernment, anti-Democrat tide.

The administration seemed increasingly weak. In July 1979, as the economy got worse, President Carter delivered his most infamous address (later dubbed "the malaise speech"). "The gap between our citizens and our government has never been so wide," declared Carter. The president tried to seize control of events by blasting his cabinet for disloyalty and firing five members. All along, reported one administration staffer in an interview, "it was an open question whether the Cabinet or the White House was in charge."[68] Four months later, in November 1979, an Islamic rebellion swept across Iran and toppled the Shah. Militants stormed the American embassy, took over 70 hostages and held them for 444 days.

The administration's health policy makers struggled on. They finally released a national health insurance proposal (in June 1979) and eventually managed to hammer out a deal with Senator Kennedy. The Democrats agreed on a plan that combined public and private sector action—not unlike the Nixon proposal.

Congressional hearings began at the end of November, entirely overshadowed by the Iran Hostage Crisis and the upcoming presidential election (primaries would start in four months). Neither one last attempt at hospital cost containment nor the administration's half-hearted national health insurance ever came close to passing—the latter, in particular, was far too little much too late.

Political scientist Richard Neustadt would later comment, "Watching President Carter in 1979, sparked the question: Is the Presidency possible?" The answer, we would learn during the next administration, was decidedly yes. But Carter left two great warnings about the office:

- First, there is no getting around the Washington establishment. The White House is responsible for running the government machinery. And that takes care, skill, talent, and experience.

- Second, you can go to the people with a large vision. But the president's ideals have to be clear, simple, and popular. Carter's scattershot—energy legislation, welfare reform, hospital cost containment, deficit reduction—would become a model of what not to do.

Still, President Carter left behind two health care legacies. First, he turned health care cost control from *an* issue to *the* issue.

Second, Jimmy Carter pushed the Democratic party to embrace a Nixon style private–public partnership. Future liberals might tout a public national health insurance based on the Medicare model. But the idea now fell out of the Washington health care mainstream. After Carter, the old liberal model would bear that ultimate political stigma: it became "unrealistic."

Ronald Reagan (1981–89)

Ronald Reagan won a landslide 44 states and swept the Republicans back to power in the Senate for the first time in a quarter century. In its first year, the new administration racked up a series of large victories highlighted by a $750 billion tax cut and more than $35 billion in domestic program reductions. The Reagan administration removed 400,000 people from the food stamps program, closed the public health service hospitals (which dated back to 1798), eliminated grants to HMOs, cut most of the funding for social science research, and combined 21 separate grant programs into four large block grants that reduced both federal discretion and budget commitment. In a harbinger of things to come, the Reagan administration did tuck a new item into the budget—$10,000 for a chastity center.[69]

The Reagan winning streak came to an abrupt end when the administration took on Social Security. The administration proposed steep cuts, watched Reagan's approval rating plunge 16 points, and retreated to the safe ground of a bipartisan National Commission. In January 1983, the Commission released a compromise.

Congress approved the Social Security changes and quietly slipped a momentous Medicare change into the bill. Medicare had traditionally paid hospitals on what was called retrospective fee-for-service—any reasonable fee the hospitals charged after providing the service. The more services the hospital performed, the more they were reimbursed. While the media glare focused on Social Security, the administration and Congress quietly agreed to use a new hospital a payment method known as Diagnostic Related Groups (or DRGs). The DRGs set hospital rates in advance ("prospectively") by the diagnosis. The new scheme flipped the incentives—since hospitals were paid the same amount (depending on the patient's diagnosis) regardless of the services they actually provided, hospitals would now make more money by providing less care.[70]

Nixon had declared a Medicare costs a crisis and Carter had made hospital cost containment his health care grail. In vivid contrast to the earlier battles, the DRG proposal passed unnoticed. Even Lyndon Johnson—fretting over those dead cats stinking up the porch—had never managed so large a health care change with so little fuss.

The great Republican innovation lay in focusing only on Medicare costs. The previous efforts—like Carter's cost containment—had applied to all payers. Now, each payer would worry only about its own payments. Hospitals would try to keep up their income by shifting the costs from payers who effectively reduced their hospital payments (like Medicare) to those who failed to find a way to squeeze. The American hospital system entered a new era of cost-shifting (from payer to payer), competition (between payers), and bargaining (between payers and the hospitals). The payers' quest for cost control would lead directly to the managed care revolution.[71]

Three years later, the Reagan administration came up with another health care surprise. By now, the administration was mired by scandals, a stalled domestic agenda and a rising budget deficit. In November 1986, the Democrats regained the Senate. The Reagan administration needed a win.

Two days after the 1986 midterm loss, Reagan gave his cabinet a pep talk and pointed to a major new domestic initiative. Secretary of HHS Otis-Bowen was "finalizing his proposal on [Medicare] catastrophic health insurance."[72] Over the next three months, the rest of the cabinet argued vociferously against expanding Medicare. Despite considerable acrimony, the administration submitted the plan that the president unveiled during a weekly radio address in February 1987.

The original draft of the radio address promised to "provide direct assistance to Americans 65 and over who find themselves in need of medical care." Beryl Sprinkle, Chairman of the Council of Economic Advisors and still implacably opposed, scratched out "assistance" and scrawled in the margin, "*assistance is incorrect. The insurance is supposed to be self-financed.*" Reagan's address followed the economist's instructions and promised to "make available catastrophic medical insurance."[73]

Sprinkle's change signals something distinctive—something Republican—about the proposal: classic social insurance redistributed wealth. The young and old, the sick and the healthy all chipped in to fund the benefits. Not this time. Medicare beneficiaries would fund their own benefits.

The original proposal had focused on covering hospital costs. The Democratic Congress added prescription drugs, skilled nursing facilities, hospice, home health care, and other benefits. By July, President Reagan was back on the radio charging that

Congress had taken his "sound, sensible program," "more than tripled the costs," and "threatened . . . the entire Medicare trust fund."[74]

However, both parties in Congress supported the legislation. Democratic leaders negotiated a compromise with the White House and the bill passed easily. That didn't end the negotiations in the White House. T. Kenneth Cribb, Reagan's top advisor for domestic affairs, advised that the presidential remarks during the signing ceremony "should distance the president" from the legislation.[75] In a gloomy address, Reagan followed the advice and offered "a word of caution." Since "the program . . . is to be paid for by the elderly themselves, noted Reagan, "This could be more than a budget problem; it could be a tragedy."[76] Still, President Reagan signed the bill surrounded by beaming Democrats.

Ronald Reagan consciously set out to replace the old New Deal order with a robust market vision. He disparaged social welfare ideals and celebrated, in their stead, images of individualism, markets, and get-ahead. The difference can be seen in the Reagan health programs—even when they increased federal control (hospital payment) and expanded federal benefits (catastrophic coverage). The administration cast aside the great web of cross subsidies that animated earlier programs. Cost containment would only apply to federal payments—and let the devil take the hindmost payer. Medicare beneficiaries would, for the first time, pay for their own benefits. The era of social welfare and common security was over.

Inspired by Reagan, conservatives would move to conquer the rest of the political establishment in the next decade. Democrats would fight back and try to restore their own coalition. The great battle for control over American politics would turn on health care policy. That contest would arise during the George H.W. Bush presidency and come to a head in the 1990s with Bill Clinton in the White House.

George H.W. Bush (1989–93)

A pre-inaugural memo neatly summed up the spirit of the Bush domestic agenda: "Premises: 1) Virtually no money. 2) Deficit will dominate discussion.

3) Congress . . . will definitely vie for control." The administration was further hamstrung by a poor economy and by the memorable pledge Bush made during the Republican national convention: My opponent won't rule out raising taxes. But I will. The Congress will push me to raise taxes, and I'll say no, and they'll push, and I'll say no, and they'll push again, and I'll say to them, "Read my lips: no new taxes."[77]

Every discussion of domestic policy raised the same flurry of memos pointing to the same bottom line: there was no money. The administration sat on the sidelines during the one great health care drama that embroiled Congress. Seniors rebelled against the Medicare surtax imposed by the Catastrophic Coverage Act. A grassroots organization, Seniors Coalition against the Catastrophic Coverage Act, claimed to have over 400,000 signatures demanding repeal. At the heart of the protest lay a sense of injustice. The federal government subsidized farmers and bailed out the savings and loans industry; other groups did not pay surtaxes when they got help from government, why should seniors?

The rebellion came to a head just 13 months after Ronald Reagan had signed the package. Representative Dan Rostenkowski met with disgruntled constituents. After the meeting—with news cameras rolling—a crowd of seniors blocked his car, pounded on the windows, and banged on the hood with picket signs. Rostenkowski had nothing to say. His colleagues soon filled the silence. "The elderly were ungrateful," said Henry Waxman, "so let them stew in their own juices." The pictures of elders attacking Rostenkowski made the cover of *Time Magazine* and became the icon of catastrophic health care.[78] "I hate to place the blame," said Otis Bowen later, "but President Bush remained totally silent, made no effort whatsoever to keep the bill." In November, the House and Senate voted overwhelmingly to repeal the entire program.[79]

Bush's silence was not coincidental. Neither he nor his advisors favored large health care programs. There was one exception to this general passivity on health care issues: the problem of costs. The administration strategy focused on malpractice litigation

and what one staffer called "the new paradigm health issue"—prevention.[80] As President Bush explained, "It's not complicated. Eat sensibly. Exercise. Wear seatbelts. Don't smoke, and if you do smoke, stop. Don't abuse alcohol, and don't use illegal drugs."[81]

The White House staff treated these modest reforms as a bully way to deflect calls for broader health care action.[82] However, the calls for national health insurance were beginning to proliferate. Congressional proposals filled the hopper and pollsters warned the administration that the issue had grown hot. In late spring 1991, the Senate Democrats released a proposal that required employers to play (insure their workers) or pay (taxes) for an *Americare* program that would cover all uninsured Americans.

The Bush administration scrambled to catch up. The *Washington Post* noted that the White House was "feeling the heat on health care" and quoted sources "close to Bush as saying that he genuinely cares about the issue but is unfamiliar with it is and getting his legs on this issue."[83]

The rising importance of health care reform seemed confirmed in November 1991, when Pennsylvania held a special election to replaced Senator John Heinz who had died in an airplane crash. Former Governor Dick Thornburgh stepped down as Bush's Attorney General and entered the race as a prohibitive favorite—three months before the election he had a 40-point lead. Harris Wofford, who had been appointed to fill Heinz's seat, staked his election on universal health insurance. In their first debate, Wofford waved a copy of the Constitution and launched his celebrated slogan: "If the Constitution guarantees criminals the right to a lawyer, shouldn't it guarantee working Americans their right to a doctor as well?" Wofford got everyone's attention when he won by 10%. National health insurance landed solidly on the national agenda.[84]

Four days later, at a press conference in Rome, President Bush told reporters, "I'd like to have a comprehensive health care plan that I can vigorously take to the American people."[85] Two months later, deep in the policy "spinach" portion of the presidents 1992 State of the Union Message—the sixth domestic item—he called for health reform: After mocking the Democrat's for their "pay or play" proposal, Bush laid out his plan: a health insurance tax credit for low income families; insurance market reforms; malpractice reform; and health information technology.

The plan itself was hastily thrown together, released, and then withdrawn for last minute revisions. The Bush administration never managed to find a way to fund their tax credit or to convinced a skeptical press that it was offering a serious plan. Nor did President Bush ever seem personally invested in the issue. During the plan's two-day roll-out in February 1992, he toured a neonatal intensive care unit in California to generate media visuals. A pool reporter overheard his *sotto voce* murmur: "What am I doing here?"

By the time the plan appeared, the primary elections had begun. The Democratic Congress had little interest in the bill. And the president himself seemed more animated when he was attacking the Democratic plan than when defending his own.

The Democratic candidate, Bill Clinton, hired Harris Wofford's campaign team, which tacked a now celebrated axiom to the wall of the election war room: "*It's the economy stupid! And don't forget about health care.*" When the Democrats won the presidency and retained both houses in Congress, health reform seemed like a winner.

Through the prism of health care, the Bush experience was anomalous. Every other modern president shaped the way Americans thought about health care and health reform. Even presidents who failed to win their reforms left their mark on the debates. In contrast President Bush found himself chasing a popular wave and still looking for health care "sea legs" two years after taking office.

It is unusual to see major health reform develop such velocity without a national champion. Most reforms leap up the agenda thanks to an advocate in the oval office. In the early 1990s, health care seemed to develop a life of its own. The prospects for national health insurance had rarely—perhaps never—been better as the Clinton administration came to power.

Still, President Bush left a mark. His administration generated proposals that would become part of the conservative health care legacy: malpractice reform, a commitment to disseminating health information technology, small group market reforms, and the use of tax credits to help poor Americans purchase private insurance. The effort to make health care markets work arose under Nixon, was revived by Reagan, and now got another boost from President Bush.

Bill Clinton (1993–2001)

Withering Republican fire—big government, big payroll taxes, heavy regulation—had made Democrats anxious about "pay or play." During the second presidential debate, Clinton announced a new health care strategy, managed care. This was a much refined variation of Richard Nixon's (1971) proposal. Clinton added all kinds of bells (a national health budget) and whistles (state flexibility for experiments) but the essential logic remained: HMO-type organizations would compete to sign up customers. The whole business was perfect for the election campaign: it sounded good and was hard to pin down. "It all sounds to me like you're going to have some government setting prices," groped President Bush in response, "I want competition." Here was the beauty of the Democratic strategy. Managed competition promised . . . competition.

Five days after the inauguration Clinton announced his health care team. The first lady, Hilary Clinton, would chair a task force managed by Ira Magaziner, an old friend and business consultant from Rhode Island. Victory seemed likely. Democrats had won two surprise victories—first Wofford, now Clinton—thanks, in good measure, to health care. The first reaction to the task force was respectful, even enthusiastic. Republicans began drawing up their own health care alternatives—a trusty gauge of political expectations.

Ira Magaziner plunged into work on the health care task force. He gathered 630 health policy experts (including one of the authors of this chapter), huddled with them over four months, and hashed out an intricate plan. The effort reflected Magaziner's own style: brilliant, workaholic, out of the box, and politically naïve.

The Clintons had planned to cram their reform into the first budget package and pass the whole gigantic bill. Under Senate rules, budget reconciliation is debated for just 24 hours and then—no filibusters permitted—gets voted up or down. Fifty votes—with vice president Al Gore to break a tie—would win Senate approval of the most important domestic legislation in decades. (The Democrats controlled 56 seats.) However, in early March, Senator Robert Byrd (D-WV), the powerful chairman of the Senate Appropriations Committee, spiked the Clinton strategy. This "very complex, very expensive, very little understood piece of legislation" should be debated out in the open. As a philosophical position, Byrd was right, but the political ramifications were devastating. Magaziner had not designed a robust plan well geared for the political scrum of Washington politics.[86]

A second fatal error followed directly: delay. Clinton's health care team—new to Washington—did not realize how swiftly the reform moment would pass. "Overconfident about the momentum of reform," wrote presidential health advisor Paul Starr, "we misjudged the health care politics of 1993 as a change in the climate when it was only a change in the weather."[87] A series of delays squandered their opportunity.

Bruising battles over bitter policy medicine like deficit reduction and the North American Free Trade Agreement (NAFTA) left the Democratic base weary and disgruntled. Meanwhile, opponents sharpened their knives. The Health Insurance Association of America (HIAA) hired savvy Bill Gradison out of the House of Representatives to lead the attack. The HIAA aired television advertisements featuring a couple—dubbed Harry and Louise—discussing the president's ill conceived concoction and concluding in exasperation, "there has to be a better way."

Finally, on September 22nd, 1993, President Clinton unveiled his proposal in a masterful prime time address to a joint session of Congress.

It's hard to believe that there was once a time . . . when retirement was nearly synonymous with poverty . . . and older Americans died in the street. That's unthinkable today, because over a half a century ago Americans had the courage . . . to create a Social Security System that ensures that no Americans will be forgotten in their later years. Forty years from now, our grandchildren will also find it unthinkable that there was a time in this country when hardworking families lost their homes, their savings, their businesses, lost everything simply because their children got sick or because they had to change jobs.[88]

The next day, the president's pollster reported that fully two thirds of the public was behind him. The president should have heeded LBJ: "For god sakes, don't let dead cats stand on your porch . . . . you call that son of a bitch up before they can get their letters written."

But the bill was still not ready. Congress would not begin deliberations until the following year, in January 1994. Rather than looking back at the Democratic victories of 1991 and 1992, Congress would be looking ahead to the elections later that year. Republicans had originally prepared to negotiate. Senator John Chafee (R-RI) co-sponsored a health bill with Senate Minority Leader Robert Dole. As Chafee himself described the progress of their plan, Dole went from calling it "my plan" (when Clinton's reform seemed inevitable) to "the Chafee–Dole plan" (as reform teetered) to "that god damn plan of Chaffee's" (as Republicans united against it).[89] In December, strategist William Kristol advised Republicans to kill the Clinton reform. Winning health care, he warned, "would revive the [Democrat's] reputation . . . as the generous protectors of middle class interests."

Clinton used his State of the Union message in January 1994 to pump up his reform. Dole used the Republican rejoinder to introduce a bewildering organizational chart that illustrated—vastly exaggerated, as described by Democrats—the sheer complexity of the government effort. Criticism appeared on every side—fair and unfair. The vagueness of managed competition now proved a liability, popular support fell, allies never mustered for the fight.

Through the spring and early summer, health reform made its way through a thicket of Congressional committees that mark the modern Congress[90]: House Health and Environment subcommittee (stalemate, no bill); House Energy and Commerce committee (one vote short, no bill); Health subcommittee of the Ways and Means (strong version of the Clinton Plan); House Ways and Means Committee (chairman Rostenkowski indicted in the process); Labor and Human Resources (a strong bill by a healthy majority); Senate Finance (a weak bill); Senate Majority Leader George Mitchell's "rescue bill"; House Speaker Tom Foley's last ditch bill. Increasingly weaker compromises followed one another.

On August 25th, after exhausting rounds of negotiation, nose counting, and rewrites, the Democrats gave up. A famous *New York Times* report quoted Senator Bob Packwood (R-OR) at a closed door Republican strategy session: "We've killed health care reform, now we've got to make sure our fingerprints are not on [the body]." Republicans, pointing to health care as another example of "Big Government Democrats Gone Wild," captured both houses of Congress and came to power on every level of government.

In the aftermath, private payers seized on the key element in the president's plan, managed competition. The Clinton reformers took a conservative nostrum—failed to harness it to broad social reform—and essentially publicized it as a cost control mechanism. Stripped of its public framework, the plan became a crude way for payers to limit their costs by limiting services. Managed care rapidly spread across the American health care system.

All the underlying problems of the health care system remained—indeed, they got worse. Complexity, costs, gaps in coverage, inequality, miserable aggregate health data. Before long, some international surveys were ranking the United States 28th (for women) and 31st (for men) in life expectancy.[91] However, the old, fervently prescribed solutions had vanished. Conservatives long believed that a solid dose of competition would cure the system's ills. Liberals, of course, had their national health insurance dreams. After the Clintons' failure and the private sector's unhappy experience with managed care, the traditional solutions lost their allure.

The most important political legacy of the entire Clinton effort lay in the aftermath: Republican's controlled the historical spin. There was no shame in losing health reform—Clinton got much deeper into the Congressional process than, say, Harry Truman. But Truman never abandoned the ideal. He kept roasting opponents long after his reform was dead and buried. Truman left office a deeply unpopular president, but his reform survived him thanks to the boundless energy of his defense.

Contrast Clinton. "I was . . . disappointed," he wrote mildly in his memoirs, "and I felt bad that Hilary and Ira Magaziner were taking the rap."[92] No memory now of "hardworking families [who] lost their homes, their savings, their businesses, lost everything simply because their children got sick or because they had to change jobs." The fire of September was out and forgotten by the following August.

Clinton would hold off the Republican majorities, win an easy reelection victory and rack up very high approval ratings by the end of his term. But, in exchange, he backed off his own program and permitted the Republicans to control the history. The Republican strategists had originally read Clinton's plan and concluded that, if it passed, the program might "revive" the Democrats reputation as "the generous protectors of the middle class." Conservatives feared precisely what Clinton predicted: this would be seen as a second social security.

Yet everyone now "knows" that naïve liberals designed a foolish plan—overly complicated (true enough), overly ambitious (debatable), a disaster that the Republicans helped America avert (not even the Republicans believed that at the time). A Harry Truman would have challenged that story, he would have kept fighting, he would have left his lost reform on the American agenda. Another kind of politician would have seized the bully pulpit and blamed opponents for betraying America. Clinton,

Magaziner, and the liberals ruefully accepted the Republican narrative: Democrats had overreached and paid the price.[93]

Bill Clinton aspired to more and yet—ironically—left less on the political table. He would continue to chip away at health problems. However, in contrast to almost every other modern president he would leave no large idea behind, no health care ideal to rally for, no grand aspiration to inspire future generations. Truman's reform now seemed to slip into history. At the end of Clinton's tenure, the Democrat's were out of power, out of ideas, out of time.

CONCLUSION

Our reading across seven decades suggests a different way to understand the presidency. Rather than simply measuring success in winning programs, consider how each administration reshaped the health care debates. Presidents introduce ideas, redefine problems and propose solutions. Each changes the way Americans think and talk about health care.

Harry Truman, for example, left an enduring mark, not by winning—he never came close—but by fiercely championing an idea that the Roosevelt administration had half heartedly passed down to him. His fight inspired liberal reformers for generations. Richard Nixon plucked the idea of health care competition out of the policy stream; although his proposals never get very deep into the legislative process, he fundamentally reorganized the debate by championing both competition and public private partnerships. Even liberal plans would soon reflect the Nixon approach. And Bill Clinton changed the future, not by losing but by walking away from his own reform, by letting his opponents re-imagine the plan as a close brush with policy disaster.

Every president—enthusiastically or grudgingly—has joined the health care battle. Every modern president has contrived a plan. But presidential efficacy in this domain requires passion and a willingness to take major risks for an uncertain goal. It requires enormous presidential skill as both politician and policy maker. Health care is in many ways the ultimate domestic test of presidential effectiveness, which is perhaps why so few appear to have succeeded in achieving their health care goals.

What advice can we offer after our survey of the presidents and their efforts to extend health benefits to Americans? Of course, the context is always crucial and ever changing. Still, across all the differences, we find the same patterns.

Move Fast, Act Early

The day after the presidential election, the savvy health policy analyst ought to slip his president-elect a message: Hurry up, you're almost out of time. Administrations begin spending their political capital from the moment they take office and they rarely acquire more. Health care, in particular, requires every shred of capital a president can muster. Clinton is the great example. After two underdog victories by Democrats touting health care, national health insurance seemed irresistible—even Republicans were signing on to a plan. By the following year, Congress was maneuvering for advantage over the next election. The reform moment slipped away before a bill even appeared in Congress.

Lyndon Johnson offers the corollary. Historians look at that 1964 landslide, count the votes on the Ways and Means Committee and conclude that Medicare enjoyed, in Theodore Marmor's memorable phrase, the "politics of legislative certainty." Medicare proved a certain winner partially because Johnson hustled the bill through both House and Senate while the November vote count was still warm. Not only did he move his favorite bills through early, he demanded speed throughout the process. As he warned his colleagues—in that inimitable Texas style—delays permit opponents to recoup and strike. Johnson spoke a political lesson for the ages: "For god sake, don't let dead cats stand on your porch . . . they stunk and they stunk and they stunk . . ."

Master the Legislative Process

Modern presidents have extraordinary resources at their disposal. Yet, many administrations have been maladroit at managing the congressional process.

As Tip O'Neil told Jimmy Carter, "Pennsylvania Avenue is a two way street." There is no escaping the duet. President and Congress "legislate together," as political scientist Mark Peterson put it. If the president is not effective at working the other end of Pennsylvania Avenue, he needs to find skillful staff members to do the job.[94]

Master the White House

When Franklin Roosevelt came to power, he could sit down with his entire staff in the Oval Office. Over time the White House Staff grew until hundreds of staff members (thousands if you count the larger EOP) encircle the president. There is always an economic advisor buzzing in the president's ear. The policy detail can be overwhelming. The president has to constantly focus on the big picture while mastering enough detail and information to keep the big picture grounded. President Jimmy Carter famously lost sight of the former, President George W. Bush the latter.

Big picture aside, the presidential office takes management. Here, for the most part, Republicans have been more skillful than Democrats. Democrats keep imagining that they can leash the creative chaos of a Franklin Roosevelt or a Lyndon Johnson. They cannot—not any more, not today. In fact, President Johnson could not do it like Johnson for very long and had to impose a more orderly process on his White House. There are plenty of ways to keep the windows open to new ideas. But the modern presidency needs careful organization around a nimble and experienced chief of staff.

Beyond the simple pressures of smooth organization lies a formidable political question. The president has his own White House advisors, directs the EOP, and leads the sprawling executive branch of government. What is to be the relationship between these institutions? Some presidents, most famously Richard Nixon, try to run the country from the White House; others (like Ronald Reagan) carefully placed loyalists in the cabinet agencies and turned decisionmaking over to them. The Carter administration never quite sorted out the relationship between White House and cabinet—which led to

friction, faction, and firings. The key is not finding the perfect alignment—each model has strengths and weaknesses—but making the three pieces of the executive branch work together smoothly. Or put more realistically, the administration must manage the executive branch's inherent tendency to chaos.

What's the Big Thing?

Presidents can normally win only a few big things. Each administration has to focus on a few important objectives if they're to win their agenda. Jimmy Carter lined up his do-good reforms, "bumper to bumper," and lost most of the big ones. Clinton complained that events constantly distracted him and knocked him off his main concerns. Presidents do well to keep their big idea—health care for Truman, reducing government for Ronald Reagan, homeland security for George W. Bush—at the center of their attention. To succeed, first focus—then push, push, push.

This rule can also inform voters as they judge candidates. The key test of any president is very simple and often overlooked: What does this man or woman care intensely about? What's the passion? Voters should take the candidate's gut deep obsession seriously because that is what they are most likely to achieve. Voters who care about health care should not expect much from presidents who lack passion on the issue. The issue is too tough and too risky. The fate of health care reform is sealed, in many respects, on election day.

The Power of Ideas

We often score presidents by how many bills they get through Congress. Presidency watchers publish "scorecards" with their success rates. But the deepest power of the office lies in the ideas that the president promotes. Harry Truman or Ronald Reagan succeeded more at projecting a set of ideals than in crafting laws or winning programs. The presidency is, of course, a bully pulpit. It is the one institution in American life that is geared for projecting ideas to the country and the world. One of the great health care legacies for any president is the power to imagine a new health care idea, to leave his successors a new set of options.

Lessons of History

Before coming into office, Reagan administration officials carefully studied what their predecessors, had done right and wrong. From the start, they organized their administration around the history lessons. Every administration is a learning process, each holds important clues about running an effective White House.

One classic mistake is to simply react against the errors of the last administration—especially if the other party held the office. However, every administration, no matter how troubled, does something well. Every administration, no matter how successful, offers warnings about things to avoid.

Of course, administrations learn. Presidents and their advisors often grow into their roles. By the time they do, they've lost that early advantage. Moving fast and early means working the White House—working the government machinery—smoothly right from the start. The best way to do that is to master the lessons of the past administrations: How did they organize the White House? The relations with the cabinet agencies? With Congress? With the media? Each prior administration is rich in do's and don'ts. An incoming administration ignores them at its peril. Successful administrations examine the health legacies of previous administrations without the blinders of political distaste or personal pique for predecessors. Clinton's faith that he could design a new proposal that was fundamentally better than anything to come before may have sunk his program, his party (for more than a decade), and even the idea of national health insurance (perhaps for even longer). In contrast, President Johnson's willingness to embrace the Kennedy legacy gave him a huge head start: the policy work was already done.

STUDY QUESTIONS

1. What sort of circumstances often leads to an increase in presidential power?
2. How does the US Constitution contribute to the ambiguity surrounding presidential authority?
3. How does the concept of "political time" relate to presidential effectiveness?
4. Why has the expansion of health care coverage become an important issue for each successive president across several decades?
5. How did the timing of President Clinton's health care reform plan affect its fortunes in Congress?
6. What were the political circumstances immediately leading up to the American Medical Association's decision (in 1938) to endorse private health insurance?
7. Why did President Truman's plans for national health insurance fail to come to fruition?
8. What was the Eisenhower administration's chief contribution to the national health care debate?
9. How did President Johnson overcome the resistance of two powerful congressional figures—Rep. Wilbur Mills and Sen. Harry Byrd—to get Medicare passed?
10. How did the specter of Watergate affect President Nixon's HMO-based health care reform plan?
11. What was President Reagan's contribution to health care cost control?
12. What political event brought comprehensive health care reform back to the top of the political agenda in the early 1990's?
13. Which party has, over the long term, proven more successful at "mastering the White House," and why?
14. The authors end with six lessons from history. Describe any three. Which of the six do you think are most important? Why?

NOTES

1. Dallek, 1996. xii, xiii.
2. Ibid.
3. The Constitution of the United States of America, Amendment #10.
4. Henry David Thoreau, 1848. The quote is often mistakenly attributed to Jefferson. President Ronald Reagan's 1st inaugural address.

5. Bryce, Vol. I: 83–4.
6. Alexander Hamilton, *Federalist* #70.
7. James Bryce, I: 83–4.
8. Schlesinger, 1973.
9. Franklin D. Roosevelt, 1933. For a perspective that emphasizes the talents of the presidents themselves see Landy and Milkis, 2001.
10. See Skowronek, 1993; Skowronek 2006.
11. Kingdon, 1994.
12. President and Mrs. Reagan, 1986. Morone, 2003, pp 466–8.
13. Lyndon Baines Johnson, *The White House Tapes.* Lyndon B. Johnson Presidential library. C.7024-7025 Hubert Humphrey. March 6, 1965. 11:25 AM.
14. The quote, from historian Doris Kearns Goodwin, is reprinted in Weissert and Weissert, p 75.
15. Johnson Library, C.7141 John McCormack, March 23, 1965. 4:54 PM.
16. Light used data from 1960 through 1977. Some recent studies have questioned his findings though for health care they hold up extremely well (Light, 1982); Johnson quoted by Burns, p 83.
17. Jacobs, 2006; Shapiro and Jacobs, 2000.
18. See Dickerson, 2005.
19. Fraser, 2005; Roosevelt, 1933.
20. For citation and discussion, see Morone, 1990, p 258.
21. Roosevelt, October 2, 1936. Quotation from shorthand record of delivered speech. Roosevelt Archives.
22. J. Hamilton Lewis, 1937; *Time Magazine,* 1937.
23. Telegram from Corning, 1938.
24. Roosevelt, 1939.
25. Harris, 1966, p 30.
26. Truman Presidential Library, October 5, 1953.
27. Truman, November 19, 1945. The draft data gathered in considerable detail in Papers of Samuel I. Rosenman.
28. Harry Truman Library. Papers of Samuel I. Rosenman.
29. US Senate, National April 2–16, 1946, 47 ff. For discussion, see Starr, p 283.
30. McCullough, 1992, p 473.
31. Milkis and Nelson, p 299.
32. Greenstein,1982.
33. Quoted in Milkis and Nelson, p 299.
34. Dwight David Eisenhower, January 1954. The insurance data from Quadagno, 2005, p 52, covers the period from 1946–57. See Hacker, Chapter 10.
35. Harris, 1966, p 66.
36. Quoted in Quadagno, p 46.
37. Eisenhower, 1960.
38. Southern Democrats had fought this same fight over the Aid to Families with Children (or welfare) in the Social Security Act. Southern Democrats refused to permit federal funds to go directly to poor, black families and substituted welfare programs run by the states.
39. Milkis and Nelson, 312–13; Lowi, 1985.
40. Quoted in Milkis and Nelson, p 310.
41. Arthur Schlesinger, 1965, p 651
42. *New York Times*, February 10, 1961, 1:1. Emphasis added.
43. For a fine account of the legislative (and committee) politics, see Theodore Marmor, 1971.
44. *New York Times*, May 21, 1962, 1:8; see also the related article on 1:4.
45. Quoted in Harris, 1966, p 143.
46. Kennedy quoted in *New York Times*, July 18, 1962, 1:8, 14.
47. The comment quoted by Arthur Schlesinger (1965, 652). At the time Schlesinger thought the comment "bizarre." But it vividly illuminates the future of American politics. As the Republicans came to power, this Congressman's attitude turned to a red hot resentment of liberal elites and rose to power in the 1980s and 1990s.
48. Lyndon B. Johnson Library, *White House Tapes*, Citation 3642 Wilbur Mills June 9, 1964, 9:55 AM. (telephone); Citation 3686 Larry O'Brien June 11, 1964, 3:55 PM.
49. Lyndon B. Johnson Library, *White House Tapes*, Citation 5444 Myer Feldman September 3, 1964, 11:14 AM.
50. Richard Harris, 1966, pp 187, 188.
51. Lyndon B. Johnson Library, *White House Tapes*, C.7141 John McCormack March 23, 1965, 4:54 PM. Rayburn, Johnson's mentor, had died four years earlier in November 1961.

52. LBJ Library. Lawrence F. O'Brien Oral History. Interview XI. July 24, 1986. By Michael L. Gillette. Internet Copy. Full quotation in Richard Harris, 1966, pp 190–1.
53. LBJ Library. Lawrence F. O'Brien Oral History, pp 24–5.
54. Wilbur Mills, Oral History, March 25, 1987.
55. Lyndon B. Johnson Library, *White House Tapes*, C.6718 Edward Kennedy January 9, 1965 11:32 AM.
56. Iserman and Kazin, p 109.
57. Richard M. Nixon, 1969.
58. Richard M. Nixon, 1971, Special Message to Congress Proposing a National Health Strategy.
59. For an outstanding account of HMOs in this period, see Brown, 1981.
60. December 21, 1976 memo from Pat Caddell.
61. Jimmy Carter, April 16, 1976.
62. Califano, 1981, p 98.
63. Califano, 1981, p 106.
64. Carter, April 25, 1977.
65. Quadagno, p 127.
66. Jimmy Carter, 1979.
67. WHCF Insurance, Box IS-2 Folder IS 1/20/77-1/20/81.
68. Interview conducted by the authors.
69. Lynn Etheridge, 1983.
70. For a description of DRGs see Morone and Dunham, 1985.
71. Cost shifting data from Oberlander, p 125.
72. President Reagan's talking points: p 1 [difficult session], 2 [lame duck], 6 [catastrophic].
73. WHOOF: Research Office. Radio Talk.
74. Ronald Reagan, July 25, 1987.
75. Sprinkle, June 15, 1988. T. Kenneth Cribb Jr, White House Staffing Memorandum. June 29, 1988.
76. Ronald Reagan, July 1, 1988.
77. Robert Grady Files. Box 14 Folder. Memoranda Concerning Various White House Initiatives Including Health Care 0A/ID 08841]; George H.W. Bush, Acceptance Speech delivered before the Republican National Convention. August 18, 1988.
78. *New York Times*, Associated Press, "House Panel Leader Jeered by Elderly in Chicago." Sunday, August 19, 1989. Stark and Waxman quoted in Quadagno, p 158.
79. Otis Bowen, 2001, p 60.
80. J. Kuttner Files. Box 28 Folder: DPC study.
81. 1992, Kuttner Files Backup {Disk: TTR-VOL0005/Director: TT-Jul006.004}. Health Care Issues. OA/ID 08768 Box 63.
82. J. Kuttner Files. Box 82 Health Care Reform—4/16/91 Kuttner, Porter Meeting on Status, Progress. OA/ID 09799.
83. Spencer Rich, *Washington Post*, September 4, 1991, A-7; Ann Devoy, *Washington Post*, September 26, 1991, 1.
84. Michael Decourcy Hinds, 1991; Hacker: p 10 (on 40 point lead).
85. George Bush, 1991.
86. Hacker, p 179.
87. Paul Starr, 1995, p 20–31.
88. William Jefferson Clinton, September 22, 1993. See the description in Clinton, 548–9.
89. Personal conversation, Senator Chaffee, March 1993.
90. In the 1970s, a reaction against the old Congressional barons like Wilbur Mills multiplied the number of committees and subcommittees and permitted action on the same bill in more than one committee.
91. Morone and Jacobs, 2005.
92. Clinton, 1994, p 620.
93. For an exception, see Paul Starr, 1995, "Was defeat inevitable? . . . I do not believe that. We had a historic opportunity and we blew it."
94. Peterson, 1990.

REFERENCES

Bryce, J. 1888. *The American Commonwealth*. London: Macmillan and Company.
Brown, L.D. 1983. Politics and Health Care Organization: HMOs as Federal Policy. Washington DC: Brookings Institution.
Burns, J.M. 2006. Running Alone: Presidential Leadership—JFK to Bush II. New York: Basic Books.
Califano, J. 1981. Governing America: An Insider's Report from the White House and the Cabinet. New York: Simon and Schuster.

Dalleck, R. 1996. *Hail to the Chief.* New York: Oxford University Press.

Dickinson, M. 2006. "The Executive Office of the President: The Paradox of Politicization," J. Aberbach and P. Peterson, eds. *The Executive Branch.* New York: Oxford University Press.

Etheridge, L. 1983. "Reagan, Congress and Health Spending." *Health Affairs* 2(1): 15–24.

Fraser, S. 2005. Every Man a Speculator: A History of Wall Street in American Life. New York: Harper.

Greenstein, F. 1982. The Hidden Hand Presidency: Eisenhower as a Leader. New York: Basic Books.

Hacker, J. 1997. *The Road to Nowhere.* Princeton: Princeton University Press.

Harris, R. 1966. *A Sacred Trust.* New York: New American Library.

Isserman, M., and M. Kazin. 2000. *America Divided: The Civil War of the 1960s.* New York: Oxford University Press.

Jacobs, L. 2006. "Communicating from the White House." J. Aberbach and P. Peterson, eds. *The Executive Branch.* New York: Oxford University Press.

Jacobs, L. and R. Shapiro. 2000. *Politicians Don't Pander.* Chicago: University of Chicago Press.

Jones, C. *The Reagan Legacy.* Chatham, NY: Chatham House.

Kingdon, J. 1984. Agendas, Alternatives and Public Policy. Boston: Little Brown.

Landy, M., and S. Milkis. 2001. *Presidential Greatness.* Lawrence: University Press of Kansas.

Light, P. 1982. The President's Agenda: Domestic Policy Choice from Kennedy to Carter. Baltimore: Johns Hopkins University Press.

Lowi, T.J. 1985. The Personal President: Power Invested, Promise Unfulfilled. Ithaca: Cornell University Press.

McCullough, D. 1992. *Truman.* New York: Simon and Schuster. p 473.

Marmor, T.J. 1973. *The Politics of Medicare.* Chicago: Aldine.

Milkis, S.M. 2003. *The President and the Parties.* New York: Oxford.

Morone, J. 2003. Hellfire Nation: The Politics of Sin in American History. New Haven: Yale University Press.

—— 1998. The Democratic Wish: Popular Participation and the Limits of American Government. New Haven: Yale University Press.

Morone, J., and A. Dunham. 1985. "Slouching to National Health Insurance: The New Health Care Politics," *Yale Journal of Regulation* II (2): 263–291

Peterson, M.A. 1990. Legislating Together: The White House and Capitol Hill from Eisenhower to Reagan. Cambridge: Harvard University Press.

Quadagno, J. 2005. One Nation Uninsured: Why the US Has no National Health Insurance. New York: Oxford University Press.

Schlesinger, A. 1973. The Imperial Presidency. New York: Popular Library.

Skowronek, S. 1993. The Politics Presidents Make: Leadership from John Adams to George Bush. Cambridge: Harvard University Press.

—— 2006. "Presidential Leadership in Political Time." M. Nelson, ed., *The Presidency and the Political System.* Washington DC: CQ Press.

Starr, P. 1982. The Social Transformation of American Medicine. New York: Basic Books.

—— 1995. "What Happened to Health Care Reform?" *The American Prospect* 20 (Winter): 20–31.

Thoreau, H.D. 1848. *On Civil Disobedience.* A lecture given at the Concord Lyceum [originally published, 1949]. Available on line at: http://www.gutenberg.org/etext/71 [last accessed March 30, 2007].

Weissert C., and W. Weissert. 1996. *Governing Health: The Politics of Health Policy.* Baltimore: Johns Hopkins.

CHAPTER 6

The Courts

Rand E. Rosenblatt[†]

Rand Rosenblatt explains how the courts fit into the American political process. He describes three different legal models that have defined both litigation and the health care system itself. Rosenblatt concludes by sketching a potential fourth model that may be emerging today.

American health law continues to be shaped largely by three familiar models. Each model was dominant in a particular historical period, although that dominance was usually contested by one or more of the other models. This chapter explores the nature and dynamics of the models with special reference to the courts. The most complete hegemony was achieved by the first model, *the authority of the medical profession*, from roughly 1880 to 1960. Under this paradigm, legal authority over virtually all aspects of health care delivery was delegated to the medical profession—indeed to individual physicians in private practice—and justified primarily by what was seen as doctors' scientific expertise.

A second model, which became dominant in health law from about 1960 to about 1980 and continues to the present, is that of the *modestly egalitarian social contract*. This paradigm holds that patients and society as a whole, as well as physicians and other stakeholders, have legitimate rights and interests in the health care system. The role of law in this model is to achieve a fair resolution of conflicting interests, especially in the light of highly unequal information and power between patients and other actors. Given this model's egalitarian values, fairness has typically been articulated as access to care largely on the basis of medical need, high quality of care, and respect for patient autonomy and dignity. By the standards of the rest of the developed world, notably western Europe and Canada, the American social contract has been limited and uneven—hence the phrase "modestly egalitarian."

A third perspective holds that however modest by international standards, the American social contract is far too regulatory and redistributive, and should be replaced by legal principles appropriate to full-fledged *market competition*. The function of law in this model is to ensure that choices about health insurance and health services are made by individuals based on their own financial resources (assuming they are above some specified minimum); some versions of the model seek to eliminate hidden "cross-subsidies"—the many ways in which wealthier (or better insured) patients pay higher prices to cover health care for poor (or uninsured) patients. Market proponents believe that individual (or aggregated individual) choice under financial constraint maximizes freedom and efficiency; people want to pay only for coverage or services that really benefit them, and providers will respond to such market pressure by economizing. The market competition model developed in the early 1970s began affecting policy very quickly and became the dominant paradigm in the 1980s and 1990s.[1]

Each of these three models continues to exercise influence in political and legal contexts. While it is unlikely that we would ever again delegate to doctors the sweeping authority they enjoyed before 1960, the ideal of the trustworthy, independent physician delivering the best possible medical care for her or his individual patients still has powerful appeal or, as some market advocates see it, pernicious influence.[2] Similarly, while the egalitarian social contract model has been subjected to relentless intellectual and political criticism, the idea of access to health care on the basis of medical need remains attractive, and the counter-vision of health care distributed according to ability to pay remains troubling for public opinion and explicit policy.[3] Yet, it is also true that many in more affluent socio-economic groups appear uncomfortable with the implications of universal coverage, and favor or at least acquiesce in some version of the market model. This is because their deepest commitment is to unrestrained access for themselves to the latest medical technology, combined with a fear that extending such access to all would be too costly and would result either in higher premiums and taxes and/or rationing applicable to everyone, including themselves.[4] The result is that all three perspectives actively contend for influence over numerous issues of health policy and law.

The struggle among the three models occurs in all the institutional and cultural venues where public policy and law take shape. While the most politically accountable branches of government—legislatures and the executive branch (including administrative agencies)—have the primary role in making law and policy, courts also play an important part. This is so for two basic reasons. First, the political branches expect and authorize the courts to make law, most obviously (in the context of health law) concerning liability for professional negligence. While legislatures could (and occasionally do) enact statutes governing this area of law, for the most part they have acquiesced in a centuries-old tradition under which judges make the substantive and procedural rules of liability in the course of deciding individual cases—what lawyers call "the common law."

Second, even where the political process has expressed itself through federal or state legislation ("statutes") or administrative regulations, the policy outcome is often ambiguous or unclear, because (1) contending political forces and perspectives are still in struggle; (2) the statute is striving to reconcile competing values (e.g., cost control versus access for underserved populations), and/or (3) the inevitably general language of a statute or regulation will have troubling or unclear implications when applied to particular situations, again reflecting the inevitable multiplicity of applicable social values, particularly in the area of health care. In short, legislative or administrative policies and rules do not implement themselves; they must be implemented by flesh and blood people in institutional roles, and in the United States the courts (together with administrative agencies) have been major places where such work is done. The legal name for this judicial function is "statutory (or regulatory) interpretation," i.e., deciding what the legislature's (or administrative agency's) law means in a particular case. To be sure, if the political branches disagree with a court's interpretation, the statute or regulation can be amended, but this requires formation of a new or clarified political consensus, which may or may not be possible.

The courts' interpretive function applies even more forcefully to cases involving the federal and state constitutions. Although the federal Constitution says nothing about health care, the broadly written guarantees of "equal protection of the laws" and no governmental deprivation without "due process of law" of "life, liberty, and property" have implications for such matters as access to contraceptives, choice regarding abortion and procreation, and the right to refuse life-prolonging care. The courts have played a central role in these matters.

In the early 21st century, it is possible that we will see a "fourth model" of health law and policy, and indeed of law and policy more generally. In part, this may be because the three major models have been unable to reconcile our society's (or at least its politically influential sectors) simultaneous and arguably contradictory values regarding health care in a credible and legitimate way: (1) solidarity and mutual aid, which in the United States is often understood as including unrestricted access to the most advanced medical technology; (2) efficiency and cost containment; and (3) no or minimal governmental interference with the ability of health care entrepreneurs, pharmaceutical companies, insurance companies, physicians, and other well-situated players to make very large incomes and profits.[5] Interacting with and transcending these conflicts are two other potential major components of a fourth model: globalization, which many see as having profound effects on the nation-state, democracy, and the feasibility and nature of a social contract; and what is known as "the biotechnology revolution," also expected to pose major dilemmas and have deep ramifications. As discussed later on the chapter, the meaning and direction of this new model is sharply contested.

Part One of this chapter explores the three major models of health law, including judicial opinions that exemplify each model's style of reasoning. Part Two considers briefly the debate about the possibilities of a "fourth model."

Two matters require some preliminary clarification. First, the term "social contract" is used in this chapter to refer to statutes and judicial doctrines that seek to articulate an explicitly social or political, as distinguished from what is known as a professional or market, conception of fairness and good policy. The phrase "modestly egalitarian social contract" emphasizes the social (primarily legislative or judicial) source of egalitarian legal norms, while not meaning to imply that the professional authority and market competition perspectives are not also socially created and authorized.[6]

Second, the notion of a model refers primarily to the assumptions, values, background norms, orientations, etc., of private and governmental decision makers. Thus, when I say that the professional authority model was dominant from about 1880 to about 1960, I mean that one can see the influence of the model in such contexts as legislation, judicial opinions, positions of the American Medical Association, and hospital bylaws and practices. Interestingly, at the time of their dominance, neither the professional authority nor social contract models generated a large and highly visible "advocacy" academic literature that sought to promote those models. In contrast, the market competition perspective has indeed generated such a literature, some of which distinguishes itself sharply from the "market model" that has actually been implemented as a matter of health law and policy.[7]

THREE MODELS OF HEALTH LAW

The Model of Professional Authority

The model of professional authority dominated health law and policy in the United States from about 1880 to about 1960.[8] During this period the main point of health law—its more or less conscious purpose—was to support the authority and autonomy of individual physicians engaged in the private practice of medicine. Thus the law allowed and even aided doctors to suppress salaried and prepaid financial arrangements, and to insist on being paid a fee for each discrete service, thereby maximizing physician control over the terms and amount of payment.[9] The law also gave doctors control over licensing standards and enforcement,[10] what patients they would accept,[11] hospital policies regarding doctors,[12] and what patients should be told about their treatment, if anything.[13] With respect to medical malpractice liability, judge-made common law defined the doctor's "standard of care" as the customary practices of the "ordinary" physician practicing in the same or similar locality.[14] In effect, a patient could only recover for injuries if a local colleague of the defendant doctor testified that he had committed negligence.[15] Needless to say, this was a requirement that usually could not be satisfied. This sweeping delegation of authority to physicians was later justified on a theory of "agency": the doctor could and should be trusted to act as the knowledgeable agent for the patient's well being.[16] At the time, the equation of the doctor's purported scientific expertise with sound public policy was so obvious as barely to merit discussion.

A paradigm case from the age of professional authority is Judge Benjamin Cardozo's 1914 opinion for the New York Court of Appeals in *Schloendorff v. Society of New York Hospital*.[17] The issue was whether the hospital had legal responsibility for an operation having been performed on a patient without her consent, despite the patient having made several efforts to explain to the resident physician, the nurse preparing her for the procedure, and the physician administering the anesthetic, that she was consenting only to an "examination" and not to an "operation."[18] While Judge Cardozo famously articulated the patient's right to decide what should happen to her own body,[19] the issue of *hospital* liability was a different matter.[20] Cardozo could imagine only one theory that supported hospital liability: that the hospital was the employer ("master") who controlled everyone involved in the treatment process, including the eminent surgeon who performed the operation. Since this seemed starkly contrary to actual fact—no hospital administrator (who in those days was typically not even a physician) would presume to "control" an eminent surgeon in the details of his work—it must follow that the hospital had no responsibility at all for any part of the process, including the alleged failure of the nurse (who was indeed the hospital's employee) to inform the surgeon of the patient's wishes.[21] Similarly, when a for-profit corporation established a low-cost clinic in Chicago in the 1930s where salaried and licensed physicians could treat patients, the Illinois

Supreme Court granted a request for an injunction by the Attorney General to shut the clinic down, on the theory that the corporation was practicing medicine without a license (and, of course, was not eligible to obtain a license, which could be granted only to individuals). The court summarily dismissed the corporation's argument that the corporation itself was not practicing or purporting to practice medicine, but only providing a place where the doctors would practice (and provide services at lower cost to patients who likely could not afford the charges of fee-for-service medicine).[22]

Strikingly absent in these "all or nothing" opinions is the possibility of shared or overlapping responsibility, so evident to modern eyes accustomed to looking at complex institutional structures and relationships. That a judge as thoughtful as Cardozo could not see this is a testament to the power of the professional authority model of health law. So strong was the belief in, and commitment to, the physician's authority over patient care, that any suggestion that the authority be shared was perceived as a complete denial of the physician's authority, and hence, unthinkable.

While providing doctors with sweeping control over health care, the professional authority model also set the limits of the problems it could solve, and therefore contained the seeds of its own fall from dominance. Three issues in particular were beyond its ken. The first was access to adequate (or any) care for people who could not afford fee-for-service medicine (which included most of the aged) and/or faced barriers such as race, ethnicity, and geography. "Charity" by hospitals and individual physicians was supposed to meet this need, but evidently could not, and even those who were served often received strikingly inferior care.[23] "The purpose of publicly sponsored and charitable health services . . . was primarily to protect the healthy, well-off population from the contagiously ill or socially disruptive poor, and to provide teaching material (in the form of patients) for medical education. '[The] health of the individual was secondary, if not incidental.'"[24] A huge number of people were effectively excluded from care, resulting in shock when the nation had to mobilize for

World War II and found that about 40% of the young men called were physically unfit to serve.[25]

Second, physician "self regulation" could not reliably achieve quality of care, or even police the most egregiously incompetent or impaired physicians. The mechanisms of self-regulation—professional and industry-administered accreditation standards and internal peer review by the hospital's medical staff—generated vague standards of care, poorly defined procedures, and overlapping and rotating committees that diffused responsibility.[26] To expect physicians who had bonded together during intense training, depended on each other for patient referrals and the financial viability of their hospitals, and shared a strong professional culture of perfectionism and resistance to criticism to police each other aggressively was fantasy on its face. The consequences could be extreme. For example, a hospital medical staff permitted a charming doctor to do complex spinal surgery for which he was totally unqualified. He persuaded patients who did not need the surgery to undergo it, paralyzed them through his incompetence, and then falsified the hospital records to hide his responsibility. The hospital's defense was that it had followed the standards and practices of the accreditation and peer review process designed and administered by the hospital industry and medical profession through the private Joint Commission on the Accreditation of Hospitals. Perhaps not surprisingly, a California trial judge found the system of professional authority inadequate in light of the socially defined standard of reasonable care.[27]

Third, the professional authority model had no internal mechanism for controlling costs, other than the vague and voluntary norms of professionalism. To be sure, as long as patients had to pay for most care out of their own pockets, their ability to pay operated as a check on doctors' fees. But as private health insurance, fueled by federal tax exemption, union contracts, and corporate desire to maintain employee loyalty spread during the 1940s and 1950s, patients' ability to pay was no longer limited by their immediate incomes. Thus, doctors' fees and hospitals' costs were free to, and did, rise sharply,

especially after the enactment of public health insurance (Medicare and Medicaid) in 1965.

The Model of the Egalitarian Social Contract

From the perspective of the modestly egalitarian social contract, unreviewable physician authority is seen as potentially dangerous and self-interested. To achieve fairness in health care access, quality, and financing in a context of inequality between patients and other actors (doctors, hospitals, insurance companies), the law must be able to define and enforce a "social contract," and thereby override professional and industry custom, practices, and contractual arrangements. To be sure, in many contexts professional or private standards or contracts would remain enforceable under this model, but only if they were seen as consistent with standards of need and fairness defined by courts, legislatures, and administrative agencies. For example, many state legislatures enacted laws requiring health insurers to cover the costs of at least some mental health care, thereby overriding the companies' private contracts that excluded it from coverage.[28] Similarly, in many states common law judicial doctrines, following the social contract model, have redefined informed consent in terms of what a reasonable patient would want to know, rather than what a reasonable physician would consider appropriate.[29] Other major components of the social contract model include the federal statutes creating social insurance for the elderly (Medicare) and a substantial number of the poor (Medicaid),[30] judicial doctrines recognizing legal rights for patients and providers in these programs,[31] and laws prohibiting discrimination in health care on the basis of race, gender, and disability.[32]

A number of paradigm cases, primarily in the 1950s and 1960s but extending both earlier and later, held that contrary to *Schloendorff*, hospitals may in appropriate cases share responsibility with physicians for quality of care and liability for negligence in treating patients.[33] The reasoning of these opinions both reflected and helped constitute the emerging social contract model of health law. Many factors contributed to this shift in the perspective of judges and other policy makers. For example, focusing only on health care delivery, the growth of Blue Cross and other forms of private health insurance, notably for hospitalization, from the mid-1930s onward transformed many formerly charity or near-charity patients into paying customers, giving hospitals a financial base for expansion and transformation. The federal Hill-Burton Act, which provided over four billion dollars in public funds for construction of public and private non-profit hospitals between 1946 and 1972, highlighted the societal importance of adequate hospital facilities and services.[34] Hospitals themselves, through the American Hospital Association and its state organizations, and (after 1951) through the Joint Commission on the Accreditation of Hospitals (JCAHO), issued standards and guidelines that proclaimed the "public service" nature of hospitals as institutions, and their corporate mission of providing high quality care.[35]

Perhaps equally important were the jurisprudential legacy of Legal Realism and the political legacy of the New Deal. Legal Realism encouraged judges to break out of the all-or-nothing categories of traditional legal doctrine, look at how institutions were actually functioning, and craft more flexible legal principles.[36] The political legacy of the New Deal included the view that liberty (and indeed democracy) were threatened when private markets did not enable people to meet basic human needs; that the inability to meet these needs on a large scale was not simply aggregated individual failing or the inescapable logic of the market, but was rather the product of an interdependent society, and that government could and should intervene in markets and institutions whose workings threatened fundamental well-being.[37] In 1957, the New York Court of Appeals overruled its *Schloendorff* precedent for these reasons. First, wrote Judge Fuld in *Bing v. Thunig*, hospitals had been transformed from arguably fragile charities to large, business-like institutions.

They regularly employ on a salary basis a large staff of physicians, nurses and internes

[sic], as well as administrative and manual workers, and they charge patients for medical care and treatment, collecting for such services, if necessary, by legal action. Certainly, the person who avails himself of 'hospital facilities' expects that the hospital will attempt to cure him, not that its nurses or other employees will act on their own responsibility.[38]

Second, social expectations about due care and fairness had changed. The idea that certain kinds of institutions and actors should be flatly immune from damages, and could cause harm without recourse, violated basic concepts of due care and accountability. "The rule of nonliability is out of tune with the life about us, at variance with modern-day needs and with concepts of justice and fair dealing."[39] Or, as the California Supreme Court stated in a 1963 opinion, a hospital's demand that patients sign a release from liability for future negligence as a condition of admission is unenforceable. "[T]he hospital cannot claim isolated immunity in the interdependent community of our time. It, too, is part of the social fabric, and prearranged exculpation from its negligence must partly rend the pattern and necessarily affect the public interest."[40]

Change in the common law liability of hospitals was only a small part of the social contract phenomenon. The crisis of western capitalism in the 1930s, the rise of fascism, and the defeat of and exposure to the horrors of Nazi Germany in World War II, among other large-scale factors, led to major changes in political and legal consciousness. There was widespread conviction, embodied in such diverse forms as the National Labor Relations Act of 1935, Universal Declaration of Human Rights of 1948,[41] the expansion of the European social welfare systems, and the movements to dismantle the European empires in Asia and Africa, that predatory hierarchies of many sorts were no longer acceptable. "Human rights" and "social rights," so long reserved primarily for the well-off and educated members of the (largely white and male) "political class," now had to be extended much more widely, although exactly how widely remained a matter of bitter contention. In the United States these trends found expression in the African American civil rights movement of the 1950s, 1960s, and beyond, the movements of other racial and ethnic groups, and the legal services, welfare rights, women's rights, disability rights, and gay rights movements of subsequent years. Judicial opinions, statutes, regulations, and legal scholarship using the social contract model in many areas were inspired by these social movements, and several generations of lawyers and legal academics, myself included, were mobilized into the field of health law through them.

The legacy of the egalitarian social contract can be found in a paradigm case from the United States Supreme Court which, though not itself about health law, established the principle that the rule of law applied to federal social welfare legislation generally, including (as held in subsequent cases) medical assistance for the poor (Medicaid).[42] In *Rosado v. Wyman*,[43] a bipartisan six-justice majority[44] opinion by then-considered conservative Justice John Marshall Harlan, stood for three important principles. First, statutes dealing with complex social policy issues (in *Rosado*, about cost-of-living adjustments to welfare eligibility standards) should be interpreted if at all possible as sources of meaningful law. Implicitly acknowledging the tendency of the political branches of government to underenforce and ignore legal provisions benefiting the poor and other politically weak groups, Justice Harlan said that courts (and agencies) should avoid reading statutes in ways that make them "a futile, hollow, and indeed, a deceptive gesture"[45]—laws that seem to promise something for the poor, but "really" mean nothing more than formal assurances and empty bureaucratic labels. Second, the statute may contemplate not a clear rule or benefit, but a process of structured or bounded discretion, in which a federal or state agency is supposed to take certain information and values into account. Such a "consideration rule" gives rise to a right of the ultimate beneficiaries to have that consideration take place. Third, statutes such as these, even when framed as conditions on federal funding to the states, can be treated as individual (and, through class actions, group) rights, enforceable in court directly against the relevant state decision

makers. Congress's delegation to a federal agency of authority to define and enforce these statutory conditions did not preclude direct judicial action against the states, unless Congress had clearly indicated such preclusion. This was particularly true where neither Congress nor the agency had given beneficiaries access to the administrative process or effective administrative remedies. "We are most reluctant," wrote Justice Harlan, "to assume that Congress has closed the avenue of effective judicial review to those individuals most directly affected by the administration of its program."[46]

The *Rosado* case reveals how different models or background assumptions about law (including the health law models that are the theme of this chapter) operate through interpretive norms such as "clear statement rules." Prior to the welfare rights developments of the late 1960s, the courts' background interpretive norm was that if a statute did not explicitly create a legal right for beneficiaries of government "privileges" (itself a loaded term, which included professional and industry licenses, government contracts and employment, and transfer payments such as cash and medical assistance), no legal right existed, and government had virtually unreviewable discretion to deprive the individual of what was often a critically important benefit or relationship. In other words, the "clear statement rule" of this sort disfavored implied legal rights in the context of government action, and required a "clear statement" by the legislature if a right were to be recognized. Such a norm was not politically "neutral"; it reflected the view that only interests created in the market (contract and property rights) deserved full legal protection. *Rosado* and its companion cases changed this background norm; market-based rights continued to receive full protection, but the new norm added that the needs and interests of the beneficiaries of government programs (often recognized in some way in the statutes) should be considered sources of legal rights and standards to the extent possible, and a new "clear statement rule" required Congress to state clearly that it did *not* want to recognize rights of a program's beneficiaries.[47]

The social contract model speaks to most areas of health care delivery, ranging from financing and access to the meaning of quality and the nature of the physician-patient relationship. It does not provide formulas or easy answers; on the contrary, it asserts that these are matters of social and political choice broadly understood, informed by expertise and values relevant to health care delivery, but not to be resolved solely by the purportedly simple (but actually quite contested) metrics of "medical expertise" or "efficiency." In particular, the social contract model tends to see health insurance as social insurance, i.e., as a means of meeting the basic human need for health care with funds derived from the society or some large subgroup within it. The financial burden of health care is inevitably distributed unevenly, with sick or injured people facing far more costs than others.[48] In the social contract view, the goal of health insurance is to spread these costs as broadly as possible, so as to lower the per capita financial impact, reduce administrative expenses (no need for risk selection), and provide as many people as possible with reasonably-priced access to health insurance and health services against the largely random risks of illness and injury. To achieve this kind of universalism, or what Deborah Stone calls the "logic of solidarity" and mutual aid (see Chapter 1), payments into the system (through taxes, premiums, and patient out-of-pocket cost-sharing) have to be generally equal and affordable (and thus subsidized for lower-income enrollees), and benefits have to be as much as possible available to all on the basis of medical need, with minimal influence of "ability to pay, past consumption of medical care, or expected future consumption."[49]

Like the professional authority model before it, the social contract model, as it emerged in American health law and policy, was unable to solve three major, related problems. First, because of the considerable political power of the hospital industry and organized medicine, the major federal health insurance programs enacted in 1965—Medicare and Medicaid—had to acquiesce to hospital control of prices through payment of dramatically misnamed "reasonable costs," and (for Medicare) physician

control of prices through fee-for-service payment for "reasonable," "customary," or "prevailing" charges."[50] These mechanisms, which were substantially in place until the early 1980s, the absence of a strong constituency for restraint, and the high political costs of "control[ling] the incomes of all those with interests in the health care industry,"[51] made it impossible for the social contract model to constrain very rapid increases in prices and overall health expenditures. Second, as medical and pharmaceutical technology continued its explosive development, many began to believe that there needed to be some way to regulate or restrain use of the most expensive (and often experimental or at least not clearly proven beneficial) treatments. But the increasingly entrepreneurial and income-driven culture of doctors and hospitals precluded low-visibility rationing, and the framers of thesocial contract (political leaders and, to a lesser extent, judges) could find no acceptable political or legal basis for rationing.[52] Third, political leaders working with the social contract model were unable to devise a method of redistribution that would fund universal access and be politically acceptable to those who already had private health insurance—much of the middle class (including unionized blue-collar sectors) and more affluent socio-economic groups. Instead, programs such as Medicare and Medicaid had to rely primarily on relatively regressive tax bases—the federal payroll tax and out-of-pocket cost-sharing for Medicare, and (for the nonfederal share) state sales and income taxes for Medicaid. These limitations guaranteed various inadequacies in coverage and provider payment in both programs, as well as leaving over forty million people without health insurance. President Clinton attempted to solve these problems with a national health insurance proposal that ingeniously combined the social contract, market competition, and professional authority models, but was unable to mobilize the political support needed to overcome intense opposition.

The Market Competition Model

Advocates of market competition rose to prominence in the 1970s by launching two major attacks on the previously dominant professional authority and social contract models. First, they argued that both the scientific justification for professional authority and the public interest justification for the social contract were largely illusory, particularly as expressed in actual American health care policy. Most health care services were not matters of immediate life-and-death, nor scientifically validated as "necessary," but rather were matters of comfort and convenience, and should be properly treated as discretionary consumption.[53]

The asserted logic of solidarity or mutual aid largely functioned as a cover for self-interested and powerful groups to grab a monopolistic (in the case of doctors and hospitals) or otherwise unfair share of common resources. Hence, the profound inequity of tax-subsidized, employment-based health insurance, which allows the upper-middle class to avoid paying taxes on lavish employer-provided health insurance policies, while providing no benefit to low-wage workers whose employers offer no health insurance at all, and, according to Professor Clark Havighurst, provides much less benefit to lower-income insured workers who often lack the upper-middle class's social connections with elite doctors and aggressive sense of entitlement.[54] Second, the market advocates argued, in the classic fashion of all conservative arguments against equality and mutual aid,[55] that the egalitarian social contract model led to perverse and dysfunctional results, notably unrestrained cost increases and misallocation of resources. By severing the demand for health services from the individual's obligation to pay, tax subsidies and social insurance (including its private American version, community-rated Blue Cross/Blue Shield) supported consumption of decreasingly beneficial services, while denying desperately needed care to those with inadequate economic and political power to secure the benefits of politically-structured solidarity.

More generally, the market advocates denied that government regulation could provide any solution to the problems of equity and cost containment. Governmental or (as in the case of Blue Cross/Blue Shield) private nonprofit financing and regulatory programs are notoriously subject to "capture" by

powerful and well-organized interests (in this context, doctors and hospitals), as the history of Blue Cross/Blue Shield, Hill-Burton, Medicare, and Medicaid seemed to confirm. Moreover, governmental agencies lack the technical skills and political authority to influence the powerful forces of economic self-interest that operate in the health care industry. The market advocates proposed to solve two of the three problems that bedeviled the social contract model: cost containment and rationing. Both would be accomplished in the only way that, in this view, was politically acceptable to most Americans as well as pragmatically feasible: the market, which constrains costs through the pressures of competition and rations through the magic of "voluntary" consumer choice in response to price signals.[56] The third problem—universal access or health insurance—admittedly could not be solved through purely market means, because some redistributive mechanism had to be built in to subsidize access for low-income people. Even here, though, market advocates claimed that a dominant market principle would help. Once the market had achieved cost containment and rationing for most of the population, the redistributive task would be smaller and less politically controversial.

As with the earlier emergence of the social contract model, the political and intellectual rise of the market competition model was due to factors both internal and external to health care delivery. The inability of the social contract model to restrain annual double-digit increases in health care spending, epitomized by the Carter administration's proposal of and failure to enact hospital price controls, strongly reinforced a broader deregulatory movement in the health care context among economists, other policy experts, and politicians away from "command and control" approaches and in favor of market mechanisms.[57] The promarket, antigovernment phenomenon, like the social contract model before it, was also connected to larger and deeper forces. Such phenomena as suburbanization, the decline of manufacturing and organized labor, the reaction of many Americans against the movements for African American civil rights, feminism, and gay rights, the Watergate crisis, the cultural ferment of the 1960s and 1970s, and the deregulation of international finance and trade formed a complex brew in which a new conservative political coalition would arise that linked, more effectively than ever before, laissez-faire capitalism and social traditionalism (including religious fundamentalism and significant support for hierarchies of race, gender, and sexual orientation).

An idea critical to the market model is that the individual health care consumer experiences the true costs of her or his choices. The social insurance model wants to separate the consumption of health care as much as possible from the individual's ability to pay, and regards linking the two as largely irrational. The market competition model wants to intensify the connection. Thus two prominent law professor advocates of the market competition model, Clark Havighurst and James Blumstein, state that the appropriate test for evaluating a health care financing system's performance is whether "it give[s] reasonable individuals what they want *and only what they want*, in the sense that, understanding the alternatives, they would purchase it for themselves assuming their income is not below a certain level, perhaps the median in the population."[58]

The problem, according to the market advocates, is that the failure to tax employment-based health insurance or deduct its cost from employees' wages gives employees the false impression that both the insurance and health services are "free," thereby leading to inefficient overconsumption of health insurance and health care services. In terms of Havighurst's and Blumstein's criterion above, this overconsumption means that millions of Americans are receiving more health insurance and more health care services than they "really want," because what they "really want" can only be determined by how they would spend their money if they had to buy health insurance and health services with their own after-tax dollars. The goal of market reform is to reduce or eliminate the current tax exclusion of health insurance, and thereby drive middle-income people's insurance down to the level where it should properly be—at the level they will choose when they pay for it with their own after-tax dollars. They would then

experience individual responsibility for, and freedom of, their choices.[59] Of course, better-off people would be free to buy better insurance and services.

Having (by hypothesis) created millions of cost-conscious consumers searching for the best health insurance "deal," what kind of competition among insurers should be encouraged or required by law and policy? Interestingly, two of the most prominent academic market advocates—Alain Enthoven and Havighurst—reject what Enthoven calls "a completely free market" in favor of "rules to channel the competition along socially desirable lines,"[60]—a policy structure widely known as "managed competition."[61] Although Enthoven and Havighurst appear to differ somewhat on the relative roles of government and private entities, they both endorse standardized health insurance policies with a few tiers of benefits and co-payments, so that consumers can easily compare options and prices.[62] Both plans try to address a perverse incentive in health care markets: Competing health plans have a strong incentive to sign up healthier patients who will require fewer medical services permitting the plans to offer lower premiums. Enthoven would have government mandate open enrollment and community rating, so as to "require all insurers (or at least all those whose policies are eligible for tax subsidies) to accept the bad risks (the old, the sick, and the poor) along with the good risks (young, healthy, and affluent), and to charge them the same premium."[63] Havighurst would pursue somewhat similar goals through predominantly private "plan sponsors" (e.g., a large employer or coalition of smaller employers) operating under government-designed market incentives. In particular, Havighurst wants health plans to offer moderate income consumers something less than "first-class, state-of-the-art, American style medical care," which he refers to as a "health care Cadillac,"[64] and to encourage moderate income patients (through price reductions) to waive many or most of their legal rights under tort and contract law, as a way of further lowering the plan's price and freeing providers to engage in economizing practice styles.[65]

The market competition model has played out rather differently in the real world of health law and policy. One of the key components of Enthoven's and Havighurst's vision—the deterrence of preferred risk selection and channeling of price competition into some version of quality and efficiency—was not enacted into law and has otherwise largely failed to take place. On the contrary, the for-profit health insurance industry eagerly pursues low risk groups; risk selection, medical underwriting, and experience rating are the essence of a properly functioning market.[66] Health insurance is not seen as a social mechanism for paying for the health care needs of a population. Rather, insurance is seen as a transaction between two economically "rational" actors—an individual (or group of aggregated individuals) and an insurance company. Each of these actors is trying to achieve maximum economic utility. The individual (or group) wants the lowest possible price for the desired insurance coverage. The insurance company wants the maximum profit. The logic of this perspective leads to market fragmentation, the exact opposite of the universalism and solidarity of social insurance. In the market, individuals want to associate themselves with the lowest possible risk group, and exclude people with serious illnesses or other high cost characteristics. Insurance companies want to segregate risk pools as much as possible—the industry term is "actuarial fairness"—so as to charge low competitive prices to healthy groups and high, actuarially "appropriate premiums" to people with high-cost characteristics.[67]

A paradigm case for the market competition model of this sort is *McGann v. H. & H. Music Co.*[68] John McGann, an employee of H & H Music, discovered that he was afflicted with AIDS in December 1987 and soon submitted his first claims for reimbursement under the company's group health insurance policy, which provided for lifetime benefits up to one million dollars. In July 1988, the company informed its employees that it was not renewing its group health insurance policy, and that its new self-insured health plan included a $5,000 lifetime cap on benefits payable for AIDS-related (but no other) illnesses.[69] McGann sued H & H Music under section 510 of the federal Employee Retirement Income Security Act (ERISA),[70] arguing

that the $5,000 AIDS cap was directed specifically at him in retaliation for exercising his rights under the company's then-existing plan. To understand how the courts decided this case, some background about the very important ERISA statute is needed.[71]

Enacted in 1974 after a decade of congressional consideration, ERISA's primary focus was improving the security of retirement pension benefits for private (nongovernmental) employees. The ERISA statute also sought to improve the security of other types of employment fringe benefits, including health care, by requiring those administering such plans to act as "fiduciaries" for the plan's beneficiaries. Under this legal concept, those with discretion to invest or allocate plan resources must avoid self-enrichment and imprudent actions, and comply with the terms of the plan. The ERISA statute permitted individuals to appeal benefit denials to the federal courts, and recover the amounts that a court found to be due under the plan. The ERISA statute did not, however, require employers to offer a health (or any other) plan, nor (aside from pensions) specify what benefits had to be included. ERISA's remedy provisions were also (ambiguously) limited to "benefits under the plan," i.e., only the benefits provided in the plan itself. For pension benefits this might be an adequate remedy in most instances, but with respect to health care it was not; wrongly withheld health benefits can result in severe injury or death, after which providing the original benefit (e.g., a surgical procedure or hospital stay) is both irrational (a dead patient does not need the surgery) and inadequate.

In addition to the goal of improving employees' rights and security, a second policy agenda was added late in ERISA's legislative process. In the early 1970s, some state insurance departments had attempted to regulate and/or tax certain kinds of pension plans as a form of insurance, and a coalition of large corporations and unions sought federal preemption (i.e., prohibition) of state regulation. After the complex ERISA bills had passed the House and the Senate, and differences were being adjusted in Conference Committee, the bill's preemption provisions were greatly expanded. The Conference Committee's revised bill was then voted on by both

houses within ten days, with little discussion or understanding by most members of these momentous
changes. The result was that the final ERISA law had
a deeply schizophrenic quality: on the one hand,
promising to expand employees' rights and protections (and to some extent doing so), and on the
other hand, seeming (with considerable ambiguity)
to displace large areas of state law, regulation, and
remedies that actually provided protection.

Against this background, the employer's argument defending the $5,000 cap on AIDS-related
treatment was straightforward. The company conceded that the benefit reduction was prompted by
knowledge of McGann's illness and that McGann
was the only covered person then known to have
AIDS. Section 510 of ERISA indeed prohibited a
plan or employer from retaliating or discriminating
against an employee for exercising his rights *under
a plan*, but, the argument went, ERISA placed no
restriction on the employer *changing the plan*. Once
an employer had changed a plan in a procedurally
correct manner (as H & H Music had done, ERISA
requiring almost no procedure to complete the
change), employees no longer had any rights other
than those specified in the new plan, which, in this
case, included the AIDS cap. For the federal trial
and appeal courts, this was an easy case in the company's favor.

In fact, the case appeared easy only because of
the influence of the market competition model in
the minds of the judges. As suggested above, the
actual text of the statute and legislative history
was deeply ambiguous; on the one hand, pro-
claiming an expansion of employees rights and referring to the federal courts developing a federal
common law of fiduciary duty and equitable relief; on the other hand, setting forth seemingly
limited federal remedies and (ambiguously) pre-
empting much of state law. Judges using an egalitarian social contract approach would have given
priority (as the Supreme Court did in the *Rosado*
case) to the protective goals of the statute, and
could have interpreted the previously-existing
health plan (with the million dollar lifetime cap
for all illnesses) as containing an implied promise

not to "deselect" a known employee from the insurance pool, at least not without very clear notice
to the contrary—i.e., an egalitarian clear statement rule of the sort discussed above in connection with *Rosado*.[72]

But the Fifth Circuit Court of Appeals explicitly
stated that ERISA embodied the model of market
competition, in that "courts have no authority to
decide which benefits employers must confer upon
their employees; these are decisions which are
more appropriately influenced by forces in the marketplace and, when appropriate, by [other] federal
legislation."[73] Under this approach, the ERISA
statute's limited explicit requirements and remedies are given decisive weight, and the broader
phrases and goals are discounted, i.e., a "clear
statement" rule of the opposite sort that finds the
statutory language limiting rights and remedies
quite clear, and the broadly worded protective
goals legally insufficient.

A second paradigm case of the market competition model is *Corcoran v. United Health Care*.[74]
In this case, a physician recommended that a
woman be hospitalized for the final weeks of her
high-risk pregnancy, but a utilization review sub-
contractor (United Health Care) of the employer's
self-insured health plan refused payment approval, and authorized part-time at-home nursing
care instead.

This appears to be the kind of health insurer
cost–benefit discretion that Havighurst has in
mind. Hospitalization is obviously a very expensive
way to control for the risk of fetal distress. If there
were no scientific cost–benefit studies validating
hospitalization over less expensive part-time at-
home nursing care, the insurer should have the authority to pay only for the less expensive care so as
to keep premium costs within the employees' collective budget. The fact that while the patient was
at home and not attended by the nurse the fetus
went into distress and died is simply the incidental and voluntarily chosen result of the family's
limited resources, the legitimacy of which is
not (by hypothesis) challenged. It would be equivalent to someone dying in an automobile accident

"because" they were driving a lightweight, low-cost automobile, which was all they could afford. As long as the automobile had passed the standards of state safety inspection, no one could complain that their legal rights had been violated because others, with more money, could afford heavier and safer vehicles.[75]

To be sure, Havighurst strongly advocates contractual candor about the health plan's authority to make such decisions, so as to make higher risk contracts politically legitimate and legally enforceable (as they indeed turned out to be in *Corcoran* even with debatable candor).[76] Much to Havighurst's frustration, insurers seem to regard this as advice to commit marketing, liability, and provider-relations suicide.[77] Moreover, many moderate or lower-income people do not seem to accept riskier health care with the same grace that they appear to accept riskier automobiles.[78] The Corcorans' state law suit for damages claimed that United had been negligent in performing its role, which raised important questions about the nature of United's duty of care to patients, the applicable standard of care, and the qualifications of and procedures and criteria used by the personnel who denied authorization for the hospital stay.

The Fifth Circuit framed the key legal issue as whether United was making "medical decisions" about the care to be provided a particular patient or "benefit determinations" about what the plan would pay for.[79] Plan publications stressed both functions, and repeatedly stated that utilization review was based on "nationally accepted medical guidelines" and was "independent, professional review" that works "together with your doctor . . . to assure that you and your family receive the most appropriate medical care."[80] The Fifth Circuit reasoned that while United did make medical decisions, it did so "incident to benefit determinations," and therefore ERISA preempted any state-law damage action against it.[81] To allow such actions would impose costs varying among states on health plans using utilization review to achieve cost containment, thereby "decreasing the pool of funds available to reimburse participants" and contravening Congress's purported judgment

that state law not "interfere" with ERISA's "carefully constructed scheme of federal regulation."[82] The *Corcoran* court acknowledged that ERISA itself does not provide for any damages for "medical malpractice committed in connection with a plan benefit determination,"[83] and that therefore "the Corcorans have no remedy, state or federal, for what may have been a serious mistake."[84] The court found this "troubling for several reasons," notably that it eliminated a financial incentive for ERISA plans "to seek out the companies that can deliver both high quality services and reasonable prices,"[85] thereby implicitly encouraging health plans to use utilization reviewers who were dangerously committed to denying care. A judge following the egalitarian social contract model would very likely have said (as did Justice Harlan in *Rosado*) that Congress could choose such a dangerous policy, but that the courts would not interpret ERISA's ambiguities as meaning that Congress had done so—in short, a patient protective clear statement rule. In contrast, the Fifth Circuit held that the ERISA law was indeed sufficiently clear to block all remedies for a potentially serious wrong, and that any needed changes were up to Congress to make.[86] More than a decade after the *Corcoran* opinion, Congress, whose majority now appears quite committed to the market competition model with no regulatory safeguards, has not acted.

Like the other two models, the market competition model has been able to address some problems better than others. Its managed care dimension is widely credited with temporarily restraining increases in health care costs during the 1990s. Whether this can be accurately attributed to "market competition" is debatable; certainly the vision of numerous insurer-provider entities supplying consumers with elaborate information and cost-effective choices has not come to pass. What did happen was a shift in bargaining power, with physicians and hospitals losing power to relatively concentrated insurer-managed care entities who aggregated large numbers of "covered lives" and were, therefore, able to drive hard bargains over price and (to a less clear extent) utilization controls.[87] But while this version of market competition was able to implement some forms of cost containment and rationing, it was not able to convince the American people that these steps were legitimate. This was partly because the process was fragmented among numerous companies, often poorly administered and explained, and largely secret. In addition, the adamant refusal of managed care entities to subject themselves to legal accountability, while victorious in cases such as *Corcoran*, was disastrous from a political/public relations point of view, with audiences cheering negative portrayal of HMOs in popular movies such as the 1997 film *As Good As It Gets*.[88] Moreover, the most powerful argument for rationing—that it transfers resources from low-value (or even wasteful) to higher-value health care interventions[8]—could not be credibly made, because American law imposed no restraints on how the funds saved by rationing should be used, a phenomenon made clear by the high incomes paid to the leaders of the newly entrepreneurial health care "industry."[90]

In many respects, the academic versions of the market competition model have not been realized. In addition to the many reasons discussed by Havighurst and others, another is worthy of note: there is a political contradiction within the market model itself—the extensive regulation of the market needed to achieve the social values of managed competition, and the proposed subsidies for lower-income patients, are inconsistent with the laissez-faire political values and interests associated with a promarket regime. These values and interests oppose redistributive subsidies and pro-consumer market regulation and favor unprecedented tax cuts and redistribution upwards to the wealthy.[91] Indeed, this is the version of "market competition" that has been implemented: a considerable shift of wealth and power from physicians and hospitals to employers, managed care entrepreneurs, and others imposing cost containment, while denying hospitalization to some patients who need it,[92] and denial of most or all coverage to some easily targeted high cost patients with serious illnesses, disabilities, and chronic conditions.[93] As numerous analysts have observed, the future of managed care is quite unclear—indeed, it has been widely pronounced "dead"[94]—and some observers expect it to be replaced, at least for significant

numbers of employees, with "consumer-driven" health coverage characterized by some combination of high deductibles and cost-sharing, defined contribution by employers, and employee web-facilitated choice among price tiers of coverage and providers.[95] These mechanisms will almost certainly further "separate[e] the fates of people in society on various bases, including wealth, age, employment status and geography," "impai[r] the movement toward systemic improvement of health care [quality],"[96] and diminish our experience of compassion and social responsibility.[97]

A FOURTH MODEL FOR HEALTH LAW?

Recent developments within American health care delivery seem to point in two different directions. The failure to achieve a socially-responsible versions of managed competition—informed and (where needed) subsidized consumers choosing among plans competing (under public or private "regulation") over quality and efficiency—may well lead to a far less structured and egalitarian, and hence more dangerous, market. Poorly subsidized, perhaps risk-selected, and financially stressed consumers must then "accept" high cost sharing, crudely-framed benefit exclusions, and low-cost providers with little understanding of what they are getting. Alternatively, as sharply rising health care (notably pharmaceutical) costs and health insurance premiums,[98] as well as massive losses of well-paid jobs with benefits,[99] push many lower-middle and middle-middle class citizens into the ranks of the uninsured or underinsured,[100] the political demand for governmental action of an egalitarian and regulatory sort may intensify.

The sense of a great fork in the road between hyperindividualism and unrestrained competition, on the one hand, and some way of reconstituting solidarity and associated social policies, on the other, is also reflected in the great uncertainty about the complex forces known in shorthand as "globalization." For many, globalization is seen as embodying and validating market competition and raising it to a level of awesome, unprecedented power. In one starkly stated version, internationalized markets in capital and production, together with internationalized culture and communications, are said to have made the classic "nation-state," democratic politics, social welfare policies, and law itself virtually obsolete.[101] National governments can no longer enforce policies to better the economic welfare of their citizens; protectionism, high wages, taxes, and transfer payments are, the argument goes, subject to effective veto by capital, which can move itself and jobs to other nations with great speed.[102] Moreover, even aside from capital's "exit" option, governmental regulation and transfers have lost much of their policy credibility, as the advocates of the market revolution in health care argued in the 1970s and 1980s. Thus, there is little for politics or law to decide, because "supporting the market" is the only policy that is both empirically feasible and consistent with the new transcendent value of "individual liberty." In this view, then, there is no distinct fourth model of health law or anything else; the market competition model has triumphed decisively.

The market forces associated with globalization are undeniable, although their actual extent and impact, particularly in the United States, are open to much debate. More fundamental is the question of how political and legal systems can and should try to interact with those forces.[103] It is evident even to celebrators of globalization's benefits, such as Thomas L. Friedman of the *New York Times*, that pure markets are incoherent and self-destructive; left to their own logic, they cannot create the social cohesion, long-term investment in human capital, and rule of law that they need for their own survival and flourishing. Visiting post-genocide Rwanda in 1996 with then-US ambassador to the United Nations Madeleine Albright, Friedman

started to get mad . . . about the budget debate that was then going on in the U.S.

Congress. . . . [W]hen I listened at that time to the infamous 1994 class of freshmen Republicans, I heard mean-spirited voices . . . voices for whom the American government was some kind of evil enemy. I heard men and women who insisted that the market alone should rule, and who thought it was enough to be right about the economic imperatives of free trade and globalization, and the rest would take care of itself. I heard lawmakers who seemed to believe America had no special responsibility for maintaining global institutions, such as the UN, the World Bank, and the IMF, which are critical for stabilizing an international system from which America benefits more than any other country. . . .

[The freshmen Republicans] should come to war-torn Africa and get a real taste of what happens to countries where there is no sense of community, no sense that people owe their government anything, no sense that anyone is responsible for anyone else, and where the rich have to live behind high walls and tinted windows, while the poor are left to the tender mercies of the marketplace.

I don't want to live in such a country, or such a world. It is not only morally wrong, it will become increasingly dangerous.[104]

Those who struggle against the unregulated market vision hope that globalization can develop as a kind of extended postmodernism that will undermine not only national boundaries, but all sorts of familiar categorical oppositions, including "state regulation" and "free markets." If "government" is indeed morphing into a branch of "the market," so are "markets" morphing into government, with for-profit companies running public schools, prisons, military logistics, and much of the health care system, including a considerable portion of Medicare and Medicaid.

Proponents of a new, what I would call "fourth model," of health law and policy argue that the true logic of globalization should not be understood as unregulated market competition, but as a much more interesting, creative, and sophisticated mix of market techniques, institutional interaction, and democratic participation.[105] Thus Carolyn Hughes Tuohy explores in the health care context (albeit with substantial reservations) new techniques known as "governance" in which "government actors exercise influence not through command and control but through negotiation and persuasion" "in the context of complex organizational networks."[106] James A. Morone and Elizabeth H. Kilbreth argue that "[a] changing social environment—marked by globalization, immigration, a culture war, and managed care—could be addressed by robust, local, democratic health reforms."[107] William M. Sage sees the health care delivery system as characterized by "incomplete transformations"—"to industrial organization, informed consumerism, and universality," and, therefore, driven to policy outcomes in less than optimal litigation and judicial decisions.[108] In these circumstances, Sage suggests empowering "various subsystems of 'cabined discretion' apart from the courts."

These would be decision-making bodies in institutions, geographic areas, or subject matters whom users would value for their judgment and virtue as well as their expertise. No single entity would dictate overall policy, and each entity would be influenced by some combination of user exit and user voice in addition to the decision maker's loyalty. An entity charged with establishing a schedule of damages to be paid on a no-fault basis for avoidable injuries in lieu of malpractice litigation would be a good test of this model.[109]

Whether any of these or other innovations is pursued evidently depends on initiatives and developments at all levels of politics and society.

The existing and still-to-come biotechnology revolution underscores in the most dramatic way the need for new frameworks of social conversation and choice. Genetic privacy, access to health and life insurance, and employment discrimination raise serious issues.[110] The prospect of well-off members of society purchasing for themselves or their children genetically or chemically-enhanced health, beauty, athletic ability, intelligence, memory, and the like—something that of course already exists in a number of ways—raises profound issues of equality, freedom, and democracy, as well as our experience of "human nature."[111] Some advocates of free market or "entrepreneurial" globalization see our government and society as being constituted in a new form—a "market-state"—characterized by "sublime indifference" to "who should be allowed to grow taller or be endowed with perfect pitch . . . ."[112]

> [T]he basis for human assessment in the various competitions of the meritocracy [is shifting] from a passive acceptance of inherited abilities to a quest for the enhanced, or engineered, faculties made possible by molecular biology. Here, too, the market-state's apparent indifference to the state's role in ensuring justice fits the new, wide-open landscape of apparent opportunity. A State that tried to sort out who [should have access to biological enhancement] would soon find itself hopelessly overcommitted financially or the center of group warfare. . . . The market-state, with its sublime indifference to such questions and its refusal to guarantee outcomes, is more survivable in the new world of genetic technologies. These technologies have the power to enhance autonomy as never before, freeing men and women from their own genes, and providing choices only dreamt of until now.[113]

Since Bobbitt assumes that we cannot afford to grant this revolutionary new autonomy to everyone, and accepts with enthusiasm that it should be distributed according to the market, i.e., ability to pay, this freedom is that of the privileged to become stronger and more privileged in the most profound ways. Perhaps needless to say, such a vision is disturbing not only to political liberals who value equality and democratic participation, but also to many political conservatives who favor traditional liberties, and who oppose human intervention in what is regarded as the natural order, on religious or other grounds. Thus Francis Fukuyama, once considered a leading "neo-conservative" who celebrated the triumph of capitalism over the Soviet Union as "the end of history,"[114] has now decided that history is not quite over.

We do not have to accept any of these future worlds [e.g., "far more hierarchical and competitive," or a "soft tyranny envisioned in *Brave New World*"] under a false banner of liberty. . . . We do not have to regard ourselves as slaves to inevitable technological progress when that progress does not serve human ends. True freedom means the freedom of political communities to protect the values they hold most dear, and it is that freedom that we need to exercise with regard to the biotechnology revolution today.[115]

The biotechnology revolution will thus pose for us with stark consequences the question that "the market revolution" in health care thought it had already answered: do we as a "political community" have values that we "hold most dear," and what are they? Or are we primarily (exclusively?) an aggregation of individuals for whom the meaning of freedom is choice within the scarcity of each person's "own" resources? The fact that we are, or will be, facing this question is itself a remarkable commentary on our recent history. The courts will presumably not be the primary arenas in which the battles over these issues will be fought, but as the institutionalized embodiment of our traditional values (themselves contested) associated with the rule of law, fairness, and individual integrity, they may well play a significant role.

STUDY QUESTIONS

1. What are the three historical periods in health law?
2. Which model do you find most desirable? Why?
3. What factors led to the "downfall" of each model?
4. What evidence points to the emergence of a fourth phase in health law? What might this new model look like?
5. Describe one decisive court case from each of the models. Describe either how the case shapes health policy in the United States or how it illustrates the model of the era.
6. What is the role of the judicial branch been in the formation of health policy, as compared to the other two branches (legislative and executive)?
7. How have broader societal and intellectual trends shaped developments in health law?

NOTES

† Professor of Law, Rutgers University School of Law—Camden. Some of this material was published as "The Four Ages of Health Law," *Health Matrix* 14: 155 (2004).

1. For my own earlier discussions of these models, see Rand E. Rosenblatt et al., 1997, pp 2–3, 24–35, 131–5, 823–4; Rand E. Rosenblatt, 1998, p 147 *passim*; Rand E. Rosenblatt, 1988, p 489. For structures that are conceptually similar, see Einer Elhauge, 1994, pp 1451, 1452; James A. Morone, 1993, pp 723, 723; *Cf.* M. Gregg Bloche, 2003, pp 247, 253–4; Mark A. Hall, 2002, pp 463, 465–6.

2. For example, Clark C. Havighurst, 2002, pp 72–3.

3. On recent public attitudes, see Elizabeth A. Pendo, 2004, p 267. In addition, Alain Enthoven, a prominent advocate of a market competition approach to health care delivery, wrote in 1980 that "[m]ost Americans consider access to a decent level of medical care to be part of the right to 'life, liberty, and the pursuit of happiness.' Thus we are not willing to leave the distribution of medical purchasing power to the market and other forces that determine income distribution." Alain C. Enthoven, 1980, p 81. See also Timothy

Stoltzfus Jost, 2003, pp 23–109 (2003); Deborah Stone, 1999, pp 1213, 1214–7.

4. See, e.g., James A. Morone, 1999, pp 887, 891. See also David J. Rothman, 1997, pp 4–6.

5. *See generally* Robert G. Evans, 1997, p 427; Mark V. Pauly, 1997, p 467; Robert G. Evans, 1997, p 503. For a pervasive sense of political and policy complexity, drift, denial, and paralysis in the health care sector (albeit with some contributors perceiving or advocating various ways forward), see *Special Conference Issue: Who Shall Lead?*, 2003, pp 181–24.

6. See, e.g., Stone, *supra* note 3, at 1216–7; Karl Polanyi, 1944; David M. Frankford, 1992, pp 1, 9–10 [hereinafter *Privatizing Health Care*].

7. See, e.g., Havighurst, *supra* note 2, at 72–4; James Maxwell and Peter Temin, 2002, p 5.

8. For a comprehensive and brilliant presentation of the origins and rise of this model see Starr, *supra* note 6, at 79–378.

9. *See* Paul Starr, 1982, pp 198–34.; People *ex rel.* Kerner v. United Med. Service, Inc., 200 N.E. 157 (Ill. 1936) (ordering closure of for-profit clinic that wished to employ doctors on a salaried basis).

10. E.g., Rosenblatt et al., *supra* note 1, at 968–9.

11. See *Hurley v. Eddingfield*, 59 N.E. 1058 (Ind. 1901) (holding that neither state licensure nor the common law limits a physician's freedom to refuse to render services to any person seeking to employ the physician).

12. See, e.g., *St. John's Hosp. Med. Staff v. St. John Reg.'l Med. Ctr.*, 245 N.W.2d 472, 473–4 (S.D. 1976) (finding bylaws created and passed by the medical staff could not be altered by the hospital's board of directors without the consent of the medical staff).

13. E.g., Rosenblatt et al., *supra* note 1, at 890–1 (listing sources).

14. See, e.g., *Small v. Howard*, 128 Mass. 131, 132 (1880), discussed in Rosenblatt, et al., supra note 1, at 843–4.

15. See Jon R. Walz, 1969, pp 408, 410–11.

16. See, e.g., Carolyn Hughes Tuohy, 2003, pp 195, 197.

17. 105 N.E. 92 (1914). Judge Cardozo was one of the greatest American common law judges and several of his opinions from the early 20th century remain keystones of contemporary first year legal education.

18. The patient's allegations were not surprisingly contested by the doctors and nurses, but since the hospital had won in the trial court under a procedure that assumed the truth of the patient's allegations, the appeals court also had to assume their truth. *Id.* at 93.

19. "Every human being of adult years and sound mind has a right to determine what shall be done with his own body; and a surgeon who performs an operation without his patient's consent commits an assault, for which he is liable in damages." *Id.*

20. The statement in note 24, *infra*, evidently contemplates potential liability for the surgeon, but there is no discussion in Cardozo's opinion of any lawsuit against or settlement with the surgeon who performed the operation. If indeed the surgeon was not sued, one can speculate about the reasons, including the possibility that the patient may not have spoken directly to the surgeon, and therefore was relying on hospital employees such as the nurses, or on arguable agents of the hospital such as the anesthetist, to convey her message.

21. See *id.* at 94–5.

22. People ex rel. Kerner v. United Med. Service, Inc., 200 N.E. 157, 163–4 (Ill. 1936).

23. See generally Starr, *supra* note 6, at 262.

24. Rand E. Rosenblatt, 1975, pp 643, 644.

25. See Rand E. Rosenblatt, 1978, pp 243, 264–5.

26. See Rosenblatt et al., *supra* note 1, at 927–8, 933–4; K. J. Williams, 1976, p 401.

27. *Gonzales v. Nork*, No. 228566 (Super. Ct. Cal. Nov. 19, 1973), reprinted, in part, in Sylvia Law and Steven Polan, 1978, pp 215–45.

28. See, e.g., *Metro. Life Ins. Co. v. Mass.*, 471 U.S. 724 (1985) (holding that a Massachusetts state statute mandating coverage of mental health benefits in health insurance contracts is not preempted by ERISA); *UNUM Life Ins. Co. of Am. v. Ward*, 526 U.S. 358 (1999) (holding

that a state judicial doctrine that permits insurers to deny claims on grounds of lateness as defined by the policy only if they can show actual prejudice not preempted by ERISA).

29. E.g., *Canterbury v. Spence*, 464 F.2d 772, 780–3 (D.C. Cir. 1972).

30. See, e.g., Rosenblatt, Law, and Rosenbaum, *supra* note 1, at 14–16, 368–410 (Medicare), 410–66 (Medicaid).

31. See, e.g., *Duggan v. Bowen*, 691 F. Supp. 1487 (D.D.C. 1988) (Medicare); *Wilder v. Virginia Hosp. Ass'n*, 496 U.S. 498 (1990) (Medicaid). See generally Rand E. Rosenblatt, 1993, p 439; Sara Rosenbaum and David Rousseau, 2001, p 7.

32. See, e.g., *Bryan v. Koch*, 627 F.2d 612 (2d Cir. 1980); Sara Rosenbaum and Joel Teitelbaum, 2003, p 215; *Newport News Shipbuilding & Dry Dock Co. v. EEOC*, 462 U.S. 669 (1983) (applying the Pregnancy Discrimination Act, 42 U.S.C. § 2000e(k)); *Olmstead v. L.C.*, 527 U.S. 581 (1999) (applying the Americans with Disabilities Act, 42 U.S.C. §§ 12101–12213).

33. In addition to *Bing v. Thunig*, 143 N.E.2d 3, 8–9 (N.Y. 1957), see *President and Dir. of Georgetown Coll. v. Hughes*, 130 F.2d 810 (D.C. Cir. 1942) (abolishing charitable immunity for hospitals); *Darling v. Charlestown Cmty. Hosp.*, 211 N.E.2d 253, 260 (Ill. 1965) (applying corporate liability to hospital); *Thompson v. Nason Hosp.*, 591 A.2d 703, 708 (Pa. 1991) (same).

34. See Rosenblatt, *supra* note 30, at 264–70.

35. See Rosenblatt et al., *supra* note 1, at 917, 931.

36. See Rand E. Rosenblatt, 1970, pp 1153, 1165–72 (1970) (discussing Legal Realism).

37. See, e.g., *West Coast Hotel v. Parrish*, 300 U.S. 379, 391 (1937) (upholding State's minimum wage for women as a valid constitutional restriction of contractual liberty, because "the liberty safeguarded [under the Due Process Clause of the 14th Amendment] is liberty in a social organization which requires the protection of law against the evils which menace the health, safety, morals, and welfare of the people");

Franklin D. Roosevelt, 1995, pp 290, 294–5 ("We have accepted, so to speak, a second Bill of Rights . . . . [a]mong these [rights] are: [t]he right to a useful and remunerative job . . . ; [t]he right to earn enough to provide adequate food and clothing and recreation . . . ; [t]he right of every family to a decent home; [t]he right to adequate medical care and the opportunity to achieve and enjoy good health; [t]he right to adequate protection from the economic fears of old age, sickness, accident, and unemployment; the right to a good education.").

38. 143 N.E.2d 3 (N.Y. 1957)

39. *Id*. at 9.

40. *Tunkl v. The Regents of the Univ. of Cal.*, 383 P.2d 441, 449 (1963).

41. Article 25(1) of the Declaration provides that "Everyone has the right to a standard of living adequate for the health and well-being of himself and his family, including food, clothing, housing, and medical care and necessary social services, and the right to security in the event of unemployment, sickness, disability, widowhood, old age or other lack of livelihood in circumstances beyond his control." For discussion of this Article and the movement for international human rights as it relates to health care, see Farmer, *supra* note 7, at 213–46.

42. See, e.g., *Bass v. Rockefeller*, 331 F. Supp. 945 (S.D.N.Y. 1971) (holding that the Social Security Act protects Medicaid recipients from state modifications that would reduce benefits without federal approval); *Bass v. Richardson*, 338 F. Supp. 478 (S.D.N.Y. 1971) (holding that the state could not cut Medicaid benefits without showing that § 1902(d) has been met); *Wilder v. Virginia Hosp. Assn.*, 496 U.S. 498 (1990) (holding that mandatory provisions of the Medicaid Act create rights enforceable under 42 U.S.C. § 1983).

43. 397 U.S. 397 (1970).

44. Justice Harlan's opinion was joined by his fellow Republican Potter Stewart, liberal Democrats William Douglas, William Brennan, and Thurgood Marshall, and conservative Democrat Byron White. New Deal Democrat

Hugo Black and Republican Warren Burger dissented. There were eight justices on the Supreme Court at that moment rather than the usual nine.

45. *Rosado,* 397 U.S. at 415.

46. *Id.* at 420 (finding that state welfare provisions are judicially reviewable). For additional discussion of the *Rosado* principles, their incorporation into social welfare and health law, and the attack on them by Chief Justice Rehnquist and his colleagues, see Rand E. Rosenblatt, 1993, p 439.

47. For more on these developments, see Rand E. Rosenblatt, 1990. Egalitarian clear statement rules have been challenged and cut back by the Supreme Court under Chief Justice Rehnquist. See Rosenblatt, *supra* note 38.

48. *See* Jost, *supra* note 3, at 8–9.

49. Deborah Stone, 1993, pp 287, 290.

50. See, e.g., Starr *supra* note 6 at 374–8; Theodore Marmor, 1973, 85–6.

51. Starr, *supra* note 6, at 412.

52. For examples and discussion of judicial and political reaction to insurers' efforts to deny payment for expensive care of an arguably debatable benefit—high dose chemotherapy with autologous bone marrow transplants for various stages of breast cancer—see Rosenblatt et al., *supra* note 1, at 224–37, 251–61 and Rosenblatt et al., 2001–02, pp 196–213.

53. See Charles Fried, 1983, pp 527–9; Clark C. Havighurst and James Blumstein, 1975, pp 6, 12.

54. See Havighurst, *supra* note 2, at 86–7, 92–4.

55. See *generally* Albert O. Hirschman, 1991.

56. See Enthoven, *supra* note 3, at 102–3, 111–13.

57. See, Starr, *supra* note 6, at 412–13; Enthoven, *supra* note 3, at 97–101. S*ee also* Clark C. Havighurst, 1995, p 98 [hereinafter *Health Care Choices*]; *cf.* Robert Kuttner, 1996, pp 34–37. Detailed accounts of the rise of the market competition perspective can be found in Gail B. Agrawal and Howard R. Veit, 2002, pp 11–36, and James C. Robinson, 2003, pp 341–46.

58. Havighurst & Blumstein, *supra* note 63, at 15–16 (emphasis in the original).

59. See Fried, *supra* note 63, at 529–30. For a critique of this vision of freedom, see *Privatizing Health Care*, *supra* note 12, at 10, *passim*.

60. Enthoven, *supra* note 3, at 78. See also Clark C. Havighurst, 1976–7, pp 471, 490–1.

61. "Managed competition" must be distinguished from the similarly-named "managed care." As explained above in the text, "managed competition" is the effort to "structure" competition among health plans and providers through rules or law to achieve specified goals or values. "Managed care" is a more fluid term that generally refers to the effort to structure the clinical relationship between providers and patients to achieve specified goals, often cost containment.

62. Enthoven, *supra* note 3 at 127–9; Health Care Choices, *supra* note 69, at 26.

63. Enthoven, *supra* note 3 at 80.

64. Health Care Choices, supra note xx, at 104.

65. *Id.* at 266, 303–19.

66. See generally Stone, *supra* note 57; see also Deborah Stone, 1990, pp 385, 388–91 [hereinafter *Rhetoric of Insurance Law*].

67. Stone, *supra* note 57, at 290. For arguments in favor of risk rating, see *Rhetoric of Insurance Law*, *supra* note 84, at 392–3; Kenneth J. Arrow, 1963, pp 942, 963–4. For arguments against risk rating, see David M. Frankford, 1993, pp 351, 365–71 [hereinafter *Neoclassical Health Economics*]); Bryan Ford, 1994, pp 109, 110–20. See also, Mark V. Pauly, 1992, pp 137.

68. 946 F.2d 401 (5th Cir. 1991), *cert. denied*, 506 U.S. 981 (1992).

69. Other changed characteristics of the new plan included "increased individual and family deductibles, elimination of coverage for chemical dependency treatment, adoption of a preferred provider plan and increased contribution requirements." *Id.* at 403 n.1.

70. ERISA, 29 U.S.C. § 1140 (2000) (prohibiting discrimination against a participant or

beneficiary who exercises any right she is entitled to under an employee benefit plan).

71. The following discussion of ERISA is drawn from Rosenblatt et al. *supra* note 1, at 159–61, 173–7, 196, and sources cited therein.

72. To understand this argument, imagine that before McGann accepted the job with H & H Music, he had asked about the health benefits. Assume that the company spokesperson had replied: "You will have one million dollars in lifetime health coverage, except if you develop an unusual and expensive condition we may re-design the plan to limit severely your benefits for that condition." McGann and many other prospective employees might have refused such job conditions, and the company's failure to make this clear may have helped induce McGann to accept these conditions unknowingly.

73. *Id.* at 407 (quoting *Moore v. Reynolds Metals Co. Ret. Program for Salaried Employees,* 740 F.2d 454, 456 (6th Cir. 1984)). Arguing (successfully) against Supreme Court review, the Solicitor General stated that while ERISA did not regulate employers' design of plan benefits, the Americans with Disabilities Act (ADA), 42 U.S.C. §§12101 et seq. (enacted in 1990 and hence not applicable to the events in *McGann*) could resolve the problem. See Robert Pear, 1992, A18. While the Equal Employment Opportunity Commission indeed interpreted the ADA as prohibiting disease-specific caps in most circumstances, see 1993 Daily Lab. Rep. (BNA) 109 d22 (June 19, 1993), the federal courts have rejected this view on the ground that the ADA's provisions that seem to regulate insurance policies are not sufficiently clear, i.e., an antiregulatory or anti-egalitarian clear statement rule. See, e.g., *Doe v. Mutual of Omaha Ins. Co.,* 179 F.3d 557 (7th Cir. 1999). .

74. 965 F.2d 1321 (5th Cir. 1992), *cert. denied,* 506 U.S. 1033 (1992).

75. *See* John A. Siliciano, 1991, pp 439–40.

76. Havighurst, *supra* note 2, at 96–100.

77. *Id.* at 100. Havighurst also criticizes the managed care industry for not having been candid

with and for not having educated consumers during the more politically favorable 1980s when cost savings were also much easier to achieve. *Id.* at 74–7.

78. Havighurst sees consumers' false consciousness on this point as based on their continued insulation from the actual costs of their care, and hence neither their economic nor political choices "reveal their true preferences." *Id.* at 78.

79. *Corcoran,* 965 F.2d at 1329–31.

80. *Id.* at 1323–4.

81. *Id.*

82. 965 F.2d at 1331.

83. *Id.* at 1333. The argument that tort damages for seriously injured patients must be precluded so as to preserve the limited pool of available funds was previously used to bar charitable patients from recovery under the doctrine of charitable immunity for hospitals. For reasons why this doctrine was abandoned, see *President and Dir. of Georgetown Coll. v. Hughes,* 130 F.2d 810, 822–3, 827 (D.C. Cir. 1942). For reasons why ERISA's express preemption provision, ERISA §514, should not be regarded as "carefully constructed," see, e.g., Rosenblatt, Law, and Rosenbaum, *supra* note 1, at 173–7. For reasons why ERISA's remedies provisions, notably ERISA §502, as interpreted by the Supreme Court, are widely regarded as conceptually erroneous and a policy disaster, see, for example., *Cicio v. Does,* 321 F.3d 83, 106 (2d Cir. 2003) (Calabresi, J., dissenting in part).

84. Corcoran, 965 F.2d at 1333.

85. *Id.* at 1338.

86. *Id.* at 1338.

87. *Id.* at 1338–9.

88. See Havighurst, *supra* note 2, at 58–64. See also Agrawal and Veit, *supra* note 69, at 41–42 who argue that managed care slowed health care spending, particularly from 1993 to 1998 (but not thereafter), reduced hospital lengths of stay, encouraged more outpatient procedures, and held down payments to providers.

89. See Clark C. Havighurst, 2001, p 395; Pendo, *supra* note 3 who describes audience response

to *As Good As It Gets* and extensively analyzes the films *Critical Care, The Rainmaker,* and *John Q.* for their portrayal of managed care, the accuracy of the portrayals, and the individualistic solutions arrived at in each film.

90. David M. Eddy, 1994, pp 817, 818.

91. See Havighurst, *supra* note 2, at 75— "[C]onsumers could not see HMOs' vaunted accomplishments. Reported cost savings, for example, appeared to accrue only to employers, plan shareholders, or well-paid CEOs— even when they were in fact passed on, unlabeled (and therefore taken for granted), in higher take-home pay." See also George Anders, 1996, pp 55–73 which details HMO executives' extravagant financial compensation.

92. For a prediction of exactly these sorts of political values associated with an emphasis on market competition, see Rand E. Rosenblatt, 1981, pp 1067, 1108–15.

93. See, e.g., *Batas v. Prudential Ins. Co. of Am.*, 724 N.Y.S.2d 3 (N.Y. App. Div. 2001) (analyzing a situation where the insurer's nurse-reviewer, without consulting treating physician, refused to grant extended hospitalization to pregnant patient with Crohn's Disease). The patient could not afford to self-pay and "elect[ed]" early discharge, only to return to hospital seven days later with high fever and severe pain. Two days later while waiting for pre-authorization for exploratory surgery, patient's intestine burst and required emergency removal of part of her colon; four days later, on the basis of "Milliman & Robertson Guidelines," insurer's nurse-reviewer demanded that the patient be discharged. According to the Milliman and Robertson Website in 2001, http://www.milliman-hmg.com/publications/hmg/hmgqa.html, the guidelines are "a set of optimal clinical practice benchmarks for treating common conditions for patients who have no complications." Batas, 724 N.Y.S.2d at 9 n.1.

94. See, e.g., *Bedrick v. Travelers Ins. Co.*, 93 F.3d 149 (4th Cir. 1996) (ruling that the insurer's reviewing physician's criteria for denial of on-going coverage for most physical, occupational, and speech therapy prescribed for infant with spastic quadriplegia were neither stated nor referenced in the insurance contract, nor were they present in the insurer's own guidelines, and holding that the denial of coverage was in violation of applicable ERISA procedures and in violation of reviewing physician's duty as ERISA fiduciary to provide "full and fair hearing").

95. Jacobson, *supra* note 113, at 365; Jacobi, *supra* note 113, at 398, 400. See also James C. Robinson, 2001, p 2622.

96. Jon R. Gabel, et al., 2002.

97. Jacobi, *supra* note 113, at 407–8.

98. *Cf.* Deborah A. Stone, 1999–2000, pp 11, 16.

99. See Pugh, *supra* note 81 reporting a survey by the Kaiser Family Foundation and the Health, Research and Educational Trust that "the typical family policy for all types of health plans averaged $9,068 a year in the spring of 2003, compared with $7,954 in the spring of 2002."

100. See, e.g., Louis Uchitelle, 2003, p A20. "[T]he high-end estimate comes from Mark Zandi, chief economist at Economy.com, who calculates that 995,000 jobs have been lost overseas since the last recession began in March 2001. That is 35 percent of the total decline in employment since then. While most of the loss is in manufacturing, about 15 percent is among college-trained professionals." *Id.*

101. E.g., Robert Pear, 2003, p A1.

102. See Philip Bobbitt, 2002, pp 213–42. For a positive review of this book, see Dennis Patterson, 2003, p 2501. For a critique, see Rand E. Rosenblatt, *Constitutional Interpretation and the Dynamics of World History* (in progress).

103. See Bobbitt, *supra* note 131, at 220–1. See also Uchitelle, *supra* note 128.

104. As an empirical matter, free trade and unregulated markets were not in fact the dominant basis of economic success for newly emerging national economies from the 1950s through

the 1980s. Indeed, the Asian "economic miracles" of Japan, South Korea, Taiwan, Malaysia, and Singapore were based on "government leadership in industrial planning, a high degree of financial leverage, and some degree of protection for the domestic economy, as well as the ability to control wages," George Soros, 1998, p 110—the latter meaning in some countries authoritarian and violent suppression of labor movements. In addition to organized governmental violence, the lack of social protection demanded by market theory and practice gives rise to what Third World health activist Dr. Paul Farmer terms "structural violence." Farmer, *supra* note 7, at 40. See Amartya Sen, 2003, Forward to Farmer, *supra* note 7, at xii–xvi.

105. Thomas L. Friedman, 2000, pp 435–6.

106. For examples of a rapidly-growing literature of this sort (whether or not explicitly focused on globalization), see, for example, Jody Freeman, 2003, p 1285; Archon Fung and Erik Olin Wright, 2001, p 5; Charles F. Sabel and William H. Simon, 2004, p 1015; Joshua Cohen and Charles Sabel; Andrew Gamble, 1996, pp 117, 128–30; Michael C. Dorf and Charles F. Sabel, 1998, p 267. For an example of this general perspective applied to health policy, see Mary Ruggie, 1996, Realignments in the Welfare State: Health Policy in the United States, Britain, and Canada, pp ix–xi, 1–27, *passim*.

107. Tuohy, *supra* note 21, at 202.

108. James A. Morone and Elizabeth H. Kilbreth, 2003, pp 271.

109. William M. Sage, 2003, pp 387, 414.

110. *Id.* at 414–5.

111. See, e.g., Lori B. Andrews, Maxwell J. Mehlman, and Mark A. Rothstein, 2002, pp 592–734.

112. See, e.g., Francis Fukuyama, 2002, pp 4–17, 216–8 (depicting a world where people have all their desires realized but, as a result, cease to be human beings); Andrews, Mehlman, and Rothstein, *supra* note 135, at 281–98.

113. Bobbitt, *supra* note 131, at 232.

114. See Francis Fukuyama, 1989, p 3 (arguing that the end of the Cold War is signaling the end of history as we know it and beginning "the final form of human government"); Francis Fukuyama, 1992.

115. Fukuyama, 2002, *supra* note 141, at 218.

REFERENCES

Agrawal, G.B., and H.R. Veit. 2002. "Back to the Future: The Managed Care Revolution," *Law & Contemporary Problems* 65 (Autumn): 11–36.

Anders, G. 1996. Health Against Wealth: HMOs and the Breakdown of Medical Trust. Boston: Houghton Mifflin Company, pp 55–73.

Andrews, L.B., M.J. Mehlman and M.A. Rothstein. 2002. *Genetics: Ethics, Law and Policy.* Eagan, MI: West Law School, pp 592–734.

Arrow, K.J. 1963. "Uncertainty and the Welfare Economics of Medical Care," *American Economic Review* 53: 942, 963–4.

Bloche, M.G. 2003. "The Invention of Health Law," *California Law Review* 91: 247, 253–4.

Blumstein, J., and C.C. Havighurst. 1975. "Coping with Quality/Cost Trade-Offs in Medical Care: The Role of PSROs," *NorthWestern University Law Review* 70: 6, 12.

Bobbitt, P. 2002. The Shield of Achilles: War, Peace, and the Course of History. New York: Knopf pp 213–42.

Cohen, J., and C. Sabel. *Directly-Deliberative Polyarchy.* Available at: http://www2.law.columbia.edu/sabel/papers/DDP.html. [Most recently accessed, 12, September, 2007].

Dorf, M.C., and C.F. Sabel. 1998. "A Constitution of Democratic Experimentalism," *Columbia Law Review* 98: 267.

Dormandy, T. 2001. *The White Death: A History of Tuberculosis.* London: Hambledon & London, pp 78, 224.

Dubos, J., and R. Dubos. 1987. *The White Plague: Tuberculosis, Man and Society.* Piscataway: Rutgers University Press, p xxxvii.

Eddy, D.M. 1994. "Rationing Resources While Improving Quality: How to Get More for Less," *Journal of the American Medical Association* 272: 817, 818.

Elhauge, E. 1994. "Allocating Health Care Morally,"
    California Law Review 82: 1451, 1452.

Enthoven, A.C. 1980. Health Plan: The Only Practical
    Solution to the Soaring Cost of Medical Care
    Indianapolis, Indiana: Addison Wessley.

Evans, R.G. 1997a. "Going for the Gold: The
    Redistributive Agenda behind Market-Based Health
    Care Reform," *Journal of Health Politics Policy &
    Law* 22: 427.

—— 1997b. "Response: Coarse Correction – And Way
    Off Target," *Journal of Health Politics Policy & Law*
    22: 503.

Farmer, P. 2003. Pathologies of Power: Health, Human
    Rights, and the New War on the Poor. San Francisco,
    University of California Press.

Ford, B. 1994. "The Uncertain Case for Market Pricing
    of Health Insurance," *Boston University Law Review*
    74: 109, 110–20.

Frankford, D.M. 1993. "Neoclassical Health Economics
    and the Debate Over National Health Insurance:
    The Power of Abstraction," *Law & Society Inquiry*
    18: 351, 365–71.

—— 1992. "Privatizing Health Care: Economic Magic
    to Cure Legal Medicine," *Southern California Law
    Review* 66: 1, 9–10.

Freeman, J. 2003. "Extending Public Law Norms Through
    Privatization," *Harvard Law Review* 116: 1285.

Fried, C. 1983. "Health Care, Cost Containment,
    Liberty," in J. Arras & R. Hunt, eds., *Ethical Issues
    in Modern Medicine.* New York: McGraw-Hill,
    pp 527, 527–9.

Friedman, T.L. 2000. *The Lexus and the Olive Tree.*
    New York: Anchor Books, pp 435–6.

Fukuyama, F. 2002. *Our Posthuman Future: Consequences
    of the Biotechnology Revolution.* New York: Farrar
    Straus & Giroux, pp 4–17, 216–18.

Fukuyama, F. *The End of History and the Last Man.*
    New York: Free Press, 1992.

Fung, A., and E.O. Wright. 2001. "Deepening Democracy:
    Innovations in Empowered Participatory Governance,"
    Politics & Society 29: 5.

Gabel, J.R., et al. 2002. "Consumer-Driven Health
    Plans: Are They More Than Talk Now?," *Health
    Affairs* Web Exclusives W395, http://www.
    healthaffairs.org/WebExclusives/Gabel_Web_Excl_1
    12002.htm. November 20.

Gamble, A. "The Limits of Democracy," in P. Hirst and
    S. Khilnani, eds., *Reinventing Democracy.* Oxford:
    Blackwell Publishers, pp 117, 128–30.

Hall, M.A. 2002. "Law, Medicine and Trust," *Stanford
    Law Review* 55: 463, 465–6.

Havighurst, C.C. 1976–77. "Controlling Health Care
    Costs: Strengthening the Private Sector's Hand,"
    Journal of Health Politics, Policy & Law 1: 471,
    490–1.

—— 1995. *Health Care Choices.* Washington DC, AEI
    Press, p 98.

—— 2001. "The Backlash Against Managed Health
    Care: Hard Politics Make Bad Policy," *Indiana Law
    Review* 34: 395.

—— 2002. "How the Health Care Revolution Fell
    Short," *Law & Contemporary Problems* (Autumn):
    55, 72–3.

Hirschman, A.O. 1991. The Rhetoric of Reaction:
    Perversity, Futility, Jeopardy. Cambridge: Belknap
    Press.

Jost, T.S. 2003. Disentitlement?: The Threats Facing
    Our Public Health – Care Programs and a Rights-
    Based Response. New York: Oxford University
    Press, pp 23–109.

Kilbreth, E.H., and J.A. Morone. 2003. "Power to the
    People? Restoring Citizen Participation," *Journal of
    Health Politics, Policy & Law* 28: 271.

Konner, M. 1993. Medicine at the Crossroads: The
    Crisis in Health Care. New York: Pantheon, p 82.

Kuttner, R. 1996. *Everything for Sale: The Virtues and
    Limits of Markets.* Chicago: University of Chicago
    Press, pp 34–7.

Law, S., S. Rosenbaum and R.E. Rosenblatt. 1997. *Law
    and the American Health Care System.* Eagan, MI:
    Foundation Press, pp 2–3, 24–35, 131–5, 823–4.

Marmor, T. 1973. *The Politics of Medicare.* [New York:
    Aldine Publishing Company, pp 85–6.

Maxwell, J., and P. Temin. 2002. "Managed Competition
    Versus Industrial Purchasing of Health Care
    Among the Fortune 500," *Journal of Health Politics,
    Policy & Law* 27: 5.

Morone, J.A. 1993. "The Health Care Bureaucracy:
    Small Changes, Big Consequences," *Journal of
    Health Politics, Policy & Law* 18: 723.

—— 1999. "Populists in a Global Market," *Journal of
    Health Politics, Policy & Law* 24: 887, 891.

Patterson, D. 2003. "The New Leviathan," *Michigan
    Law Review* 101: 2501.

Pauly, M.V. 1992. "Risk Variation and Fallback Insurers
    in Universal Coverage Insurance Plans," *Inquiry:
    Journal of Health Care Organization Provision &
    Finance* 29: 137.

Pauly, M.V. 1997. "Who Was that Straw Man Anyway? A Comment on Evans and Rice," *Journal of Health Politics, Policy & Law* 22: 467.

Pear, R. 2003. "Big Increase Seen in People Lacking Health Insurance," *New York Times,* September 20: A1.

Pendo, E.A. 2004. "Images of Health Insurance in Popular Film: The Dissolving Critique," *Journal of Health Law* 37: 267.

Peterson, Mark, ed., 2003. "Special Conference Issue: Who Shall Lead?" *Journal of Health Politics, Policy & Law* 28: 181–24.

Polanyi, Karl. 1944. *The Great Transformation.* New York: Farrar and Rhinehart.

Robinson, J.C. 2001. "The End of Managed Care," *Journal of the American Medical Association* 285: 2622.

—— 2003. "The Politics of Managed Competition: Public Abuse of the Private Interest," *Journal of Health Politics, Policy & Law* 28: 341–46.

Roosevelt, Franklin, Delano. 1944. State of the Union Message to Congress (January 11). http://www.presidency.ucsb.edu/ws/print.php?pid=16518 [Last assessed 12, September, 2007].

Rosenbaum, S., and D. Rousseau. 2001. "Medicaid At Thirty-Five," *St Louis University Law Journal* 45: 7.

Rosenbaum, S., and J. Teitelbaum. 2003. "Civil Rights Enforcement in the Modern Healthcare System," *Yale Journal of Health Policy, Law & Ethics* 3: 215.

Rosenblatt, R.E. 1988. "Conceptualizing Health Law for Teaching Purposes: The Social Justice Perspective," *Journal of Legal Educaion* 38: 489.

—— Forthcoming. Constitutional Interpretation and the Dynamics of World History.

—— 1970. "Note, Legal Theory and Legal Education," *Yale Law Journal* 79: 1153, 1165–72.

—— 1975. "Dual Track Health Care—The Decline of the Medicaid Cure," *University of Cincinnati Law Review* 44: 643, 644.

—— 1978. "Health Care Reform and Administrative Law: A Structural Approach," *Yale Law Journal* 88: 243, 264–5.

—— 1981. "Health Care, Markets, and Democratic Values," *Vanderbil Law Review* 34: 1067, 1108–15.

—— 1993. "The Courts, Health Care Reform, and the Reconstruction of American Social Legislation," *Journal of Health Politics, Policy & Law* 18: 439: 147–171.

—— 1998. "Health Law," in D. Kairys, ed., *The Politics of Law: A Progressive Critique* (3d ed.). New York: Basic Books,

—— "Social Duties and the Problem of Rights in the American Welfare State," in D. Kairys, ed., *The Politics of Law* (rev. ed.). New York: Pantheon, p 90.

—— 2004. "The Four Ages of Health Law," *Health Matrix* 14: 155.

Rosenblatt R.E., et al. 2001–02. *Law and the American Health Care System.* Eagan, MN: Foundation Press, pp 196–213.

Rosner, D. "Twentieth Century Medicine," in R.W. Bulliett, ed. *The Columbia History of the 20th Century.* New York: Columbia University Press, pp 483, 504.

Rothman, D.J. 1991. Strangers at the Bedside: A History of How Law and Bioethics Transformed Medical Decisionmaking. Piscataway: Aldine Transaction, pp 1–4, 70–84.

Rothman, D.J. 1997. Beginnings Count: The Technological Imperative in American Health Care. New York: Oxford University Press, pp 4–6.

Ruggie, M. 1996. Realignments in the Welfare State: Health Policy in the United States, Britain, and Canada. New York: Columbia University Press, pp ix–xi, 1–27.

Sabel, C.F., and W.H. Simon. 2004. "Destablization Rights: How Public Law Litigation Succeeds," *Harvard Law Review* 117: 1015.

Sage, W.M. 2003. "Unfinished Business: How Litigation Relates to Health Care Regulation," *Journal of Health Politics, Policy & Law* 28: 387, 414.

Siliciano, J.A. "Wealth, Equity, and the Unitary Medical Malpractice Standard," *Virginia Law Review* 77: 439, 439–40.

Soros, G. 1998. *The Crisis of Global Capitalism: Open Society Endangered.* New York: Public Affairs Press, p 110.

Starr, P. 1982. *The Social Transformation of American Medicine.* New York: Basic Books, pp 180–97.

Stone, D. "Managed Care and the Second Great Transformation," *Journal of Health Politics, Policy & Law* 24: 1213, 1214–17.

—— 1990. "The Rhetoric of Insurance Law: The Debate Over AIDS Testing," *Law & Social Inquiry* 15: 385, 388–91.

—— 1993. "The Struggle for the Soul of Health Insurance," *Journal of Health Politics, Policy & Law* 18: 287, 290.

—— 1999–2000. "Beyond Moral Hazard: Insurance as Moral Opportunity," *Connecticut Insurance Law Journal* 6: 11, 16.

Tuohy, C.H. 2003. "Agency, Contract, and Governance: Shifting Shapes of Accountability in the Health Care Arena," *Journal of Health Politics, Policy & Law* 28: 195, 197.

Uchitelle, L. 2003. "A Statistic That's Missing: Jobs That Moved Overseas," *New York Times* October 5: A20.

Walz, J.R. 1969. "The Rise and Gradual Fall of the Locality Rule in Medical Malpractice Litigation," *DePaul Law Review* 18: 408, 410–11.

Williams, K.J. 1976. "The Quandary of the Hospital Administrator in Dealing with the Medical Malpractice Problem," *Nebraska Law Review* 55: 401.

CHAPTER 7

Federalism*

Frank J. Thompson and James Fossett

The balance of power between federal and state government always ebbs and flows. In this chapter, Thompson and Fossett describe the dynamics of federalism, reflect on the main features of contemporary federal–state relations, and explain the significance for health politics and policy.

In late December 2003 Governor Rod R. Blagojevich of Illinois petitioned the federal government for permission to buy prescription drugs from Canada. With drug prices from 30% to 50% lower in Canada than in the United States, Blagojevich estimated that the Illinois state government could save over $90 million a year in drug purchases for state employees and retirees if it could facilitate imports from Canada. Federal officials promptly denied the governor's request warning about the potential for false labeling, counterfeiting, and poor quality. Nonetheless, Blagojevich, a Democrat, and Governor Tim Pawlenty of Minnesota, a Republican, moved to sponsor a governors summit on this topic early in 2004 and to press for change in federal policy. Subsequently, various states and localities found ways around the national government's prohibitions on pharmaceutical purchases from Canada.[1]

While the founding fathers of the United States would be surprised at the magnitude of government and the intricacies of health policy at the dawn of the 21st century, they would certainly recognize this episode as a natural outgrowth of an institution they established—federalism. Writing over 200 years ago in support of the new Constitution, James Madison in the *Federalist Papers* observed that the founders were calling for "neither a national nor a federal Constitution, but a composition of both." Madison understood that the system forged in 1787 would in many ways preserve the "faculty" of national and state governments "to resist and frustrate the measures of each other."[2]

It would, of course, be a mistake to portray issues of federalism and health policy as a saga of unremitting contention and conflict between the national government and the states. The two levels of government often collaborate and forge productive partnerships to address health problems. But even in programs marked by substantial cooperation between the federal government and the states, differences of perspective often surface. These differences fuel an elaborate intergovernmental politics that involves legislative bodies, courts, administrative agents, and others. This politics yields a balance of power between the national government and the states that ebbs and flows and shapes who gets what, when, and how from government's health policies.

Federalism animates the behavior of a wide range of health policy stakeholders, jockeying for advantage. Hence, positions on the appropriate balance of power between the federal government and the states generally flow less from abstract political theories than from concrete interests and preferences. In recent years, for instance, leading Democrats have generally seen the states as less sympathetic to the interests of low-income citizens than the national government; Democrats have resisted many Republican proposals to devolve more responsibility over health programs to the states. But both parties often shift their stance on federalism depending on the issue and the circumstances.

American federalism not only features an ever-changing balance of power between national and state officials, it also plays a catalytic role. When the federal and state governments team up to share the cost of a health program, it may lead government in general to be more dominant vis-à-vis the private sector than would be the case if either level of government had to absorb all of the costs of the program.

In seeking to describe the complexities of federalism, observers have turned to cakes for useful metaphors. Some people have seen federalism as a three-layer cake with federal, state, and local governments each having distinct, clearly defined responsibilities. In earlier periods of the nation's history, the crisp division suggested by this metaphor at least partly captured political reality. However, political scientists today generally hold that federalism has become more like a marble cake—with rules, regulations, responsibilities, functions, and funding all blurred and intermingled.[3]

Federalism intersects in myriad ways with efforts to enhance the nation's health. Some important intergovernmental initiatives have little to do with the delivery of health care. Various preventive policies seek to head off death, disease, disability, and discomfort by reducing hazards in the environment and by encouraging personal lifestyles conducive to health. For instance, government efforts to assure that citizens have safe drinking water, minimize their exposure to asbestos, and cut down on their smoking all feature a fascinating politics of federalism.[4] In this chapter, however, we confine our focus to the intergovernmental dynamics shaping the *delivery* of health care services. Within this context, we target one very important policy tool that has loomed especially large since World War II—federal grants to state and local governments. National policy makers have repeatedly employed this tool to induce states to address some health challenge—constructing hospitals, educating health professionals, assuring access to medical care for women and children, providing nursing services for the elderly, and much more. The politics of these intergovernmental grants has profoundly shaped the balance between access, cost, and quality in the American health care system.

This chapter opens with a brief historical sketch of federalism and health care pointing in particular to the 1960s as a watershed. The second section plumbs key features of the intergovernmental grant system. It emphasizes the substantial bargaining power and discretion of the states, the rise of executive federalism over the last two decades, and the fiscal dimensions of intergovernmental politics especially as pertains to state entrepreneurship and the difficulties of targeting federal funds. The third and fourth sections assess devolution, a concept that sparked intense debate in the 1990s and 2000s. This debate centers on whether the national government should shift more authority over health care policy to the states. Proponents of devolution frequently build their case on optimistic assessments of the growing capacity and commitment of state governments. Our analysis suggests that these favorable assessments are at times overblown.

HISTORICAL SNAPSHOT: THE SIXTIES AS WATERSHED

In broad historical perspective, issues of federalism and health policy sort themselves into three general periods. The *minimalist period* ran from the founding of the republic in 1789 until the end of the Civil War. During this period grand issues of federalism revolved around basic questions of whether the federal government could move into certain policy arenas (e.g., establish a national bank, fund public infrastructure like roads and canals), whether states could overtly nullify legislation approved by the national government within their geographic boundaries, and whether states could secede from the union. To the degree that any level of government did much about public health, local governments tended to be in the forefront though the federal government provided some health care to soldiers and veterans and some states operated mental institutions.

The *emergent period* extends from the end of the Civil War to 1965. Both federal and state governments became increasingly involved in the health arena. By the late 19th century, the development of a better underlying science rooted in the germ theory of diseases fueled the creation of government institutions committed to fostering public health through sanitation, immunization, and health education. In 1869, Massachusetts developed the first viable state health board. States also became increasingly active in licensing medical professionals, in operating laboratories to deal with epidemics and disease, and in funding medical schools.[5] Intergovernmental grant programs for health care also began to develop. Of particular note, Congress approved the Sheppard-Towner Act in 1921—a grant program to the states designed to promote the health and welfare of mothers and children. Following World War II, national policy makers approved the Hill-Burton program, which provided federal grants

to stoke the construction of local hospitals. In these and many other ways, the federal and state governments became active on the health stage.

The *contemporary period* of health policy and federalism commenced in 1965 and continues to the present. It features massive increases in public funding for health care services to a substantial segment of the population. In 1965, President Lyndon B. Johnson signed two landmark measures into law—Medicare, a program for the elderly operated by the national government, and Medicaid, a federal grant program to the states that provides health services to low-income individuals. Medicaid has had a profound impact not only on health policy but also on the fabric of federalism. During the contemporary period, the image of federalism as "marble cake" with no neat horizontal stratification of functions surged to the fore. The birth of Medicaid in 1965 and the subsequent proliferation of federal grant programs further mingled national and state officials in efforts to ameliorate health problems. An intergovernmental politics featuring conflict and cooperation between the national government and the states flourished.

GRANT PROGRAMS AND THE FABRIC OF FEDERALISM

The core of contemporary health care federalism is the intergovernmental grant. These grants feature a mix of incentives and regulation. To entice states to ameliorate some health problems national policy makers promise to pay a percentage of the costs of a program (the federal match), leaving states to pick up the tab for the rest. States do not have to participate in these programs but they usually find the money irresistible. In exchange for the subsidy, national policy makers typically impose rules (whether in the statute or via administrative regulation) that reflect their own preferences and constrain state discretion. While state leaders welcome federal dollars, they often chafe under the requirements ("red tape" in their eyes) that limit state discretion.

By the year 2000, the federal government operated over 650 grant programs to states and localities. Dozens of these programs focused on health. Many of the health grants claim a small share of the federal purse and target specific groups or diseases. For instance, the federal Centers for Disease Control provide monies to states to support early detection programs for breast and cervical cancer. At the other end of the scale stands Medicaid, a major open-ended entitlement program that funds a broad range of health services for low-income people and consumes a major share of federal and state budgets.

Over the past four decades, intergovernmental health grants have grown in importance. The dollars associated with these grants not only increased rapidly in the period from 1965 to 2005, they soared as a proportion of all grant monies. As Table 7-1 indicates, all grants to state and local governments in 2005 were almost 40 times greater than in 1965; in contrast, health grants were over 325 times greater in 2005 than in 1965. At the inception of Medicaid, health programs consumed 6% of all federal grants to states and localities. By 2005, this share had grown to 48%.

Within the health sector, Medicaid loomed increasingly large. By the year 2000 it consumed well over 90% of all health funding that the national government provided via intergovernmental grant programs. Moreover, its fiscal importance relative to the country's other major public health insurance program, Medicare, had increased. When President Lyndon Johnson signed both Medicare and Medicaid into law in 1965, many observers saw the latter as a program afterthought. Medicare captured the spotlight with many seeing it as the template for subsequent movement to national health insurance for all. By the end of the 20th century, however, the staying power of Medicaid had become evident. In 1970, expenditures for Medicaid from all sources amounted to just over two-thirds of what the federal government spent on Medicare. In 2002, Medicaid expenditures from all sources were 94% (over $250 billion)

Table 7-1 Federal Outlays for Grants to State and Local Governments

Health and Other (in millions of dollars)

Year	All Grants	Health	Health Percentage of All Grants
1965	10,910	624	6%
1970	24,065	3,849	16%
1980	91,385	15,758	17%
1990	135,325	43,890	32%
2000	284,659	124,843	44%
2004	406,330	189,883	47%
2005*	425,793	203,253	48%

SOURCE: US Office of Management and Budget, Historical Tables, Budget of the United States Government, Fiscal Year 2006.

*Estimate

of the sum spent on Medicare (some $267 billion).[6] To a remarkable degree, efforts to provide public health insurance to the populace had become an exercise in federalism.

State Discretion and Bargaining Power

In broad terms, national policy makers make decisions on how much discretion they want to give states when they decide whether to work through a *categorical* or a *block grant* and whether to make the program an *entitlement* or one dependent on a *fixed budget*. According to the US General Accounting Office (GAO), "the typical categorical grant permits funds to be used only for specific, narrowly defined purposes and populations and includes administrative and reporting requirements that help to ensure both financial and programmatic accountability." In contrast "block grants award funds to state or local governments, to be used at their discretion to support a range of activities aimed at achieving a broad national purpose." Block grants tend to have "limited administrative and reporting requirements."[7] While useful conceptually, the distinction between categorical and block grants is much fuzzier than these definitions imply. For instance, many block grants spin a regulatory web on participating states.

Not surprisingly, state officials usually prefer generously funded block grants. National policy makers, in contrast, go through cycles. They often pursue their own policy goals through narrowly defined categorical grants. The resulting administrative complexity leads to spasms of support for combining existing categorical programs into block grants. For instance, Congress moved in this direction in the early 1980s under the Reagan administration. But after periods of consolidation the desire to control programs and to win credit from constituents for fighting a specific problem (like AIDS) tends to lead members of Congress to create a new generation of categorical grant programs.[8]

Whether or not a grant is an entitlement or has a fixed budget also affects state discretion. Medicaid, the king of the hill in the intergovernmental arena, is an entitlement. Once a state decides to make certain individuals eligible for specific services (e.g., podiatry, prescription drugs) under this program, they must provide them to all individuals in that category regardless of the immediate budget implications. While state officials can try to predict their Medicaid expenditures for a year based on past patterns, they cannot formally cut off funded services if the demand from beneficiaries exceeds expectations, at least without drafting a major policy revision and submitting it to the national government for approval. The federal government also has an open-ended commitment to bankroll state Medicaid costs according to the state's particular match rate.

In contrast to Medicaid, states that established a freestanding State Children's Health Insurance Program (SCHIP) after passage of this federal law in 1997, operate under fixed budgets. The federal government commits a specific sum of money; in response, states budget particular amounts depending on their respective match rates. If states experience cost overruns they can suspend enrollments in SCHIP until their fiscal fortunes improve.

Although federal grants constrain state discretion, they by no means eliminate the ability of states to shape who gets what, when, and how from their health programs. States continue to possess considerable discretion even when federal policy appears to be quite directive. Prior to the Civil War, one of the great federalism debates revolved around the issue of nullification—whether state legislatures could nullify federal laws within their jurisdictions. While the Civil War effectively ruled out such action, states in many respects possess de facto nullification powers at least over the short term in their role as implementing agents of the federal government. Without officially challenging the law, states can drag their feet and take other action to nullify federal intent in the implementation process. The image of states as puppets with the federal government pulling the strings almost never applies even in the case of entitlements and highly specific categorical programs. For instance, the Early, Periodic, Screening, Diagnostic and Treatment Program, a federal Medicaid initiative approved in 1967, required participating states to provide preventive care and treatment to poor children. Over subsequent decades, however, the states delivered these mandated services to less than half of the intended beneficiaries.[9]

The symmetrical power relationships between the national government and the states in intergovernmental grant programs spring from several sources. Federal administrators often lack enough information about state program activities to know whether they are efficiently, effectively, and lawfully implementing federal policy. The national government's paltry staff and inadequate information systems frequently make monitoring state behavior difficult. A substantial lag in acquiring data from state officials often exacerbates problems. By the time an issue finally shows up on the federal radar screen, state officials can claim they have long since dealt with it.

The sanctions that the national government possesses to compel state compliance are often difficult to employ. For instance, the law generally authorizes federal administrators to withhold funding from errant states, but such action is seldom appealing because it would often hurt the very people national officials wish to help (e.g., low-income citizens in need of health care). More calibrated sanctions (e.g., smaller penalties) may be easier to impose but do not necessarily provide states with enough incentive to mute their resistance to federal directives. Moreover, efforts to impose sanctions can ignite lobbying efforts by state officials directed at Congress and the White House who may in turn put pressure on federal administrators to back off.

Federal officials also know that state failures often stem less from willful resistance than from flawed national policy or state incapacity. The national government may not offer sufficient revenue for states to achieve the ambitious goals embedded in federal legislation. Or the law itself may rest on a mistaken theory about how to ameliorate some health problem. Finally, the enduring view that states have a special constitutional position and that the national government and states ought to be "partners," not adversaries, can undercut aggressive action by federal administrative agencies.

All of this is not to suggest that states can blithely ignore the law and preferences of federal officials. Executives in the national bureaucracy are generally committed to the objectives of their health programs and will seek to prod laggard states into implementing them. At times they can turn to supporters in the White House, Congress, and the states for assistance. Furthermore, private advocacy groups frequently use federal statutes as the basis for suits to require states and local officials to do a better job of implementing a program. These groups have constituted a kind of unofficial enforcement arm of the federal government. In the late 1990s, for instance, the Giuliani Administration in New York City adopted enrollment procedures designed to discourage people from applying for public assistance. Among other things, intake workers as a matter of routine accepted an application for Medicaid only after an individual visited the office a second time. Aware that this practice violated federal regulations, the Legal Aid Society joined other advocates for the poor to sue the city. Subsequently, a federal district

judge sided with these advocates. City officials responded by bringing their intake practices into compliance with federal and state law.

On balance, however, the power resources of the federal government seldom permit it to secure state compliance through "command-and-control" behavior. Power relationships and approaches tend to vary from one intergovernmental grant program to the next. But in general, the management of these programs tends to be a matter of bargaining and negotiation between the national government and the states.[10]

The Administrative Presidency and State Discretion: Waivers

States form an intergovernmental lobby in the nation's capital that constantly seeks to bolster their discretion in grant programs. States pressure Congress to enact legislative changes conducive to this goal. They strive to influence the federal bureaucracy when it promulgates important rules interpreting a law in the *Code of Federal Regulation*. Moreover, and of special importance in recent years, states often petition the executive branch for waivers. Major statutes often contain provisions empowering the national bureaucracy to grant waivers to states that think "outside the box" and seek to pursue alternative approaches. These waivers are part of the toolbox of an administrative presidency—resources that a particular presidential administration can employ without seeking congressional approval.[11] The willingness of the White House and executive agencies to grant waivers can markedly affect the ability of the states to shape their federally subsidized health programs. The waiver process itself typically features a pervasive characteristic of intergovernmental politics—extended, often intense, negotiation and bargaining between federal and state officials.

Medicaid provides particularly vivid examples of the use of waivers. Section 1115 of the Social Security Act authorizes the federal bureaucracy to approve comprehensive waivers for innovative approaches (known as demonstration projects) proposed by the state.[12] Prior to the 1990s, the federal government

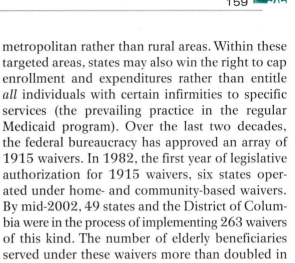

had been extremely reluctant to approve these comprehensive waivers, doing so only for Arizona in the early 1980s. The arrival of the Clinton presidency in 1993 marked the abandonment of this stringent approach. While President Clinton successfully fought the efforts of a Republican Congress to convert Medicaid to a block grant (Medigrant), he did empower the states through the comprehensive waiver process. Under President Clinton, federal officials quickly began to entertain and endorse 1115 waivers that promised a dramatic restructuring of state Medicaid programs. Officials in Tennessee, for example, won approval for a plan called TennCare that pledged to open the Medicaid gates to at least a half million new enrollees and to place primary responsibility for service delivery in the hands of managed care organizations. By the end of the Clinton administration in January 2001, 21 states had won approval of their 1115 waiver requests.[13] Upon taking office in 2001, President George W. Bush continued the emphasis on 1115 waivers. Under the banner of an initiative called Health Insurance Flexibility and Accountability (HIFA), the Bush administration endorsed an array of 1115 waiver requests from the states. As of December 2003, the states had submitted over 15 waiver requests under HIFA to the Department of Health and Human Services and nine had been approved.[14]

While 1115 waivers provide opportunities for the bold and sweeping exercise of state discretion, other statutory provisions open the door to more modest but nonetheless significant initiatives. For example, Section 1915 of the Social Security Act allows states to petition for Medicaid waivers to provide home- and community-based services to elderly and disabled individuals who would otherwise be placed in nursing homes or other long-term care institutions. These waivers empower states to provide services not routinely covered by Medicaid, such as installing a wheel chair ramp in a disabled person's home, training family members to be caregivers, and paying workers to perform heavy household chores like washing floors and windows. They permit states to limit these services geographically, say to

metropolitan rather than rural areas. Within these targeted areas, states may also win the right to cap enrollment and expenditures rather than entitle *all* individuals with certain infirmities to specific services (the prevailing practice in the regular Medicaid program). Over the last two decades, the federal bureaucracy has approved an array of 1915 waivers. In 1982, the first year of legislative authorization for 1915 waivers, six states operated under home- and community-based waivers. By mid-2002, 49 states and the District of Columbia were in the process of implementing 263 waivers of this kind. The number of elderly beneficiaries served under these waivers more than doubled in the period from 1991 through 1999 growing from about 155,000 to over 377,000.[15]

Not surprisingly in a political system marked by a constitutional separation of powers, Congress has at times expressed concern about waivers. In December 2001, for instance, the Bush administration approved a Section 1115 waiver sought by Arizona officials to use federal funds to expand coverage to low-income uninsured adults. The state proposed that at least part of the funding for this initiative come from unspent SCHIP funds. However, Congress had created SCHIP in order to provide care to children. The GAO, an analytic arm of Congress, reported that the Bush administration's approval of this waiver may well have violated legal requirements under the SCHIP law by shifting funds from children to adults.[16] The legislation creating SCHIP in 1997 provides incentives to the states to implement the program vigorously by requiring that any federal monies that a state fails to spend on SCHIP be reallocated to states that have used all of their federal allotment. The GAO contended that by letting Arizona keep unspent SCHIP funds and allocate them elsewhere, the executive branch had undercut a key component of this incentive system. The GAO report in July 2002 prompted Senators Charles Grassley (R-IA), the ranking Republican on the Senate Finance Committee, and Senator Max Baucus (D-MT), the ranking Democrat, to write the Secretary of Health and Human Services, Tommy Thompson, indicating that he should desist from approving waivers that shifted SCHIP funds to childless adults. Several members of Congress submitted legislation to prevent such action by the bureaucracy. But these proposals made no headway in congress and an additional GAO report to the Senate Finance Committee in January 2004 reported that the Department of Health and Human Services continued to approve 1115 waivers that ran counter to congressional intent.[17] In the face of executive branch recalcitrance, Congress finally inserted a provision in the Deficit Reduction Act of 2005 that prohibited the Centers for Medicare and Medicaid Services CMS from granting any new 1115 waivers that reallocated SCHIP funds in this way.

This pattern and comparable developments at the state level point to the rise of "executive federalism."[18] Top federal executives and state governors negotiate significant changes in state programs through the waiver process. Congress and the state legislatures typically watch from the sidelines at least initially and may have little influence. This development has made grant programs more malleable; program innovations can diffuse more rapidly in the states. At the same time, however, executive federalism in some cases erodes checks and balances within both the national and state governments. A complex pattern of policy innovation unfolds without much visibility or public debate.

Federal Grants: Targeting and Entrepreneurship

Federal grants rest on the principle that dollar incentives can entice states to pursue health goals espoused by national policy makers. The first question is how much money the federal government needs to put up to induce the states to act. Is a 50% match rate enough? Or does the federal government need to provide 65% of the funds to assure that states will seek to solve a health problem? In addition to this issue, policy makers face other challenges including those related to targeting and state entrepreneurship.

Targeting refers to federal efforts to funnel funds to states or jurisdictions in greatest need of assistance.

One form of targeting involves the provision of more generous subsidies to poorer states. Political dynamics make highly calibrated targeting difficult. Building broad supporting coalitions for health programs across many congressional districts often leads policy makers to allocate substantial resources to less needy states. Again, Medicaid provides a useful example. In forging this program national policy makers attempted to compensate for disparities in wealth among states through a formula that increases the match rate for states with lower per capita incomes. However, it also sets some basic limits on targeting by promising that the federal government will pay no less than 50% and no more than 83% of a state's Medicaid costs. The Medicaid formula has drawn criticism from those who favor more finely honed targeting. For instance, the GAO argues that targeting would improve if Congress eliminated the 50% floor on the federal match and adopted a more refined measure of state fiscal capacity.[19] In this regard, the GAO contends that state per capita income suffers from many limitations as an indicator and should be replaced by more sensitive measures (specifically the US Treasury Department's data on a state's total taxable resources adjusted for poverty rates and the price of health care in a state). Use of this alternative formula and elimination of the 50% floor on the Medicaid match would do more to assure that the federal government allocated funds to states in greatest need.

But members of Congress know that almost any effort to modify an existing funding formula opens a political can of worms. Notions of targeting collide headlong with the desires of Senators and Representatives to protect the amount of funding flowing to their particular jurisdictions. The constitutional guarantee that each state have two Senators assures that even formula changes that would benefit the most populous states face difficulties. For instance, the modification in the Medicaid formula recommended by GAO would benefit the four most populous states—California, Florida, New York, and Texas.[20] United, the congressional delegations from these states possess substantial clout in the House of Representatives with nearly one-third of all members coming from these states. In the Senate, however, these four states are much weaker with only 8% of the membership.

Federal grants often become an invitation to *fiscal entrepreneurship* by the states especially in the case of an open-ended entitlement program like Medicaid. Such entrepreneurship flows from the interest states have in increasing the share of their costs borne by the national government.[21] One type of entrepreneurship, fiscal substitution, occurs when states shift the cost of health services they had previously funded out of their own budgets to the federal government. For instance, changes in Medicaid law in the early 1980s allowed states to reapportion the costs of many services for the developmentally disabled (such as assistance with the basic tasks of living) from their own budgets to Medicaid.

A second kind of fiscal entrepreneurship involves the outright manipulation of the federal match rate. In this regard, many states have used "free money" to comply with federal Medicaid cost-sharing stipulations. The case of West Virginia is illustrative. Faced with acute budget problems in the mid-1980s, Medicaid officials in that state persuaded hospitals to "donate" (in fact loan) some $22 million to the program. This donation became part of the state Medicaid expenditures which justified matching federal dollars. Because West Virginia has a low per capita income and hence a more generous federal match rate, this move generated over $60 million in federal Medicaid funds. Once they had the federal dollars, West Virginia officials found a way to return the $22 million to the hospitals that had donated this sum. The state used the remaining federal money to support various Medicaid services. Other states soon followed West Virginia's lead. By 1990, all but six states operated a donation or provider tax program designed to inflate the federal match rate via the use of free dollars at the state level. The effect on the federal purse was substantial. Under Medicaid law, the overall federal share of Medicaid costs is supposed to approximate 57% of total program costs. By 1992, the federal government's

proportion of the Medicaid tab had, by one estimate, climbed to over 65%.[22]

The extraordinary entrepreneurship of the states did not escape the attention of federal policy makers and they responded with proposals to curtail it. When the National Governors Association and other elements of the intergovernmental lobby complained that the proposed changes would hurt the poor, Representative Norman Lent, a Republican congressman from New York, retorted that these claims were akin to catching a bank cashier embezzling funds to support his wife and children: "Should he be allowed to do it for another year lest we lower the standard of living for his family?"[23] Given strong lobbying from the governors and a divided government (the president was Republican and the congress Democratic), it was not until 1991 that the federal government approved a law that closed many of the loopholes that had allowed states to inflate their match rates.

While these and related measures constrained state fiscal entrepreneurship to a degree, they by no means eradicated it. By the turn of the decade, many states had once again managed to elevate the federal Medicaid match rate by exploiting payment provisions for hospitals that disproportionately serve low-income people as well as other regulations governing nursing home payments. Intergovernmental transfers of funds between state and local governments or between state agencies provided the mechanism for this manipulation. For instance, local governments involved in nursing home care might transfer funds to the state. Officials would then apply the monies to the state Medicaid match. Having used the transfers to obtain federal dollars, the state would then find a way for the local governments to recoup much or all of their transfers. By one estimate, state exploitation of intergovernmental transfers had raised the effective federal match for the Medicaid program by three percentage points as of the early 2000s.[24] These practices prompted the administration of George W. Bush to promise new steps to fight fiscal manipulation by the states in the early 2000s. However, the underlying issue endures: with health program costs relentlessly rising, both federal and state officials face constant pressure to limit their own expenditures—and shifting costs to another level of government is the most alluring and painless way to do so.

THE DEVOLUTION DEBATE

The last two decades have witnessed substantial debate about the virtues and defects of devolution—of shifting greater responsibilities from the national government to the states. Two major factors have fueled this development. First, policy makers and others have become increasingly impressed with the capacity of state governments. Supreme Court decisions insisting that legislative districts at the state level reflect the principle of one-person, one-vote and the passage of civil rights laws in the 1960s helped remove the taint of racism and undemocratic governance from the states. Moreover, observers began to highlight the steps states had taken to enhance the capacities of their legislative, judicial, and executive branches. The fact that many states had steadily bolstered these institutions long before the 1960s mattered less than the growing perception that the states had scored a major breakthrough. Meanwhile, the national government increasingly fell on hard times in public esteem. This government had inspired confidence in fighting the great depression, World War II, and, however belatedly, racial segregation in the South. However, during the 1970s it suffered through defeat in Vietnam, the Watergate scandal, a humiliating hostage crisis in Iran, and a decade of low economic growth coupled with high inflation. These circumstances, among others, eroded public trust.[25] By the 1980s states were, as one observer put it, no longer perceived as "no-talent spear carriers worthy only to serve the federal prima donna, they were moving to center stage and winning an unaccustomed share of the limelight."[26]

Second, the power of the Republican Party in national and state governments has assured that issues of devolution hover near center stage in health policy. The Republican Party has traditionally paid greater

homage to the role of the states in the federal system. Its takeover of both houses of Congress in 1994 and the election of George W. Bush in 2000 fueled interest in devolution. So too did Republican breakthroughs in gaining control of a majority of governorships and increasing their representation in state legislatures in the 1990s and early 2000s. The Republican tide led to two major devolution proposals between 1995 and 2005—both focused on the Medicaid program.

Proposals to shift greater responsibility to the states revolve around two major dimensions—the degree to which the federal government seeks to direct and regulate the states and the extent to which it provides funding to them. Given these dimensions, at least two types of devolution quickly come to mind. *Empowering devolution* features a relatively generous national government sustaining or increasing funding for a health program while granting states more flexibility to choose policy ends, means, or both. The 1115 waivers that the federal bureaucracy grants to states for their Medicaid programs tend to fall into this category. States sustain and even enhance their federal subsidies as they launch these bold initiatives. In contrast, *retrenching devolution* involves a trade-off for the states. It promises to give them more discretion over their health programs but also to provide less federal financial assistance.[27]

Retrenching devolution is most radical when the national government decides to terminate a program and leave the issue entirely to the states. Consider the Sheppard-Towner Act, which had provided federal grants to the states to foster the health of mothers and children. Signed into law by President Warren Harding in November 1921, the program provided a steady stream of grants to the states throughout the 1920s. All but three states participated. When the program came up for renewal toward the end of the decade, however, it encountered stiff opposition from the American Medical Association and others. With President Calvin Coolidge announcing that he welcomed the withdrawal of the federal government from this and other "state-aid projects," the program died in 1929. Faced with federal withdrawal, about one-third of the states managed to find funding from their own coffers to sustain the maternity and infancy programs of Sheppard-Towner. But the Great Depression soon vitiated fiscal support for these activities among even the most committed states.[28] The case of Sheppard-Towner plays to the views of devolution skeptics. They contend that radical devolution will almost surely lead to diminished government effort on behalf of health objectives.

Radical retreat, however, tends to be the exception rather than the rule at least in the case of larger grant programs. Instead, federal policy makers more typically propose initiatives that feature some diminution of federal funding in exchange for greater state discretion over how to spend it. Often, the national government provides a sweetener, promising states more money initially and then reducing federal financial support over the longer term. In 1995 and 1996, for instance, a Republican Congress led by Representative Newt Gingrich attempted to convert the Medicaid program from an open-ended entitlement to a fixed annual block grant that would give the states more flexibility. Concerned that the measure would rip holes in the health safety net President Bill Clinton vetoed the measure. While the quest for retrenching devolution did not surface again in the 1990s, the election of George W. Bush pushed the issue to the fore in the early 2000s.

Retrenching Devolution and the Bush Administration

President George W. Bush's first term illustrates some of the political dynamics unleashed by proposals for retrenching devolution. Presidents over the last 30 years have often entered office touting their version of a "new federalism." President Bush did not explicitly articulate such a vision. Nor in his election campaign did he go as far as most presidential candidates in sketching an ambitious agenda for health policy. But the general thrust of his presidency has strongly tilted toward retrenching devolution where the overall objective is clear: reduce the federal dollars that flow to the states in intergovernmental health programs. As a secondary (but only a secondary) priority, the Bush administration has at times sought to expand state discretion over the use of federal grants.[29] This approach has been most evident in its stance toward the towering giant of intergovernmental health programs, Medicaid.

Two major events have established the context for the Bush administration's commitment to shifting greater fiscal and programmatic responsibility to the states. The first is the president's obeisance to a hard-core conservative dictum: "starve-the-beast" ("beast" here being the government). This strategy, which the Republican Party has exploited with great electoral success since 1980, features three central components: cut taxes substantially, strongly oppose efforts to offset this drain in government revenues, and use the resulting fiscal stress (as manifested, for instance, in skyrocketing budget deficits) to justify cutting federal support for health and other domestic programs. Upon coming to office in 2001, President Bush soon succeeded in gaining congressional approval for massive tax cuts that would help create this climate of fiscal stress. By 2004, the projected federal budget deficit had grown to nearly a half trillion dollars. A second major event also intruded to displace most health care programs as a domestic priority, the tragic events of September 11, 2001 and President Bush's quest both at home and abroad to wage a "war against terrorism." This war necessitated growing expenditures for the military and for homeland security. It heightened the incentive for the Bush administration to save money elsewhere in the federal budget including intergovernmental health programs.

In 2003, the Bush administration set off in pursuit of cost savings and devolution by proposing a voluntary block grant for Medicaid. Under the proposal, states could elect to accept Medicaid and SCHIP funds through two allotments—one for ordinary medical services and one for long-term care. The proposal counted on the states to take a short-term perspective. It promised to treat them more generously in the early years of the program than the existing Medicaid program would. Over the longer term, however, the initiative would provide fewer federal dollars to the states than Medicaid. In addition to front-loading federal money, the president tried to make the proposal attractive to the states by granting them more flexibility to define the population groups they would cover and the services beneficiaries would receive. It also opened the door for states to levy higher co-payments and deductibles on enrollees. While the additional discretion granted to the states would be less than that found in the Medigrant legislation President Clinton had vetoed in the mid-1990s, it would be a significant step toward freeing the states from federal requirements.

The White House launched an aggressive lobbying campaign aimed at persuading the National Governors Association and others to back the plan. Sensing some resistance, it worked through several governors in an abortive attempt to have the executive director of this association fired. Despite this arm-twisting and extensive negotiations, however, the great majority of governors (including many Republicans) refrained from endorsing the Bush proposal.[30] While governors welcomed the increased flexibility embedded in the president's initiative, most of them were skittish about the financial terms involved in converting the program from an entitlement into a block grant. Instead, facing acute fiscal stress brought on by a sluggish economy, the governors pressed their case in Congress for additional federal financial support for Medicaid. Congress ultimately responded by temporarily increasing the federal share of total Medicaid spending by approximately $10 billion.

Stymied by Congress the Bush administration increasingly came to see the tools of the administrative presidency as a more promising vehicle for the reforms it sought. Early in 2004, top Bush officials announced plans to offer waivers to states that wished to restructure their programs and accept a federal spending cap as part of the bargain. Federal officials also upped the ante for states that did not seek such waivers by promising to intensify federal oversight of their Medicaid programs through more vigorous administrative review and budget audits. In doing so, federal officials took aim at an old nemesis—fiscal entrepreneurship by the states.[31] Federal administrators promised to crack down on state schemes to obtain a higher federal match rate through complex spending maneuvers including intergovernmental transfers. The Bush administration asserted that this aggressive supervision of state Medicaid spending would allow it to save more than $23 billion over a ten-year period. Many governors and advocacy groups criticized the Bush administration for these steps. By mid-2004, the administration at least temporarily retreated, announcing that it would not push the states to accept spending caps.[32] But President Bush continued to espouse aggressive federal supervision of the states to achieve cost savings after his reelection later that year.

State Response to Federal Retreat?

The experiences of the Gingrich-led Congress in 1995 and President George W. Bush in 2003 indicate that proposals for retrenching devolution face serious political obstacles, at least in the case of Medicaid. But the ballooning federal debt, budget pressures emanating from the country's war on terrorism, and the growing cost of health care grants make it likely that proposals for such devolution will repeatedly surface. Republican dominance of the national government would heighten prospects for the eventual approval of such a proposal. However, even Democratic-led Congresses face the crunch imposed by both deficits and wartime spending. Given this fiscal setting, it is important to assay possible state responses to retrenching devolution. In this regard, assessments of state capacity and commitment loom especially large. Do states have the governing and fiscal capacity to cope with reduced federal funding and greater freedom to design their programs? Would they have the political will, or commitment, to sustain or enhance an intergovernmental health program in the face of federal retreat?

State Governing and Fiscal Capacity

Proponents of devolution frequently tout the growing capacity of the states to deal effectively with health policy issues. In their assessments, two forms of capacity stand front and center. First, they point to the *governing capacity* of the states—their ability to formulate coherent, creative, plausible, responsive policy and to implement it efficiently, effectively, and accountably. Second, but to a lesser degree, they suggest that states have increased their *fiscal capacity*—their total taxable resources and their formal rights to tap these resources for public purposes.

No handy scorecard exists that allows us to define, measure, and track trends in state governing capacity with precision. On balance, however, a strong case exists that most states can under the right circumstances effectively shoulder considerable responsibility for implementing major programs. Or, stated differently, they stand at least as good a chance of doing so as the federal government. (In part, this view reflects the distinct possibility that the last three decades have featured the erosion of administrative capacity at the national level.)[33]

While states have probably increased their governing capacity, certain factors caution against exuberance in assessing their ability to take on new responsibilities. First, assessments of governing capacity need to acknowledge more fully its fluidity and potential for backsliding. Arguably, the 1960s and 1970s featured a great leap forward in state governing capacity. The period after that presents a more mixed picture. For instance, the success of the term limits movement has undercut and in some instances derailed efforts to foster legislative professionalism. The increased use of mechanisms of direct democracy (the initiative and the referendum) in states like California has led to a jumble of laws that foster policy incoherence, fuel gridlock, and give pause to those who favor deliberative democratic institutions. Moreover, the ideology of bureaucratic downsizing (which at times might more aptly be termed "dumbsizing") and, in many states, the

economic troubles of the early 2000s have eroded government workforces and the administrative infrastructure needed to implement public programs efficiently and effectively. In these and other ways, one cannot assume a steady march toward greater governing capacity among the states.

Second, assessments of state capacity need to consider the challenge of rising expectations. The critical issue is not so much whether state capacity has increased, but its status relative to the policy promises being made. Consider, for instance, the expansion of state initiatives to enroll more Medicaid recipients in managed care. The administrative challenges of managed care systems tend to exceed those that states faced under the old fee-for-service system where they paid the bills submitted by providers. Some states have been up to the challenge of building their capacity to be prudent purchasers of managed care while others have not.

Finally, the Employment Relations and Income Security Act (ERISA) continues to undermine state capacity. Approved by federal policy makers in the 1970s, this law effectively curtails the options states can pursue in health policy. Among other things, ERISA exempts companies that self-insure their employees from state regulation. Eager to escape state control, many large companies have rushed to self-insure. This makes it difficult for states to address the problems of the uninsured by passing laws requiring all employers to provide a specific health benefit package to their workers. It also allows certain employers to dodge reporting requirements that might enable states to formulate and implement more effective health policy.[34] Devolution of a grant program that also included reform of ERISA would be a significant step toward enhancing state flexibility and governing capacity. But business and union opposition make such reform unlikely.

The devolution debate also intersects with issues of state fiscal capacity. The taxable resources available to all levels of government have increased over the last decade largely because the economy grew. But this rising economic tide has not eradicated substantial variation among states in the taxable resources they have available to fund health programs. In 2001, for example, total taxable resources per capita ranged from approximately $26,800 in Mississippi to $56,500 in Connecticut.[35] Unless a proposal for retrenching devolution employs highly calibrated matching rates to offset variations in state wealth, citizens in less affluent states will, other things being equal, tend to receive fewer benefits. As discussed earlier, political dynamics often make it difficult to target federal funds to the neediest states.

The fiscal capacity of a state not only reflects the total taxable resources within its borders; it also derives from procedures it applies to taxing and spending decisions. As the 21st century opened, over half of the states had added tax or expenditure limitations to their constitutions or statutes. These provisions come in many guises, but all of them make it harder for policy makers to fund public programs. Some of the provisions seek to remove fiscal decisions from the realm of majoritarian politics by requiring legislative supermajorities to approve tax boosts. For instance, California requires a two-thirds majority in both houses of the legislature to raise taxes. Others require voter approval of certain tax hikes. Whatever the precise form, these fiscal rules make it harder for many states to increase their tax and expenditure effort in response to retrenching devolution in the health arena.

The antitax provisions that flourished in the last decades of the 20th century have reinforced another institutional factor that has traditionally placed states at a fiscal disadvantage relative to the national government. States cannot as easily run budget deficits to ride out economic downturns as the federal government can. When the economy sours, federal policy makers often see continued public spending and deficits by the national government as a way to counteract the slump. Nearly all states, in contrast, face requirements to balance their budgets even if it means slashing public programs. To be sure, states do find ways to borrow money and many employ an arsenal of fiscal gimmicks in an effort to mute the need for budget cuts. Upon winning a recall election in 2003, for instance, Governor Arnold Schwarzenegger's main response to the fiscal crisis of California was a

proposal to borrow some $15 billion through a special bond issue. Nonetheless, states tend to have less fiscal capacity during recessions than the national government. To the degree that proposals for retrenching devolution fail to take into account the limits to state capacity in fiscal downturns (e.g., by increasing the federal match during these periods), the constancy of state funding may well suffer.

State Commitment

Where there is a way, there may not be a will. Retrenching devolution also tests the commitment of states to health programs. Will policy processes in a state yield the kind of effort needed to overcome the loss of federal dollars so that health programs can be sustained and even enhanced? States may be able to compensate for reduced federal support in one of several ways. First, they may become more efficient or cost-effective in achieving health goals. Many proponents of devolution believe that narrow categorical programs that constrain state discretion breed inefficiencies. They contend that states can do the same or more with less if they are freed from federal rules. Second, state officials may mute the pain of federal retrenchment through heightened fiscal entrepreneurship. They may, for instance, "Medicaid" certain services that had previously been subsidized exclusively from the state's own treasury. Or they may come up with new gimmicks to increase the federal match per dollar of state expenditure. Third, policy makers at the state level may replace the lost federal dollars by shifting resources from other policy spheres to the health arena. As Colleen Grogan shows in Chapter 15, the interest groups supporting a health program such as Medicaid (e.g., nursing home providers, hospitals, advocates for disabled middle class children, unions) may be much more potent than those found in other policy arenas, such as higher education or welfare.

Fourth, states may be able to compensate for retrenching devolution through greater tax collection. Economic growth may allow this to occur painlessly by increasing the flow of revenues into state coffers. Other political developments may yield a windfall for the states. For instance, the signing of an historic Master Settlement Agreement between the tobacco companies and 46 state governments in November 1998 has been a fiscal godsend. (Four other states had reached a settlement with these companies earlier.) Under the terms of the agreement, major United States tobacco companies agreed to provide states with an estimated $206 billion over 25 years in exchange for agreements by state officials to hold them harmless for past and future medical claims related to tobacco use.

While states may prefer to deal with retrenching devolution in politically painless ways, they will at times face a difficult test—whether to let the health program erode or whether to raise taxes. In general, the greater the cuts in federal funding, the greater the likelihood that states will face this unpleasant choice. Some observers contend that the forces of competitive federalism especially as they pertain to economic development will tilt states toward reducing health benefits rather than enhancing their tax effort. Some even predict that states will race to the bottom in cutting health services.[36] This view in part rests on notions about the willingness of the affluent and business firms to vote with their feet. Presumably, greater tax effort on behalf of health care programs for low-income citizens would tend to trigger the departure of firms and the well heeled to lower-tax states with more business-friendly climates. This development could erode a state's fiscal capacity. The pessimistic perspective on state commitment also springs from the idea that generous health benefits could cause the state to become a magnet for low-income people living elsewhere. Fiscal pressure on the state would thereby grow as out-of-staters moved in and signed up for program benefits. To stem this tide, state policy makers would presumably move to lower benefit levels.

The exact degree to which these forces of competitive federalism will cause states to choose health program erosion over greater tax effort in the face of retrenching devolution remains an open question. Clearly, certain underlying assumptions of this perspective should be taken with a grain of salt. For instance, one can find little hard evidence to support the view that low-income people base geographic decisions on their calculations of the health program benefits a state offers. Moreover, political forces within a state may unleash substantial pressures on policy makers to preserve program benefits. Nonetheless, one cannot dismiss the possibility that, other things being equal, states face more pressure to resist greater tax effort to support health program benefits than the federal government does. In an era when labor and capital are increasingly mobile, state policy makers have valid reasons to fear that greater tax effort to compensate for diminished federal funds will fuel the flight of business and the well-off.[37] Moreover, despite the absence of supporting evidence, state policy makers often cling to the view that generous benefits serve as a magnet for low-income individuals in other states.

Whatever the precise damping effect of these factors on state commitment to their health programs, one thing is clear: states vary greatly in their willingness to fund them. In the case of Medicaid, for example, great differences exist in the propensity of states to allocate their own resources to the program. In 2000, for example, Medicaid expenditures per $1,000 of total taxable resources (with adjustments for cost differences among states) ranged from a high of $18.16 in New York to a low of $3.74 in Utah. Among the ten most populous states, New York exerted over three times more effort than Texas, the least committed state in the top ten. (Texas spent $5.58 on Medicaid per $1,000 of its total taxable resources.)[38]

Hence, state responses to retrenching devolution seem sure to vary considerably. An array of factors internal to state policy processes helps explain these differences including the degree to which citizens of the state are politically liberal and degree to which interest groups supporting health programs are present. In the case of New York, for instance, health care providers (hospitals, nursing homes), unions representing health workers, and advocacy groups (e.g., parents with disabled children) routinely band together to fight cuts to the Medicaid program. Nor can one dismiss the preferences of key policy makers and executive branch administrators as independent sources of support for health care programs for low-income people. Hence, a committed governor in a relatively conservative state, Tennessee, fought successfully for a 1115 waiver under Medicaid to establish TennCare, one of the most comprehensive state programs in the country for reducing the ranks of the uninsured.

Finally, shifting funding responsibilities to the states also shifts the tax burden onto different shoulders. In part because they rely on sales and property taxes as well as relatively flat income taxes,[39] state and local revenue systems are more regressive than that of the national government. They end up taking a higher percentage of income from middle- and low-income families than from the affluent. Moreover, state policy makers over the decade of the 1990s and early 2000s approved changes in tax law that made state financing even more regressive.[40] Hence, to the degree that states cope with retrenching devolution through higher taxes, prospects increase that lower and middle-income people will bear more of the costs. Ironies sometimes underlie this pattern. Many states have opted for a highly regressive excise tax on tobacco in no small part as a public health measure. The tax to some degree deters smoking, but the hard truth remains that smokers disproportionately tend to be less educated and less affluent. While evidence suggests that low-income smokers are as likely to try to quit as those further up the socioeconomic ladder, they succeed less often than their more affluent counterparts.[41]

Overview of State Response

The heady talk of the resurgent states that became common after the 1960s has considerable basis in reality. States have bolstered their governing capacity and in many cases enjoy increased fiscal capacity as well. Many of them have repeatedly demonstrated their commitment to providing health care to needy citizens. But this does not mean they will hold programs like Medicaid harmless in the face of retrenching devolution. Many states have slipped backward in their capacity. Moreover, a constellation of forces, such as interstate economic competition and political ideology, place firm constraints on the willingness of

states to preserve health programs in the face of diminished federal subsidies. Clearly, the fiscal specifics of any proposal for retrenching devolution matter greatly. Other things being equal, the larger the cut in federal support the greater the likelihood that state health programs will erode.

CONCLUSION

In forging a constitution aimed at strengthening the national government, the founding fathers recognized that states would play an enduring role in American governance. Yet it was not until the 20th century that the states and the federal government became major actors on the health stage. Those who prefer a neat division of labor between the national government and the states would be sorely disappointed as the century unfolded. After World War II and especially after the advent of Medicaid in 1965, grants from the national government to the states became a core theme in the story of federalism and health policy.

Some see the rise of these intergovernmental grant programs as a sign of growing federal power at the expense of the states. Without question, these national programs shaped the health policy agendas of the states. The federal regulations that accompanied grants constrained state leaders in framing the goals and means of health policy. But states are not timorous servants of the federal government. Since state monies flow into these programs as well, states have had considerable leverage in negotiating with the federal government—they partially pay the piper, they partially call the tune. Moreover, the intergovernmental lobby, including such groups as the National Governors Association, often shape grant legislation in the first place. Then too, the central government cannot easily coerce states into vigorously implementing federal requirements with which they disagree. States can in critical respects practice de facto nullification of federal mandates through the implementation process at least over the short term.

Furthermore, focusing on the balance of power between the national government and the states makes it easy to overlook the way federalism enhances the role of both levels. The fact that one level of government can pursue health policy initiatives confident its partner will pick up part of the tab often empowers both levels of government vis-à-vis the private sector.

Over the last two decades, the issue of devolution to the states has become central to health policy debates. Devolution proposals involve both fiscal and programmatic issues. How much money does the federal government plan to provide to the states under a given proposal over the short and long term? How much discretion over goals and means does it intend to grant them in spending those dollars? Answers to these questions can help us distinguish between retrenching and empowering devolution. The devil is always in the details. The consequences of a devolution proposal for health care access, quality, and cost will vary depending on specifics. For instance, no amount of happy talk about the growing capacity and commitment of state governments should mask the negative consequences that would ensue if the national government puts a much greater financial burden on the states to pay for health care programs. The critical programmatic question about devolution revolves around the degree to which federal policy makers should grant states greater discretion over goals and means. Canada, for example, gives its provinces substantial discretion over their health care programs but insists on a goal—that all provinces provide universal health insurance to their citizens.

Political differences over the appropriate balance of power between the national and states governments in the health care arena will no doubt persist. The dimensions and outcomes of this struggle will partly depend on which political party prevails. If the Republican Party controls all three branches of the national government, retrenching devolution driven by "starve-the-beast" fiscal policies becomes more likely. For instance, the quest to convert Medicaid from an entitlement to a less generously funded block grant would sporadically surface. Despite fierce state resistance, substantial middle class opposition to program cuts and the propensity of Republican policy makers to run up the public debt rather than reduce federal spending, this quest might at some point succeed. If the Democratic Party comes to dominate the agenda, health care reform may very well be one of its signal issues. Democrats may succeed in shoring up support for intergovernmental health programs though this party will also face pressures to deal with massive federal budget deficits.

While the electoral fortunes of the two major political parties will do much to shape the future of federalism and health policy in at least one respect the parties have converged over the last decade. Both President Bill Clinton and President George W. Bush have effectively used the tools of the administrative presidency, specifically waivers, to foster significant programmatic devolution to the states. In this sense, devolution—and federalism more generally—has become centered more in the executive branch at both the national and state levels.

STUDY QUESTIONS

1. A famous cake metaphor illustrates differing conceptions of American federalism. Describe it.
2. How does the federal government induce state action on health care through the issuance of intergovernmental grants? What is the difference between a *categorical* and *block* grant?
3. What are some of the ways by which states can effectively nullify pieces of federal legislation? What allows states to 'get away with it'?
4. What is an executive waiver? What are the factors limiting the success Congress in challenging executive waivers?
5. What kinds of recent trends suggest an erosion of state governing capacity?

6. What is ERISA? How has ERISA limited state autonomy in the field of health policy?

7. What are some of the ways in which further devolution in health policy could affect program execution?

NOTES

* We thank Martha Derthick, George Greenberg, and James Morone for perceptive comments on an earlier draft. We alone remain responsible for any lingering defects.

1. Davey, 2003; Weissert and Miller, 2005.
2. Hamilton, Madison, and Jay, 1964 (No. 39), p 246 and (No. 46), p 295. For a contemporary overview of federalism, see Derthick, 2001.
3. Grodzins, 1960.
4. See, for example, Scheberle, 2004.
5. Starr, 1982, p 184.
6. Katharine Levit et al., 2004.
7. US General Accounting Office, 1998, p 3.
8. Posner, 2003.
9. Sardell and Johnson, 1998.
10. For another perspective on this relationship, see Gormley and Boccuti, 2001.
11. Nathan, 1983.
12. States submit their proposals to the Centers for Medicare and Medicaid Services, which is part of the federal Department of Health and Human Services. Prior to 2001, the agency was called the Health Care Financing Administration.
13. US Department of Health and Human Services, 2003.
14. US General Accounting Office, 2002; 2004.
15. US General Accounting Office, 2003a, pp 11–12.
16. US General Accounting Office, 2002.
17. US General Accounting Office, 2004.
18. Gais and Fossett, In press.
19. US General Accounting Office, 2003b.
20. US General Accounting Office, 2003b.
21. For a more detailed assessment of these practices, see Gilman, 1998, pp 155–86; and Thompson, 1998, pp 36–41.
22. Gilman, 1998, p 159.
23. Quoted in Thompson, 1998, p 39.
24. Coughlin, Bruen, and King, 2004.
25. Nye, Jr., Zelikow, and King, 1997.
26. Teaford, 2002, p 225.
27. While not discussed here, a third type of devolution deserves note. Under directive devolution, the national government shifts at least some of the burden for funding programs to the states but provides virtually no regulatory relief.
28. See Skocpol, 1992, pp 480–524.
29. On other occasions President Bush worked to strip states of discretion. The president's program to provide seniors with prescription drugs under Medicare threatens to curtail state innovation in the operation of their pharmacy assistance programs. The new law also imposes "clawback" payments on the states. Since the federal government will cover some of the drug costs for the elderly previously subsidized by state Medicaid programs, the national government has initially required the states to remit 90% of their savings to the federal treasury. See Weissert and Miller, 2005.
30. Goldstein, 2003.
31. Pear, 2004a.
32. Pear, 2004b. In October 2005, however, the Governor of Vermont and federal officials reached agreement on a waiver that would impose a cap on Medicaid expenditures in that state. "Vermont Deal Seeks to Curb Medicaid Costs," 2005.
33. See, for instance, Light, 2003.
34. See Zabawa, 2001.
35. US General Accounting Office, 2003b.
36. For a more general statement of this argument not specifically focused on health care, see Peterson and Rom, 1990.
37. Donahue, 1997, pp 171–82.
38. US General Accounting Office 2003b, pp 44–5.
39. A pure flat tax imposes one rate. While many states have a graduated income tax where the more affluent pay a higher percentage, the top rate often clicks in at a relatively low income level. Hence, the affluent and people of much more modest means are often taxed at the same rate.

40. McIntyre et al., 2003.
41. Barbeau, Krieger, and Soobader, 2004; Remler, 2004.

REFERENCES

Barbeau, E.M. N. Krieger and M-J. Soobader. 2004. Working Class Matters: Socioeconomic Disadvantage, Race/Ethnicity, Gender, and Smoking in NHIS 2000. *American Journal of Public Health* 94 (2): 269–78,

Coughlin, T.A., B.K. Bruen and J. King. 2004. States' Use of Medicaid UPL and DSH Financial Mechanisms. *Health Affairs* 23 (2): 245–57.

Davey, M. 2003. Illinois to Seek U.S. Exemption to Buy Drugs from Canada. *New York Times* December 22: A27.

Derthick, M. 2001. Keeping The Compound Republic: Essays on American Federalism. Washington DC: Brookings Institution.

Donahue, J.D. 1997. *Disunited States*. New York: Basic Books.

Gais, T., and J. Fossett. In press. *Federalism and the Executive Branch*, ed. J.D. Aberbach and M.A. Peterson. New York: Oxford University Press.

Gilman, J.D. 1998. *Medicaid and the Costs of Federalism, 1984–1992*. New York: Garland Publishing.

Goldsmith, A. 2003. Governors Cool on Medicaid Initiative. *Washington Post* February 24: A21.

Gormley, W.T., and C. Boccuti. 2001. HCFA and the States: Politics and Intergovernmental Leverage. *Journal of Health Politics, Policy and Law* 26 (2): 557–80.

Grodzins, Morton. 1960. The Federal System. *Goals For Americans: The Report of the President's Commission on National Goals*. Englewood Cliffs, NJ: Prentice Hall.

Hamilton, A., J. Madison, J. Jay. 1964. *The Federalist Papers,* ed. C. Rossiter. New York: Mentor Books.

Levit, Katharine R., et al. 2004. Health Spending Rebound Continues in 2002. *Health Affairs* 23 (1): 147–59.

Light, P.C. 2003. Measuring the Health of the Federal Public Service. In *Workways of Governance,* ed. R.H. Davidson. Washington DC: Brookings Institution, pp 90–120.

McIntyre, R.S., et al. 2003. *Who Pays? A Distributional Analysis of the Tax Systems in All 50 States*. Washington DC: Institute on Taxation and Economic Policy, second edition.

Nathan, R.P. 1983. *The Administrative Presidency*. New York: Macmillan.

Nye, J.S. Jr., P.D. Zelikow and D.C. King, eds. 1997. *Why People Don't Trust Government*. Cambridge: Harvard University Press.

Posner, P.L. 2003. *Federal Assistance: Grant System Continues to be Highly Fragmented*. Washington DC: General Accounting Office, GAO-03–718T.

Pear, R. 2004a. All Governors to be Asked to Back Bush on Medicaid. *New York Times* February 16: A1.

—— 2004b. Medicare Nominee Backs Drug Imports. *New York Times*. March 9: A22.

Peterson, P., and M. Rom. 1990. *Welfare Magnets*. Washington DC: Brookings Institution.

Remler, D.K. 2004. Poor Smokers, Poor Quitters, and Cigarette Tax Regressivity. *American Journal of Public Health* 94 (2):225–9.

Sardell, A. and K. Johnson. 1998. The Politics of EPSDT Policy in the 1990s: Policy Entrepreneurs, Political Streams, and Children's Health Benefits. *The Milbank Quarterly* 76 (2): 175–205.

Scheberle, D. 2004. *Federalism and Environmental Policy* (2nd ed.). Washington DC: Georgetown University Press.

Skocpol, T. 1992. *Protecting Soldiers and Mothers*. Cambridge: Harvard University Press.

Starr, P. 1982. The Social Transformation of American Medicine. New York: Basic Books.

Teaford, J.C. 2002. *The Rise of the States*. Baltimore: Johns Hopkins University Press.

Thompson, F.J. 1998. The Faces of Devolution. In *Medicaid and Devolution: A View From the States*, ed. F.J. Thompson and J.J. DiIulio, Jr. Washington DC: Brookings Institution, pp 14–55.

US Department of Health and Human Services. 2003. www.cms.hhs.gov/medicaid/1115/ statesum.pdf. August 28.

US General Accounting Office. 1998. Design Features Shape Flexibility, Accountability, and Performance Information. Washington DC: GAO/GGD-98–137.

—— 2002. Medicaid and SCHIP: Recent HHS Approvals of Demonstration Waiver Projects Raises Concerns. Washington DC: GAO-02–187.

—— 2003a. Long-Term Care: Federal Oversight of Growing Medicaid Home and Community-Based Waivers Should Be Strengthened. Washington DC: GAO-03–576.

—— 2003b. Medicaid Formula: Differences in Funding Ability among States Are Often Widened. Washington DC: GAO-03–620.

—— 2004. SCHIP: HHS Continues to Approve Waivers That Are Inconsistent with Program Goals. Washington DC: GAO-04–166R.

"Vermont Deal Seeks to Curb Medicaid Costs." 2005. *New York Times* October 3: A15.

Weissert, W.G., and E.A. Miller. 2005. Punishing the Pioneers: The Medicare Modernization Act and State Pharmacy Assistance Programs. *Publius* 35 (1): 115–42.

Zabawa, B.J. 2001. Breaking Through the ERISA Blockade: The Ability of States to Access Employer Health Plan Information in Medicaid Expansion Initiatives. *Quinnipiac Health Law Journal* 5 (1): 1–33.

CHAPTER 8

State Governments:
E Pluribus Multa*

Howard M. Leichter

The state governments influence almost every feature of our health care system. This chapter describes state governments—the similarities between them, the differences among them, and the problems that these "laboratories of democracy" all face.

There is a crisis in American health care. The nature of the crisis is as clear as it is alarming. First, an unacceptably large number of Americans—more than 45 million in 2005, or over 15% of the population under age 65—have no health insurance. Second, the United States spends 134% more on health care than any of the 30 industrialized nations in the Organization for Economic Cooperation and Development. Moreover, the rate of health care cost increases has exceeded overall inflation for nearly every year in the last 30. Third, despite this huge investment in health, Americans are no healthier than people in other countries which spend far less of their national resources on health care. In fact, in 2000 the United States ranked 72nd among the 191 nations surveyed by the World Health Organization in "level of health," defined as "a health system's ability to make the health status of its [citizens] as good as possible over a life cycle, including life expectancy."[1]

As revealing and disturbing as these statistics are, they actually obscure more than they reveal about both the health status of Americans and the nature of our health care system. There is enormous variation across the states in the availability, accessibility, affordability, quality, and financing of health care, as well the health status of Americans. Furthermore, many of the most important decisions affecting our health and health care are made within the states. Must a child be immunized before he or she can attend a public school? Can a poor, undocumented, and uninsured Hispanic woman get prenatal care? Does a teenage girl have access to birth control pills at a school or public health clinic? Does the owner of a small business receive a subsidy to help pay health insurance premiums for his or her employees? Can a person who is a high medical risk purchase health insurance? Is there adequate planning for a major disease outbreak or a biochemical terrorist attack? All

173

things these things do or do not happen because of some state law, regulation, or practice. To understand health care in America, one must understand that we have not one, but 50 health care systems.

In this chapter, I examine the role played by the states in the nation's health care system. I begin with the point that the states differ, significantly and dramatically, in terms of population structure, health care problems, services and facilities, as well the capacity and willingness of their people and policy makers to address outstanding problems through the use of government. Next I review the actual health and health care responsibilities of the states. From the perspective of state governments, health care is of extraordinary fiscal and political importance; nearly one-third of all state revenues are devoted to health programs. For the average American, virtually every facet of our involvement in the health care system is in some way influenced by state law, whether it is the safety of the food and water we consume, or if our private health insurance must cover the cost of contraceptive devices, or if our children must wear safety helmets when they ride their bicycles.

The importance, and impact, of health care policy on state governments is in no small measure a reflection of one program in particular, Medicaid, including the 1997 addition to that law, the State Children's Health Insurance Plan (SCHIP). Medicaid alone consumes one-fifth of most state budgets and is second in cost only to K–12 education in terms of state dollars spent. This program has come to occupy a disproportionate share of the time, energy, and resources of state governments and is the subject of the penultimate section of the chapter.

Lastly, I turn to the implications of the diversity that exists among the states, and the apparent disparities that exist among various groups within the states—a recent Institute of Medicine panel found that blacks and other minorities were less likely to get proper heart medication, heart bypass surgery, kidney dialysis, and organ transplants than whites. This diversity, and these disparities, raise a question that has both theoretical and practical implications for the health care policy debate. The question is whether the health care needs of Americans are best served by state flexibility or federally imposed uniformity? On one side there are those who believe that because of the diversity among the states, each should be given maximum flexibility and autonomy in fashioning its own health care policies. What works in Mississippi or Texas, politically, fiscally, and culturally, is unlikely to work in, or even be acceptable in, Oregon or Vermont. Others argue, however, that the states do not have the administrative or political capacity to undertake significant reform beyond incremental changes to specific problems. Furthermore, they believe that while we tolerate disparities among the citizens of different states in some policy areas (e.g., public transportation or agricultural extension services), health-related inequalities or disparities should be intolerable. Medicare, they argue, has flourished as a national program, despite the cultural differences between Mississippi and Oregon. Hence, system reform should be a federal responsibility, assuring all Americans, wherever they live, the health care they need.

DIVERSITY WITHIN AND AMONG THE AMERICAN STATES

American states are extraordinarily diverse in ways that influence both the scope and nature of health issues with which they must deal, and the political and material resources available to deal with them. An analysis of four of the factors that influence health problems and policies among the states will illustrate the nature and implications of state diversity. They are: the composition of the population; the nature of the health problems; the availability of health care resources; and the political culture of the state.

The Population

The demographic composition and socioeconomic status of a state's population shapes the nature of the health problems the state will face—and its fiscal capacity to deal with these problems. Included among the health-related population characteristics are: race and ethnicity, degree of poverty, age, and residential living patterns. States with large African American populations, such as Mississippi (36.9% of the total population), Louisiana (32.9%), South Carolina (30.0%), Georgia (28.7%), Maryland (28.1%), and Alabama (26.4%) are likely to face a different set of health problems than Montana, North and South Dakota, Idaho, and Vermont where blacks make up less than 1% of the population.[2] Race and ethnicity influence disease patterns and health problems in a variety of ways. Blacks, for example, have a higher rate or incidence of obesity, diabetes, smoking, teenage births, low-birth weight infants, and mothers receiving late or no prenatal care than non-Hispanic whites. In addition, black women are twice as likely to get and die from breast cancer as white women, and the black infant mortality rate is more than double that of whites. Clearly the health problems, and the health policy agendas, in Mississippi, South Carolina, and Louisiana differ from those in Montana and North Dakota.

Many of the same health-related disparities exist between Hispanic and non-Hispanic white populations. As a result, states with large Hispanic populations, such as New Mexico (43.2% Hispanic) California (34.3%), and Texas (34.2%), face problems similar to those in states with large African American populations. Hispanic women, for example, are more likely to receive late or no prenatal care (5.5%) than whites (3.1%), a problem that is compounded by the fact that Hispanic births constitute about one-half of all births in the three states. The problem is further complicated by the fact that Hispanics have the highest uninsured rate of all racial/ethnic groups (see Figure 8-1). One result is that Hispanics are more likely to rely on state-funded community and public health clinics than any other group: 20% of all Hispanics use these clinics as their regular source of health care compared to 9% of non-Hispanic whites.[3]

Poverty, which is highly correlated with race and ethnicity, is another key predictor of both the nature

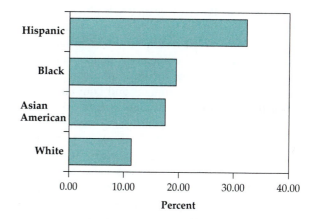

Figure 8-1 Percentage of Americans under 65 without Insurance

SOURCE: Doty, Michelle M. 2003.

Table 8-1 Percent of Population in Poverty: 2003 (National Rate = 12.1)

1.	Arkansas	18.5
2.	New Mexico	18.0
3.	Mississippi	17.9
4.	Louisiana	16.9
5.	West Virginia	16.9
45.	Connecticut	7.9
46.	Delaware	7.7
48.	Maryland	7.7
49.	Minnesota	7.1
50.	New Hampshire	6.0

a state's health problems and the resources available to deal with these. Here, too, there are extreme differences among the states (see Table 8-1): Arkansas's poverty rate is more than three times higher than New Hampshire's. Most troubling, however, is the state-by-state variation in poverty among children. Although the national average in 2002 for childhood poverty was 17.3%, the rate in New Hampshire was just 7.8%, while that in Mississippi was almost four times higher (28.3%). Poverty is related to health and health care in at least two ways. First, because eligibility in most publicly funded health insurance programs is largely determined by income, states with high poverty rates have large Medicaid populations (e.g., one of every five Mississippians and Louisianans are enrolled in Medicaid). Second, states with high poverty rates are likely to have high rates of natal-related health problems, such as births to teenage mothers, infant mortality, and mothers who receive late or no prenatal care. These states also have significant proportions of their population who engage in health-endangering lifestyle choices. Arkansas, for example, the state with the worst poverty rate in the nation, has the highest death rate from cerebrovascular disease, the second highest death rate from lung cancer, the eighth worst death rate from injuries, and the fifth worst highway fatality rate.

Although not as important as poverty or race, generational differences among states also influence health policy and politics. States with large 65-year-old or older populations, such as Florida (17.0%), Pennsylvania, West Virginia, North and South Dakota, Iowa, Maine, and Rhode Island (each with about 14%), are likely to devote a larger proportion of their health care resources to the treatment of chronic illnesses and the provision of long-term care facilities than Alaska (with only 6.3% of its population over 65), Utah (8.6%), Georgia (9.5%), or Colorado (9.7%). On the other hand, states with an older population are relieved of a significant portion of their health care responsibility because of Medicare, the federal health insurance program which covers older Americans. The reverse side of the generational coin also influences the health policy agenda. States with relatively young populations, such as Utah, Texas, and Alaska, each of with a school-age population of over 20% of its total population, will have different priorities (e.g., immunization and school-lunch programs, school-based clinics, etc.) than states with older populations (e.g., Florida and West Virginia).

Lastly, states differ with regard to dominant residential living patterns, which can be characterized in at least two ways: percentage of population living in metropolitan areas, and population density. For example, over 95% of the people in New Jersey, California, Connecticut, and Massachusetts live in metropolitan areas, whereas only one-third or fewer of the people in Wyoming, Montana, North and South Dakota, and Vermont live in such areas. A somewhat different, but related, way of viewing the distribution of state populations is in terms of population density. States like New Jersey (1,173 people per square mile), Rhode Island (1,034), and Massachusetts (818), have quite high concentrations of population, compared to much less densely populated states like Montana (6.4), Wyoming (5.2), and Alaska (1.1). What does all this have to do with health? For one thing it may help determine the accessibility of certain kinds of health services and facilities. For example, as many as three-fourths of the people living in Wyoming do not have adequate mental health practitioners "within reasonable economic and geographic bounds." Similar access problems exist in Idaho, Alabama, New Mexico, and Arkansas. This compares to Massachusetts, Connecticut, and Delaware in which 98% or more of the people have geographic access to mental health services.

States, then, differ in terms of what their populations look like, and these differences, in turn, influence health and health care issues. States also differ in terms of the nature of their health problems.

The Health Profile of States

Patterns of poor health and poor health habits do not occur randomly. Consider, for example, Kentucky and West Virginia, both of which are major tobacco producing states and rank first and second respectively in terms of the percent of adults who smoke (30.8% in Kentucky and 27.4% in West Virginia compared to the national average of 22.1%). Not surprisingly, both states were among the top three for estimated rates of new lung cancer cases in 2005: West Virginia ranked first with 88.7 new cases per 100,000 people and Kentucky third with 84.2 per 100,000, compared to the national average of 55.7 per 100,000. Furthermore, the high lung cancer rate has contributed to an overall high death rate in each state. In 2002, West Virginia had the worst death rate in the nation (1,166 deaths per 100,000 population), and Kentucky had the eighth worst rate (994.3 deaths per 100,000), both well above the national average of 847.3 deaths per 100,000 people.

Just as there are states that are characterized by poor health indicators, there are some in which good health and healthy lifestyles tend to cluster. A recent study by the United Health Foundation (UHF), used nine health risk factors, including risk of heart disease, adequacy of prenatal care, childhood poverty, and the prevalence of smoking, along with eight health outcomes (e.g., cancer deaths, infant mortality, infectious disease) to rank the 50 states. The states with the most positive health profiles, in rank-order, were Minnesota, New Hampshire, Vermont, Hawaii, and Utah.[4] The UHF results roughly correspond to a 21-factor ranking in the 2005 edition of *Health Care Rankings* which annually awards a "healthiest state" designation. The top five states in this ranking were Vermont, New Hampshire, Massachusetts, Minnesota, and Maine. Vermont's ranking is based, in part, on the fact that it had the best percentage rate of children covered by health insurance in the nation, the second best rates of teenage birth and infant mortality, the third best rates of mothers receiving first trimester prenatal care and fully immunized children, and the fifth best rate of adults who get regular, vigorous exercise.

The point here is that from a public health perspective, it is less meaningful to talk about the teen pregnancy rate in this country, than it is to note that Mississippi has a teen birth rate of 70.5 births per 1,000 women between 15 and 19 years old, the highest in the nation, and New Hampshire the lowest rate at 20.2 births per 1000 women. Why this important public health difference exists has very little to do with what happens in Washington DC and a great deal to do with what happens, or does not happen, in Concord and Jackson.

State Variations in Access to Health Care

A state's health problems, and the health status of its people, are the result of a variety of demographic and socioeconomic factors. They are also a function of the availability and accessibility of health care itself. Here, too, there is considerable state-by-state variation. We have already seen that virtually everyone in Delaware is at least within geographic proximity of mental health care whereas two-thirds the people in Wyoming are not. Although variation in access to primary care, something which affects everyone, is not as dramatic it is still problematic: about 25% of the people of Mississippi, New Mexico, Alabama, and Missouri lack either economic or geographic access to primary care, while this is a problem for roughly 5% of the people of Massachusetts, Hawaii, New Jersey, and Vermont. The issue of accessibility to primary care is at least in part a function of physician availability. State-by-state differences range from a high of over 400 physicians per 100,000 people in Massachusetts, New York, and Maryland to approximately one-half that number in Wyoming, Nevada, Mississippi, Oklahoma, and Idaho.

Variation also exists among the states with regard to the how well the health care needs of pregnant women and young children are being met. For example, over 7% of the pregnant women in Nevada and New Mexico received either late or no prenatal care in 2002 compared to less than 2% in Vermont, Maine, New Hampshire, and Rhode Island. In addition, 80% or more of children ages 19 to 35 months in Connecticut, Massachusetts, South Carolina, Rhode Island, and Virginia were fully immunized compared to fewer than 60% in Wyoming and Washington

Adequate health care facilities and services may be available and accessible in a state but will be of little use if people cannot afford to purchase them. Nearly 85% of non-elderly Americans pay for their health care primarily through some form of public or private health insurance. And, of those who are insured, the majority (60%) are covered through their employer. Like everything else related to health care in America, however, there is considerable variation among the states: about 70% of those in New Hampshire, Minnesota, Maryland, and Ohio had employment-based insurance in 2002, compared to less than 52% in New Mexico, Montana, and Arkansas.

For those non-elderly Americans who do not have private health insurance, the state and federal Medicaid programs provide the second most likely source of health insurance, covering 42.7 million Americans or 14.4% of the population in 2003. (The total cost of Medicaid in 2003 was $280 billion of which the states paid $120 billion.) As Colleen Grogran describes in Chapter 15, the federal government sets policy with regard to certain groups of people who must be covered by Medicaid (the "categorical" populations such as children under age 19, pregnant women, and persons with disabilities); however, each state decides how much of its own money to spend, the income cut off for noncategorical people, whether the Medicaid population must be enrolled in managed care or fee-for-service, what benefits they can receive, and what efforts are made to actually enroll eligible citizens into the program. We have already seen that one in five Mississippians and Louisianans are enrolled in Medicaid in large part because of the high incidence of poverty and low rates of private health insurance in these states. By way of contrast, Tennessee (22.3%) and Vermont (21.2%) have high rates of Medicaid enrollment largely because of their generous eligibility requirements. Vermont's Medicaid program, for example, is open to children below age six in families up to 225% of the federal poverty line (FPL) ($41,400 for a family of four), while its SCHIP program is open to those with family incomes up to 300% of the poverty line ($55,200 for a family of four). In the case of Tennessee, its highly acclaimed TennCare Medicaid program has no income eligibility threshold, although people with incomes above the FPL must pay premiums, deductibles, and copayments.

States also differ in terms of how much of their own money they spend on each Medicaid client—the states choose the level of spending on each client and the federal government matches with a payment between 50% and 77% of the cost. (The minimum federal match is 50% in high per capita income states such as Colorado, Connecticut,

Delaware, and Illinois and the maximum match is 77% in Mississippi, the state with the lowest per capita income.)[5] New York is by far the most generous state spending $1,895 of its own money for each Medicaid recipient in 2002 compared to just $372 per person in Nevada (the national average was $852).

Although the largest item in every state's health care budget, Medicaid is not the states' only health care responsibility. States (and localities) fund public health clinics, immunization and health education programs, operate medical schools, license and monitor the professional competence and ethical behavior of health care providers, and perform health and safety inspections. We can gauge the fiscal commitment of states to the health care needs of their citizens in two ways. The first is per capita state government spending for health programs (see Table 8-2); the second is health care expenditures as a percent of gross state product (see Table 8-3). Tables 8-2 and 8-3 list the five highest and lowest spending states in each category. As Table 8-2 indicates, there is a considerable difference in commitment in terms of per capita spending, ranging from a high of $319 per person in Hawaii to just $70 per person in Colorado and Nevada. In terms of health care spending as a percentage of

Table 8-2 Per Capita State Government Expenditures for Health Programs in 2001 (National Per Capita = $153)

Rank	State	Per Capita ($)
1.	Hawaii	319
2.	Delaware	305
3.	Massachusetts	283
4.	Michigan	272
5.	Montana	258
46.	North Dakota	79
47.	Idaho	78
48.	Iowa	76
49.	Colorado	70
50.	Nevada	70

Table 8-3 Health Care Expenditures as a Percent of Gross State Product in 1998 (National Percent = 11.6% of Total Gross Product)

Rank	State	Percent
1.	West Virginia	18.0
2.	North Dakota	15.7
3.	Maine	15.2
4.	Mississippi	14.6
5.	Florida	14.5
46.	Virginia	9.7
47.	Delaware	9.4
48.	Nevada	8.7
49.	Alaska	8.5
50.	Wyoming	8.5

Gross State Product, West Virginia spends more than twice the percentage (18%) as Wyoming, Alaska, and Nevada (about 8.5%).

Another way of capturing a state's commitment to public health has been developed by the UHF in their "support for public health" index, which they define and explain as: "A ratio of health care expenditures to low-income population. This is an indication of whether a state's budget priorities reflect the public health care needs of the population."[6] The calculation of public health care support produces a considerably different ranking than those in Tables 8-2 and 8-3. West Virginia, for instance, ranks first in the nation in terms of health care expenditures as a percentage of gross state product but is tied for 43rd place, with Alabama, on the UHF Index. The point is less which of these measures best captures a state's commitment to the health care needs of its population than the fact that states have very different levels of commitment. This is especially relevant to the most vulnerable citizens in a state, who rely heavily on public programs for their health care. From a public health perspective, according to the UHF, being poor in New Hampshire, New Jersey, or Minnesota, which have the highest levels of support for public health, is quite different in terms

of health care needs met than being poor in Oregon, Wisconsin, or New Mexico with the lowest levels of support.[7]

State Capacity for Dealing with Health Problems

The ability of a state to respond to the health care needs of its people is, to begin with, closely tied to the wealth of its citizens and taxpayers, as measured by per capita personal income. In 2003, state personal income ranged from over $40,000 per capita (e.g., Connecticut and New Jersey) to under $25,000 (Arkansas, West Virginia, and Mississippi). In fact, Connecticut's per capita income of $43,292 was nearly twice that of Mississippi's $23,343. Despite having the nation's highest teenage birth rate and second highest infant mortality rate, Mississippi's ability to respond to these problems, assuming there is the political will to do so, is limited by the revenues at its disposal.

Fashioning policies that address the health care needs of its citizens is not merely a matter of the availability of public and private resources but also a willingness of a state's political leaders to use government to solve social problems. In this regard it is important to understand that some states have political traditions and cultures that support active involvement of government in addressing social issues, including health problems. States such as Wisconsin, Minnesota, Vermont, Maine, Massachusetts, Oregon, and Hawaii have long traditions of innovative social policies—and often moderate to liberal politics—and a willingness to use government to address serious social problems. And, indeed, each of these states has been at the forefront of health care reform in the last few decades. By way of contrast, some states have political traditions that are much less supportive of activist government. One such example is Arizona, which was the last state to establish a Medicaid program, *17 years* after passage of the law in 1965. Arizona's political leadership continued to be skeptical about federal involvement in the health care of Arizonians when its legislature initially rejected participation in the

SCHIP, claiming that it was federal interference in the state's business. The state legislature ultimately agreed to participate but refused to allow public schools to receive contracts to enroll students in the program, thereby limiting the outreach effort and, presumably, enrollments in SCHIP. Other states that have shown a similar reluctance to rely on government, federal or state, to deal with health care access issues are Mississippi, Alabama, Texas, Arkansas, Louisiana, and South Carolina. One private health care foundation officer in Texas explained his state's poor performance in encouraging participation in SCHIP by noting that: "There are elements [in the state] who think this is the thin edge of the wedge of socialized medicine."[8]

The willingness of a state's leaders and people to seek public solutions to health problems is, in part, a function of what Daniel Elazar identified some years ago as the political subculture or tradition of the state. Elazar identified three ideal or pure subcultures—moralistic, individualistic, and traditional. The subculture type that is most supportive of activist government is the *moralistic* tradition which, according to Elazar,

> emphasizes the commonwealth conception as the basis for democratic government. Politics, to the moralistic political culture, is considered one of the great activities of humanity in its search for the good society. . . . Consequently, in the moralistic political culture both the general public and the politicians conceive of politics as a public activity centered on some notion of the public good and properly devoted to the advancement of the public interest.[9]

Among the moralistic states Elazar counted were Oregon, Minnesota, Wisconsin, Michigan, Vermont, and Maine; sure enough, each has been at the forefront of health care reform during the last decade. Most recently, as Elizabeth Kilbreth describes in Reflection 2, Maine enacted a program called Dirigo—after the state motto which in Latin means, "I lead." Dirigo combines an expansion of MaineCare, the state's Medicaid and SCHIP program, and a subsidized public/private health insurance plan for small businesses (i.e., 2–50 employees), self-employed, unemployed, and part-time workers. When fully implemented in 2009, Dirigo will result in universal access to health care through health insurance.[10] Dirigo joins the innovative programs in other "moralistic" states, such as the Oregon Health Plan, MinnesotaCare, BadgerCare, and Vermont's Dr. Dynasaur for children.

Elazar characterizes the other two cultural types as much less supportive of activist government. In *traditionalistic* cultures, people expect government to maintain the status quo and not engage in innovative and costly social experiments, while those in *individualistic* cultures support the notion that government spending should be limited to basic services. He categorizes New Mexico, Texas, Oklahoma, Kentucky, and West Virginia as traditionalistic-individualistic states and, indeed, none of these has been particularly innovative in its health policies. On the other hand, one might not expect much health policy innovation from Hawaii which, according to Elazar, has an individualistic–traditionalistic culture. Yet Hawaii, the only state in the nation to require employers to provide health insurance (a policy known as an "employer mandate"), is often viewed as a model of statist activism. The apparent inconsistency between a politically antistatist dominant culture and policy activism can be explained by Hawaii's unique history. At various times in its history, the Aloha State has been politically dominated or heavily influenced by a benevolent monarchy, Christian missionaries, plantation owners, and a strong labor union movement, all of whom took a paternalistic, and self-serving, attitude toward providing subjects/believers/workers health care.

A more recent and empirically based effort to characterize states values, and one which actually closely parallels the Elazar study, was a survey of the American electorate done in 2004 by The Pew

Research Center for the People and the Press. The Center asked a series of social values questions about "homosexuality, acceptable content for school libraries, the role of women, the issue of day care, AIDS, family and marriage, and ideas of good and evil." The study then ranked the most traditional (Mississippi, South Carolina, Kentucky, Oklahoma, Tennessee, North Carolina, Alabama, West Virginia, Ohio, Indiana, Louisiana, and Georgia) and least traditional states (Maine, New Hampshire, Vermont, Rhode Island, Massachusetts, Connecticut, New York, California, New Jersey, Oregon, Minnesota, and Washington.)[11] The list, with some exceptions in both categories (e.g., Tennessee and New Hampshire) corresponds closely to both what Elazar found and what we have seen here with regard to state health policy. The list of least traditional states bears remarkable resemblance to the states that I have identified as policy innovators and reformers.

In short, states differ in how they define the role of government in addressing social problems and issues. Two different states may have similar populations, share common health problems, but follow decidedly different public health policies. Consider, for example, the comparison of California and Texas. Both are large, Sunbelt states, with rapidly growing populations, and a large agricultural sector. Both have large uninsured populations—Texas ranks first and California fourth in rates of uninsured—and the second (California) and third (Texas) largest Hispanic populations in the country. Yet California is, in contemporary political parlance, a "blue (Democratic) state" and Texas a "red (Republican) state." California ranks first in the nation in terms of the percentage of its population receiving public aid (6.4% in 2002), Texas ranks 25th (3.6%); California ranks eighth in terms of per capita state government expenditures for health ($280 per person in 2002), Texas 40th ($124); Texas ranked fifth worst for the rate of mothers receiving late or no prenatal care in 2002 (5.0%), while California was 10th best (2.6%). No one, in short, would confuse the health politics and policies of California and Texas despite the similarities between the two states.

THE HEALTH ROLE OF THE STATES: A NEW AND EXPANDING MANDATE
Protecting the Public's Health

"The preservation of the public health is among the most important goals of government."[12] Beginning in 1855 with the establishment of the first state public health office in Louisiana, state governments—along with their city and county partners—have played a major role in protecting the public's health by monitoring the health status of the population, and controlling or eradicating the microbial and man-made conditions that pose hazards to the community. Historically this has meant surveillance and control of sexually transmitted (e.g., syphilis and HIV/AIDS), infectious and communicable diseases, ranging from typhoid, typhus, and yellow fever in the 19th century, to West Nile and SARS in the 21st century. State health departments are also responsible for enforcing laws concerning food handling, immunizations, air and water safety, and public sanitation.

Beyond their historical public health role, states perform an enormous range of health care-related functions. They are, for example: the primary regulators of the health care industry, licensing physicians, nurses, pharmacists, and other health professionals; regulating insurance companies, nursing homes, and hospitals; setting rules governing workers' compensation; and, establishing standards for controlling environmental pollution. Lastly, like so much else in America, September 11, 2001 altered, and expanded, the public health function of the states. The terrorist of attacks of 9/11 "followed closely by the anthrax scare . . . turned bioterrorism preparedness into the overwhelming focus of many public health departments."[13] Today the states are a key player in protecting Americans from the health consequences of any terrorist attack.

The traditional public health role of the states has also been expanded to include regulating lifestyles.

Beginning in the late 1970s, and accelerating during the next decades, health care professionals, and public policy makers, adopted what has been termed a "new perspective on health." This perspective held that improved health status could be achieved principally through reducing self-indulgent, health-endangering personal behavior. Because health promotion and disease prevention traditionally have been the primary responsibility of state and local governments, adoption of the new perspective has placed the states at the very center of trying to modify people's lifestyles. The states have adopted legislation restricting the sale, promotion, advertisement, and use of tobacco and alcohol, facilitating or opposing the distribution of free condoms and clean hypodermic needles, and regulating the behavior of motorists and their passengers (e.g., seatbelts, car seats, motorcycle helmets). Most recently the states have weighed in on yet another public health epidemic, namely obesity. An estimated 31% of Americans are obese, up from 23% in 1990, costing the nation about $93 billion, or roughly equal to the costs associated with smoking. And, according to the Centers for Disease Control, about five times as many Americans die from obesity-related conditions as from infectious diseases each year.[14] Since state governments pay a large part of the bill for over-weight- and obesity-related illnesses (e.g., diabetes and hypertension), through the Medicaid and SCHIP programs, the states and localities have been forced to address the issue. Some states (e.g., New York and California) and localities have debated, or enacted, bans on soft drinks and other junk food from school premises, and more will be debating such actions in the future.

Purchasers and Providers of Health Care

Today state governments go far beyond their historical role as protectors of the public's health and have taken on new, costly, and often controversial health care responsibilities. To begin, the states are the largest purchasers of personal health care services in the country. In this capacity, they provide health insurance for state employees—as of March 2004 there were about 4.2 million full-time state employees—as well as funding so-called safety net providers, such as community, rural, and school-based clinics, and state hospitals. For some populations, such as the homeless, non-English speakers, immigrants, and the working but uninsured poor, these clinics and hospitals are the major providers of health care. One recent study of California found that although no one seems to know precisely how many Californians rely on these safety-net institutions and providers, estimates range from 25% to 40% of the entire population.[15]

Perhaps more significantly, in the last decade or so state governments have been forced to confront one of the nation's most compelling, and seemingly intractable, health policy problems; namely, the large and growing number of uninsured Americans. Between 1992 and 2005 the number of people without health insurance grew from 35 million to 45 million. State governments have responded to the access problem through innovative and creative uses of joint federal–state programs, such as Medicaid, and the State Health Insurance Program (SCHIP). SCHIP was created in 1997 to help states extend health insurance protection to children under age 19 whose families earned too much to qualify for Medicaid, but not enough to afford private health insurance. States had the option of choosing to expand coverage through Medicaid, create a separate SCHIP program, or do a combination of both. Over one-half of the states chose to expand Medicaid. Whichever approach, states receive federal matching funds.

States apply for waivers to set aside certain federal Medicaid rules and regulations in order to experiment with their program. Many states have applied to the federal government for various Medicaid/SCHIP waivers that enable them to expand these health insurance programs to non-categorical populations. Several states, including Maine, Michigan, and New Mexico have received waivers to provide Medicaid or SCHIP coverage to low-income, childless adults, a group not normally covered by either program. In addition, over one-half of the states have received Section 1931 Medicaid waivers that allows them to disregard certain sources of income or assets, making it easier to qualify financially for Medicaid: Arkansas, Maryland, and New Hampshire, for example, allow applicants to disregard 20% of their income when calculating their financial status. Another waiver option, used by Maryland, Massachusetts, Rhode Island, Virginia, and Wisconsin is to use SCHIP funds to help subsidize families who wish to purchase employer-based insurance. Thus, under Wisconsin's BadgerCare program, families with incomes between 185% and 200% of FPL ($34,040 to $36,800 for a family of four) can get SCHIP dollars to purchase private employer-provided health insurance. Lastly, Connecticut, Florida, New York, and North Carolina allow families with incomes of between 200% and 300% FPL ($36,800 to $55,200 for a family of four) to purchase health insurance for their children through SCHIP, although the parents receive neither state nor federal funding. (For a complete accounting of waiver options see http://www.statecoverage.net/Medicaid.)

A number of states have also established state-only programs to help expand access to groups ineligible for Medicaid, and because of their health status, low income, or lack of employer-offered coverage have been unable to purchase private health insurance. About 15 states provide tax incentives, in the form of a deduction or credit, to either individuals or employers in small businesses to help reduce the cost of purchasing health insurance. Typically, those eligible may deduct 100% of their premium costs from their tax bill. In addition, about one dozen states "provide direct, major-medical health insurance coverage, or premium assistance for private insurance coverage, through programs that are state designed and state funded (without federal financial support)."[16] California, for example, has Access for Infants and Mothers (AIM), which provides health insurance to pregnant women and children up to age two, with family incomes between 200% to 300% FPL. Participating families must contribute 2% of their income and pay $100 per child in the second year.

Examples of more ambitious state programs to cover the uninsured are: Pennsylvania's "adultBasic"

health plan which provides insurance to 19–64 year olds with incomes below 200% FPL and who are ineligible for Medicaid; and Oregon's Family Health Insurance Plan, an employer buy-in, aimed at low income (up to 185% FPL) working Oregonians and their dependents who have been uninsured for at least six months. The plan pays between 70% and 95% of the cost of any qualifying commercial health plan, depending upon family income and size.

Several states have also enacted laws that allow people with serious health conditions to purchase insurance coverage. In the last decade about three-fourths of the states have created high risk insurance pools for individuals who, because of preexisting medical conditions (the so-called medically uninsurable), either face prohibitively high health insurance premiums or have been denied coverage altogether. Typically states create a non-profit association that, through a contracted insurance carrier, sells health insurance policies to those with preexisting conditions, collects premiums, and pays claims. These programs are typically financed by state funds and an assessment on insurers.

The largest group of uninsured Americans is those who work for small businesses (i.e., those with fewer than 100 employees), whose employers do not provide employment-based insurance and whose employees cannot afford to purchase individual policies on their own. State governments, which regulate the insurance industry, have enacted a number of reforms intended to lower insurance costs for both employers and employees. Several states, including California, Florida, and Connecticut have established health insurance purchasing alliances that allow groups of small businesses to pool their resources and thereby spread the experience risk, and lower premium costs. As a Rand study noted: "In principle, alliances have lower administrative costs and give small groups collective purchasing power to negotiate lower rates from insurance carriers and plans." Unfortunately, the Rand researchers found that alliances do not achieve the stated goals of increasing the percentage of small businesses offering health insurance or reducing small group insurance premiums.[17]

Medicaid: The 900-Pound Gorilla of State Health Policy

For all the range, diversity and importance of state health care policies, one program stands out. James Fossett of the Rockefeller foundation calls Medicaid the "900-pound gorilla of health care" and former Oregon governor Neil Goldschmidt tags it "the monster that ate the states." Medicaid is not only the largest item in state health budgets, but also the most problematic.[18] It is impossible to overstate the impact Medicaid has on in the policy calculations of state law makers, not just in health policy, but also in state public policy.

Looking back over the past 20 years or so, students of state health care politics and policy can not help but be reminded of the aphorism by the great New York Yankees' catcher, and ersatz social philosopher, Yogi Berra: "It's like déjà vu all over again." In a 1983 article in the journal *Health Affairs,* two officers of the Robert Wood Johnson Foundation wrote of the "hard times" facing state and local governments as a result, in part, of the "nationwide economic recession." In an effort to cope with the fiscal crisis at that time, and especially exploding health care costs, "state and local governments have been grappling with the problem of how to trim expenditures while still maintaining [health] services and programs."[19] Medicaid, which already accounted for over one-half of all state and local health care spending, was at the heart of the problem.

Two decades later a team of researchers for a Robert Wood Johnson Foundation-sponsored program, "State Coverage Initiatives," issued their *State of the States* report for 2003. The report began: "In 2003, states struggled for the third consecutive year to remain solvent in the face of falling revenues and budget-breaking expenditures."[20] And, once again, Medicaid was the primary culprit. As the State Coverage Initiatives' annual report noted: "States also struggled in 2003 to keep Medicaid and the State Children's Health Insurance Program (SCHIP) affordable despite difficult budgetary times, greater demand for coverage, and increasing cost of services."[21]

State governors agree: "Nothing concerns state governors more these days than their state budgets, and nothing is driving their deficits deeper, they say, than rising Medicaid costs."[22]

Like the periodic and predictable return of the cicadas, a Medicaid crisis seems to visit itself upon the states with remarkable regularity. The economy turns bad, Medicaid enrollments soar, and state budgets buckle under the burden of increased health care costs. As the National Association of State Budget Officers concluded in their 2002 "State Expenditure Report," "The fiscal dilemma states currently face is strikingly similar to their experiences in the early 1980s and 1990s."[23] The dilemma grows out of the fiscal impact that Medicaid has on state governments. Currently Medicaid accounts, on average, for 22% of state budgets, although in some states it is around 30% (e.g., Missouri, Pennsylvania, Maine, New York, and Illinois), and in one, Tennessee, it represents one-third of the state budget. The problem for state governments lies not merely in the fact that Medicaid consumes so much of their resources, and thereby limits their ability to fund other programs, but that the costs are increasing at, in the words of the National Governors Association 2002 report, an "unsustainable" rate.[24] Consider the fact that while overall state general fund spending in FY 2002 increased 1.3%, Medicaid spending increased 11.9% in 2000–02. Furthermore, in the last several years Medicaid costs have grown at a rate that has exceeded growth rates of overall inflation, and state domestic product, and population increases. As a result, between 2002 and 2004 almost all the states had to reduce Medicaid costs or face the prospect of raising taxes. Predictably, most chose the former. Cost containment measures included cutting or eliminating optional benefits (e.g., dentures, eyeglasses, hospice care), freezing or reducing provider reimbursement rates, tightening eligibility requirements (e.g., raising the income threshold, or including non-income assets), dropping some optional groups (e.g., severely disabled children whose families do not qualify for Medicaid), increasing co-payments, and controlling drug costs (e.g., limiting the number of prescriptions, increased use of prior authorization, seeking deeper discounts, or rebates from drug manufacturers).[25]

Medicaid casts such a large shadow over the state policy landscape not only because of its impact on state budgets, but because it is so important to so many Americans—51 million in 2003 relied on Medicaid for their health care, up from 21 million in 1983. It is the largest health insurance program in the country, exceeding Medicare, covering 24 million children, 14 million adults, and 13 million disabled and elderly people.[26] The role of Medicaid in the nation's health care system is underscored by some telling facts about the program. Consider, for example, these facts about Medicaid: it covers over one-fourth of all children in the country; pays for nearly 40% of all births, over one-half of all HIV/AIDS care, and two-thirds of all nursing home patients, and; accounts for 17% of the total personal health care, hospital care, and prescription drug spending in the country.[27]

Although the federal government establishes broad Medicaid guidelines, there is a great deal of discretion left to state policy makers—and that means large differences from state to state. According to the Centers for Medicare & Medicaid Services, "[E]ach State (1) establishes its own eligibility standards; (2) determines the type, amount, duration, and scope of services; (3) sets the rate of payment for services; and (4) administers its own program."[28] Take the seemingly straightforward issue of eligibility. Medicaid is routinely described as health care coverage for "poor" or "low-income" people. And, in fact, there are certain categories of low-income people who *must* be covered, including children and pregnant women with family incomes below 133% of the federal poverty line, and children under the age of 19 with incomes below the poverty line. States, however, have the option of providing Medicaid and SCHIP to non-categorical groups as well. We have already seen, for example, that several states have received Section 1115 Medicaid or SCHIP waivers to cover populations normally ineligible under federally prescribed guidelines. Some examples of programs covering non-categorical groups are: (1) MinnesotaCare—parents up to 275% of the

poverty line and children under age 19 with incomes up to 280% FPL ($50,500 per year for a family of four); (2) the Oregon Health Plan—everyone under age 65 who falls below 100% FPL ($8,980 for a one person); (3) New York's Family Health Plus—parents up to 150% FPL ($26,600 for a family of four) and childless adults up to 100% FPL, and; (4) Wisconsin's BadgerCare—uninsured children and parents up to 185% FPL ($34,040).[29]

States not only have considerable flexibility in who they cover but also how aggressively and creatively they enroll eligible adults and children in the Medicaid and SCHIP programs. Thus they can facilitate and encourage participation through simplifying administrative requirements, such as: replace face-to-face qualifying interviews with mail-in applications; have annual rather than semi-annual or quarterly eligibility reapplications; and, market the program in schools, shopping centers, and community clinics, or through such organizations as the Boy and Girl Scouts. Alternatively, when hard economic times arrive and states seek ways to reduce costs, they can make it more, not less, difficult to find out about and enroll or reenroll in these programs. "Mississippi, Nebraska and Washington have recently [2003–04] added more rigorous documentation requirements for reporting income, while Connecticut, Indiana, Nebraska and Washington did away with the guarantee of 12 months of uninterrupted coverage."[30] In addition, Idaho cancelled its contract with Head Start and the Girl Scouts to promote SCHIP, and Kentucky now requires parents to show up in person once a year to reenroll children.[31]

Nearly two-thirds of the benefits provided under the Medicaid and SCHIP are optional—each state decides whether to offer them. The 34 optional Medical services include occupational, physical and speech therapies, transportation services, dental, chiropractic, podiatry, and optometrist services, long-term home and community care, as well as prescribed drugs and prosthetic devices.[32] As a result, the breadth of coverage under Medicaid is, to a considerable extent, dependent on where a person lives: Medicaid clients in Alabama have dental benefits, those in Texas do not; Oregonians on Medicaid can get organ transplants, those in Wyoming cannot.

The state fiscal crisis that followed the dot.com bust, corporate scandals, and 9/11, resulted in reduced state revenues, increased unemployment, a burgeoning uninsured population—and more people eligible for and in need of Medicaid. Faced with these demands, state governments had few options with regard to Medicaid/SCHIP: cut benefits, place a cap on or drop recipients, or reduce payments to providers. With regard to provider reimbursement, states enjoy considerable autonomy in setting Medicaid fees, both in terms of how much, and on what basis reimbursement will be made. (In practice, states determine the rate of most Medicaid provider reimbursement and submit a justification or a rationale for the rates to the Centers for Medicare and Medicaid Services—the federal agency which oversees the program—as part of the state's Medicaid plan.) Most states got on the managed care bandwagon, moving from the fee-for-service payment that dominated the program since 1965, to a per capita, managed care fee system. Indeed, many states used the promise of cost savings from managed care as a bargaining tool to win Medicaid waiver approval from the federal government. Oregon, for example, got a Medicaid waiver for its innovative plan to expand health care to all persons under the poverty lines without increasing costs (which would, of course, increase the federal government's costs) by promising to save money by prioritizing or rationing health services, and by the promised discipline of managed care. Today 38 state Medicaid programs have 50% or more of their Medicaid clients in managed care—a dramatic change from 1990 when the number was less than 10%.

States have used another, blunter cost-containment tools, namely, to reduce provider reimbursements—or fail to increase them, which given the perennially high rate of medical inflation, has the same practical effect. Although this approach may save state governments dollars, it has also had the effect of driving some physicians from the Medicaid program. The director of government relations for the California Medical Association, not an unbiased source on the

subject to be sure, was reported to have said that, "Doctors [in California] are fleeing the program because of historically low payments."[33] In fact, reimbursement rates have been the source of conflict between providers and state officials for years. Hospital administrators and physicians complain that Medicaid clients are typically more costly to treat than non-Medicaid patients because they often miss appointments or fail to show up for follow-up appointments, and are unreliable in taking prescribed medications. In addition, they often require additional non-medical administrative support services such as bilingual staff, childcare, and transportation. Doctors in virtually every state complain of inadequate Medicaid reimbursement, and anecdotal data suggest that many—although no one knows exactly how many—refuse to accept, or eventually drop, Medicaid patients.

Finally, with some exceptions dictated by federal law (e.g., "pregnant women, children under age 18, and hospital or nursing home patients who are expected to contribute most of their income to institutional care"), states may require copayments, coinsurance, or deductibles from Medicaid clients to help offset the burden on state Medicaid budgets."[34] In response to the fiscal crisis in 2002, 17 states initiated new or increased beneficiary copayments and 21 states indicated that they intended to do so in 2004.[35]

For a long time, the conventional wisdom among academics was that state Medicaid activities were essentially administrative; that is, the states were little more than administrative field offices for the federal government. That view is no longer warranted—if it ever was. To be sure, the states must work within guidelines laid out in the federal Medicaid law. But to view the states' Medicaid/SCHIP role as simply administrative is to miss not only enormous variation among the states but also extensive experimentation and creativity. States may expand access to health insurance through programs that involve only state money, or they may expand access to non-categorical groups through the Medicaid program. Both approaches require a political decision to commit state funds to expand access to health care. Today the state role is at least as important as that of the federal government when it comes to who will be covered, how long they will be covered, what will be covered, the prospect that people will be enrolled and the likelihood that physicians will participate in Medicaid/SCHIP. And when the economy turns sour, as it did beginning in 2001, Medicaid becomes almost exclusively a state, not a federal, problem because it consumes such a large—and ever growing—portion of the state budget.

FEDERALISM AND HEALTH POLICY

In September 2003, a delegation of Hawaii state legislators traveled over 5,100 miles to Augusta, Maine to study that state's law-making low-cost prescription drugs available to Mainers who did not have drug coverage. Under the law, state officials negotiate discounts with manufacturers to purchase drugs for an estimated 275,000 people, a number large enough to give them considerable bargaining leverage. Maine State Senator Michael Brennan (D-Portland) spoke for his colleagues from around the country when he observed that, "If we wait for Washington [to act on prescription drug costs], the citizens of our states would be waiting a long time." A decade earlier Booth Gardner, then governor of Washington State, argued that the states should take the lead in health care reform because: "We can't wait for the federal government in Washington, D.C. to act. Only if we push, and push hard, will we get reform to move forward. And we can do that best by demonstrating in the states that health care reform is viable."[36] Senator Brennan and Governor Gardner articulated one side of a debate that has been around since the Founding. What is the appropriate division of labor in our federal system between the national and state governments? It is a question that Woodrow Wilson once called "the cardinal question of our constitutional system."[37] While the basics of

American federalism were introduced in the last chapter, here we take up one key issue for the study of states: Should the health care of the American people be primarily entrusted to the national government insuring uniformity (the federal solution) or should it be left up to the states, allowing flexibility and diversity (the state solution)? Who, in short, should take the lead in health care reform and control the health care system, the states or the federal government?

The Case for National Leadership

A decade ago, when the nation was engrossed in a debate over universal access to health care, academics asked the question: "Can States Take the Lead in Health Care Reform?"[38] The preponderance of academic sentiment then, and now, is blunt: "no" they cannot and should not. This view in part reflects a skepticism, outdated in most instances, about the political commitment and progressive inclinations of some states to undertake major reform, as well as the fiscal and administrative capacity to pull it off. It also reflects faith in, and preference for, federal leadership.

The case for federal leadership in health care reform is compelling and has been implicit in much of what I have said. To begin, it will strike many as politically unjust and morally unconscionable that, for example, the likelihood of being uninsured in this country is in large part a function of where you live. Texans are two and one-half times more likely to be uninsured than people living in New Hampshire; New York spends nine times as much on Medicaid as Nevada; pregnant women in Rhode Island are far more likely to get prenatal care than women in New Mexico. We, of course, tolerate differences in other areas of public policy, such as in vocational training or land use planning, but health and health care are more central to our effective functioning as political, social, and economic actors than if a state has urban growth boundaries. Health disparities are far less tolerable than differences in these other policy areas. Only the national government can assure uniformity in health care access across all the states, much as it guarantees roughly equal protection from external enemies, or of civil rights, or of air traffic safety.

Second, not only is the national government in the best position to ensure equality of access but it is more administratively competent and fiscally capable than the states in devising, implementing, and funding what would be an extraordinarily complex and costly social undertaking such as national health insurance. Although state governments have made great strides over the last few decades to become more modern (e.g., greater use of computer technology, more sophisticated and efficient administrative procedures), more professional (e.g., larger number of full-time legislators, revised or new state constitutions, longer terms for governors, etc.), and more democratic (e.g., court imposed reapportionment ensuring one person–one vote in both houses of state legislature), they still lag behind the federal government in the resources and skills needed to run the $1.6 trillion enterprise that is our health care system. In fact, the political competence of the states to undertake reform has been eroded since almost one-half the states have adopted term limits for state legislators, virtually guaranteeing periodic depletion of policy expertise.

Third, and related to this point, although several states (e.g., California, Colorado, Florida, Hawaii, Iowa, Maine, Maryland, Massachusetts, Minnesota, New Jersey, New York, Oregon, Tennessee, Vermont, and Washington) have been willing to tackle issues such as cost containment and expanding access, most states have really done very little. The reasons are not hard to find. "Some may not see it as a priority; others may be unable to reach consensus, particularly if they have diverse populations; others may not have the money."[39] At least one scholarly study lends support to the charge that some states would find expanding coverage difficult at best. Marquis and Long found that the states with the highest levels of uninsured were also those with the lowest taxing capacity. They concluded by noting that: "there is a serious geographic disparity between the distribution of uninsured persons and the distribution of ability to finance subsidized health insurance

coverage for them. In addition, the cost of reform is significant relative to current tax effort. We seriously doubt the states, left to their own resolve, will solve the problem."[40] Although Connecticut and Massachusetts might be able to afford to extend health insurance coverage to most or all their citizens, it is doubtful that Mississippi, New Mexico, and a score of other states have the resources to do so. By way of contrast, the federal government clearly has the fiscal capacity to undertake a major health care expansion. "The federal government's deep pockets come from the lack of governmental competition at the national level, progressive taxation, large-scale operations, and the ability to print and borrow money and hence continue spending even in deficit."[41]

Federal leadership in health care policy also recommends itself because it eliminates the possibility of people and companies shopping around to find those states which impose the least burden on wealthier citizens. This dilemma is two-fold and is characterized as either a "race to the bottom"— reduce health care benefits, taxes and regulations in order to attract wealth to your state; or as "the welfare magnet" problem in which a state's generous benefit package might attract too many poor people (and thus create more needs, require higher taxes and drive wealthier people and businesses to another state). During his tenure as governor of Vermont, Howard Dean explained his concerns about his state's leadership in health care reform in precisely these terms. "My principle concerns are that we not drive small business across the border, based upon the financing package [of our plan to adopt universal access to health care] and that New Hampshire's uninsured poor not seek care in Vermont for free."[42]

Another reason for state hesitancy in health care reform has to do with legal constraints imposed by the federal government on the states. As we saw in Chapter 6, one recurring nightmare for state policy makers who wish to pursue state health care reform is the 1974 federal ERISA. Initially intended to protect the pensions of retired workers from fraud and mismanagement, ERISA has been interpreted by the courts to prohibit states from regulating the benefits of self-insured companies. Since about two-thirds of all companies, and about one-half of all companies with more than 50 employees, choose to self-insure, ERISA severely limits the ability of states to adopt comprehensive reforms. States may seek a federal waiver or exemption from ERISA, but thus far only one state, Hawaii in 1983, has received such an exemption.

In summary, social justice, administrative competence, fiscal capacity, economic competition, federal law, and concerns with political equity all demand federal leadership in reforming the nation's health care system.

The Case for the States

There is an equally convincing case, at least in the minds of some, to be made for state leadership in health care reform. First, we have already seen the incredible diversity of the states. It is difficult to imagine more different political, geographic, and economic circumstances than those that exist, say, between Vermont and Mississippi, or California and North Dakota. Advocates of state leadership in health care reform argue that public policy must spring from and accommodate that diversity. "One size does not fit all" in health care policy. And, as researchers from the Urban Institute explain in summarizing, but not endorsing, the case for states, the need for local autonomy "is especially true in health care, where health care institutions, medical practice patterns, referral networks, and provider markets are local."[43] Some years ago Emily Friedman illustrated this point when she noted that: "Reforms based on managed care are a comfortable fit in Hawaii, Minnesota, and Washington, and would be in California; but there are no health maintenance organizations in Alaska or Wyoming, and fewer than 1% of the residents of Mississippi and North Dakota belong to one."[44] The general point about the organization and operation of health care institutions remains valid—although in this case the facts have changed in ways that demonstrate the limits of the argument—today, about 40% of the people in Wyoming are in managed care, compared to 95% in California.

Second, Americans, to the extent that they accept government involvement in their lives at all, prefer it be geographically proximate. This is, in part, based on the belief that locally made policy is more likely be sensitive and responsive to local values, resources, and problems. It also allows citizens to monitor the activities of state policy makers more closely—and hold them accountable for their actions. As Rachel Block, former executive director of the Vermont Health Care Authority, has argued: "Just as health care cannot be effectively managed on a long distance basis, neither can the political consequences of health care reform be effectively handled through a toll-free hotline to an anonymous federal bureaucrat."[45] Americans, in fact, tend to place greater faith in their state and local governments than in the national government. A July 2000 Pew Charitable Trust study found that 29% of Americans reported that they "always" or "most of the time" trusted the federal government "to do the right thing," while 39% indicated greater trust in both the state and local governments.[46]

Some advocates of state health care reform leadership suggest that the states today are the most dynamic players in our federal system, willing to tackle highly charged health policy issues. In a comment that is as relevant today as it was a decade ago, the national political commentator Joe Klein argued that: "The governors have been the most creative players in American politics for the past 20 years. They tend to be more moderate, pragmatic, frugal—and less ideological—than legislators (especially those who reside in Washington)."[47] The same may be said of state legislators and legislatures. According to William Pound, executive director of the National Conference of State Legislators, "Today, state legislatures are among the most revitalized and changed institutions in America, with a vastly increased capacity to govern," and state law makers "are better educated, more diverse and more representative than at any time in history."[48]

In fact, recent state activity adds credence to this faith in state governments. In view of the persistent inability of the federal government to reach agreement on several critical health issues, including malpractice insurance and prescription drug costs and access, the states have stepped in to fill the political void. For example, anyone following the recent national debate—some would say debacle— over a prescription drug benefit for Medicare recipients, might be interested to learn that Pennsylvania has been making affordable prescription drugs available to its seniors for three decades. In 1974, Pennsylvania enacted a program for low-income seniors called the Pennsylvania Pharmaceutical Assistance Contract for the Elderly (PACE). For $6 copay per prescription, seniors receive all their prescription medication. The program is funded by Pennsylvania lottery money.[49] Today about one-half of the states have prescription drug plans that address both cost and access issues for various groups: the elderly, the poor, and others without drug coverage. As of 2004, over one-half of the states had programs providing subsidies for certain groups, while 16 states had discount or bulk purchasing programs. The most recent state to join the fray is Hawaii, inaugurating the "Hawaii RxPlan" on July 1, 2004. Passed by Democratic controlled legislature and signed by a Republican governor, the program allows state residents who have no drug benefit or inadequate coverage, and who do not qualify for Medicaid, to purchase drugs at Medicaid prices. State officials estimate that this will save participants between 9% and 20% of cost depending on the particular drug. To qualify for the program, people must have a household income of 350% of FPL or below ($37,464 for a single person or $75,888 for a family of four).

Finally, several states, including Massachusetts, Minnesota, Iowa, Illinois, and Michigan have attacked the cost and access problem, and infuriated the pharmaceutical industry, by proposing to import prescription drugs from Canada, where costs are 30% to 75% lower than in the United States. Although the status and legality of these proposals are unclear as of this writing—federal law prohibits importation of drugs by anyone except a pharmaceutical company—they illustrate the willingness of the states to deal with pressing social problems, especially in the absence of federal action.

The states have also taken the lead in addressing the issue of malpractice insurance reform. Although it is unclear how much malpractice settlements and premiums really contribute to health care costs, policy makers sense that they undermine the system in two ways—by driving costs up, and by driving physicians (especially obstetricians and neurosurgeons) and insurers away. Whatever the facts, the impression among policy makers is that there is a malpractice insurance crisis in the United States. Here, too, the federal government, despite at least a decade of trying, has been unable to act. And, here too, the states have stepped up to the plate. The main, and most politically controversial, approach to dealing with the escalating size of damage awards and the concomitant rise in insurance premiums has been to place a cap on malpractice awards for non-economic damages. In fact, this is exactly what California did 30 years ago when, in 1975, it limited non-economic damage awards to no more than $250,000. The result, applauded by insurers and providers, condemned by attorneys and advocates for people severely injured by medical malpractice, has been to reduce jury awards by 30%.[50] The National Council of State Legislatures reported that in 2003, 34 states considered tort reform and 11 of them actually enacted legislation setting caps.[51] Other states, including Arkansas, Florida, Maryland, and Wisconsin have similar laws, and legislation is certain to be adopted in many others as well. Another state approach to the malpractice problem eases the financial burden on doctors and insurance companies by setting up special funds either to create a special insurance company that provides medical practice insurance (e.g., West Virginia's Physicians Mutual Medical Malpractice Insurance Company which is funded by a $1,000 assessment on each physician) or to provide a financial backup to insurance companies who face serious loses due to large settlements (e.g., New Jersey's Medical Malpractice Reinsurance Association).

Lastly, the states continue to grapple with the problem of the uninsured. We have already seen that Maine, through its recently enacted Dirigo program, hopes to achieve universal access to health care by

2009. In addition, in 2003 Californians adopted a so-called play-or-pay law, in which employers must either offer health insurance to their employees (play) or pay a fee into a statewide insurance pool. The employer mandate, if it survives court scrutiny over the ERISA issue, will be phased in over several years. By January 1, 2006 employers with 200 more employees must provide a health benefit to their employees and dependents; employers with 50–199 employees must do so by the following year. In each case employers pay 80% of the costs and employees 20%. Employers with 20–49 employees will only have to provide insurance if, and when, the state can provide a tax credit to ease the financial burden on the mandated benefit. Employers with fewer than 20 employees are exempt from the program.

These efforts to fill the gap left by the lack of a federal solution to the access problem underscore a third reason why the states are looked to as leaders in health care reform, namely their historical role as "laboratories of democracy." This notion was first articulated by the late Supreme Court Justice Louis Brandeis in 1932: "It is one of the happy incidents of the federal system that a single courageous state may, if its citizens choose, serve as a laboratory; and try novel social and economic experiments without risk to the rest of the country."[52] Throughout our history, the states have experimented with social policy including unemployment insurance, child labor and minimum wage laws, as well as environmental protection laws, all of which ultimately were adopted at the national level.

In the absence of a national consensus over what should be done to solve the cost and access crisis in American health care, and in light of the ideological sclerosis that has gripped national politics and prevented major health care reform for more than two decades, "Why not then let states choose how to reform American health care? If it is uncertain how any new proposal would work out in practice, why run a single experiment, which might fail, on the whole country at once?"[53]

Fourth, even when state governments are unwilling or unable to institute innovative health care programs, it is still possible in 17 of the states for the people to take matters into their own hands through the initiative process. Oregonians, for example, voted to allow people with terminal illnesses to choose to end their own lives, and created a commission to ensure quality home care services for the elderly and disabled; Texans agreed to set a $250,000 cap on malpractice claims; people with certain medical conditions in California, Oregon, Alaska, Nevada, Washington, Maine, and Colorado are allowed to grow and/or purchase marijuana for medical purposes; Floridians voted to protect people in the workplace from second-hand smoke. In addition, citizens in several states have approved initiatives that have required state governments to use tobacco settlement money for specific health programs (e.g., smoking education, subsidizing health care for the poor, or school health centers).

In sum, the demographic, economic, and political diversity of the nation, the strong attachment to the states as political and cultural units, the proven ability of many state governments to "get things done," the role allocated to the states as laboratories of democracy, and the opportunity in 17 states for direct citizen health policymaking through the initiative process all support the notion that the states, not the federal government, are the best managers of the nation's health care system.

CONCLUSION

Most Americans will find the debate over federal versus state leadership in health care policy reform a bit beside the point. Despite greater confidence in their own state government than the federal government, I suspect that Americans, especially those who have no health insurance or live in fear of losing it, care less about where to locate responsibility for health care than they do about results. As researchers from the Urban Institute recently noted, ". . . most Americans are pragmatists. When they see a problem, they will turn to whichever level of government they believe will do the best job."[54] In fact, the state responsibility for protecting public health is so historically and politically entrenched that it is sheer fantasy to imagine states abandoning this vital functions. Nevertheless, two critical health policy problems remain unresolved, as they have for decades—millions of Americans have no health insurance and the cost of care is unsustainably high and rising. We are left to face the question of the relative roles and responsibilities of the federal and state governments in dealing with these problems.

Having rejected a national solution to universal access and affordable health care in 1993–94, we have opted, by default, for a collaborative federal–state approach. The federal government, through increased flexibility of Medicaid and SCHIP waivers, has allowed the states to incrementally expand access to government provided health insurance for certain vulnerable groups. And many states have taken advantage of these opportunities. In addition, several states, on their own, have created subsidy programs for some groups outside the health insurance safety net, such as the working but uninsured poor; states have lowered financial barriers to health insurance for other groups, such as small businesses and people with preexisting medical conditions. Despite these efforts, the basic structure of the American health care system, a highly fragmented, employment-based, private health insurance covering about 70% on the non-elderly population, remains intact—as does the fact that more people are uninsured in 2005 than there were in 1995. What also remains is the blunt fact that the likelihood of being uninsured is at least in part a function of the state in which you live.

Meanwhile, the states continue as laboratories of reform, testing various programs, hoping, in the absence of systemic national reform, to incrementally expand access to health care to as many of their citizens as possible. Hawaii, in the 1980s, came closest to realizing the goal near-universal access, when its uninsured population fell below 5%, the lowest in the nation. But Hawaii is unique in being the only state to have an ERISA waiver. It is also, unfortunately, an example of the difficulty individual states face in sustaining success. By 2005, Hawaii's uninsured rate

had climbed to about 10%. (Faced with rising health care costs, Hawaii's employers have gotten around the mandate that they provide health insurance for all employees who work 20 hours per week or more, by replacing full-time employees with part-time employees who work less than 20 hours per week). Similar tales of initial success followed by backsliding can be told of Oregon, Tennessee, Minnesota, Florida, and other states. State efforts "to do the right thing" are simply too vulnerable to the vagaries and vicissitudes of economic and fiscal cycles. Yet the states, as Maine's Dirigo program suggests, persist in their efforts. In the absence of a national solution to the access problem, states like Maine and California have no choice, politically or morally, but to continue to experiment.

Similarly the states have no choice but to continue to try and slow the rise in health care costs. Nowhere is the notion that state lawmakers cannot wait for the federal government more applicable than in the area of costs. States are staggering under the burden of the increasing cost of health care, and unlike the national government 49 of the 50 states—Vermont is the exception—cannot run budget deficits. States have taken the lead in expanding managed care, imposing caps on malpractice claims, and seeking ways to hold down prescription drug costs. No one suggests that the states, individually or collectively, can solve either the cost or access crisis in American health care; but no one can plausibly suggest that a solution from the federal government is imminent. Health and health care will continue to be a joint federal–state responsibility.

STUDY QUESTIONS

1. How do disparities in poverty rates across the states help determine health outcomes?
2. How do experts measure health spending on the state level? How do the indicators differ?
3. The chapter describes three kinds of political subculture—moral, traditional, and individual.

Describe them. Explain how they affect state health policy.

4. Which of the subcultures do you find most attractive? Why?

5. How have the states expanded, or altered, Medicaid programs in recent years?

6. Why is the Medicaid program so significant for the states?

7. What are the arguments in favor entrusting health care to the federal government?

8. What are the arguments in favor of leaving health care to the states?

9. What is your view of the preceding two questions? Should the federal government or the states take the lead in health care policy? Why?

NOTES

* The phrase "e pluribus, unum," out of many, one seems inappropriate to describe the American health care system. In its place I suggest "e pluribus, multa," "out of many, many."

1. Sipkoff, 2004.
2. Unless otherwise indicated, the data for this section comes from: Morgan and Morgan, 2004a; and Morgan and Morgan, 2004b. Data is from most recent year available, which is typically between 2000 and 2004.
3. Doty, 2003.
4. United Health Foundation, 2004.
5. Iglehart, 2003, p 2142.
6. United Health Foundation, 2003, p 17.
7. United Health Foundation, 2004.
8. Yemane and Hill, 2002, p 16.
9. Elazar, 1984,, p 114.
10. State Coverage Initiatives, 2004, p 13.
11. Pew Research Center, 2004.
12. Gostin, Burris, Lazzarini, and Maguire, 1998, p 5.
13. Governing, 2004, p 3.
14. Easterbrook, 2004, p 5.
15. Leichter, 2004, p 181.
16. State Coverage Initiatives March, 2004.
17. Rand Health, 2004, p 2.
18. Leichter, 1997, p 15; Barrett and Mariani, 2004, p 2.
19. Altman and Morgan, 1983, p 8.
20. Folz, 2004, p 1.
21. Ibid., p 4.
22. Janofsky, 2003.
23. National Association of State Budget Officers, 2002, p 4.
24. Quoted in Pear, 2002, p 14.
25. See Smith, et al.,2004.
26. Iglehart 2003,p 2140; Grogan, this volume.
27. Smith, 2003.
28. Centers for Medicare and Medicaid Services, 2003, p 1.
29. State Coverage Initiatives, 2004.
30. Governing.com, 2004a.
31. Ornstein, 2002.
32. Centers for Medicare and Medicaid Services, 2003.
33. Ornstein, 2001, p 2.
34. Centers for Medicare and Medicaid Services, 2003, p 4.
35. See Smith et al., 2004, p 6. The results taken from The Kaiser Commission on Medicaid and the Uninsured.
36. Gardner, 1992, p 27.
37. Wilson, 1908, p 684.
38. Moon and Holahan, 1992.
39. Friedman, 1994, p 876.
40. Marquis and Long, 1997, p 517.
41. Bovbjerg, Wiener, and Housman, 2003, p 45.
42. Quoted in Friedman, 1994, p 877.
43. Holahan, Weil, and Weiner, 2003, p 6–7.
44. Friedman, 1994, p 876.
45. Block, 1994, p 45.
46. Pew Charitable Trust, 2000.
47. Klein, 1994, 35.
48. National Conference of State Legislatures, 1997, p 5–6.
49. *State Coverage Initiatives,* July 2000, 3.
50. Girion, 2004.
51. Folz, 2004, p 21.
52. *New State Ice Co. v. Liebmann,* 1932.
53. Mashaw, 1993–94, p 12.
54. Holahan, Weil, and Weiner, July 2003.

REFERENCES

Altman, D.E., and D.H. Morgan. 1983. "The Role of State and Local Government in Health." *Health Affairs* Winter: 7–31.

Barrett, K., R. Greene, and M. Mariani. 2004. "A Case of Neglect: Why Health Care is Getting Worse, Even Though Medicine is Getting Better." Governing.com. (February). Retrieved from http://www.governing.com/gpp/2004/intro.htm

Block, R.1994. "Navigating Health Care Reform: Why States Should be Captains of the Ship," in F.P. Chisman, L.D. Brown, and P.J. Larson, editors. *National Health Reform: What Should the State Role Be?* Washington DC:National Academy of Social Insurance: 41–6.

Bovbjerg, R.R., J.M. Wiener, and M. Housman. 2003. "State and Federal Roles in Health Care: Rationales for Allocating Responsibilities," in J. Holahan, A. Weil, and J.M. Wiener, *Federalism & Health Policy*. Washington DC: The Urban Institute Press.

Centers for Medicare and Medicaid Services. 2003. *Medicaid: A Brief Summary*:1–7.

Doty, M.M. 2003. "Insurance, Access and Quality of Care Among Hispanic Population." The Commonwealth Fund for the National Alliance for Hispanic Health Meeting. October 15–17.

Easterbrook, G. 2004. "All This Progress is Killing Us, Bite by Bite," *The New York Times* 14 March:p 5.

Elazar, D.J. 1984. *American Federalism: A View From the States*. New York:Harper & Row.

Finkelstein, E. 2003. "National Medical Spending Attributable to Overweight and Obesity: How Much, and Who's Paying?" *Health Affairs* web exclusive. May 14: W3–219–W3–226.

Folz, C. (ed.). 2004. *State of the States: Cultivating Hope in Rough Terrain*. Washington DC: Academy Health.

Friedman, E. 1994. "Getting a Head Start: The States and Health Care Reform," *Journal of the American Medical Association* 271 (16 March): [875–8].

Gardner, B. 1992. "Health Care Reform: The State Perspective." *Intergovernmental Perspective* (Spring): 27–9.

Girion, L. 2004. "Damage Cap Hits Some Hard."*Los Angeles Times.com*. 13 July. Retrieved from http://www.latimes.com/business/la-fi-malpractice13jul13,1,7501163.story.

Gostin, L.O., S. Burris, Z. Lazzarini, and K. Maguire. 1998. "Improving State Law to Prevent and Treat Infectious Disease." New York: Milbank Memorial Fund.

Governing.com. 2004. "Public Health:Costs of Complacency." The GovernmentPerformance Project. Retrieved from http://www.governing.com/gpp/2004/public.htm.

Governing.com. 2004a. "Public Health: Children's Health." Retrieved from http://www.governing.com/grp/2004/child.htm.

Holahan, J., A. Weil, and J.M. Weiner. 2003. "Which Way for Federalism and Health Policy," *Health Affairs* Web Excluisve (16 July). Retrieved from http://www.healthafairs.org/WebExclusives/Holahan_Web_Excl_071603.htm.

Holahan, J., A. Weil and J.M. Wiener. 2003. "Federalism and Health Policy: An Overview," in *Federalism & Health Policy*. J. Holahan, A. Weil, and J.Weiner. Washington DC, The Urban Institute Press: 1–23.

Iglehart, J. 2003. "The Dilemma of Medicaid." *New England Journal of Medicine* 348 (21): 2140–8.

Janofsky, M. 2003."Governors Unite to Urge Shifting Cost of Medicaid." *The New York Times* 18 August: 1.

Klein, J. 1994. "Let the States do it." *Newsweek*: 35.

Leichter, H.M. 1997."Health Care Reform in America:Back to the Laboratories," in Howard M. Leichter.*Health Policy Reform in America:Innovations From the States*. Armonk, NY:M.E. Sharpe: 3–28.

—— 2004. "Ethnic Politics, Policy Fragmentation, and Dependent Health Care Access in California." *Journal of Health Politics, Policy and Law* 29: [177–201].

Mashaw, J.L. 1993–94. "Taking Federalism Seriously: The Case for State-Led Health Care Reform," *Domestic Affairs* 2: (Winter)pages].

Marquis, S.M., and S.H. Long. 1997. "Federalism and Health System Reform: Prospects for State Action," *Journal of the American Medical Association* 278 (13 August): 858–863

Moon, M., and J. Holahan. 1992. "Can the States Taken the Lead in Health Care Reform," *Journal of the American Medical Association* 268 (23/30 September): 1588–4.

Morgan, K. O'Leary and S. Morgan, eds. 2004a. *Health Care State Rankings, 2004: Health Care in the 50 States*. Lawrence, KS: Morgan Quinto Press.

Morgan, K. O'Leary, and S. Morgan, eds. 2004b. *State Rankings 2004: A Statistical View of the 50 United States*. Lawrence, KS: Morgan Quinto Press.

National Association of State Budget Officers. 2002. *State Expenditure Report*. Washington DC:

National Conference of State Legislatures 1997. "Time Enough? States Respond to Term Limits," a report by the National Conference of State Legislatures and the Milbank Memorial Fund.New York: Milbank Memorial Fund.

Ornstein, C. 2002. States Cut Back Coverage for Poor. *Los Angeles Times* 25, February: 1.

Ornstein, C., and S. Bernstein (2001). "Spiraling Medicaid Costs Putting States in a Bind." *Los Angeles Times* 24, November 24:1.

Pear, R. 2002. "Governor's Say Medicaid Needs More Federal Help to Control Rising Costs." *The New York Times* [25 February: A14.

The Pew Research Center for the People and the Press. 2000. Retrieved from http://www.npr.org/ programs/specials/poll/govt/summary.html.

The Pew Research Center for the People and the Press. 2004. "The 2004 Political Landscape:Evenly Divided and Increasingly Polarize." Retrieved from http://people-press.org/reports/display.php3?/ PageID+749.

Rand Health. 2004. "State Efforts to Insure the Uninsured: An Unfinished Story," Rand Health/Research Highlights (July). Retrieved from http://www.rand.org/publications/RB/ RB4558.1/.

Sipkoff, Martin. 2004."Do We Really Have Best Health Care in the World?" *Managed Care Magazine*. Retrieved from http://www.magagedcaremag. com/archives/0404/0404.worldbest.html.

Skocpol, T. 1994. "The Nation and the States in U.S. Social Policy: Lessons from the Past" in F.P. Chisman, L.D. Brown, and P.J. Larson, eds. *National Health Reform: What Should the State Role Be?* Washington DC: National Academy of Social Insurance, p 71–5.

Smith, V., R. Ramesh, K. Gifford, E. Ellis, V. Wachino, and M. O'Malley. 2004. States Respond to Fiscal Pressure: A 50-State Update of State Medicaid Spending Growth and Cost Containment Actions. Kaiser Commission on Medicaid and the Uninsured. January. Retrieved from http://www.kff.org.

Smith, V.K. 2003. "The Future of Medicaid: State Responses in a Time of Budget Stress and the Outlook for the Future," for Midwestern Legislative Conference, Council of State Governments, 25 August. Retrieved from Vsmith@healthmanagement.com

State Coverage Initiatives. 2004. "State-Only Coverage Program," http://www.statecoverage.net/ coverageprogram.htm, retrieved 5/12/04. Information was updated March 2004.

State Coverage Initiatives. 2000. "States Extend Pharmaceutical Coverage." July (No. 2). Retrieved from http://www.statecoverage.net.

United Health Foundation. 2004. *America's Health: State Health Rankings*. Retrieved from www. unitedhealthfoundation.org.

United Health Foundation. 2003. *America's Health: State Health Rankings*. Retrieved from www.unitedhealthfoundation.org.

Wilson, Woodrow. 1908. "The States and the Federal Government," *North American Review* CLXXXVII (May): [684–701].

Yemane, A., and I. Hill. 2002. "Recent Changes in Health Policy for Low-Income People in Florida, The Urban Institute. *State Update* 16 (April): 1–29.

Elizabeth Kilbreth

In this section, Elizabeth Kilbreth illustrates the themes of the preceding two chapters, Federalism and state health politics, by describing Maine's effort to achieve universal coverage.

Americans attempt health care reform only when the status quo exceeds our pain threshold. The problem is, like the proverbial frog in the pot of heating water, we grow more tolerant of pain with increased exposure. Once, 30 million uninsured seemed intolerable, now we live comfortably with 47 million uninsured neighbors. Once, 11% of the GDP seemed an excessive amount to spend on health care, now we have reached 16% and are still growing.

Maine is the nation's most recent laboratory for health reform efforts because its burden of pain recently increased more dramatically than other states—enough to make the frog jump. Maine's personal health care spending rose faster than any other state over the 1990s and its average health insurance premiums are among the highest in the country. The arithmetic of such high premium costs in a low-wage state has produced a politically explosive and economically unsustainable environment. Maine's average total family coverage premium for employer benefit plans is greater than 25% of average household income—about the same amount families expect to spend on housing costs. Both employers and employees feel the strain. Small business employers in Maine, in particular, have been begging for relief. In just two years, the number of Mainers covered through small group plans shrank by 19% (between 2001 and 2003).

In 2002, Maine's new governor came into office with a sense of urgency about the need to address both health care costs and access barriers. The administration put forward a comprehensive reform package that gained bipartisan support in the legislature and become law in 2003. Much of the legislation will be familiar to observers of earlier federal and state reform efforts. But the Maine strategy is unique in its effort to tackle health care costs and access simultaneously, and to make these two aspects of the reform mutually dependent.

To extend access to health coverage, Maine expanded eligibility to the Medicaid program and authorized a new state agency to implement state-sponsored health insurance—the Dirigo-Choice plan—with sliding scale subsidies based on household income for small businesses, sole proprietors, and some individuals. (Dirigo—Latin for "*I lead*"—is the Maine state motto.) The plan emphasizes preventive care with full coverage of well-baby visits, physician recommended screening tests, and smoking cessation programs. In a unique design feature, plan deductibles and out of pocket maximum payments, in addition to premiums, are reduced on a sliding scale. The subsidies extend to households with incomes up to 300% of the federal poverty level. Persons with income above this level can enroll at full cost. Employers are required to contribute a minimum of 60% of employees' premium costs—the employee share and costs of dependents are subject to the subsidy program.

The administration agreed to fund the first year of the new program with a one-time general fund appropriation of $53 million. But, determined not to stimulate a new inflationary spiral in the health care system, policy makers structured *future* funding of the program to draw on "recycled" moneys derived from savings in the health care system. Initially, the administration proposed a global spending cap on hospital costs. In addition, new capital expenditures within the health care system would be capped. Under this proposed model, DirigoChoice would be funded through an assessment on all private health insurance—an assessment that would be offset by savings from the cost containment measures and the reduction in bad debt and charity care expected to result from enrollment of the uninsured into the Dirigo-Choice program. To assure that the savings accrued to policyholders, not insurance companies, the legislation proposed a mandate requiring insurers to absorb the assessment and not reflect it in premium increases.

In the political battle that ensued, the hospitals successfully beat back the administration and legislature on the global spending cap. Arguing that hospitals have no control over volume, their spokespersons frightened communities and employees with visions of massive hospital lay-offs and closures. Legislators were inundated with calls from alarmed constituents. Voluntary constraints on cost increases and hospital margins were substituted for the mandatory limits on spending. The prohibition on a pass-through of the insurance assessment was lifted. In its place, the legislation specified that the State could levy an assessment of up to 4% only if the Dirigo Board could demonstrate system savings in an amount that offset the assessment.

Maine was left with a grand experiment. Could greater transparency and voluntary efforts, with regulatory constraints only on capital expen-

ditures, cool the over-heated state health economy? Would savings specifically earmarked for coverage expansions result in a realignment of incentives for consumers and employers to pressure health care providers for greater savings? The first test came near the end of the first year of DirigoChoice operations. After 10 months, the plan had enrolled about 8,300 members representing 711 small businesses, close to 1,400 sole proprietors, and 1,400 individual enrollees. The heaviest enrollment was among the most deeply discounted income groups. In an adjudicatory hearing before Maine's Superintendent of Insurance, the Dirigo Agency presented evidence of system savings based on analysis of four year's of hospital cost reports and insurance company filings. The hearing was a circus of lawyers, with the Maine Association of Health Plans, the Chamber of Commerce, and other employer associations intervening to challenge the Dirigo Agency filing, and a consumer advocacy group intervening in support of the Dirigo Agency. The superintendent ruled that the Agency had reasonably documented $44 million in savings, in large measure derived from the hospital voluntary actions and in smaller measure from the DirigoChoice program's impact on bad debt and charity care. Based on this ruling, the Dirigo Agency levied an assessment of approximately 2.3% on insurers and employer benefit plans. Insurers and several large employers immediately notified their policyholders that the assessment would be passed through to their premiums and sought to reverse the ruling in court. Despite the fact that Maine won its case in both the state court and the Law Court, more suits and appeals are in the pipeline.

Maine's unique program funding mechanism sustained the program for two years, but the vindication by the courts and the early application of the strategy proved to be a pyrrhic victory. The Savings Offset Payment, as it was called, generated so much political animosity from employers and insurers that support for the program in the legislature wavered and divided along party lines. The Governor caved to political pressure and proposed abandoning the Savings Offset Payment in favor of dedicated sin taxes.

Then everything was complicated by a citizen tax revolt. A tax cap referendum was narrowly defeated in 2006 but it reverberated through Maine politics. The 2007 legislature struggled mightily with tax reform legislation but could not build a bridge across the chasm that separated the tax philosophies of the Democrats and Republicans. When tax reform went down to defeat, the prospect of *any* new tax—even for a popular program—was unthinkable. So, in 2007, all legislation related to the DirigoChoice Program was tabled without action. The original funding mechanism remained in place but currently generates insufficient funds to sustain program growth. As of July, 2007, new enrollment is closed until new funds can be secured. Although, coverage continues for currently enrolled businesses and individuals, and any new dependents or employees who apply through an existing account.)

The jury is still out on the ultimate success or failure of Maine's reform efforts. Nevertheless, some lessons are already clear. Maine's legislature diffused significant political opposition during the debate over the original legislation by leaving the crucial question of how to fund the program ambiguous. Proponents saw a clear source of funds that killed two birds with one stone—reining in health care spending and recycling dollars to expand access. The designated payers assumed that savings would not materialize or could not be proven, and that they were off the hook. The legislature's compromise only delayed the inevitable political battle over program funding, when payment came due. That's always been the great snare for state level health reform. Everyone wants universal coverage, but everyone wants someone else to pay for it. The "cash flow" issue creates particular strains in poor states like Maine, where state revenues are scant and the demand for social pro-

grams is high. Policymakers have observed for some time, that the US spends more on health care than any other country, and that, with significant improvement in efficiency, we ought to be able to provide decent health coverage to all our citizens without spending even more. Maine tried to come up with a formula to make that concept a reality. Reality, however, turns out to be both more and less complicated than flow charts. The complexity arises from the fact that measurement of savings is against what *would have* been spent in the absence of reform—always a debatable number. Furthermore, savings in the health delivery system do not translate into savings to payers, except through renegotiated reimbursement rates or reduced utilization, a step that requires payers to have some leverage and to bargain hard with providers. The simple reality that foils reform efforts time and again is that, regardless of system savings, funding for expanded health coverage is a redistributive effort that takes from the "haves" and gives to the "have-nots." The pain from rapidly escalating health care costs opened the door to reform efforts in Maine. But that same pain—the burden faced by employers and citizens in meeting their own coverage needs—increased rather than lessened their resistance to "sharing" the costs associated with those reform efforts.

Maine was first out of the box, in the new millennium, with an effort to respond to the health system crisis. It was soon followed by Massachusetts, Vermont, California and others. Maine's early experience offers a sober lesson to other states on the frailty of the political coalitions that, on rare occasions, come together to make significant reform legislation possible. When legislation channels resources from powerful stakeholders to new programs, enactment is only the call to battle, not the end of the war.

The Maine experience raises a sharp question for health care reform: Is it possible to sustain in all but the most exceptional states? Is it possible on the state level at all? Stay Tuned!

SNAPSHOTS OF A STATE HEALTH CRISIS

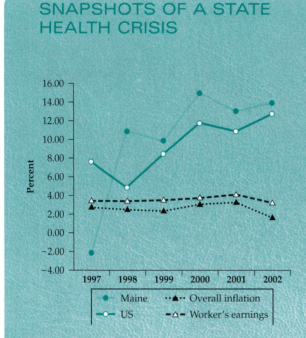

Increases in Health Insurance Premiums Compared to Other Indicators, 1996–2003

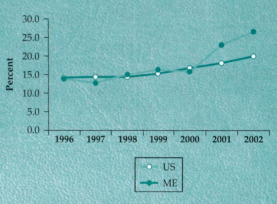

Maine and U.S. Family Premiums as % of Median Household Income, employers with fewer than 50 employees

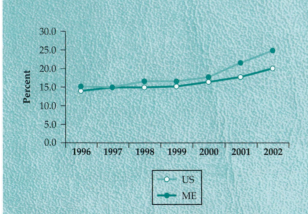

Maine & U.S. Family Premiums as % of Median Household Income, all employees

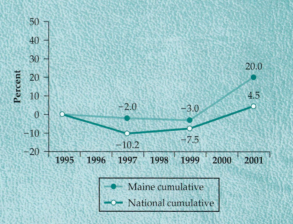

Biennial Cumulative Changes in Per Capita Inpatient Care Costs Maine Employer Benefit Plan Study Group and National Privately Insured, 1995–2001

(Continued)

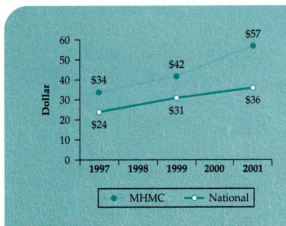

**Estimated National Average Commercial Plan
PMPM for Hospital Outpatient Services, Compared
to MHMC Experience, 1997–2001**

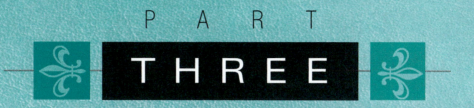

THREE

The Health Policy Process: Interest Groups, Stakeholders, and Public Opinion

Privatizing Health Politics: The Origins—and Enduring Dilemmas—of America's Public–Private Insurance Framework

Jacob S. Hacker

Jacob Hacker describes the rise of the private, employee-based health insurance system in the United States. He explains how public policies firmly guided the benefits into place. And how the system of employee benefits, in turn, fundamentally shaped—and continues to shape—the politics of health care.

It was late on November 21, 2003, and House Majority Leader Tom DeLay—the ultraconservative Texas Republican, legendary for hardball politics (and soon forced from his leadership post by legal charges against his fundraising practices)—was doing something he was unaccustomed to: racing to round up more Republican votes for a high-profile bill backed by President George W. Bush. The unprecedented three-hour scramble provided plenty of drama—including, it would later become known, credible evidence of Republican attempts at bribery—but what made it particularly jarring was the cause for which DeLay was desperately campaigning: the addition of drug coverage to Medicare, the massive health

insurance program for the aged that conservatives so love to hate.[1]

To be sure, the Medicare expansion that Bush and his allies were seeking introduced some challenges to the existing Medicare framework. Ignoring charges that they wished to privatize the program, Republicans insisted that prescription drug benefits be handled by private companies and that the legislation include generous new incentives to move seniors out of traditional Medicare and into Medicare-overseen private health plans. Still, at the eleventh hour, the hold-outs on whom DeLay was focusing his threats and promises were not Democrats, but conservative Republicans who accused their leaders of selling out for political gain. Representative Charlie Norwood of Georgia, for example, derisively called the bill the "Medicare Missed Opportunity and Open-Ended Entitlement Act"—"poorly packaged, fiscally irresponsible and just plain dangerous."[2]

In the end, DeLay prevailed. After House and then Senate passage, President Bush triumphantly signed the bill into law in early December. Because the new benefit was not scheduled to take effect until 2006—and, indeed, would not be fully implemented until 2010—virtually none of its ultimate effects were clear in the wake of its passage. But whatever its eventual consequences, the law and its genesis stand out as a revealing marker of two great intertwined movements in modern US health policy, movements usually seen as separate from each other. The first is the rise of the activist welfare state, embodied in and symbolized by programs like Medicare. The second is the dramatic expansion of private health insurance in response to government laws and subsidies. The Medicare fight was so contentious, in large part, because it centered on the oldest struggle in American health care politics: the balance between public and private insurance in providing health security. In a deeper sense, however, the Medicare battle was atypical, for it signaled a broad bipartisan recognition that the private sector, even with public subsidies, could not care for the needs of vulnerable Americans on its own. As we shall see, that recognition is far from broad or bipartisan in other realms of US health policy.

The Medicare fight is also notable for what it reveals about the development of America's jerry-rigged structure of social welfare provision. Even in an era of budgetary austerity and antigovernment ideology, Republicans could not halt the tide in favor of expanded Medicare protection. They were, however, able to channel it into reforms that make Medicare more dependent than ever on the private sector while showering generous largesse on private companies that have an increasingly powerful vested interest in a partially privatized Medicare system. This largely untold story—of popular demands parlayed by conservatives into private sector responses that create enduring private enrichment and entrenchment—is not a new one. As will become clear, it is the grand narrative behind the rise of America's peculiar public–private insurance complex.

AMERICA'S PUBLIC–PRIVATE INSURANCE FRAMEWORK

The United States stands apart from other affluent western nations in many spheres. Its military dwarfs that of other nations. Its aggregate economic production is unrivaled. Its ideals of equality and liberty are beacons on the global landscape. Yet among the most distinctive and least recognized features of the contemporary US social order is the unparalleled reliance of Americans on the private sector for basic protection against what President Franklin Roosevelt once called "the hazards and vicissitudes of life." This reliance is so extensive, so embedded, and so ubiquitous it is often overlooked. But even a glance at Figures 9-1 and 9-2 demolishes any suggestion that the American social policy model is the international norm.

Figure 9-1 tells the first half of the story: As a share of the economy, US public social expenditures are much, much lower than those of other affluent western democracies. Indeed, at 17.1% of GDP in 1995, US spending is not merely the lowest in the group; it is barely more than half the average level of the other nations. As Figure 9-2 shows, however, the story is not quite so simple once two basic adjustments are made to the traditional spending tallies. The first is to account for relative tax levels across nations. Through the tax code, many nations "claw back" a large share of the benefits delivered through direct social spending. What they giveth they also taketh away. Adjusting for taxation thus markedly increases the social spending total for nations with low tax rates, of which the United States is the preeminent example.

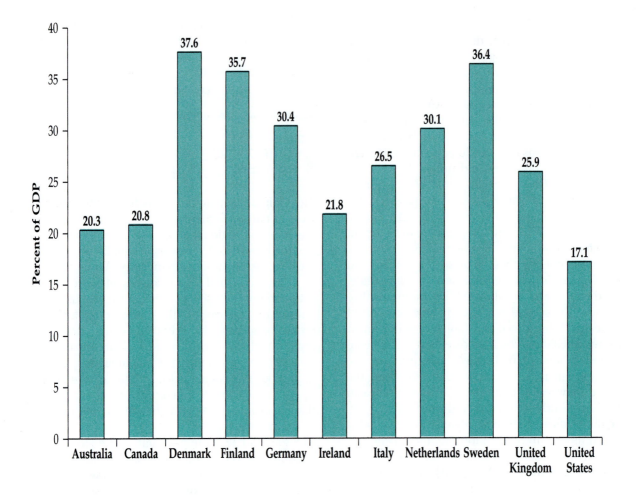

Figure 9-1 Public Social Welfare Expenditures as a Percentage of GDP in 11 Nations, 1995

SOURCE: Calculated from Willem Adema, "Net Social Expenditure," *Labour Market and Social Policy-Occasional Papers No. 39* (Paris: OECD, August 1999), 30.

NOTES: Public social welfare expenditures exclude education. They include cash benefits for a wide range of social contingencies—disability, old age, death of a spouse, occupational injuries, disease, sickness, childbirth, unemployment, poverty—as well as spending on housing, health care, services for the elderly and disabled, active labor-market policies, and other similar social benefits.

The second adjustment is to include in the social spending column benefits that are provided by employers and non-governmental organizations, so long as these benefits are (a) similar in structure and function to public social benefits and (b) actively subsidized and regulated by the government. In the absence of broad comparative data on such private social benefits, the figures here are essentially limited to private employment-based health and pension plans—which, in the United States, are generously

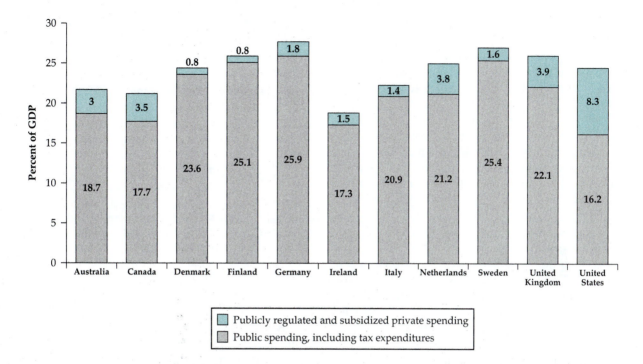

Figure 9-2 After-Tax Public and Private Social Welfare Expenditures as a Percentage of GDP in Eleven Nations, 1995

SOURCE: Calculated from Willem Adema, "Net Social Expenditure," *Labour Market and Social Policy-Occasional Papers No. 39* (Paris: OECD, August 1999), 30.

NOTES: Public social welfare expenditures exclude education. They include cash benefits for a wide range of social contingencies—disability, old age, death of a spouse, occupational injuries, disease, sickness, childbirth, unemployment, poverty—as well as spending on housing, health care, services for the elderly and disabled, active labor-market policies, and other similar social benefits. Private social welfare expenditures are payments for the same purposes made by employers and other non-governmental organizations, provided that such benefits are mandated, subsidized, or regulated by government. To prevent double-counting, tax breaks for private benefits are not included in the public spending estimate.

subsidized through the tax code and heavily regulated by the federal government. But the massive numbers involved are eye-opening even on this narrow definition. In the United States, private social benefits represented more than 8% of GDP in 1995—an amount slightly more than half as large as US public social spending in that year.

Looking across all eleven nations, these two simple adjustments produce striking results. The United States, we have seen, ranks last according to direct social spending—the traditional measure of social welfare effort. But once we adjust for relative tax burdens and publicly subsidized private social benefits, the United States rises to the middle of the pack. In fact, its net public and private spending, at 24.5% of GDP, is above the average for all 11 nations (24%). No less striking is how exceptional the American sphere of private social benefits looks in comparative perspective. Private social benefits in the United States represent more than 34% of net public and private spending. In contrast, they represent an average of less than 9% of net spending in the 10 other nations. In no other nation does private social welfare spending comprise even half as large a share of total social spending as it does in the United States.

All this may seem dry and technical. Yet its importance cannot be overemphasized. Properly measured, the United States does not devote a markedly smaller proportion of national resources to social services and transfers than do other affluent democracies. Not only does the United States tax public benefits more lightly than do other nations, it also uses the tax code more aggressively to provide benefits and underwrite their private provision. Moreover, the United States hosts a far more sizable sphere of private social benefits than do other nations. American social provision is exceptional, in sum, not because social spending is istinctly low in comparative perspective, but because so much of that spending comes from the private sector.

It is comforting to conclude from this that America's social welfare framework is functionally equivalent to the state-oriented frameworks found abroad—that the United States does just what other nations do, only through different (and, to the many who doubt government's capacity, presumably better) means. Yet treating public and private benefits as identical is as misdirected as ignoring private benefits altogether. The United States may spend as much as many European governments when private benefits and tax policy are taken into account, but the distribution of these benefits is fundamentally different. For one, the *vertical* distribution of benefits—up and down the income ladder—is much less favorable toward lower-income citizens. Employment-based benefits are much more prevalent and generous at higher ends of the wage scale, as Table 9-1 demonstrates, and tax subsidies for private benefits, because they forgive tax that would otherwise be owed, are generally worth the most to taxpayers in the highest tax brackets. For another, the *horizontal* distribution of benefits across similarly situated workers is also much less equal. Employers decide whether to

Table 9-1 Share of Non-Agricultural Private Workers Receiving Health and Pension Benefits, by Earnings, 1998

Wage Quintile	Pension Benefits	Health Benefits
Lowest	15.7%	23.7%
Second	34.1	44.5
Third	52.3	59.4
Fourth	63.9	67.3
Highest	72.1	68.8

SOURCE: James Medoff and Michael Calabrese, "The Impact of Labor Market Trends on Health and Pension Benefit Coverage," Preliminary Report of the Center for National Policy, September 2000, Tables H25 and P18. I am grateful to the authors for providing me with this unpublished report, which is based on Census data.

provide benefits, and there are whole industries and categories of employment where they are quite rare. Overall, only about two-thirds of workers receive health insurance through employment, and fewer than that have a pension plan at work, much less contribute to it. Perhaps not surprisingly, then, comparative figures on redistribution suggest that US social policies reduce inequality significantly less than do social policies in any other rich democracy.[3]

And these are just the distributional differences. Private social benefits—and the government subsidies that encourage them—also differ from public social programs in other crucial ways. They are, in the first place, considerably less visible in public debate and discussion. All of us know about Medicare and Social Security. But few Americans know that the federal government spends about as much as it does on Medicare to subsidize private pension and health benefits through the tax code—and fewer still understand the complex web of regulations that shape the character and distribution of these benefits. This lack of visibility may be why the huge distributional inequities that characterize private benefits are not only tolerated, but actively promoted by federal policy (through, for example, tax breaks that are worth the most to the best off). Is it

Table 9-2 Average Tax Subsidy for Health Insurance Received by Families, by Income, 1998

Family income	Average subsidy per family
Less than $15,000	$71
$15,000–$19,999	296
$20,000–$29,999	535
$30,000–$39,999	847
$40,000–$49,999	1,195
$50,000–$74,999	1,684
$75,000–$99,999	1,971
$100,000 or more	2,357

SOURCE: Jon Sheils and Paul Hogan, "Cost of Tax-Exempt Health Benefits in 1998," *Health Affairs* 18, no. 2 (1999): 180.

conceivable, for example, that elected politicians would promote a new health insurance program that delivered a few hundred dollars a year to lower-income families but showered five or ten times that on better-off citizens? Perhaps not, but that, as Table 9-2 shows, is exactly what the special tax treatment of employment-based health benefits does. And, if anything, the tax treatment of health insurance is *less* imbalanced than other tax breaks. The Treasury Department estimates, for example, that *fully 80%* of the $100 billion or so spent each year to subsidize private pensions and retirement accounts goes to the richest 20% of Americans.[4]

Finally, and for many of the same reasons, private social benefits also differ *politically* from public social programs. Policies that encourage and shape private benefits, unlike public social programs, are more likely to emerge through a "subterranean" political process in which interested parties, like employers and insurers, dominate deliberations and the general public has little or no involvement or awareness. Similarly, policies encouraging private social benefits—again, unlike public social programs—are likely to start small and grow big, as employers and insurers take advantage of new government subsidies. They are also likely to gain the enthusiastic support of political conservatives who are otherwise

hostile to an active government role in the social welfare field. Across a range of features, then—the scope of conflict, the character of development, the constellation of supporters—the politics of private benefits is an almost mirror image of our received view of social welfare politics.

And yet, despite all these differences, there is one crucial similarity between public and private benefits: Once they are enjoyed by large swaths of citizens, they are very, very hard to change. Social Security and Medicare are usually seen as "third rails" in American politics—"touch and die." But when private social benefits become a core source of protection for Americans, they are also very difficult to challenge. For this reason, whether publicly subsidized private benefits gain a secure foothold before viable movements for government social programs emerge is often crucial in determining whether Americans end up relying on the public or private sector for primary protection against key social risks. To use the language of business economics, in the world of social policy, the "first mover"—whether private benefits or public programs—often enjoys tremendous political advantages in the struggle over how society should deal with pressing problems. In fact, it is precisely *because* private benefits are so hard to displace once they are widely distributed that private interests and conservative politicians so aggressively promote them. By embedding private solutions, they hope to head off public ones.

Exhibit A for all these conclusions is American health insurance. In other social policy areas, such as retirement pensions, private benefits rest atop a core program of government protection—in the retirement field, Social Security. The exact opposite is true of American health insurance. Although US health spending is by far the highest in the world, less than half of that spending comes from public sources, compared with an average of almost three quarters in the other nations (see in Table I–1 for the exact figures). Moreover, much less than half of the population in the United States is eligible for public insurance coverage, compared with an average of 98% of the population in the other nations.

Most Americans, in short, get health insurance from their employer, or do not get health insurance at all.

And not coincidentally, the United States is also the only advanced capitalist democracy in which a sizable number of residents—in 2004, some 46 million—are without health insurance and therefore must go without care or rely on family funds or charity. The vast majority (85%) of those without health insurance live in families headed by at least one worker, and nearly three-fifths of the uninsured lack coverage for two years or more. They are also more than four times as likely to say they do not have a regular source of care, more than three times as likely to say they postponed care or went without needed care because of the cost, and two to three times as likely to say that when they received care, it posed a financial hardship for them. Indeed, almost a quarter of the uninsured say they have been contacted by a collection agency about unpaid medical bills, and, strikingly, roughly half of the more than 1 million individuals and families that file for bankruptcy each year do so because of financially debilitating medical costs.[5]

So why does the United States lack national health insurance? This is among the oldest and most debated questions in the study of US social policy, and commentators have fingered many culprits, from the medical profession to political conservatives to America's fragmented political institutions. The bewildering array of arguments belies the stunningly obvious answer: *The United States lacks national health insurance because Americans have come to rely on other, predominantly private, means for health security.* Most Americans have health coverage. If they are workers, they are likely to receive insurance as a benefit of employment—an arrangement that has been heavily subsidized through the tax code and extensively encouraged by public policy. If they are older than 65 or very poor, they are covered by public health programs that fill the gaps in employment-based coverage. To be sure, private coverage has contracted in recent decades and many Americans who have insurance are insufficiently protected or risk losing coverage. Nonetheless, private health insurance reaches still more than two-thirds of

non-elderly Americans, overwhelmingly through employment. And this means, in turn, that proposals for government-sponsored health insurance face singular hurdles—not just the opposition of a huge and resourceful private medical industry, but also the fears of insured Americans about threats to their existing coverage. This is the essential dilemma faced by health reformers in the United States.

For all the fascination with the puzzle of why the United States lacks a national health program, students of US health policy have paid surprisingly little attention to the corollary question of why the United States relies so heavily on private employment-based health insurance. Their not-unreasonable assumption seems to be that this unusual state of affairs is merely the flip-side of the absence of a universal government program. This reasonable assumption is wrong. Understanding the peculiar public–private character of US health policy requires a convincing political and historical explanation of the rise of employment-based health plans as a viable alternative to national insurance—an outcome that was neither foreordained by America's antigovernment culture nor an inevitable byproduct of the early defeats of public insurance. Endemically prone to failure, the health insurance market had to be actively constructed by private leadership and public policy, which came together at critical junctures to bolster private institutions as a bulwark against direct state intervention.

EARLY POLITICAL DEFEATS AND THE EMERGENCE OF PRIVATE INSURANCE

In the United States, "compulsory health insurance" (as government insurance was initially called) first became a prominent political issue during the early 1910s. Although Theodore Roosevelt campaigned on a third-party platform that endorsed compulsory insurance in 1912, his defeat left the mantle of reform in the hands of the American Association for

Labor Legislation (AALL), an association of reform-minded philanthropists and academics. The AALL pledged in 1916 to lobby for the passage of compulsory programs at the state level, modeling its campaign closely on its earlier successful legislative drive for the enactment of workers' compensation laws in numerous states. Indeed, this previous success left members of the AALL confident that they would have little trouble convincing state leaders to pass health programs, which they believed was much more urgently needed than the workers' compensation laws had been.

But the success of workers' compensation was not a good benchmark for the likely fate of compulsory health insurance. The former had been supported by corporations tired of expensive litigation over accidents; the latter was unambiguously opposed by employers and "involved a proud profession, not simply the writing of checks for disability pensions."[6] Although the AALL started impressively, its campaign soon stalled and opponents quickly throttled AALL proposals in state after state. Although much has been made of the ineptitude of the AALL and the stridency of the rhetoric surrounding the debate, it is hard to see how either mattered very much given the political–institutional constraints the AALL faced. The members of the AALL were not, as were European reformers at the time, powerful leaders within a centralized national state. Nor were they representatives of disciplined political parties. Instead, they were forced to act as independent policy activists trying to raise simultaneous interest in reform in as many states as possible while overcoming state politicians' fears that a new program would hurt their state's ability to attract and retain business. Perhaps if World War I had not interceded, the AALL campaign would have fared better. But, considering that no other major social programs passed at the state level during this period, this is highly unlikely.[7]

Still, the inglorious demise of the first campaign for compulsory health insurance did not leave the political terrain unaltered. The AALL's abject failure predictably soured reformers on the prospect of touching the hornet's nests of organized interests again. Immensely more important, the debate helped unite and define the interests of a constellation of groups that might otherwise have found themselves in conflict—employers, insurers, and doctors. The most well organized of these groups was the medical profession, which emerged from debate over compulsory health insurance bristling with confidence and vigilant against future threats. Insurers and employers, however, were far more important to the rise of private protections. Ironically, if the AALL had succeeded in demonstrating anything during its futile march, it was the growing need for insurance against the costs of sickness—a need that insurers increasingly felt they could meet. Beginning around 1910, carriers started to write life insurance policies not on an individual basis, as had been the practice before, but rather by contracting with large groups of employees within a single firm or industry.[8] The advantages of group underwriting were profound. First, it spread costs and risks across myriad workers, allowing carriers to offer coverage at reasonable rates without inquiring into the health status of every enrollee. The second advantage was administrative. Although policies still had to be sold and administered, the cost of doing so dropped dramatically as the insured workforce grew.

The employment group thus came to be the cornerstone of the new structure of commercial insurance—a position freighted with future significance. In the philosophy of group insurance, American employers were to be the repositories of tiny social insurance systems that spread risks and benefits within, and only within, the universe of their workers. In other nations, the state encouraged voluntary organizations involved in social provision, but the employment group did not take on such a prominent role in many of them.

For employers, the motives for installing group health plans went beyond concerns about the stability of benefits to include the less lofty goal of resisting union encroachments, an aim that became more pressing with the labor upswing of the 1930s. Not surprisingly then, "industries that faced the most active union organizing efforts—autos, paper, and rubber—show remarkable rates of private health coverage."[9]

If the response of employers and commercial insurers to the threat of compulsory insurance helped set the stage for the rise of group health insurance, the spur that would ultimately become most critical originated elsewhere—in the intersection of business and benevolence at Baylor University Hospital in Dallas, Texas. There, in 1929, the model of hospital coverage that would evolve into Blue Cross was born, earning a modest hospital plan for school teachers a permanent place in the annals of private welfare leadership.

From the beginning, Blue Cross was an unusual amalgam of civic and business principles—an institution situated in both the commercial sector and "civil society," that domain of social life governed neither by the coercive power of the state nor the profit motive of the market. The early Blue Cross plans were founded by community notables and progressive businessmen who aimed to deliver broad social rewards as well as immediate economic benefits. Crucially, the Blue Cross leadership also demanded—and, in state after state, received—special enabling legislation that exempted plans from taxation while giving them special operating charters. These special state charters "were originally conceived and passed specifically because of the non-profit and social character of the plans. This social characteristic anticipated the enrollment of low-income members of the community and their being provided with protection equal to that received by the more affluent community members at a lower cost. The implication, if not the stated goal, of this element . . . was that Blue Cross would serve as an income redistribution device, a role customarily reserved for governmental action."[10] The private sector would do what the public sector could not.

A SECOND DEFEAT AND THE EXPANSION OF PRIVATE PROTECTION

The Great Depression transformed the balance of partisan power in American politics and shifted the institutional locus of US social policymaking from the states to the federal government. As dramatic as the upheaval was, however, the opportunities it created were not unlimited. Although Democrats decisively controlled Congress, the party was split between its Northern and Southern wings. And within Congress, Southern Democrats benefited the most from their party's gains in the 1930s. Most came from safe one-party states and districts, and the seniority system in Congress ensured that they occupied powerful positions within the congressional hierarchy, allowing them to resist any challenge to the white power structure and low-wage economy of the South.

The members of the Committee on Economic Security (CES) were well aware of these constraints. Although they studied the feasibility of including compulsory health insurance in the Social Security Act, they ultimately decided against it in the face of fierce protests from the AMA. It is important to emphasize that health insurance was not postponed because the New Dealers believed that private alternatives were sufficient. The 1935 report of the CES stated categorically (and wrongly) that "voluntary insurance holds no promise of being much more effective in the near future than it has been in the past."[11] Although some opponents of government action were touting voluntary health insurance, a leading CES policy expert recalled that "[t]his was pipsqueak stuff . . . . That argument was advanced, but there was no substantial supporting ground for it in going operations." [12] The best estimates from the early 1930s indicate that no more than 2 to 3 million workers and their dependents enjoyed any health insurance protection.[13]

Although the need for health insurance was real, the goal suffered from the lessons and legacies of the first campaign for compulsory health insurance less than two decades before. In the wake of the AALL's defeat, health insurance had faded from the wish list of progressive reformers. At the same time, the health insurance campaign mobilized a formidable core of interest group resistance that new reform efforts would have to overcome, including the AMA. Ironically, then, health insurance faltered during the

New Deal not because it had arrived too late as a compelling issue, but because it had arrived too early. If it had percolated upwards from continuing state-level agitation without the baggage of prior defeat, perhaps there would have been greater social pressure and elite-level commitment in favor of action—and a less cohesive and resourceful opposition lying in wait.

One conclusion, however, is unmistakable: The decision to leave health insurance out of the Social Security Act represented a turning point in the fortunes of private health protection. Scattered and still scarce, private health insurance was not a major stumbling block for the Roosevelt administration when it considered government health insurance. In the wake of the Social Security Act, however, the seeds sown during the 1920s and early 1930s burst into flower. With medical providers, employers, and insurers all pushing for private alternatives, a rapidly increasing proportion of corporations enrolled their workers in group hospital and physician plans. By the end of World War II, private health insurance would enjoy a formidable presence on the American welfare landscape and reformers would be forced to rethink the wisdom of their elusive goal once again.

As Figure 9-3 demonstrates, the growth of voluntary health insurance during the late 1930s and 1940s was certainly remarkable. And although national health insurance continually failed, federal law was not immaterial to these developments. One spur was favorable tax law. Although Congress never addressed the tax treatment of private health insurance before the 1950s, the IRS in effect "treated employer contributions for the accident and health insurance as non-taxable fringe benefits from the inception of the income tax in 1913."[14] Nonetheless, deep uncertainties about the treatment of health benefits remained through the 1940s, and IRS precedents applied only to group health insurance, not individual union or company plans. In 1954, however, President Eisenhower successfully pressed Congress to use the tax code to encourage "insurance and other plans adopted by employers to protect their employees against the risks of sickness . . . by removing the present uncertainties in the tax law."[15]

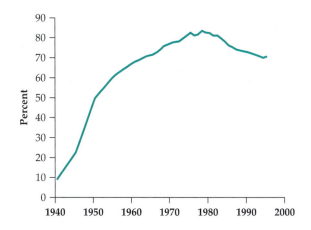

Figure 9-3 Share of U.S. Population with Private Health Insurance, 1940-1995

SOURCE: Health Insurance Association of America (HIAA), *Source Book of Health Insurance Data* (Washington, D.C.: HIAA, 1996), 41.

Today, all health benefits are exempt from taxation as employee income as well as deductible by corporations—a policy that costs more than $100 billion annually.

Make no mistake, tax breaks for health insurance are a form of spending—big spending. But in 1954, they were not treated as such and no one professed to know how much they would cost. Nor was there much mention of the distributional consequences of channeling subsidies through the tax code—despite the reality that the resulting distribution comported with no known theory of tax equity, much less any articulated philosophy of social justice. The tax exclusion for employer-provided health insurance, after all, benefits only those who have workplace coverage, and its value is vastly greater for those with higher incomes because they pay taxes at higher marginal rates. And while tax-favored private pensions are subject to modest rules requiring a modicum of equal distribution, health plans are (and have always been) essentially exempt from these requirements.[16]

The expansion of private health insurance was further encouraged during World War II by the exclusion of fringe benefits from wage and price controls. Given the tight conditions of the labor market, firms were already under heavy pressure to attract and retain workers. But a decision by the War Labor Board to exempt health and pension benefits from price controls highlighted the use of fringe benefits as a management tool and gave corporations an additional incentive to adopt them. The fastest growth occurred in Blue Cross plans, the membership of which increased at an average annual rate of 23% between 1943 and 1946, when the exclusion was in effect.

For all these policy incentives, the most fundamental reason for the rise of employment-based coverage in the 1940s was raw political self-interest. Amid the battle over government insurance, a range of groups—doctors, hospitals, insurers, employers—came to see private protections as a way of achieving not just their own organizational imperatives, but also larger political goals. Out of the crucible of prior failed reform efforts emerged a route of escape from the looming threat of government action, one that also delivered important benefits to those who adopted and championed it, from employee goodwill to the stabilization of income. Private health insurance began as an uncertain commitment viewed with ambivalence by nearly all the actors involved in its creation and growth. By the mid-1940s, however, it was an organizational reality backed by powerful interests and invested with larger strategic aims—and one that, as events would soon reveal, would make national health insurance a nearly impossible goal.

THE PRIVATE INSURANCE TRAP

The years after World War II seemed auspicious for the completion of the unfinished business of the New Deal. Wartime expansion vastly increased the power of the state and polls taken in the 1940s showed upwards of 85 % of Americans supporting a national health program based on Social Security.[17]

Yet hopes for national health insurance went unfulfilled. After a quixotic postwar crusade by President Truman to enact national health insurance ended in failure, Truman's successor, Dwight Eisenhower, worked to put government squarely behind private health insurance. As employment-based coverage spread like wildfire through the workplace, reformers struggled to craft a new reform approach that would work around the burgeoning system of private insurance rather than supplant it. They succeeded, but the twin programs that they eventually passed in 1965—Medicare and Medicaid—would prove to be the first and last massive expansions of government health insurance in the 20th century.

The contemporary diagnoses of this persistent stalemate were many: the recalcitrance of the AMA, public fears of "socialized medicine," legislative missteps by reform advocates. But two causes—one obvious at the time, one less so—stand out in broad historical and comparative perspective. The first was the enduring barriers encountered by those seeking to construct proreform majorities in America's fragmented political context. As private insurance expanded, however, a second critical constraint came to dominate: the increasingly privileged place of publicly regulated and subsidized private insurance in American medical finance. This distinctive position was sustained not only by powerful vested interests in the employment-based system, and not only by the continued decomposition of the potential constituency for reform. It was also anchored by the very division of public and private duties in health care, which made public officials acutely sensitive to the effect of government action on private coverage and yet gave them few instruments for controlling spending or expanding public insurance. Much as changes to established public programs entailed massive transition costs and salient losses to organized groups, changes to the private core of American health insurance posed a test that reformers found themselves repeatedly unable to pass.

Today, we see the principal barrier to expanding public coverage as money—specifically, where government will get it. Yet during the rosy era of postwar growth, the influential consideration was not the expense of public action, but the growing reach of voluntary insurance. Private insurance had not been central in previous battles over public coverage, for the simple reason that it had not been central in American medical care. But in the late 1940s it was both, and the opponents of national health insurance called attention to its promise as never before. After the obligatory salvos against "socialized medicine" had been launched, the critics of government insurance always turned to the same battle-tested line of defense: Voluntary health insurance was solving whatever problems of access there were in America's otherwise idyllic medical system.

No better evidence of this shift can be found than the evolving strategy of the AMA, the most visible and vocal foe of national health insurance. During the debate over the Truman plan, the AMA made voluntary health insurance the foundation of its bitter assault on government insurance. The most ubiquitous advertisement in the AMA's campaign featured a famous 19th century Fildes painting, *The Doctor*, in which a compassionate physician ministers to a sick child as her grief-stricken parents hover nearby. In the AMA ad, the painting is ringed by the words: "Voluntary Health Insurance—The American Way Will KEEP POLITICS OUT OF THIS PICTURE."[18] The advertisement were the product of the husband-and-wife public relations firm, Whitaker and Baxter, who emphasized that "[y]ou can't beat something with nothing." "We want everybody in the health insurance field selling insurance as he never sold it before," declared Whitaker in a speech before the AMA in February 1949. "If we can get ten million more people insured in the next year and ten million more in the next year, the threat of socialized medicine in this country will be over."[19]

Although the AMA was the most prominent group touting the virtues and potential of private insurance, it was hardly alone. Health insurers were obviously on board, and so too was corporate America. The same, however, was not true of organized labor. American unions were at the height of their organizational strength in the 1940s, and they placed national health insurance near the top of their legislative priorities. Yet it became increasingly clear

that unions would either wrest concession from employers or go without health benefits altogether. As early as 1946, United Auto Workers (UAW) President Walter Reuther declared, "There is no evidence to encourage the belief that we may look to Congress for relief. In the immediate future, security will be won for our people only to the extent that the union succeeds in obtaining such security through collective bargaining."[20] Reuther's prediction was prescient. In the decade after 1945, organized labor negotiated health benefits in industry after industry. In 1946, negotiated health plans covered fewer than a million workers and their dependents. Between 1948 and 1950, however, the number rose from 2.7 million to more than 7 million, and by 1954, it had reached 27 million—one-fourth of all health insurance in the United States.[21]

This had important implications for labor views of national health insurance. For as employee health insurance spread through the workforce, it could not help but reduce the interest of unions and covered workers in a government program of protection.[22] A confidential memo prepared by the UAW in 1949, for example, strongly emphasized the continuing need for national health insurance but warned that "labor leaders will be forced by their constituents to support collective bargaining programs, rather than government programs, if the proposals for government programs provide for too heavy a levy on earnings."[23] In the early 1950s, the Committee on the Nation's Health, a proreform organization with close ties to the Truman administration, lamented "a tendency on the part of many unions to lose effective interest in national health legislation even though they may continue to give it verbal support in convention resolutions."[24]

Equally revealing was labor's stance toward the favorable tax treatment of health insurance, which as discussed earlier was codified in 1954. When the Eisenhower Treasury Department announced it was reviewing the tax treatment, the Congress of Industrial Organizations (CIO—later, through a merger, the AFL-CIO) submitted a frank memo on behalf of "five million wage earners" stating that a "change in the rules of the Bureau of Internal Revenue or a specific amendment to the Internal Revenue Code to define such employer payments as taxable income to . . . employees would be both inequitable and impracticable."[25] The CIO pointed out the huge costs and dislocations that would result if health benefits were taxed. It closed, however, by appealing directly to Eisenhower's conservative instincts: "One last point—the significance of which cannot be overemphasized—which must be considered by the Treasury Department, is the harmful effect which a reversal of the present tax ruling would have on the growth of voluntary hospitalization and medical plans."[26] The same CIO that had stated in 1949 that "[t]he voluntary groups are limited by their very nature from providing comprehensive care to everyone" now criticized any action that would "adversely affect the continued growth of voluntary prepayment plans and their development as a mechanism for providing comprehensive health services to the American people."[27]

The clearest sign of the changing fortunes of national health insurance was the changing strategy of its strongest supporters: the Truman administration executives who had pushed for reform in the 1940s. In 1950, administration officials bowed to the inevitable and began to search for a more limited legislative alternative that would still retain the contributory social insurance structure of Social Security. The proposal that eventually emerged focused on the aged alone, promising up to 60 days of hospital treatment annually to Social Security recipients, their spouses, and their survivors.

The new proposal was a major strategic retreat for the advocates of national health insurance, incomprehensible without an appreciation of the stunning rise of private health security. The elderly were, after all, the most identifiable and clearly "deserving" group left out of employment-based coverage. Poorer and sicker than the rest of the population, they rarely enjoyed health insurance after retirement, and few could obtain affordable insurance because the problem of adverse selection was too great. The proposal would be cast as simply extending accepted insurance practices to the aged.

In return for these rhetorical advantages, however, advocates inevitably made significant concessions. Gone from the reformers' rhetorical arsenal was the principled indictment of voluntary insurance that had been so central to their campaign in the late 1940s. Instead, reformers would now argue that their plan "would not adversely affect existing insurance plans," because it "would not invade a field of substantial interest to private insurance, non-profit or commercial."[28] Arthur Hess, a deputy commissioner of Social Security, noted that the argument for government action was increasingly a narrow pragmatic one: "[I]t was just in terms of, 'Everybody accepts the insurance type mechanism as the answer here, and the extent that it works in voluntary hands and works well, the government can't do it any cheaper. To the extent that it doesn't work in voluntary hands, somebody's got to step in.'"[29] Of course, claiming that private health insurance worked for most Americans weakened the case for the national health program to which Social Security executives were still deeply committed. But it strengthened the case for a national hospital program for aged Americans left out of workplace insurance.

Opponents of national health insurance recognized well that the weaknesses of the private system threatened past victories. Moderate conservatives who had worked to encourage private insurance in the early 1950s continued to entreat the private sector to extend coverage on its own. Yet all these efforts came to naught, and in 1965, a window of opportunity for major reform opened in the wake of President Lyndon B. Johnson's landslide victory. The 1964 sweep meant that Medicare was a "legislative certainty."[30] The question was what form it would take. What eventually emerged was Medicare and Medicaid—a federal hospital insurance plan for the aged based on payroll taxes (Medicare Part A) coupled with a physicians' insurance plan financed mainly by general income tax revenue (Part B) and a federal–state program for the poor (Medicaid).

Medicare was a reflection of the constricted political opening through which it passed. The bill itself promised that "nothing in this title shall be construed to authorize any federal official or employee to exercise any supervision or control over the practice of medicine."[31] Medicare allowed private insurers to act as "fiscal intermediaries" for the program. These intermediaries would pay for services at rates that were "reasonable and customary," meaning, at the outset, essentially whatever providers chose to charge. Not surprisingly, the cost of the program outstripped even the most expansive expectations voiced before passage. The federal government had first become a generous subsidizer of private health insurance, and then finally stepped in as a largely passive financier of private medical care itself. It did not at first challenge the basic structure that had arisen in the aftermath of past unsuccessful campaigns for compulsory health insurance.

THE STRUGGLES OF THE 1970s

The 1970s dawned with the widespread recognition of a "crisis" in American medicine. This was not a crisis of access or quality. It was a crisis of costs—untenable, explosive, unstoppable health care costs. The loser in this new climate was the medical profession. The expansion of private insurance had been the profession's escape from the penury of government control. But the expensive medical industry that the profession had helped construct was not the profession's alone to manage. Not only government, but also business firms and commercial insurers had their own stake in the finance and delivery of medicine, and their interest in controlling costs was not congruent with the profession's interest in maintaining income and autonomy. From the private sector, the major challenge to doctors was prepaid group practice, which doctors had fought bitterly for years. Prepaid group plans integrated the finance and delivery of care, organizing panels of doctors and paying them either a salary or a fixed fee per patient. Recast as "health maintenance organizations" (HMOs), these plans gained the support

of the Nixon administration in 1970, and a bill to aid their development passed in 1973.

While alarm about costs spurred new departures, it also briefly revived the fortunes of universal health insurance. This time, however, the president advocating reform was a Republican, Richard Nixon, and the plan he was advocating would not have created a universal government program but rather mandated employers to offer private coverage. Nixon's proposal was not greeted warmly by liberal Democrats, most of whom remained committed to a single federal insurance system and believed that Nixon would soon be forced from office by the emerging Watergate scandal. They proved correct—but with Nixon went national health insurance, and perhaps the only hope for a national health program, albeit a program based on private rather than public coverage.

The United States might have universal health insurance today if propitious political circumstances and able leadership had come together in the early 1970s before the stagflation and resurgent conservatism of that decade stalled further progress toward reform. But if a compromise had been reached, it almost certainly would not have resembled the publicly sponsored health insurance systems found elsewhere. By the 1970s, the complex legacy of past political struggles had left the United States with a costly patchwork of public and private health insurance over which no interested party could exert control. This complicated structure divided erstwhile opponents of government action, but it also divided advocates. It created new public demands for government intervention, but it also split Americans into warring factions. It moved medical costs to the center of public debate, but it gave public and private authorities few means to control them. These dilemmas bedeviled America's fragmented polity and stalemated progress toward health care reform for more than two decades.

Yet, as new antigovernment winds swept Washington, a little-noticed legislative legacy of a vanishing liberal era was rapidly reshaping the structure of private medical finance. That legacy was contained in a law of immeasurable scope and complexity: the Employee Retirement Income Security Act of 1974, or "ERISA."

Although the law aimed to regulate pensions, at the last minute and with little debate congressional sponsors included a provision that exempted corporate health plans that "self-insured" (that is, paid claims directly out of corporate coffers, rather than contracted with an insurer to pay them) from all benefit regulations passed by the states.

The ERISA "preemption clause," as this crucial provision came to be called, was originally touted as a source of uniformity in employee benefits. Its effect, however, was to further fragment the health insurance risk pool. As employers rushed to self-insure, the insurance market split ever more into self-contained risk groups, each jealously guarded from outside interference or the imposition of new costs. By encouraging self-funding, ERISA also gave corporate purchasers of health insurance new reasons to eschew collective responses and look for their own solutions to rising health care costs. By the 1980s, moreover, states had begun to experiment with limited programs designed to pool costs for high-risk populations. Yet ERISA placed self-insured employment groups beyond the reach of state law.[32] Thus national politicians not only failed to pass major insurance reforms in the 1970s, they also added new hurdles to the already formidable barriers that stood in the way of action. The forces unleashed would eventually push reform back into the spotlight, but only after two decades of stalemate allowed the troubles of American medical finance to grow much more pressing.

THE FAILURE OF THE CLINTON PLAN

Other chapters delve into the details of the Clinton reform effort of 1993–94.[33] What needs to be emphasized, however, is how deeply the political dilemmas that President Clinton faced were shaped by the failure of past political efforts to enact national health insurance in the United States. First, the very structure of Clinton's proposal represented a concession to the distinctive structure of medical finance and delivery that had arisen in the United States.[34] Clinton's Health Security plan attempted to lock into place a disintegrating private financing system while furthering the movement toward managed care that had been under way for two decades. For most Americans, insurance would be funded largely through employer contributions. Americans would choose among private health plans and be encouraged to select managed care plans. Medicare was explicitly left out of this new system, although much of the funding for the plan came through decreased Medicare payments. Very large employers would be allowed to opt out of the program if they met strict requirements, restrained their own costs, and paid an assessment designed to minimize the dumping of poor risks into the publicly overseen framework.

Ironically, the failure of the Clinton plan left the field clear for the type of radical market changes that detractors of the proposal had warned would result from its implementation. Partly in anticipation of the Clinton plan, insurers and corporations accelerated their movement toward managed care in the early 1990s, nearly doubling the number of Americans in these more restrictive arrangements between 1992 and 1995.[35] A wave of mergers and acquisitions saw for-profit hospitals and insurers sweep into the field, displacing much of the nonprofit organizational infrastructure upon which the case for public-spirited private medical care had been premised. Although this dramatic transformation did nothing to address the worsening plight of the uninsured, it did temporarily slow the rate of medical inflation and lessen cost pressures on employers and public programs. In the rest of the industrialized world, cost-containment had been spearheaded by government authorities. In the United States, responsibility for cost control fell by default to the private sector. Indeed, as private actors moved to reshape medicine, government leaders were left scrambling to respond.[36] This reversal of fortune is perhaps the strongest evidence yet that the United States has followed a fundamentally different path of health policy development than have other nations—one that will almost certainly not culminate in the passage of European-style national health insurance.

A second historically inherited constraint that stood in the way of health care reform in the 1990s was fiscal. Comparative experience suggests that a publicly financed system with clear lines of fiscal responsibility is most able to control medical costs. But adopting such a system in America would require moving a large portion of private medical spending onto the public ledger. This was not considered an option in the United States as it had been in Britain and Canada. Not only was American medicine vastly more complex and vastly more expensive as a share of the economy than British and Canadian medicine had been when national programs were introduced, but it would also have to be underwritten in a much harsher fiscal climate. In response, the Clinton administration sought to do the opposite of what Britain and Canada had done: keep as much of the cost of medical care as possible in the private sector. To do this and still restrain spending, however, the administration had to propose an elaborate regulatory apparatus centered around a network of new government purchasing agents called "Health Alliances." This regulatory framework became the central focus of the viciously effective attacks on the president's program.

Third, and most important, the Clinton administration had to navigate around the fragmented collection of private interests activated by current arrangements. These interests not only included countless interest groups that campaigned against the plan but also, and more important, various segments of the American public that differentially benefit from the present structure of medical finance. The thorny challenge Clinton confronted was to move all Americans into a new regulatory framework without appreciably harming the standing of any—a challenge analogous in many ways to the one opponents of the welfare state face when trying to move citizens out of public programs.[37]

This already daunting task was further complicated by three historically inherited constraints. First, most Americans were not aware of the full cost that they paid for health insurance through indirect subsidies, hidden taxes, and (above all) forgone cash wages. Reformers thus had to consider not merely whether Americans would really pay more for less, but whether the new burdens they would bear would be more visible than the hidden costs they already shouldered. Second, the chief beneficiaries of Clinton's proposal—uninsured Americans—were diffuse and unorganized, while the chief opponents were concentrated and well organized.[38] Finally, budgetary constraints ensured that Clinton would not be able to provide generous "side payments" to affected interests to ease them into the new system.

Finally, no other nation enacted national health insurance under the stark conditions Clinton confronted. If leaders in other countries had been faced with a medical system as costly and complex as that of the United States, if they had been forced to seamlessly move two-thirds of the public from private and public insurance plans into a common public framework, and if they had faced the challenges that all welfare states faced after the mid-1970s, then perhaps the United States would not be the only advanced industrial democracy without national health insurance. Of course, American political institutions were crucial in pushing US health policy down the ill-fated track it took. But the failure of reform in the early 1990s was as much a reflection of the inherited legacies of distant political struggles as it was of the distinctive organization of American political power.

WHITHER AMERICA'S VEXED PUBLIC–PRIVATE SYSTEM?

In the wake of the failure of the Clinton plan, incremental reforms have become the order of the day. In 1996, for example, Congress and the president agreed on a package of modest insurance reforms designed to encourage portability of group health coverage across jobs, and in 1997, a new federal

Children's Health Insurance Program (CHIP) was created to fund state programs to expand coverage among America's over 10 million uninsured children. Meanwhile, Democrats and Republicans continue to spar over whether existing state-based efforts for lower-income Americans should be expanded, and over whether new federal tax credits for the uninsured should be created.

None of these policies and proposals suggests a departure from the primary reliance on private health benefits. Instead, all represent regulatory interventions and largely indirect government supports designed to deal with the most glaring deficiencies of private insurance or to extend protection to Americans who are not expected to be included in employment-based coverage. Indeed, the bipartisan support that these policies have garnered suggests that after the Clinton reform debacle, neither side is eager to re-fight past battles over the basic division of public and private responsibilities.

It is tempting to see the failure of the Clinton plan as simply another victory for the groups that helped build up America's predominantly private system—for the medical profession, employers, and the insurance industry, and perhaps even for unionized workers who negotiated lavish benefits in the postwar years. Yet the paradox is that many of these groups are genuinely dissatisfied with current arrangements. Doctors bridle at the restrictions imposed by large health plans. Most insurers are facing tough economic times. Employers see health care costs as a continuing economic threat and an often onerous administrative burden. The Clinton reform effort failed not because it encountered unified opposition—and certainly not because of the sniping of the once-feared AMA—but because the health insurance framework that arose in the United States created nearly insuperable policy dilemmas while dividing Americans into ever smaller pools of common interest and shared risk. Only this can explain why a system so troubled and friendless has so consistently resisted major reform.

Amid the struggles over health policy of the 20th century, policy choices were made (or not made) that created dangerous traps for future reformers: a well subsidized private insurance system based on employment, a technologically intensive medical structure so costly as to stymie coverage expansions, and a framework of categorical programs that filled gaps but undermined the case for general protection. These were not accidental developments, and yet neither were they entirely chosen. They emerged from the sometimes unexpected and often subterranean interaction of public policy with the private benefit activities of employers and unions—and from the concerted attempt by the defenders of private insurance to restrict the scope of shared risk to minimize redistribution and retain autonomy over private social benefits.

But however unplanned elements of this system were, they are a pervasive feature of today's political and social policy landscape. Americans have come to depend on the private insurance system; powerful vested interest have arisen within and around it. Major legislative changes to that system—even changes that will make Americans as a whole better off—run headlong into the specific dislocations these reforms will create. The mobilization of those who stand to lose from reform only compounds the problem. As with well entrenched public programs, changing established private benefits is a political fool's errand, and all the more so in America's fragmented political context.

But there is a second and deeper reason for the embedded resistance to reform of American medical financing—one rooted in the distinctive role that employment-based health insurance has come to play. In ceding power and purpose to the employment-based system, policy makers made themselves hostage to the abilities and disabilities of the private sector. Leaders found not only that the costs of change were great, but also that the system itself created thorny problems that they could not satisfactorily resolve. Helping groups left out of the system also reduced the pressure for more systemic reform. Trying to increase coverage through increased regulation undercut the incentive for firms to provide health insurance in the first place. Providing insurance through public programs risked crowding out existing private protections.

Thus, the division of public and private responsibilities conditioned political choices and weakened policy control, placing US health policy in the hands of private actors over which public officials could exercise only limited and blunt authority. Public ends became the responsibility of private institutions, and because they did, public officials became wary of threatening arrangements that they might otherwise have challenged.

We return full circle, then, to the present moment. In the Medicare fight of 2003 that launched us on our historical journey, critics of America's cherished health program for the aged found themselves in the strange position of expanding Medicare in order to reform it—of accepting the central role of Medicare in the provision of health care for the aged, even as they tried to shift the balance *within* Medicare in favor of private health plans. Switch the names and party labels and the challenge faced by conservatives with regard to Medicare is strikingly similar to the challenge faced by liberals with regard to the embedded reliance of working-age Americans on private health benefits. If present proposals are any indication, neither the left nor the right has the power to challenge the basic division of public and private responsibilities that nearly a century of evolution and entrenchment has created. Yet the outcome of the Medicare battle also indicates that the contemporary playing field of American social welfare politics is fundamentally tilted in favor of private-sector solutions—notwithstanding the overwhelming evidence that the private sector cannot provide health security to all Americans at a reasonable cost, at least not without massive government supports that the private sector itself vehemently resists.

And this may well be the ultimate irony of a story already rich in contradiction: In the years after World War II, the rise of private health insurance made government action seem unnecessary. Now, when it is recognized by many as necessary and indeed essential, government is stalemated by the very private protections in which so much faith was once invested.

STUDY QUESTIONS

1. How does US spending on social benefits compare with other nations once private benefits and lower tax rates are taken into account?
2. Why are citizens in lower income brackets relatively disadvantaged by the unique structure of American benefits and transfers?
3. Why are private forms of social protection difficult to dislodge once enacted?
4. What are some of the challenges facing those lacking health insurance?
5. Why did the workplace, or 'employment group' become the primary unit around which health insurance policies were based?
6. Why did the exclusion of health insurance provision from the Social Security Act prove pivotal?
7. What difference did employment based insurance make during the Clinton health care reform effort?
8. What political problems does the current system pose for policy makers in the future?

NOTES

1. Hulse, 2004.
2. Norwood, 2003.
3. Hacker, forthcoming.
4. All figures in this section are from Hacker, 2002.
5. Kaiser, 2003; Jacoby et al., 2001.
6. Anderson, 1990, p 69.
7. On the fate of other social policy proposals, see Hacker and Pierson, 2002.
8. The following discussion draws on Avnet, 1944.
9. Dobbin, 1992, p 1430.
10. Hedinger, 1966, p 52.
11. Report, 1985, p 61.
12. Falk, 1876, p 41.
13. US, 1993.

14. Congressional, 1994, p 5.
15. President's, 1996, p 451, fn. 19.
16. Joint, 1954, pp 8–9.
17. Erskine, 1975, p 135.
18. The ad is reprinted in Campion, 1984, p 150.
19. Ibid., p 162.
20. Quoted in Brown, 1997–98, p 653.
21. Starr, 1982, pp 312–13.
22. See Derickson, 1994; Gottschalk, 2000.
23. Becker, 1949.
24. Gordon, 1997, p 302.
25. Memorandum, Box 4.
26. Ibid., p 19.
27. Ibid., p 22; Testimony, 1949, p 421.
28. Cohen, 1951, pp 1–2, Health, 1951–54, 1960–62; Revolving.
29. Hess, 1976, p 73.
30. Marmor and Marmor, 2000, p 59.
31. Quoted in Morone, p 263.
32. With the exception of Hawaii, which obtained a federal waiver from ERISA only because it had instituted a mandated benefits plan before the law took effect.
33. For that, see Skocpol, 1996; Broder and Johnson, 1996.
34. Hacker, 1999, pp 14–15, 58–60, 86–99, 162–70.
35. Peterson, 1997, p 297.
36. By the late 1990s, most state Medicaid programs had moved their beneficiaries into private health plans, and the proportion of Medicare beneficiaries enrolled in HMOs had reached nearly a fifth, with conservatives calling for even more aggressive contracting out.
37. Pierson, 1994.
38. On the difficulties of and preconditions for "entrepreneurial politics" of this sort, see Wilson, 1973, pp 15–16.

REFERENCES

Anderson, O.W. 1990. *Health Services as a Growth Enterprise in the United States Since 1875.* Ann Arbor: Health Administration Press, p 69.

Avnet, H.H. 1944. *Voluntary Medical Insurance in the United States: Major Trends and Current Problems.* New York: Medical Administration Service, Inc.

Becker, H. 1949. "A New Proposal for National Health Insurance," 14 February, 6, Murray Latimer Papers, Box 27, George Washington University, Washington DC.

Broder, D.S. and H. Johnson. 1996. *The System: The American Way of Politics at the Breaking Point.* New York: Little Brown.

Brown, M.K. 1997–98. "Bargaining for Social Rights: Unions and the Emergence of Welfare Capitalism, 1945–52," *Political Science Quarterly* 112 (4): 653.

Campion, F.D. 1984. *The AMA and U.S. Health Policy since 1940.* Chicago: Chicago Review Press, p 150.

Cohen, W. 1951. *Memorandum.* "Major Arguments in Favor of Providing Hospitalization Benefits for Old-Age and Survivors Insurance Beneficiaries," 16 August.

Congressional Budget Office (CBO). 1994. *The Tax Treatment of Employment-Based Health Insurance.* Washington DC: CBO, p 5.

Derickson, A. 1994. "Health Security for All? Social Unionism and Universal Health Insurance, 1935–1958," *The Journal of American History* 80 (4): *1333–1356.*

Dobbin, F.R. 1992. "The Origins of Private Social Insurance: Public Policy and Fringe Benefits in America, 1920–1950," *American Journal of Sociology* 97 (5): 1430.

Erskine, H. 1975. "The Polls: Health Insurance," *Public Opinion Quarterly* 39 (1): 135.

Falk, I.S. 1976. Interview, *Social Security Administration Project,* pt. 3, no. 156, tape recorded in 1965. New York: Columbia University Oral History Collection, p 41.

Gordon, C. 1997. "Why No National Health Insurance in the U.S.? The Limits of Social Provision in War and Peace, 1941–1948," *Journal of Policy History* 9 (3): 302.

Gottschalk, M. 2000. *The Shadow Welfare State: Labor, Business, and the Politics of Health Care in the United States.* Ithaca, NY: Cornell University Press.

Hacker, J.S. 2004. "Privatizing Risk without Privatizing the Welfare State: The Hidden Politics of Social Policy Retrenchment in the United States," *American Political Science Review* 98: 243-260.

Hacker, J.S. 1999. *The Road to Nowhere*. Princeton: Princeton University Press, pp 14–15, 58–60, 86–99, 162–70.

—— 2002. *The Divided Welfare State: The Battle over Public and Private Social Benefits in the United States*. New York: Cambridge University Press.

Hacker, J.S., and P. Pierson. 2002. "Business Power and Social Policy: Employers and the Formation of the American Welfare State," *Politics and Society* 30 (2): 277–325.

Hedinger, F.R. 1966. *The Social Role of Blue Cross as a Device for Financing the Costs of Hospital Care: An Evaluation*. Iowa City: Graduate Program in Hospital and Health Administration, University of Iowa, p 52.

Hess, A. 1976. Interview, *Social Security Administration Project*, pt. 3, no. 160, tape recorded 22 March 1966. New York: Columbia University Oral History Collection, p 73.

Hulse, C. 2004. "Inquiry Sought in House Vote on Drug Plan for Medicare," *New York Times*, 2 February.

Joint Committee on Internal Revenue Taxation and the Department of the Treasury. 1954. *Internal Revenue Code of 1954: Comparison of the Principal Changes Made in the 1939 Code by H.R. 8300 after Action by House, Senate, and Conference*, 83rd Cong., 13 August, 8–9.

Kaiser Family Foundation. 2003. *The Uninsured: A Primer*. Washington DC: KFF.

Jacoby, T.A.S., and E. Warren. 2001. "Rethinking the Debates over Health Care Financing: Evidence from the Bankruptcy Courts," *New York University Law Review* 76: 375–418.

Marmor, J.S., and T.R. Marmor. 2000. *The Politics of Medicare*, 2nd ed. London: Routledge & K. Paul, p 59.

"Memorandum of the Congress of Industrial Organizations in Support of the Principle that Employer Payments for the Cost of Group Hospitalization Medical and Like Benefits are not Taxable Income to the Employee," Office of Tax Policy, Box 4, National Archives and Records Administration, p 1.

Morone, J.A. 1990. *The Democratic Wish: Popular Participation and the Limits of American Government*. New York: Basic Books, p 263.

Norwood, C. 2003. "Norwood Skeptical About Medicare Bill," Washington DC: Office of Charlie Norwood, U.S. House of Representatives.

Peterson, M.A. 1997. "Introduction: Health Care into the Next Century," *Journal of Health Politics, Policy, and Law* 22: 297.

Pierson, P. 1994. *Dismantling the Welfare State? Reagan, Thatcher, and the Politics of Retrenchment*. New York: Cambridge University Press.

President's Budget Message of 1954. 1996. Quoted in J.A. Soled, "Taxation of Employer-Provided Health Coverage: Inclusion, Timing, and Policy Issues," *University of Virginia School of Law* 15: 451, fn. 19.

Report to the President of the Committee of Economic Security. 1935. Washington DC: US GPO, p 41, reprinted in A. Pifer and F. Chisman, eds. 1985. *The Report of the Committee on Economic Security and Other Basic Documents Relating to the Development of the Social Security Act: 50th Anniversary Edition*. Washington DC: National Conference on Social Welfare, p 61.

Revolving Files, Social Security Administration Historical Archives, Baltimore, MD.

Skocpol, T. 1996. *Boomerang: Clinton's Health Security Effort and the Turn Against Government in U.S. Politics*. New York: Norton.

Starr, P. 1982. *The Social Transformation of American Medicine*. New York: Basic Books, pp 312–13.

Testimony of James B. Carey to Subcommittee on Health of the Committee on Labor and Public Welfare. 1949. *National Health Program*, p 421.

US Institute of Medicine. 1993. Committee on Employer-Based Health Benefits., *Employment and Health Benefits: A Connection at Risk*, ed. H.T. Shapiro. Washington DC: National Academy Press.

Wilson, J.Q. 1973. *Political Organization*. New York: Basic Books, pp 15–16.

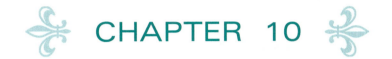

CHAPTER 10

American Health Care:
How It Became Inefficient, Inequitable, and Costly

Donald W. Light

This chapter traces the history of the American medical profession and explains how its past choices led directly to its current challenges. Light shows how physicians used both politics and science to beat their competitors at the start of the last century; however, the powerful and autonomous system that the doctors built produced the troubled system that we find today.

We have fallen into the habit of calling our medical services the "health care system," when in most cases there is no system at all and health care gets little attention. Why is this so-called system in such organizational, financial, and clinical disarray? Even the orthodox, elite Institute of Medicine has issued a stream of reports showing that American services are deeply unjust and discriminate against the vulnerable and disadvantaged.[1] The fragmented structure wastes far more than any comparable system in administration, marketing, and other non-clinical costs. Hospital care causes plane-loads of avoidable, treatment-induced deaths, injuries, and illnesses. Primary care ranks lowest among other advanced systems, and public health is weak.

Patients get patchy care, even if we put aside the one-sixth of the nation that has no insurance and the one-fifth with limited health insurance (but why should we?). While politicians gloat that we have "the best health care system in the world," a systematic review found that clinicians provide the services their own professional bodies recommend only 54.9% of the time.[2] Consistency of quality ranged from 78.7% for cataracts to 10.5% for alcohol dependence.

We keep rediscovering this harsh reality. In 1999, the Institute of Medicine found a large number of preventable deaths, injuries, and illnesses that patients in American hospitals suffer each month, a pattern that has existed at least since the 1960s.[3]

Why does "the best health care system in the world" rank below health care in every other affluent country and below several developing nations as well?[4] This chapter explains how American health care became so inefficient, inequitable, and costly. It is painful to read. Perhaps that is why so few know about it, why our leaders keep perpetuating the same mistakes, and why the result is an increasingly powerful corporate structure that makes money from fragmentation, inefficiencies, and risk selection.

This chapter provides a historical and sociological framework for understanding how mainstream American health care acquired its contemporary problems. Elementary forms of managed care and price competition arose about a century ago, were suppressed by the medical profession as they gained dominance, and then rose again as the excesses of professional dominance led major buyers to control costs and coordinate care over the objections of outraged physicians. It is a history of *countervailing powers,* of stakeholders with contrasting values and visions who vie with each other, or form alliances among each other, in order to win the kind of finances and services they desire.[5]

EARLY MARKETS AND COMPETITION

In 1912, the noted surgeon and critic, James Warbasse (1912: p 274), wrote:

> The matter with the medical profession is that the doctor is a private tradesman engaged in a competitive business for profit . . . It is difficult, nay, impossible for him to do otherwise. He is surrounded by the competitive system, and unless he conforms to the methods of warfare about him, he must go down . . .

Warbasse saw that normal price competition turned doctors from professionals into tradesmen who have to offer bargain medicine. Or they competed by promoting their special skills or new cures for a high fee. Market competition was undermining good science. Warbasse observed,

> The science of medicine has made wonderful progress in the past fifty years . . . The whole history of medicine . . . is a glorious refutation of the sophistry that competition for profit is important to human progress. The competitive system, which surrounds and harnesses medical advancement, hindered it from the beginning and retards it still . . .

Warbasse, who had published the first book entitled, *Medical Sociology* (1909), provides an apt starting point for this history of markets and health care. Most of the literature on how markets form overlooks the predatory ways in which major stakeholders get legislators and governmental agencies to make large sums of taxpayers' money available to them and to disadvantage or even eliminate rivals.

The most formative period of the modern American health care system occurred between about 1880 and 1920. In the last quarter of the 19th century, mainstream physicians faced several competitive forces which threatened their status and kept their income low.

1. Price competition among the surplus of doctors, due to scores of loosely assembled "medical schools" by physicians trying to make extra money by collecting lecture fees;

2. Competition for fees from a raft of alternative healers, often popular for their more naturalistic, gentle forms of therapy, and aided by weak licensure laws;

3. Free care at dispensaries as part of the revolutionary success of public health based on germ theory and the new science of medicine;

4. The rapid proliferation of wholesale contracts and services that threatened the autonomy and income of physicians; and

5. A proliferation of nostrums, cure-alls, and other medicines widely advertised in newspapers and magazines that substituted for seeing the doctor and competed with doctors' own concoctions made up in their offices.[6]

A Surplus of Competing Providers

The census of 1870 found 64,414 medical practitioners; by 1900 there were more than 132,000, and this did not include a large number of "irregular" practitioners using alternative methods that were popular in many areas.[7] By the 1890s, a serious surplus was widely discussed, though this might have had more to do with sharp recessions in the general economy than with the growth in medical practioners. The period also witnessed a rapid proliferation of "medical schools," so that by 1900 there were 126 "regular" schools and perhaps 40 homeopathic, osteopathic, and eclectic schools. Altogether, these schools graduated up to 5,700 new physicians a year.[8]

Initially, regular or orthodox physicians had no clear technical or therapeutic advantage, and their therapies were as likely to do harm as to do good. However, advances in scientific medicine came rapidly so that by World War I, "scientific medicine" had distinct advantages which were largely enjoyed by the medical elite who had attended the leading schools of scientific medicine in Europe. Thus, while the number of herbalists, bone setters, and healers proliferated, normal market dynamics were rewarding those with new, effective skills.

Public Health and Dispensaries

Originally created in the 18th century as a humanitarian gesture toward the sick poor, dispensaries took on a new meaning and posed a competitive threat to the rank and file profession at the end of the 19th century. That fact has profound implications for today. As scientific medicine rapidly advanced, dispensaries proliferated as the place where new specialty techniques were first tried out on "clinical material." Since the leading specialists worked and trained at dispensaries, the affluent came in disguise: "There was also the millionaire in poor clothes, the lawyer, the broker . . . fully fifty percent of 'charity' patients are persons whose financial position puts them wholly beyond the scope of charity."[9]

Dispensaries proliferated in response to the millions of new immigrants. In New York City, for example, the number of dispensaries increased from 100 in 1900 to 574 in 1910 and exceeded 700 by 1915.[10] They were considered superior to ordinary doctors because they offered a skilled team of specialists at the leading edges of scientific medicine, and the famous Boston Dispensary (affiliated with Harvard Medical School) integrated social work and a home health care plan as well as a service for detecting occupational health problems.

The leaders of major public health departments, where the greatest gains in reducing morbidity and mortality were taking place, applied scientific advances to improve the health of whole cities. They found it natural to extend their successes to the clinical diagnosis and treatment of individual patients. Nothing could have more threatened the leaders of autonomous private practice at county medical societies.

A Proliferation of Cure-Alls

As if the provider surplus and the proliferation of dispensaries were not enough, everyone had a cure for everything. Physicians made up their own cures and advertised them on their calling cards. Pharmacists made new compounds and stole the compounds of others whose prescriptions they filled. Companies sprang up with thousands of medicines. Most threatening of all was Lydia Pinkham's compound, because she in effect said, "Why go see a doctor? Write me and I will personally advise you about your health problem." Her compound cured all female ills, she claimed, and she further guaranteed that no man's eyes would see the letters of her clients.[11] Lydia Pinkham became one of the most successful businesswomen in the industry—and a serious threat to local doctors. Every letter was one less visit and one less fee for a local doctor. Patent medicines were sold at grocery, dry-goods, and hardware stores. Sales nearly doubled in five years, from $74.5 million in 1904 to $141.9 million in 1909. As one article in the *Journal of the American Medical Association* put it, ". . . as the proprietary manufacturer becomes richer, the physician becomes poorer."[12]

The manufacturers produced a plethora of prepackaged, ready-made drugs to make medical practice easy. G. Frank Lydston (1900), a prominent critic and professor at the University of Illinois School of Medicine, called such manufacturers "fakirs" and wrote a scathing commentary on the effects:

> How gently flows the current of Doctor Readymade's professional life. No more incurable cases. No more midnight oil. No more worry . . . All the doctor has to do now-a-days is to read the labels on the bottles and boxes of samples the fakir brings him. Does the patient complain of stomach disturbance? He is given "Stomachine" . . . Give him one of these pretty little tablets with a hieroglyph on it, which nobody knows the composition of . . . . (p. 1403)

Contract Medicine

Besides the relevance of Dr. Readymade to the billions spent today on commercializing prescription decisions, the other most relevant form of competition that presaged our current era was wholesale contracts to provide services to groups of employees or people belonging to an association, or union, or working for a company or a branch of government.[13] The corporate practice of medicine began during the 19th century in the railroad, mining, and lumber industries, where remote locations, high accident rates, and the

growth of lawsuits by injured workers called for companies to organize medical services.[14] They contracted for services on a retainer basis or on salary; some even owned hospitals and dispensaries for their workers. Some textile industries also established comprehensive medical services in mill towns. Thousands of doctors were involved in these contracts or worked on salary.

By the end of the 19th century, however, more and more businesses with none of these special needs also began to contract on a competitive basis for the health care of their employees. For example, the Michigan State Medical Society reported in 1907 that many companies of various sizes were contracting for the health care of their employees.[15] The Plate Glass Factory contracted with physicians and hospitals for all medical and surgical care needed by its employees and their families for $1.00 a month apiece. The Michigan Alkali Company did the same but did not include family members. Several other companies had contracts for the treatment of accidents and injuries. Commercial insurance companies of the day also got involved, putting together packages of services for a flat amount per person per year (capitation) or for a discounted fee schedule. Their profits must have been enormous and the doctors' pay low, since several reports allude to the "usual" 10% of premiums that physicians received.

More widespread than early corporate health care plans were comprehensive health care medical services offered for a flat subscription price per year to members of the fraternal orders that had proliferated rapidly during the same period. The national and regional orders of the Eagles, the Foresters, the Moose, the Orioles, as well as other fraternal associations, offered medical care at deeply discounted prices through their local lodges.[16] Various reports from Louisiana, Rhode Island, California, and New York attest to the prevalence of such plans and of "contract practice," as competitive health care was then called. A 1909 report on Rhode Island stated, "The English, Irish, Scotch, Germans, French-Canadians, and Jews have clubs employing the contract doctor. The Manchester Unity, Foresters, Sons of St. George, Eagles, Owls and others are in this number."[17]

The government also became heavily involved in organized buying at the turn of the 20th century. Most of the more comprehensive reports on contract practice describe municipal, county, and state agencies putting out for bid service contracts for the poor, for prisoners, and for government employees. At the federal level, the armed services and Coast Guard had long contracted for medical services at wholesale prices.[18] The rates for the physician varied from $1.00 to $2.50 per member per annum. A committee of physicians in 1916 reported, "[T]he growth of contract practice has been so amazingly great during the last twenty-five years as almost to preclude belief . . . Practically all of the large cities are fairly *honeycombed* with lodges, steadily increasing in number, with a constantly growing membership."[19]

Hospitals also designed prepaid insurance plans, a little-known fact that reframes the commonly held view that this did not happen before the origins of Blue Cross at Baylor Hospital.[20] "Hospital service associations" were formed and organized prepaid contract services. For example, the Hospital Service Association of Rockford, Illinois offered in 1912 hospitalization up to six weeks a year and surgery, with defined benefit ceilings, for an entrance fee of $10, an annual fee of $1, and a weekly contribution of 10 cents. A report from Chicago stated that by 1910, over 25% of hospitals in Chicago had some form of contract practice.[21]

Contract practice was considered the most dangerous threat to medicine as a profession. A typically scathing report claimed that "A certain institution which advertises as a hospital engages in wholesale contracts for an infinitesimal amount to care for its policy-holders . . . for any illness of any nature whatsoever. This institution has a dispensary where colored solutions under alphabetical labels are dispensed by an undergraduate."[22] Through contract practice, critics claimed, employers obtained the records of each worker's physical and mental condition and used it if there was litigation: "This clearly invalidates the pre-established idea that the first duty of the physician is toward his patient."[23] Despite these criticisms, there seemed to be considerable evidence that a wholesale market of volume discount plans and capitated medical services with selected willing providers were being established on several fronts and growing, long before Sidney Garfield and Henry Kaiser put together the first Kaiser plan.

A Profession in Crisis?

These five sources of competition contributed to the historically low income of physicians—about $1,200 a year, the same as skilled craft workers.[24] State medical societies reported that fierce competition had fostered backbiting, fee splitting, and open criticism between members. From their point of view, no one was in control and matters were deteriorating rapidly. However, it was a favorable situation for consumers and institutional buyers, who felt they were exercising the control they wanted in order to secure adequate services at reasonable prices.

No one had good market information about quality, so patients and payers did not know what they were getting for their money. (Fortunately, we no longer have this problem.) In a rough and ready way, however, based on hearsay and testimonials, competition was steadily favoring the new scientific medicine, and winnowing out ineffective therapies, poorly trained doctors, and inferior medical schools.

The average income of poorly trained physicians was being driven down while specialists were earning three to ten times as much, even with only the skeleton of modern licensing and with no specialty boards.[25] Their growing stature complemented the efforts by hospitals to attract middle- and upper-class patients. The proprietary medical schools, established by physicians who used lecture fees to supplement their income from private practice, were beginning to face competition from the serious, university-based schools, whose graduates were earning the respect of the marketplace.[26] Thus, quality and value were being recognized by "the market" on several fronts. Nevertheless, the organized profession campaigned hard for regulations, arguing that the public must be protected from inferior medicine.

SUPPRESSING COMPETITION

The ability of organized medicine to address the sources of "ruinous competition" both within its ranks and from outside remained weak until, in 1901, new leadership revised the American Medical Association's constitution so that medical societies became a pyramid of coherent power. The new AMA was a confederation of state medical societies, which in turn became a confederation of county societies, with delegates elected at each level to make up the committees and House of Delegates at the next level. A physician could not be a member in good standing at the national or state levels without being in good standing at the county level. Membership became the basis for hospital privileges, group malpractice insurance, and other benefits.[27] This ingenious design transformed the AMA into a pyramid of power and control. Medical societies reorganized and membership shot up from 8,000 in 1900 to 70,000 in 1910. The whole structure formed a hierarchy of networks, coordinated by small groups of influential physicians at the center of each. These networks were used to mount campaigns against competition, contract medicine, and universal health insurance.[28] A key tool was the *Journal of the American Medical Association*, whose circulation rose with membership as it became the authoritative voice of AMA leadership against "unscientific sects."

The legendary Joseph McCormick led this transformation of the AMA from a weak association to the uniting center of "organized medicine." This charismatic president traveled tirelessly across the country to attack the bitter fruits of competition and oversupply: rivalry, advertising, contract medicine, price competition, unethical behavior, and a surplus of badly trained doctors. He held out a uniting alternative: higher standards, good schools, fewer doctors, and fees set at reasonable levels.[29]

Eliminating Sects and Reducing Supply

One campaign aimed to eliminate competing sects and reduce the supply of physicians by gaining control of licensure and setting high standards based on the new scientific medicine. In the early 1900s, medical societies launched a campaign to gain influence over state licensing boards. The boards, in turn, supervised state licensing examinations; the societies' leaders constantly raised the scientific standards of the exams thus forcing other sects to convert to mainstream scientific medicine or fail the licensing exams. This reflected a strategy formulated by N.S. Davis, a founder of the AMA and its first president. The way to control the profession but avoid charges of monopoly, Davis wrote, was to make graduating from a certified medical school a prerequisite for licensure and to establish state licensing boards outside the profession, but with members chosen by the profession.[30]

Populism and a suspicion of privilege had undermined licensure in the 1830s, but it returned in the 1870s as part of a cultural celebration of science and professionalism in every endeavor: undertakers, librarians, social workers, pharmacists, dentists, accountants, social scientists, and others.[31] By 1877, the first Davis-style medical practice act was passed. "Irregular" practitioners objected that open competition based on patient choice was being replaced by one sect using state power to create a professional monopoly. They took the new laws to court, but the laws were upheld. By 1898, every state had an act and licensing board.[32]

A related AMA tactic broadened the legal definition of medicine so that all sects would be subject to the medical practice laws; they then defined "unprofessional behavior" by the new, scientific standards. By 1904, the AMA's Committee on National Legislation had lobbying organizations in every state except Nevada and Virginia, staffed by 1,940 members. In many states this political machine succeeded in obtaining single boards or increasing power over composite boards.[33]

Frank Billings, president of the American Medical Association in 1903, displayed a demographic understanding and nicely summarized the profession's campaign. There was one physician to every 600 population, and there was a net surplus of 2,000 new graduates a year "thrown on the profession, overcrowding it, and steadily reducing the opportunities of those already in the profession to acquire a livelihood."[34] Billings recommended that about three-fourths of the 156 medical schools be closed and the rest upgraded. He also sketched out the concept of special, regional hospitals, devoted to research and teaching. At the same time that Billings advocated the elimination of "unfit and irregular" doctors by training small cohorts in scientific medicine, he conceded that diagnosis amounted to little more than naming the disease and that "in the vast majority of the infectious diseases we are helpless to apply a specific cure." This is important, because today we commonly assume that mainstream medicine's therapeutic superiority justified its strong actions in the early years to eliminate competing sects and monopolize services.

In the same spirit, the profession captured or professionalized other markets. It attacked midwives, who attended one-half of all births in 1910, as the cause of high infant mortality and sought legislation outlawing them. This campaign largely succeeded, even though midwives surpassed physicians in all measures of safe birth across the country, such as puerperal fever and infant and maternal morbidity and mortality.[35] In Washington DC, infant mortality rose as the percent of physicians delivering increased. Moreover, few medical schools had a strong curriculum in obstetrics with which to prepare physicians for the responsibilities they had insisted on assuming.[36]

This massive lobbying effort to squeeze out competing sects by mobilizing the power of the state was joined by the second prong of the campaign, to drive inferior medical schools out of business and reduce the supply of physicians. As Abraham Flexner noted, "The state boards are the instruments through which reconstruction of medical education will be largely effected."[37]

The *Journal of the American Medical Association* (*JAMA*) began collecting and publishing data on the quality of every medical school in 1901, and in 1904 the AMA created the Council of Medical Education. Composed of a distinguished group of academic physicians trained at the leading centers of medicine in Europe, the Council quickly became the voice of the profession on educational matters, and that voice advocated high admission standards, long and expensive training, training in laboratories and hospitals, and tough examinations for licensure. Working closely with *JAMA*, the Council started to publish the failure rates by school of graduates taking licensing examinations. The Council established committees on medical education in the states and territories to carry out its work, and it held national conferences on medical education where it propagated its ideas about model curricula based on the new medical sciences. These efforts constituted market information on quality, and enrollments at proprietary schools with low pass rates declined. What went beyond marketing was the incorporation of the Council's model into the requirements for state board licensing examinations.

The elite members of the Council on Medical Education developed a detailed framework for quality education and began to visit every medical school in the land. It recruited state medical societies and governments along the way, and in 1907 it launched its first attack on medical schools that could not meet its high standards: a four-year curriculum of 3,600 hours. The Council launched a second inspection by Abraham Flexner at the Carnegie Foundation that led to his famously scathing report of 1910. He charged most commercial medical schools to be little more than money machines for their faculty, and he recommended that all but 31 medical schools be shut down. The Flexner report is widely regarded as single-handedly ushering in scientific medical education. In fact, however, the report was part of a systematic campaign started some years earlier by the new elite at the AMA to reduce physician supply and raise quality. The campaign championed both scientific standards and professional self interest.

The Flexner report played another important role—that of recruiting the great fortunes of Andrew Carnegie and John D. Rockefeller to the AMA's cause.[38] Between 1911 and 1938, they together gave the staggering amount of $154 million to a small circle of medical schools that agreed to install the new, costly curriculum. To this amount was added $600 million in other grants and matching funds from the fortunes of other industrialists. Historical research shows that Flexner and the foundation staff systematically disguised the degree to which they insisted that medical schools receiving their millions adhere to their model of medical education. By these means, a very small group of socially and professionally elite physicians were able to recast the entire profession in their image.[39]

This two-pronged campaign of building the new curriculum and standards into state licensure exams and giving large sums only to schools that would implement it worked. The number of graduates plummeted, from 5,440 in 1910 to 2,529 in 1922. Medical schools, which were already closing from competitive pressures before 1910, could not keep up with the rising expense of teaching the new curriculum that was increasingly reflected in state licensing exams. By 1924 there were only 80 schools left. Six of the eight "Negro" medical schools were forced to close, and quotas on ethnic groups could be found in many places.[40] Women's medical schools were closed, on the false expectation that women would be admitted to the new medical mainstream. This might be regarded as a by-product of scientific medicine, but that would ignore how few effective scientific techniques the orthodox practitioners had and how central to the campaign was the leaders' goals of reducing supply and raising incomes. Between 1900 and 1928, physicians' incomes more than doubled, even after accounting for inflation.[41]

What the Council had done with the help of Flexner and the two great foundations was to redefine professional education so that all the small, marginal, and for-profit medical schools had to close. Medical schools could only survive if they toed the line and thus received philanthropy from foundations dedicated to implementing the Council's new vision of professionalism. This might be regarded as monopoly capitalism shaping modern medicine after its own image, but the evidence supports the obverse: Leaders of professionalism mobilized monopoly capital to their goal of creating a professional monopoly.[42] Only decades later—beginning in the 1970s—did investors exploit the protected markets that the organized profession had constructed.

Eliminating Price Competition and Free Care

A third campaign which contributed to the doubling of incomes focused on minimizing the growth of free care at dispensaries, price competition among physicians, and external price competition by sponsors of contract medicine. To battle contract medicine, county and state medical societies took a number of actions.[43] They conducted studies and reported on the allegedly terrible conditions under which contract physicians worked. Strangely enough, the few times that remarks were published by physicians doing contract work, they said they liked the guaranteed income rather than having to deal with the large number of unpaid bills, often from patients who could barely make a living. County medical societies were also forced to acknowledge that a sizable proportion of their own members actively bid for contracts and did contract work.[44]

To those leading this campaign, however, complicity was reason to redouble their efforts and save their colleagues from their own bad judgment. Some medical societies drew up lists of physicians known to practice contract medicine in order to embarrass them. Others drew up "honor rolls" of members who promised to swear off competitive contracts. Committee members would ferret out every recalcitrant colleague and make group visits to pressure him to abandon contract practice. Some societies threatened to expel or censure members who did not cooperate in stamping out price-competitive medicine. On other fronts, state and county medical societies pressured departments of public health, legislators, and their members who worked at dispensaries to have public health stop where clinical medicine begins and to turn over patients with infectious diseases of concern to public health to private practitioners.

They also transformed hospitals from charitable institutions, where the local poor could receive rest and nursing, to centers of surgery and scientific technique, wooing the paying middle-class patient. Trustees of charitable hospitals reluctantly began to woo physicians in private practice, needing their well-to-do patients, yet fearing that the doctors would demand too much control in return.[45] The pursuit of paying patients changed the character of hospitals, just as trustees had feared. Historian David Rosner writes, "By 1915, doctors at many institutions had essentially wrested control from the trustees and had gained the power to make the decisions that were in their best interests, regardless of the traditional charity goals of the hospital." In changing from wards to semiprivate or private rooms and to specialized departments, the architecture and organization of hospitals reflected the new power relations and the new social composition of patients. Commercialism, Rosner points out, was also evident in the national movement to transform "the old rich charity hospitals into a 'scientifically' managed medical enterprise."[46]

By 1912, there was enough of an organized audience for a magazine called *Hospital Management*, featuring techniques to attract well-heeled customers out of the comfort of their homes and into the "superior" accommodations of the hospital for serious medical problems. Towns, counties, states, governmental departments, religious sects, labor unions, and fraternal orders built hospitals at the turn of the century; in places where no one built hospitals, doctors converted a large home to a small "hospital." By 1928, 38.9% of the 4,367 of the nongovernmental general hospitals were proprietary—a much higher percentage than in the 1980s when for profit hospital chains proliferated. They had only 16% of the beds, however, and often lost money, so that doctors were only too happy when a growing town or voluntary association supplanted them with a larger community hospital.[47]

Although organized medicine never eliminated competitive contracts entirely, it greatly reduced their numbers and shifted them from service to cash contracts. Fraternal orders did not want to cause a row with county and state medical societies, and they shifted benefits to partial payments for wages lost and reimbursement for medical bills rather than for prepaid contracted services. Reimbursement allowed doctors to set their own fees and eliminated any intermediaries setting the terms of service.

Several court decisions supported the profession's opposition to the corporate practice of medicine. In a number of states, societies persuaded state legislators to pass laws prohibiting the corporate practice of medicine or the practice of medicine by organizations run by non-physicians. They also won by prohibiting for profit medicine. Medical societies meanwhile dusted off their old fee schedules and raised their prices to a professionally respectable level.[48] Historian James Burrow observed, "Hardly had the United States Steel Corporation succeeded in its consolidation effects that raised prices of basic steel products in 1901 from 200 to 300 percent above the most competitive level of 1898, when the medical profession began its income uplift and price maintenance program."[49]

The goal of these and other efforts to gain control over the practice of medicine has not been to eliminate competition entirely but rather to keep outsiders (i.e., consumers and buyers) from setting terms, especially prices. As Max Weber understood, guilds secure a monopoly over a domain and then let members compete freely within it. By the 1920s, the medical profession had confined contract medicine to a few industries with special needs, to group purchasing of services for the poor and the military, and to a few maverick experiments on the periphery of medicine.[50]

"No Middlemen" was a call to arms by the Propaganda Department of the AMA in the 1920s and 1930s: to attack any form of "contract medicine" where packaged services (like the early HMOs) were sold at a discount. Having patients pay doctors directly was the only way to keep the profession free of commercial agents and also free to charge what they wanted. Ironically, this principle of "no middlemen" most directly links professional services to the pocketbook. The drive for national health insurance between 1910 and 1915 posed a threat, especially since the reformers advocated paying doctors by capitation. While initially attracted to the idea of universal coverage, the rank and file of medical societies made clear they would have none of it.

Reining in the Nostrums Industry

As part of the assault on competing sects, dispensaries, public health clinics, midwives, and other forms of treatment that reduced the demand for professional medical care, the AMA mounted an intense campaign against patent medicines. Many basic professional issues spurred this action. First, doctors faced relentless competition from drug salespeople, peddling their wares directly to customers and through mass advertising. Second, this $100 million industry (in 1905) promoted self-care and home remedies instead of going to the expense and trouble of seeing a doctor. Patent pharmaceutical companies not only sold drugs which they widely advertised, but they published guides for laypeople and set up advisory services such as the popular "Write Mrs. Pinkham." Third, many doctors made up their own secret remedies and promoted them as superior to others, thus tacitly undermining their colleagues. Fourth, druggists competed with the doctors by refilling prescriptions without a return visit and by stealing doctors' remedies and offering them independently. Scientifically, none of these patent medicines or doctors' remedies were tested. Starr observed, "The nostrum makers were the nemesis of the physicians. They mimicked, distorted, derided, and undercut the authority of the profession." One article estimated that the money spent on nostrums was enough in 1905 to more than double physicians' incomes.[51] Yet the medical journals were implicated, and only a few were immune from manufacturers' demands that promotions appear disguised as articles or editorials.[52]

In 1900, the AMA published an eight-part series of unsigned articles which provided an overview of issues and policies toward relations with pharmaceutical firms. The series called for drugs to have names that reflected their composition rather than their alleged healing qualities. It discussed the problem of substitution and warned against the widespread use of "polypharmacy," the combination of more than one drug in a pill or dose. It identified the pernicious pattern of companies donating drugs to hospitals and dispensaries where medical students learn, "with the result that the average medical student's ideas and experience concerning medicines are largely confined to the proprietary articles, which his 'professors' used in their demonstrations." It described the problem of secret proprietary drugs.[53]

In concert with its other actions to promote scientifically based medicine, the newly reorganized AMA created in 1905 the Council on Pharmacy and Chemistry to professionalize drugs by providing the public and its doctors with an AMA-approved list of drugs. It required a drug manufacturer to reveal the ingredients and formula of any drug submitted for the Council's review, and it set itself up as the arbiter of advertising copy in professional journals. The overall goal was to have a list of drugs that were known only to doctors and prescribed by them. It established professional rules of acceptability which included a prohibition against advertising to the public or stating on the label the diseases for which the drug was indicated. Doctors would decide that, as they often do today for disorders for which drugs have not been tested.

The AMA wished to professionalize the large and growing market of self-administered medicines. Without advertising or indications, the profession hoped that patent medicines would disappear. At the same time, the power to prescribe the more effective, AMA-tested medicines would add to the profession's powers to certify sick leaves from work and admit patients to hospitals. The AMA also established what it called the Propaganda Department to publish books and articles warning the public against patent medicines and self-diagnosis. These articles repeatedly told the public that medicine was now a complex scientific field that required years of training, and the articles reported deaths, injuries, and disabilities which patent medicines had purportedly caused. Of great assistance was an exposé by Samuel Hopkins Adams, detailing the dangers and deceptions of patent medicine manufacturers.[54] The Propaganda Department of the AMA also put pressure on lay publications to refuse ads for prescription drugs and even for patent drugs. All these efforts met with partial success, particularly in reducing the number of doctors who developed their own remedies and in stopping druggists from competing against them.

Consolidating Professional Control

By 1920, the organized profession had largely succeeded in transforming medical care from an open marketplace where providers and therapeutic schools competed on price and claims of effectiveness to a professional monopoly that claimed to end "ruinous competition," guarantee quality, and establish true patient choice. Freedom and choice were central values. But as Charles Weller has pointed out, professional "free choice" is a restraint on trade. It is *guild* free choice rather than *market* free choice, that is to say free choice within the profession's terms of training, licensure, fees, and the structure of services. Market free choice would mean competing on price as well as different kinds of services offered by competing kinds of providers.[55]

The profession had in effect created a trust during the era of trust-busting, because professions were regarded then as benevolent forms of social control as developed by E.A. Ross (1969 [1901]). His best seller, *Social Control*, helped shape efforts by community leaders to clean up corrupt political machines, monopoly trusts, and companies that would sell contaminated meat or dangerous drugs to an unsuspecting public. However, Ross noted that social control could become class control when done by a closely knit elite. They would pass laws

and regulations that appeared to treat all parties equally, yet most benefited their own class. Leaders of the medical profession did much to clean up the medical profession in ways that brought civilizing order to modern communities, and they were exempted from antitrust law. They did so, however, in ways that resembled class control more than community-based social control, especially by creating professionally controlled monopoly markets. In short, they harnessed scientific medicine—with all its indisputable benefits—and used it to monopolize alternate forms of treatment.[56]

Later, the celebrated sociologist Talcott Parsons admired the professions as viable alternatives to business but did not see the degree to which the tactics of the organized profession echoed those of business monopolies.[57] Max Weber better understood the nature of these classic guilds, which pursue quality, prestige, and profits for their members by forming an interest group and then pursuing a legal monopoly.[58] What the profession did not anticipate was the degree to which the very success of their harnessing the nostrum manufacturers would commercialize it. Many of the practices which the AMA attacked returned, but now within the professional fold.

Two theories dominate the sociology of modern medicine. The prevailing view emphasizes *professional dominance:* for most of the 20th century medical authority was rooted in internalized professional norms (based on scientific training and expertise) rather than any outside forces such as markets or politics.[59] An alternative theory, the *proletarianization* view, posits that capitalism turned medical professionals into nothing more than well paid workers—ultimately no different from any other group in the work force.[60] Both theories identify part of the whole but do not provide a comparative, historical framework.[61] The first emphasizes the rise to dominance and the other the decline to subordination, but neither explains both. The concept of countervailing powers offers a more fruitful framework, one which invites us to consider the changing stakeholder dynamics over time and across countries.[62]

The medical profession turned expertise into market power by creating a new kind of monopoly market.[63] The key was to define and defend a unique service or commodity; to standardize it and the training of professionals who provide it; to get the backing of the government in the name of safety; and thereby to exclude all other claimants. The result is a professional caste centered on autonomy and control. Ironically, the profession is "allowed to define the very standards by which its superior competence is judged . . . professionals live within ideologies of their own creation, which they present to the outside as the most valid definitions of specific spheres of social reality."[64] This monopolistic project takes place within a specific economic and institutional context which shapes the structure of professional markets.[65] This provides a framework for understanding both the ferocious campaigns to eliminate or contain other countervailing powers and the unanticipated consequences that have led to the pathologies of the health care system today.

Health care in Germany, France, England, and other industrialized countries also experienced a rise of scientific and specialized medicine. Most American observers, however, overlook the fundamental differences when professionalism is orchestrated top-down by the state (as in France) or in coordination with the state (Germany), rather than having the profession capture the state for its own interests and health care ideals (the United States). In other countries, medicine's rise to dominance, especially hospital-based specialty medicine, was framed by societal debates; state power determined the number and distribution of specialists, what they charged, and how they fit into a national system of health care.[66] Some social scientists imagine that contemporary health care delivery emerged from a long series of historical "accidents." As this history shows there was nothing "accidental" about the development of the contemporary American system and its lack of universal health coverage.[67]

The rise of professional medicine—like the rise of the great corporations in the same period—relied on political power rather than on efficiency.[68] Markets, in this view, are constructed by the participants with the cooperation of government. Control over training and licensure gave the profession property rights over medical knowledge. Of course, in retrospect the promotion of scientific medicine seems enlightened and correct. However, when the profession first used state power to control medicine, the aggressive therapies (advanced under the cover of science) were doing as much harm as good. Evidence indicates scientific medicine was rapidly winning converts on its own merits—regardless of the AMA's march to power.

THE PROFESSIONALLY DRIVEN HEALTH CARE SYSTEM

The health care system that evolved from the campaigns of organized medicine fulfilled the professional vision of what a good system should look like, a system that strives to provide the best clinical care for every sick patient who could pay, to develop scientific medicine to its highest degree, to preserve the autonomy of the physician, and to increase the dominance of the medical profession. See Table 10-1. Power centers on the profession, and the organization of work centers on physicians' choices of specialty, location, and clinical judgment. The result is a loosely linked network of autonomous offices, clinics, hospitals, and related facilities. The image of the individual is of a private person who lives as he or she sees fit and comes in for help as she or he chooses. Financing in this ideal type centers on the fees that doctors choose to charge.

The organized profession's vision of ideal health care differs dramatically from those of most governments or from the ambitions of corporate health care, as summarized in Table 10-1. Governments and legislatures want a healthy, vigorous population that is productive and thrives, but at least cost. Strong public health and primary care achieve that goal best by addressing risks and problems upstream before they develop into serious conditions. By contrast, health care corporations want to maximize sales and profits which are highest for specialized medicine that treats

Table 10-1 Contrasting Visions and Values of a Good Health Care System

The Organized Profession	Governments or Other Large Payers	Corporate Providers, Suppliers, and Middlemen
Key Values and Goals:		
To provide the best possible clinical care to every sick patient (who can pay and who lives near a doctor's practice).	To have a healthy, vigorous workforce.	To maximize market share and profits. To maximize the size, range, and expenditures of markets.
To develop scientific medicine to its highest level.	To minimize illness and maximize self-care.	To increase demand and form new markets.
To protect the autonomy of physicians and services.	To minimize the cost of medical services.	To minimize, neutralize, or circumvent regulations by government or payers.
To increase the power and wealth of the profession.	Perhaps to provide good, accessible care to all.	
Image of the Individual:		
A private person who chooses how to live and when to use the medical system.	An employee, and somewhat the responsibility of the employer.	An object of marketing to maximize expenditures.
Power:		
Centers on the medical profession, and uses state powers to enhance its own.	Centers on key governmental officials, politicians, sometimes unions.	Centers on corporate headquarters. State and profession relatively weak.
Key Institutions:		
Professional associations. Autonomous physicians and hospitals.	Departments of health, social security, and related departments.	Health care and supplier corporations. Governments and employers as sources of revenues and managers of competition.

problems far downstream. Prevention minimizes profits, unless we are talking about drugs people take for years or HMOs that get paid a flat amount per person per year. In that case, profits are maximized by spending as little on hospital or subspecialty care. Mental or behavioral health care corporations, for example, tend to minimize psychiatric care for seriously disturbed patients.

The vision of the organized medical profession had several flaws from a societal point of view. Organized medicine destroyed medical schools for women and

"Negroes," crushed midwifery and alternative sects, used scare tactics to discredit national health insurance, and cared little about patients in low income and rural areas. Its almost exclusive focus on clinical care for sick patients who can pay also prompted the historic separation of medicine from public health, even though public health achieved more spectacular successes using the same scientific foundation and discoveries, and a disinterest in prevention and primary care as low-status work of little interest. The organizational profession's vision of good medicine also lacked a sense of responsibility for communities or community health, because doing so would require forms of financing and governance that compromised professional autonomy. Concepts of interprofessional teams were resisted as threats to professional authority.

The organized profession, however, rarely behaves as a servant of humanity or public good. For that to happen, it needs a strong societal framework, precisely what other countries provided where the state constructed the modern profession or where the state and profession worked in harness as equally strong partners.[69] One cannot expect a profession to be much different from the economic, organizational, and political framework of the society in which it operates.[70] If that society sanctions a for-profit, financial system that does not reward disease prevention or care of poorer patients, and rewards hi-tech corporate specialty services, then doctors will concentrate on hi-tech specialty services.[71]

This fundamental point is illustrated by contrasting the professional ideal health care system with the societal ideal of a universal health care system and a stronger state. The societal system seeks to promote a healthy, vigorous population and to minimize illness. Medical services are therefore universal, equitably distributed, and focused on primary care and prevention. The number and distribution of specialists, hospitals, and costly technology, as well as costs, are subject to institutional rules and regulations within which the profession works. For-profit services have been rare, and for-profit suppliers are held in check. The result is comprehensive, universal health care for about half to two-thirds of the cost.

Creating Provider-friendly Insurance

Despite pressure from doctors with thousands of unpaid bills, the AMA adamantly opposed health insurance from the 1910s to the end of the Depression. This sociological interpretation makes clear why, even when millions of poor and elderly people were being impoverished and not getting needed care. When unpaid hospital bills became so great

that the American Hospital Association broke ranks with the AMA, it began the search for a non-profit, passive form of hospital insurance that would play a minimal middle-man role. The AHA discovered and shaped what became Blue Cross. Great care was taken to avoid comprehensive prepaid plans and consumer-based plans, and to endorse only private, voluntary, no-profit insurance that covered just the hospital part of the bill.[72]

The AMA's Bureau of Medical Economics remained steadfastly opposed. Insurance, its reports had maintained, depends on compensating for defined liabilities (like fires or thefts), which are impossible in medicine.[73] Service-based coverage, like Blue Cross, leads to standardized, cookie-cutter care for the wide variations among individual patients. This degrading of professional medicine was what contract medicine had brought 30 year earlier, the AMA's Bureau pointed out, and it must not be allowed again. But open rebellion among physicians during the Depression and their development of various insurance schemes led the AMA reluctantly to develop Blue Shield several years after the American Hospital Association (AHA) launched Blue Cross. Great care was taken to be sure it was pass-through reimbursement of what doctors charged, largely focused on hospital-based specialists, rather than based on a fee schedule.[74] Passive middlemen who respected physician autonomy was the key goal—not any collective sense of access or managing costs. Thus the organized profession laid the institutional and cultural foundations for private, voluntary, and pass-through approaches to covering medical bills that would ironically undermine their professional dominance.

Both of the Blues required a majority of directors to be hospital trustees, administrators, or specialists, hardly an auspicious group to restrain costs. The Blues were professionally controlled insurance organizations that covered only those who could afford to pay, and they laid the institutional foundation for commercial insurance companies to cover lower-risk groups.[75] The authoritative Louis Reed envisioned in 1947 that although most hospitals were not for profit,

. . . under a situation in which a large proportion of the population was enrolled and hospitals were paid on a cost basis, hospital administrators would wish in general to provide a more and more perfect or elaborate service, and to make this possible would ask for higher and higher rates of payment.[76]

This is precisely what happened over the next 30 years. With the enemies of professionalism vanquished and the victories won before 1920 anchored in institutional reforms, the professionally driven health care system roared ahead, magnifying its successes as well as its pathologies. Professionally designed passive insurance led to ever-higher charges for ever-more procedures and bed-days.

Professionally Crafted Public Funding

World War II produced great advances in surgery and medical science. After the war, the Public Health Service was transposed into the National Institutes of Health. Further federal support for research and academic medicine came from a realignment and expansion of the Veteran's Administration hospital system around medical schools. Hospital reconstruction received central attention through the Hill-Burton program, guided by a national commission through which the American Hospital Association outlined a huge, 40% expansion in beds. Hill-Burton regulations favored poorer and Southern states but required that community hospitals raise two-thirds of the funds for construction and be financially viable, thus favoring middle-class communities. In a carefully constructed argument, Starr demonstrates that these major infusions of public money were designed to reinforce professional sovereignty and local institutions. Requirements that recipient hospitals treat those unable to pay remained ignored for decades.[77]

Federal funds also greatly influenced the growth and shape of academic medicine. The incomes of medical schools tripled during the 1940s, more than doubled in the 1950s, and nearly tripled again during the 1960s, but largely from federal funds concentrated on research. This focus enhanced the technical prowess of American medicine, but diverted attention from organizing medical schools, the recruitment of students, and the distribution of specialists to meet the health needs of the population. It led to building academic health care "empires" that exploited the poor more than it served their considerable health care needs.[78]

In the private sector, commercial health insurance grew rapidly. The non-profit Blue Cross plans had developed a community-based ethos—all subscribers were charged a single rate. The commercially oriented insurance companies drew away the lower-risk groups (younger and healthier populations) by offering them lower premiums. This private insurance practice of risk-rating, or pursuing subscribers who were less likely to be ill, left the Blues with more unhealthy or sick members in their community-rated pools. This forced them to raise their premiums, making them less competitive with the risk-selective commercials, resulting in a hopeless spiral. Eventually they had to cave in and risk-rate too.[79] Focused on quarterly returns to investors, corporate insurers eventually turned on professional autonomy itself in order to contain costs for their true clients, the employers who hired them. Through the 1950s and 1960s, however, health insurance covered just about anything doctors wanted to order. This exacerbated the super-professionalism of academic health complexes.[80]

PATHOLOGIES OF PROFESSIONALISM

Most accounts of American health care since the 1970s describe its fragmentation, inefficiencies, run-away costs, impersonal care, maldistribution, variable quality, and over-specialization, but without acknowledging how these emanated from a professionally driven health care system operating in its own professionally constructed markets. In time, corporations realized that protected professional markets were a capitalist's dream of a market with virtually no downside risk.

Increased Specialization and Bureaucracy

After 1920, the drive to develop the best clinical medicine based on physician autonomy led quite naturally to more and more specialization. Specialists charged higher fees, and sub-specialists charged even more. Since doctors were free to choose their specialty and where they practiced, rural areas, poor neighborhoods, and primary care were all underserved. This emphasis on professional freedom contrasts with national health systems, that try to have specialized medicine proportional to the need for them, and that try to ensure medical services in poor and rural areas. By the 1970s a double crisis of uneven distribution became a central policy concern. Impersonal care was also an unanticipated consequence of specialization leading to highly bureaucratic medicine divided into narrow compartments of expertise. This problem can be overcome, but it takes a shared vision of specialty-based care that is not common.

Specialization, when combined with professional autonomy, produces fragmented care. The need for coordination fostered secondary industries of middlemen—just what the profession wanted to avoid at all costs and yet an ironic consequence of its ideal system. Another pathology resulted from presuming that quality was whatever a licensed physician did. This led to great variation in actual skills, preferences, and practices without any evidence that more costly care produces better results.[81] The whole system, as well as its hierarchy of values and prestige, centered on hospital care for the seriously ill. As hospitals grew and became elaborated, costs not only rose faster, but hospitals became large institutions in their own right, and this led to a new profession to run them: professionally trained administrators. Thus, by the 1970s, the professionally ideal health care system had led to

widespread complaints about impersonal, over-specialized, fragmented care; run-away costs; widely varying and uneven quality; and a neglect of public health, prevention, and primary care.[82]

The Golden Age or the Age of Gold?

One pathology of professionalism was to make medical care and charity less and less affordable to the poor and elderly who did not have pass-through commercial insurance. Despite these untenable gaps, the AMA fought long and hard against all efforts to provide coverage and relief. When Medicaid and Medicare finally passed in 1965, it took a form that explicitly extended the profession's ideal of autonomous physicians in private practice charging what they liked. The medical profession insisted that the government programs reimburse them for whatever they charged. Community hospitals insisted that their debt service be built into their bed-day rates, even charging for Hill-Burton assets that had been funded by taxpayers. "Community hospitals" no longer needed to appeal to their communities to raise funds, though they continued to do so anyway. All costs for medical equipment were rolled into the bed rate too, so even mistakes were fully paid for. Fledgling hospital corporations induced legislators to insert phrasing that enabled them to use taxpayers' money to develop large corporate chains. In short, the values, mind-set, and regulations built into major new public funding reflected the professional model on a binge. Physicians exercised their uncontrolled autonomy by raising their fees almost three-fold between 1965 and 1980. Hospital bed-day charges quadrupled.

Leaders and advocates of professional medicine now look back at the postwar period as "the Golden Age of Medicine";[83] however, while there were legendary individuals, the period looks more like an Age of Gold. Physicians incorporated themselves and became increasingly commercial in their approach to patient care. As early as the mid-1950s, physicians led the movement to establish for-profit hospitals and made many times more than they could in their practices. An early detailed report noted that these doctors' hospitals did not provide any community services that did not make money and used elaborate legal strategies to create interlocking sets of corporations.[84]

Leaders of the profession rarely admit that the corporatization of direct services was a natural outgrowth of the system the profession itself put in place. They do not admit that physicians commercialized themselves before corporations commercialized them. When combined with insurance that passively reimbursed charges, the professionally driven health care system was a capitalist's dream. Soon, outside investors began to realize the low-risk, high-profit character of medical services, and the corporatization of medicine moved into full swing.

Investor-owned health care corporations grew rapidly, a logical extension, I would argue, of the monopoly markets that the organized profession set up for itself in the absence of a national health care system. When O'Neil reported in 1956 that some doctors had discovered that building a private hospital pumped out more profit than having an oil well, investors would not be far behind. By 1964, the early chains and their lobbyists inserted extraordinarily profitable phrases into Medicare and the floodgates opened. In 1980, the editor of the *New England Journal of Medicine*, Arnold Relman wrote a famous article warning about the "new medical-industrial complex." Relman missed the point: What he lamented was a natural extension of the old medical-industrial complex centered on the medical profession.[85] Two years later, Paul Starr concluded a Pulitzer Prize winning history of American health care by discerning that "Medical care in America now appears to be in the early stages of a major transformation in its institutional structure, comparable to the rise of professional sovereignty at the opening of the twentieth century."[86] He predicted a shift in ownership to for-profit corporations and a concentration of ownership into conglomerates that would integrate hospitals, clinics, and physicians both horizontally and vertically.

In 1983, Howard Waitzkin famously described how a high-tech fad (coronary care units) proliferated without any evidence that it was effective, based on campaigns of academic and corporate entrepreneurs who profited from the costly fad. And when they had saturated the US market, the major corporations turned to exporting their costly product lines to countries in Latin America and Asia that have much smaller, fixed, medical budgets. American corporations smoothly persuaded government ministers to give their people "the latest" and "the best" from the global center of academic-medical capitalism.[87]

In summary, the financial, political, organizational and clinical pathologies of professionalism (Table 10-1) were built into Medicare and Medicaid and accelerated after them. It is for these reasons that I do not think a new era of American health care began with this legislation, but rather a few years later when a countervailing power—all the payers—began to revolt and launched a series of efforts to rein in costs and rationalize medicine.

THE REVOLT OF COUNTERVAILING POWERS

Unrestrained growth in utilization, variation, and charges in this age of gold for doctors and hospitals generated an intense feeling across the political spectrum that professionally driven health care had led to greed, waste, inequities, and dubious quality. Friedson's studies of the "golden age of medicine" described in detail the structural dominance of the profession in the United States and the resulting pathologies. He concluded that an organized profession could not discipline itself effectively.[88] In the 1960s, the tragic effects of thalidomide, a fertility drug that often resulted in deformed babies, documented how medical hubris could wreak havoc on the lives of trusting patients and how professional arrogance led to abuses.[89] In 1971, Dr. Robert McCleery produced a graphic report that detailed the low quality of clinical work, the injury to patients by ordinary physicians (in contrast to those celebrated in the press at the great medial centers) and the very limited ability of medical societies and state boards to do much about it. In 1972, Senator Abraham Ribicoff, who had been Secretary of Health, Education and Welfare (during the Kennedy administration), published *The American Medical Machine* and described the machine's relentless ability to generate bills. In Tulsa, Oklahoma, he found, medical debts accounted for 60% of all personal bankruptcies (Ribicoff and Dandaceau, 1972). In the same year, Senator Ted Kennedy (1972) published his critique, *In Critical Condition*, based on vivid testimony from citizens at hearings his committee held across the country.[90]

These books were widely read and discussed and set the stage for the most radical critique of all, *Medical Nemesis: The Expropriation of Health*, published in 1976 by a Jesuit priest, Ivan Illich. Drawing on research reports in the leading medical journals, Illich held up a mirror that both shocked and fascinated the public. Illich described a world of medicine gone mad, full of mistakes and iatrogenesis (or medically induced disease).[91]

Weak Regulatory Reforms

The health care payers, including Congress and state legislatures, had enough. As seen in Table 10-2, payers as the new dominant power, wanted better performance at less cost. Moreover, the state as regulator had become worried about lapses in quality; the unshakeable trust in the profession to safeguard standards of care began to crumble. During the 1970s, Congress and the states developed large-scale programs to rationalize physician referrals and hospitalization, to plan more equitable capital expenditures, to develop a comprehensive cost base for reasonable charges, to establish hospital rate-setting systems, and to establish quality review. These national and state systems and proposals were all undermined in various ways by hospitals and doctors.[92]

In the meantime, a policy entrepreneur named Paul Ellwood realized that prepaid group health

plans—formerly seen as "hotbeds of socialism" and adamantly opposed by the medical profession—could be recast as private, self-regulating health care systems in which incentives were aligned with keeping people healthy and keeping costs down.[93] These "health maintenance organizations (HMOs)" were just what the newly elected President Nixon needed: a private alternative to socialized medicine. In 1970, he gave the first speech on health care to the joint houses of Congress and proposed universal health care delivered by a national network of 1,700 HMOs. The corporate lobbies of all the suppliers, providers, and insurers opposed it.[94] What eventually came out the other end was the HMO Act of 1973, which lobbyists first tried to block and then weighed down with so many requirements that federally qualified HMOs would collapse under their weight.[95] The nation's leaders concluded that "regulation does not work," despite its working reasonably well in every other advanced medical system. A signal event occurred in 1975 when the US Supreme Court reversed the long-standing exemption of professions from antitrust regulations, on the grounds that professions were, after all, businesses. These events, despite their limitations and failures, signaled a transformation in values and vision and a new balance between countervailing powers.

Strong Corporate Reforms

With the "failure" of regulation, the stage was set for the Reagan era of market-based solutions to social problems. Employers, who had increasingly self-insured to avoid a thicket of regulations that had developed over the years, turned from years of complaining to staging what I have called a Buyers' Revolt.[96] Table 10-3 outlines the basic cultural, economic, organizational, political, and technological changes wrought by a re-balance of countervailing powers.

As employers aggressively sought ways to rein in costs, insurance companies took on a new role: aggressively seeking to control costs by developing

Table 10-2 The Buyer's Revolt: Axes of Change

Dimensions	From Provider-Driven	To Buyer-Driven
Ideological	Sacred trust in doctors.	Distrust of doctors' values, decisions, even competence.
Clinical	Exclusive control of clinical decisionmaking.	Close monitoring of clinical decisions, their cost, and their efficacy.
Economic	*Carte blanche* to do what seems best: power to set fees; incentives to specialize. Emphasis on state-of-the-art specialized intervention. Lack of interest in prevention, primary care, and chronic care. Informal array of cross subsidizations for teaching, research, charity care, community services.	Fixed prepayment or contract with accountability for decisions and their efficacy. Emphasis on prevention, primary care, and functioning. Minimize high-tech and specialized interventions. Elimination of "cost shifting" pay only for services contracted.
Organizational Political	Cottage industry. Extensive legal and administrative power to define and carry out professional work without competition, and to shape the organization and economics of medicine.	Corporate industry. Reduced legal and administrative power over professional work and also the organization and economics of services.
Technical	Political and economic incentives to develop new technologies in protected markets.	Political and economic disincentives to develop new technologies.
Potential disruptions and dislocations	- Overtreatment - Iatrogenesis - High cost - Unnecessary treatment - Fragmentation - Depersonalization	- Undertreatment - Cuts in services - Obstructed access - Reduced quality - Swamped in paperwork

techniques to monitor, and control providers. Secondary industries developed to select providers into "preferred provider organizations (PPOs)," which promised to deliver services within a fixed budget (an HMO with a loose network of providers), to screen and monitor physicians' clinical decisions for costly procedures, and to redesign health benefit plans. These new techniques and organizational forms came to be known collectively as "managed care;" the macro

theory that explained how they would achieve better value for less cost was called "managed competition." The rise of managed competition and managed care centered on the medical profession's refusal to take responsibility for the highly variable quality and rapidly rising costs that resulted from physician autonomy.

Policy entrepreneurs such as Alain Enthoven (1988), aggressively promoted managed competition as the solution to the extensive problems of market

Table 10-3 Tragic Flaws of Managed Competition/Care

The model of having self-contained HMOs (such as Kaiser) compete for quality, service, and value seems to overcome most of the serious dangers of market failure in medicine that can harm patients and exploit buyers. Yet the model has several inherent flaws:

1. Creates oligopolies, which usually minimize price competition.

2. Competitive systems require much *more* regulation (not less) than non-competitive systems.

3. The major competitors become the regulators of the market.

4. Based on a distrust of doctors but a trust of managers. (Are managers a different breed?)

5. Assumes patients will maximize value, but usually they do not.

6. Assumes efficiency gains will exceed sharp rise in administrative and marketing costs that markets require when compared to non-competitive systems.

7. Reduces provider choice by design, to choosing between plans and then providers within plans.

8. Encourages discrimination against higher risk patients.

9. Undermines a public health or community-wide agenda, because based on plans competing for market share.

10. The uncertain, emergent, contingent nature of clinical work that makes medicine so ill-suited to competition remains, only hidden within the walls of each managed care organization.

---

failure in health care. The many commentators on managed competition fail to note that deep sources of market failure remain, hidden behind the walls of the managed care organizations as they compete for contracts and market share.[97] Advocates of managed competition promote their plans by promising choice—in theory, health care consumers will chose from an array of competing plans. In reality, managed care plans restrict the most important choices—which provider a patient may choose and which procedures a provider may perform. Moreover, in most markets managed care organizations are oligopolies and oligopolies usually do not compete on price. Yet price competition is supposed to be the key goal of managed competition. Finally, managed competition presses each payer to focus on its own subscriber's health care and leaves no one responsible for common issues of public health.

Managed competition, ironically, is based on a distrust of doctors but a trust of managers. Investor-run network HMOs are in this way profoundly different from the original, non-profit, physician-run HMOs such as Kaiser. Based on the distrust of doctors—indeed, a frontal attack on the once dominant idea that professional norms should guide medicine—they

commercialize clinical decisionmaking by relying on payments and penalties. They require a great deal of regulation, for greater "efficiency" usually turns out to be the surreptitious result of enrolling fewer poor, sick, or disabled patients. In these ways, managed care corporations of various forms undermined the moral foundations on which successful markets depend.[98] Health economist Uwe Reinhardt asks another crucial question: if managed care companies require another 15% more overhead than Medicare and Medicaid and want to make at least 10% return, can they really reduce costs by 25% without cutting into needed care?

The chief result, in both Medicare and in the general markets, has been cost shifting and cost avoidance through risk selection, and these remain the more common ways to "contain costs" in a system that lacks universal coverage. Eventually, patients (as well as their doctors) rebelled.[99] Through both government regulation and popular pressure, they forced managed care organizations to relax the constraints they had placed on the practice of medicine (such as denying reimbursement for procedures that providers declared necessary). As the managed care companies partially loosened their controls at the end of the 1990s, costs began to soar yet again.

Corporate managed care profoundly altered the balance among countervailing powers. Corporate employers and public legislators developed what might be called a *managed-care industrial complex*, replete with large new secondary industries that design benefits, select providers, manage services, define outcomes, and establish systems of quality, performance, and value—precisely the functions that the profession had long promised to perform. Clinicians ". . . face an increasing set of organized stakeholders who question the content, quality, and cost of professional work, increasingly 'shop around' for the professional services they want, and otherwise act to control professional activity in ways that were unheard of as late as 20 years ago."[100] This was the result of corporations taking over health care, the last instance of a historical trend of market forces taking over every facet of society.[101]

CONCLUSION

In sum, the consequences of a professionally de-signed health care system and the efforts to deal with its social and clinical pathologies has led to the most costly, inefficient, wasteful, and inequitable health care system in the industrialized world, and to a com-plex of secondary industries that thrive on these four characteristics. Inefficiency, waste, and risk selection have become good business, and now the multibil-lion dollar beneficiaries lobby hard against efforts to reduce them.

Managed competition and managed care organi-zations arose because corporate and government buyers faced a crisis of excess created by the stake-holders of professionalized markets. They needed a new concept of how to control rising costs.[102] They sought to rein in the excesses, replace professional autonomy with accountable performance mea-sures, and reorganize the center of care from hospi-tal-based acute intervention to community-based prevention and primary care. A deep distrust and distaste for government and a belief in markets as the way to solve social problems has precluded the alternatives that employers in every other capitalist economy support. The result is socially destructive markets "designed" by legislators who take contri-butions from all the major sellers as well as the cor-porations that are supposed to manage the market. Managed care corporations, as agents for corporate employers, have designed markets in a society with few of the social protections deemed essential in other countries; as a result, "consumers" can get harmed as insurers and providers de-select costly, sick patients or shift the costs of care back to the households of sick patients. Prevention and well-ness get attention only to the extent that one can charge for them. In the current post–managed care era, corporate providers are back in full force. The organized profession is trying to restore its lost lus-ter by emphasizing "professionalism," but without admitting how professionalism contributed to many of the current problems. And employers are giving up by dropping health insurance or passing more costs on to employees. This increases discrim-ination by race and income and contributes to health disparities. A juggernaut seems at hand.

STUDY QUESTIONS

1. What were the five competitive forces that kept physicians' incomes low up until the turn of the 20th century?
2. How did the medical profession succeed in constructing an effective monopoly within the broader context of health care?
3. In what ways was the state co-opted by med-ical professionals? How does the role of the state in the 'system' differ from that in cer-tain European countries?
4. How has the medical profession's grip on the health 'market' been loosened in recent years?
5. What are some of the ways in which medi-cine has been 'commercialized' over the course of the past 30 years?
6. How did the medical profession's control over health care effectively lead to the profession's own loss of autonomy and the demise of the system they had dominated?

NOTES

1. Institute of Medicine 2001; 2003
2. McGlynn et al., 2003
3. McCleery et al., 1971; Illich, 1976, Chapter 1–3
4. World Health Organization, 2000.
5. For overviews, see Fligstein, 2001; Swedberg, 2003.
6. Starr, 1982.
7. Stern, 1945.
8. Rothstein, 1972.
9. DeVeaux, 1904.
10. Goldwater, 1915.
11. Caplan, 1981; Starr, 1982.
12. AMA Council on Pharmacy and Chemistry, 1905.
13. Wazana, 2000; Anonymous, 2003; Goodman, 2004.
14. Williams, 1932; Starr, 1982.
15. Langford et al., 1907.
16. Gist, 1937.
17. Mathews, 1909.
18. Richardson, 1945; Burrow, 1977.
19. Woodruff, 1916, p 508.
20. Richardson, 1945.
21. In Burrow, 1977, Chapter 8.
22. Haley, 1911, p 395.
23. Woodruff, 1916, p 509.
24. Burrow, 1977, p 15.
25. Stevens, 1971; Burrow, 1977; Rosen, 1983.
26. Billings, 1903; Flexner, 1911.
27. Starr, 1982, Chapter 3.
28. Quadagno, 2004.
29. Burrow, 1963; 1977.
30. Davis, 1851.
31. Bledstein, 1976.
32. Shyrock, 1967.
33. Burrow, 1963; 1977.
34. Billings, 1903, p 1272.
35. Wertz and Wertz, 1989.
36. Burrow, 1977.
37. Flexner, 1911.
38. Fox, 1980; Light, 1983.
39. Ibid.
40. Burrow, 1977.
41. Starr, 1982.
42. Navarro, 1976; McKinlay and Arches, 1985.
43. Burrow, 1977.
44. Langford et al., 1907; Haley, 1911; Woodruff, 1916.
45. Vogel, 1980; Rosner, 1982.
46. Rosner, 1982, p 121.
47. Light, 1986.
48. Schwartz, 1965.
49. Burrow, 1977, p 106.
50. Williams, 1932.
51. Starr, 1982, p 127; Caplan, 1981, p 320.
52. Young, 1961, p 207.
53. Anonymous, 1900, quoted at p 1115.
54. S.H. Adams, 1905.
55. C. Weller, 1983.
56. E.A. Ross, 1969. [1901].
57. T. Parsons, 1975; 1954. [1939].
58. Weber, 1968, pp 342–6.
59. Freidson, 1970a; 1970b; Starr, 1982.
60. Navarro, 1976; McKinlay and Arches, 1985.
61. Light and Levine, 1988.
62. Light, 1995a; 2000b.
63. Larson, 1977, p 56.
64. Larson, p xiii.
65. Larson, p 50.
66. Burrage and Torstendahl, 1990; Immergut, 1992; Light, 1994; Giarelli, 2004.
67. Touhy, 1999.
68. Perrow, 2002; Roy, 1997.
69. Roemer, 1991; White, 1995; Giarelli, 2004.
70. Light, 2000a.
71. See Emanuel, 1991.
72. Rorem, 1940; Richardson, 1945; Reed, 1947.
73. Bureau of Medical Economics, 1935.
74. Rayack, 1967.
75. Bodenheimer, Cummings, and Harding, 1974.
76. Reed, 1947, p 89.
77. Starr, 1982, pp 338–51.
78. Ehrenreich and Ehrenreich, 1976; Waitzkin, 1983.
79. Somers and Somers, 1961.
80. Ludmerer, 1999, part II.
81. Wennberg and Gittelsohn, 1982; Wennberg, 1984.

82. Cray, 1970; Kennedy, 1972; Ehrenreich and Ehrenreich, 1976; Illich, 1976.
83. McKinlay and Marcceau, 2002.
84. O'Neil, 19 56. (Dec).
85. Relman, 1980.
86. P. Starr, 1982, p 428.
87. Jasso-Aguilar, Waitzkin, and Landwehr, 2004.
88. Friedson, 1970a, 1970b.
89. Hilts, 2003.
90. Ribicoff and Dandaceau, 1972; Kennedy, 1972.
91. I. Illich, 1976. Yet as Navarro (1976: Part II) and Waitzkin (1983, ch. 8) pointed out, underlying Illich's critique was a radically conservative individualism—each person should take responsibility for his or her health and treat himself or herself—when many causes of illness as well as pathologies of the medical-industrial complex that had grown up around the profession's vision of an ideal system stemmed from a sharply inequitable class structure and a capitalist economy with fewer compensatory programs than any other advanced capitalist society (Moller et al., 2003).
92. Starr, 1982, bk. 2, Chapter 4.
93. Brown, 1983.
94. Starr, 1982, bk. 2, Chapter 4.
95. Starr, 1982; Brown, 1983.
96. Light, 1988.
97. Light, 1995b.
98. Etzioni, 1988.
99. Mechanic, 2004.
100. Leicht and Fennell, 2001.
101. Polanyi, 1920.
102. Fligstein, 1991.

REFERENCES

Adams, S.H. 1905. *The Great American Fraud*. New York: Collier & Son.

AMA Council on Pharmacy and Chemistry. 1905. "The Secret Nostrum Vs the Ethical Proprietary Preparation." *Journal of the American Medical Association* 44: 718–19.

Anonymous. 1900. "Relations of Pharmacy to the Medical Profession." *Journal of the American Medical Association* 34: 986–68,1049–51, 1114–47, 1178–9, 1327–9,1405–47, and 35: 27–9, 89–91.

—— 2003. "U.S. Promotional Spending on Prescription Drugs, 2002 ($21 Billion)." *Canadian Medical Association Journal* 169: 699.

Billings, F. 1903. "Medical Education in the United States." *Journal of the American Medical Association* 40:1271–6.

Bledstein, B. 1976. *The Culture of Professionalism*. New York: W.W. Norton.

Bodenheimer, T., S. Cummings, and E. Harding. 1974. "Capitalizing in Illness: The Health Insurance Industry." *International Journal of Health Service* 4: 583–98.

Brown, L.D. 1983. *Politics and Health Care Organization: HMOs as Federal Policy*. Washington DC: Brookings Institution.

Bureau of Medical Economics. 1935. "An Introduction to Medical Economics," rev. ed. American Medical Association, Chicago.

Burrage, M., and R. Torstendahl. 1990. *Professions in Theory and History*. London: Sage.

Burrow, J.G. 1963. *The AMA: Voice of American Medicine*. Baltimore, MD: Johns Hopkins University Press.

—— 1977. *Organized Medicine in the Progressive Era: The Move toward Monopoly*. Baltimore, MD: Johns Hopkins University Press.

Caplan, R.L. 1981. "Pasteurized Patients and Profits: The Changing Notion of Self-Care in American Medicine." PhD Thesis, Department of Economics, University of Massachusetts, Amherst, MA.

Cray, Ed. 1970. *In Failing Health: The Medical Crisis and the AMA*. New York: Bobbs-Merrill.

Davis, K., C. Schoen, S.C. Schoenbaum, A-M.J. Audet, M.M. Doty, and K. Tenny. 2004. *Mirror, Mirror on the Wall: Looking at the Quality of American Health Care through the Patient's Lens*. New York City: The Commonwealth Fund.

Davis, N.S. 1851. *History of Medical Education and Institutions in the United States*. Chicago, IL: S.C. Grigges & Co.

DeVeaux, E.P. 1904. "Free Dispensaries and Their Abuse." *Northwest Medicine* 2: 151.

Ehrenreich, B., and J. Ehrenreich. 1976. *The American Health Empire: Power, Profits and Politics*. New York: Vintage.

Emanuel, E.J. 1991. *The Ends of Human Life*. Cambridge, MA: Harvard University Press.

Enthoven, A.C. 1988. *Theory and Practice of Managed Competition in Health Care Finance*. Amsterdam, Netherlands: North-Holland.

Etzioni, A. 1988. *The Moral Dimension*. New York: Free Press.

Feder, J.M. 1977. "Medicare: The Politics of Federal Hospital Insurance." Lexington, MA: Lexington Books.

Flexner, A. 1911. "Medical Colleges." *The World's Work* 21: 1438–42.

Fligstein, N. 1990. *The Transformation of Corporate Control*. Cambridge, MA: Harvard University Press.

——2001. *The Architecture of Markets*. Princeton, NJ: Princeton University Press.

Fox, D.M. 1980. "Abraham Flexner's Unpublished Report: Foundations and Medical Education, 1909–28." *Bulletin of the History of Medicine* 54: 475–96.

Freidson, E. 1970a. *Profession of Medicine*. New York: Dodd, Mead.

——1970b. *Professional Dominance*. New York: Atherton.

Giarelli, G. 2004. "Convergence or Divergence? A Multi-Dimensional Approach to Health Care Reforms." *International Review of Sociology* 14:171–203.

Gist, N. 1937. "Secret Societies: A Cultural Study of Fraternalism in the United States." *University of Missouri Studies* 15: (entire issue).

Goldstein, A. 2003. "Medicare Bill Would Enrich Companies." *Washington Post* 24 November: A1.

Goldwater, S.S. 1915. "Dispensaries: A Growing Factor in Curative and Preventive Medicine." *The Boston Medical and Surgical Journal* 17: 613–17.

Haley, E.E. 1911. "The Evils of the Contract System." *New York State Journal of Medicine* 11: 394–6.

Hilts, P.J. 2003. *Protecting America's Health*. New York: Alfred A. Knopf.

Illich, I. 1976. *Medical Nemesis: The Expropriation of Health*. New York: Pantheon.

Immergut, E.M. 1992. *Health Politics: Interests and Institutions in Western Europe*. New York: Cambridge University Press.

Institute of Medicine. 1999. *To Err Is Human*. Washington DC: National Academy Press.

——2001. *Coverage Matters: Insurance and Health Care*. Washington DC: The National Academy Press.

——2003. *Hidden Costs, Value Lost: Uninsurance in America*. Washington DC: The National Academy Press.

Jones, E. 1921. *The Trust Problem in the United States*. New York: Macmillan.

Kennedy, E.M. 1972. *In Critical Condition: The Crisis in America's Health Care*. New York: Simon & Schuster.

Kindig, D. 1997. *Purchasing Population Health*. Madison, WI: University of Wisconsin Press.

Langford, T.S., A.S. Kimball, H.B. Garner, E.H. Flynn, and T.E. DeGurse. 1907. "Report of the Committee on Contract Practice." *Journal of the Michigan State Medical Society* VI: 377–80.

Larson, M.S. 1977. *The Rise of Professionalism: A Sociological Analysis*. Berkeley: University of California Press.

Leicht, K., and M.L. Fennell. 2001. *Professional Work: A Sociological Approach*. Malden, MA: Blackwell Publishers.

Light, D.W. 1983. "The Development of Professional Schools in America." In *The Transformation of Higher Learning: 1860–1930,* edited by K. Jarausch. Stuttgart, Germany: Klett-Cotta, pp. 345–65.

——1986. "Corporate Medicine for Profit." *Scientific American* 225 (6): 38–45.

——1988. "Towards a New Sociology of Medical Education." *Journal of Health and Social Behavior* 29: 307–22.

——1994. "Comparative Models of 'Health Care' Systems, with Application to Germany." In *The Sociology of Health and Illness*, edited by P. Conrad and R. Kern. New York: St. Martin's Press, pp 455–70.

——1995a. "Countervailing Powers: A Framework for Professions in Transition." In *Health Professions and the State in Europe,* edited by T. Johnson, G. Larkin, and M. Saks. London: Routledge, pp 25–41.

——1995b. "*Homo Economicus*: Escaping the Traps of Managed Competition." *European Journal of Public Health* 5: 145–54.

——1997. "The Rhetorics and Realities of Community Health Care: Limits of Countervailing Powers to Meet the Health Care Needs of the 21st Century." *Journal of Health Politics, Policy and Law* 22: 105–45.

——2000a. "The Medical Profession and Organizational Change: From Professional Dominance to Countervailing Power." In *Handbook of Medical Sociology*, edited by C. Bird, P. Conrad, and A. Fremont. Englewood Cliffs, NJ: Prentice-Hall, pp 201–16.

——2000b. "The Sociological Character of Markets in Health Care." In *Handbook of Social Studies in Health and Medicine*, edited by G.L. Albrecht, R. Fitzpatrick, and S. C. Scrimshaw. London: Sage, pp 394–408.

Light, D.W., and S. Levine. 1988. "The Changing Character of the Medical Profession: A Theoretical Overview." *The Milbank Quarterly* 66 (Supplement 2): 10–32.

Ludmerer, K.M. 1999. *Time to Heal: American Medical Education from the Turn of the Century to the Era of Managed Care*. New York: Oxford University Press.

Lydston, G.F. 1900. "Medicine as a Business Proposition." *Journal of the American Medical Association* 35: 1403.

Mathews, G.S. 1909. "Contract Practice in Rhode Island." *Bulletin of the American Academy of Medicine* 10: 599–603.

McCleery, R.S., L.T. Keelty, M. Lam, R.E. Phillips, and T.M. Quinn. 1971. *One Life-One Physician: An Inquiry into the Medical Profession's Performance in Self-Regulation*. Washington DC: Public Affairs Press.

McGlynn, E.A., S.M. Asch, J. Adams, and J. Keesey. 2003. "The Quality of Health Care Delivered to Adults in the United States." *New England Journal of Medicine* 348:2635–45.

McKinlay, J., and J. Arches. 1985. "Toward the Proletarianization of Physicians." *International Journal of Health Services* 15: 161–95.

McKinlay, J., and L. Marcceau. 2002. "The End of the Golden Age of Doctoring." *International Journal of Health Services* 32: 379–416.

Moller, S., E. Huber, J.D. Stephens, D. Bradley, and F. Nielsen. 2003. "Determinants of Relative Poverty in Advanced Capitalist Democracies." *American Sociological Review* 68: 22–51.

Navarro, V. 1976. *Medicine under Capitalism*. New York: Prodist.

O'Neil, W. 1956. "How to Get Rich: Own a Hospital?" *Modern Hospital* (Dec): 51–5, 134, 138, 140, 142.

——1954 [1939]. "The Professions and Social Structure." In *Essays in Sociological Theory*, edited

by T. Parsons. Glencoe, IL: The Free Press, pp 34–49.

Parsons, T. 1975. "The Sick Role and the Role of the Physician Reconsidered." In *Action Theory and the Human Condition*, edited by T. Parsons. New York: The Free Press, pp 66–81.

Perrow, C. 2002. *Organizing America: Wealth, Power and the Origin of Corporate Capitalism*. Princeton, NJ: Princeton University Press.

Rayack, E. 1967. *Professional Power and American Medicine: The Economics of the American Medical Association*. Cleveland, OH: World Publication Co.

Reed, L. 1947. *Blue Cross and Medical Service Plans*. Washington DC: Federal Security Agency.

Relman, A.S. 1980. "The New Medical-Industrial Complex." *New England Journal of Medicine* 303: 963–70.

Ribicoff, A., and P. Dandaceau. 1972. *The American Medical Machine*. New York: Saturday Review Press.

Richardson, J.T. 1945. "The Origins and Development of Group Hospitalization in the United States." *University of Missouri Studies* XX: 9–102.

Roemer, M.I. 1991. *National Health Systems of the World*. New York: Oxford University Press.

Rorem, C.R. 1940. *Non-Profit Hospital Service Plans*. Chicago, IL: Commission on Hospital Services.

Rosen, G. 1983. *The Structure of American Medical Practice, 1875–1941*. Philadelphia, PA: University of Pennsylvania Press.

Rosner, D. 1982. *A Once Charitable Enterprise: Hospitals and Health Care in Brooklyn and New York: 1885–1915*. New York: Cambridge University Press.

Ross, E.A. 1969 [1901]. *Social Control: A Survey of the Foundations of Order*. Cleveland: The Press of Case Western Reserve University.

Rothstein, W.G. 1972. *American Physicians in the Nineteenth Century: From Sects to Science*. Baltimore, MD: Johns Hopkins University Press.

Roy, W.G. 1997. *Socializing Capital: The Rise of the Large Industrial Corporation in America*. Princeton, NJ: Princeton University Press.

Sager, A., and D. Socolar. 2003. "61 Percent of Medicare's New Prescription Drug Subsidy Is Windfall Profit to Drug Makers." Boston University School of Public Health, Health Reform Program, Boston.

Schwartz, J.I. 1965. "Early History of Prepaid Medical Care Plans." *Bulletin of the History of Medicine* 39: 450–75.

Scott, W.R., M. Ruef, P.J. Mendel, and C. Caronna. 2000. *Institutional Change and Healthcare Organizations: From Professional Dominance to Managed Care.* Chicago, IL: University of Chicago Press.

Shearer, G. 2003. *Medicare Prescription Drugs.* Washington DC: Consumers Union.

Shyrock, R.H. 1967. *Medical Licensing in America: 1650–1965.* Baltimore: Johns Hopkins University Press.

Somers, H.M., and A.H. Somers. 1961. *Doctors, Patients, and Health Insurance.* Washington DC: The Brookings Institution.

Starr, P. 1982. *The Social Transformation of American Medicine.* New York: Basic.

Stern, B.J. 1945. *American Medical Practice in the Perspective of a Century.* New York: The Commonwealth Fund.

Stevens, R. 1971. *American Medicine and the Public Interest.* New Haven, CT: Yale University Press.

Swedberg, R. 2003. *Principles of Economic Sociology.* Princeton, NJ: Princeton University Press.

Touhy, C.H. 1999. *Accidental Logics.* New York: Oxford University Press.

US Department of Health and Human Services. 1982. "Health United States, 1982." Washington DC: US Department of Health and Human Services.

Vogel, M. 1980. *The Invention of the Modern Hospital.* Chicago, IL: University of Chicago Press.

Waitzkin, H. 1983. *The Second Sickness: Contradictions of Capitalist Health Care.* New York: The Free Press.

Warbasse, J.P. 1909. *Medical Sociology.* New York: D. Appleton and Company.

——1912. "What Is the Matter with the Medical Profession?" *Long Island Journal of Medicine* 6: 271–5.

Wazana, A. 2000. "Physicians and the Pharmaceutical Industry." *Journal of the American Medical Association* 283: 373–80.

Weber, M. 1968. *Economy and Society.* New York: Bedminster Press.

Weller, C. 1983. "'Free Choice' as a Restraint of Trade, and the Counterintuitive Contours of Competition." *Health Matrix* III (2): 3–23.

Wennberg, J. 1984. "Dealing with Medical Practice Variations: A Proposal for Action." *Health Affairs* 3: 6–32.

Wennberg, J., and A. Gittelsohn. 1982. "Variations in Medical Care among Small Areas." *Scientific American* 246: 120–35.

Wertz, R.W., and D.C. Wertz. 1989. *Lying-In: A History of Childbirth in America* (Expanded Ed.). New Haven, CT: Yale University Press.

White, J. 1995. *Competing Solutions: American Health Care Proposals and International Experience.* Washington DC: Brookings Institution.

Williams, P. 1932. *The Purchase of Medical Care through Fixed Periodic Payments.* New York: National Bureau of Economic Research.

Woodruff, J.V. 1916. "Contract Practice." *New York State Journal of Medicine* 16: 507–11.

World Health Organization. 2000. *The World Health Report 2000.* Geneva, Switzerland: World Health Organization.

Young, J.H. 1961. *The Toadstool Millionaires: A Social History of Patent Medicines in American before Federal Regulation.* Princeton, NJ: Princeton University Press.

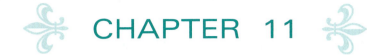

CHAPTER 11

Public Opinion and Health Policy

Mollyann Brodie and Robert J. Blendon

This chapter addresses the relationship between public opinion and health policy outcomes. Because health policy takes place within the broader political system, it is influenced by the same factors that affect policies and politics in general, including public opinion, electoral outcomes, and political-institutional structures.

Understanding the nature of public opinion in the health care context is important for a number of reasons. First, public opinion influences the outcomes of elections. Candidates who wish to be elected to public office must concern themselves with the perceived needs and preferences of the American public. Public opinion surveys capture the mood, values, and policy preferences of Americans, and therefore help predict election outcomes and set political agendas. Public opinion in the electoral context is reflected by more than just opinion surveys, however; it includes voting patterns and individual contacts with elected official (mail, telephone, and electronic technologies).

Second, studies have shown that public opinion influences political decisionmaking on many issues beyond election outcomes.[1] Public opinion is associated with Congress action, executive decisions, Supreme Court rulings, and with policy changes. Public opinion was the second most

influential factor on congressional decisionmaking in the 1993–94 health care reform debate.[2] Furthermore, the public's (in this case senior citizens') response to the increase in taxes required to pay for the expanded benefits of the Medicare program led directly to the repeal of the Medicare Catastrophic Act just one year after its passage—one of the most embarrassing outcomes in recent policy history.[3]

Third, public opinion matters because Americans have very low levels of trust in government leaders and experts. In the absence of a clear-cut legitimacy for the views of leaders and experts, political decisions to determine the direction of public policies often give substantial weight to the views of the public over those of government officials and experts. Therefore, understanding the public's policy preferences and attitudes toward decisions on the governmental agenda helps us predict trends in legislative decisionmaking.

Fourth, though public opinion does not directly influence all policy decisions, particularly those made away from the public spotlight, it is a measure of the political environment within which issues are debated and discussed. As we will show later, the mood of Americans often has a direct and profound impact on the policy solutions they will support. During periods of economic uncertainty, Americans' willingness to grant the federal government more power declines, particularly for policies that would increase government regulation in various aspects of their daily lives.

Fifth, even when political leaders have very clear policy agendas, they pay close attention to public opinion as they shape and "sell" their policies. Contemporary politicians monitor public opinion at every stage of the policy process—from the moment they first float a proposal to its final implementation.[4]

Finally, we should recognize the unique role that public opinion plays in the health field. Health care is a service industry that directly touches the lives of most Americans. Therefore, the public's views on how well the health system works or on how well doctors and hospitals serve them acts as one indicator of the success of our health policies. Cross-national studies show that Americans express a greater degree of dissatisfaction with their health care system than do the French, Germans, or British. While 65% of the French, 58% of Germans, and 57% of the British report they are satisfied with their own health care system, fewer Americans (40%) express this level of satisfaction.[5]

Interpreting the role public opinion requires some understanding of the nature of the issues involved and the context in which individuals are considering these issues. Public opinion will have a stronger influence and effect on policymaking when certain conditions are met. Public opinion is likely to be most influential in highly visible debates, for issues that could affect the outcomes of elections, and for issues decided by initiative or referendum. On the other hand, public opinion matters less in the case of more technical policymaking, where the public lacks knowledge, interest, and opinions regarding the possible policy outcomes. For example, the public's views on whether specific factors should be used in devising

the resource-based relative value scale to pay physicians for services provided to Medicare patients will be decidedly less important than their views on whether and how the Medicare program should help seniors with their prescription drug costs. Similarly, because these issues are technical and far removed from average people's lives, the public's preferences on how clinical labs should be regulated are likely to be irrelevant, whereas their views will be decidedly more influential in the issue of whether individuals should be limited in their choices of doctors.

This chapter is divided into three sections. In the first we explore some of the key principles of public opinion as it relates to health care policy. In the second section, we turn our attention to the values and beliefs that directly influence the way Americans think about health care policies and that shape the way in which they answer public opinion survey questions. These tools, underlying principles, and core beliefs, explain precisely how public opinion influences health policy; and they suggest how we can strategically respond to the dynamics of public opinion. Finally, in the third section we apply what we have learned to the case of national health insurance over the period from President Truman to President Clinton.

KEY PRINCIPLES OF PUBLIC OPINION

In order to understand the nature of public opinion on health care issues, we must first understand the key principles that underlie public opinion. Understanding these principles will make us much better interpreters of public opinion surveys and more sophisticated analysts of the health policy process.

Public Lacks Knowledge but Holds Strong Beliefs and Values

Americans do not know a great deal about the details of health policy, but they do hold a set of core beliefs and values that shape how they think about health policy choices. Given their importance and influence, the next section of this chapter explores those core beliefs in greater depth. For now, however, note that despite poor performance on knowledge-based questions, the public is able to draw clear policy preferences and exert strong opinions.

For example, although the public knew little about the key issues and terms in the 1993–94 health care reform debate, they had come to the judgment that they did not support the Clinton plan. After a year-long debate about health care reform, the public remained largely unaware of the major Democratic alternatives to President Clinton's health reform plan and even less aware of Republican options. Most Americans (73%) did not know that President Clinton was the principal sponsor of an employer mandate. Furthermore, in spite of intense media coverage, only 34% of the American public knew that most of the uninsured come from families in which someone is employed; but 35% knew that the United States spends more on health care than other countries.[6] However, polling results showed that Americans had strong policy preferences: People wanted health care reform, but a plurality (48%) opposed the president's plan—the only plan they were aware of.[7]

The Public Prioritizes Their Opinions on Issues

Because the number of issues for public debate exceeds the number of issues any individual is able to pay attention to and engage in at a given point of time, individuals prioritize their opinions on issues, with some being more or less important to them personally. The political system recognizes this and responds to public priorities. Therefore, it is crucial to understand the *salience* that the public ascribes to issues, particularly health policy issues.

Salience of a given issue is assessed in comparison to other issues. The most common method of determining how salient an issue is to ask the public an open ended question: "What do you think are the most important problems facing the country?" Or, alternatively, "What are the most important issues for government to address?" Policy makers and legislators consider the issues that rank from number one to number four as the most important issues on the public agenda and the ones most likely to influence the outcomes of elections. The highly ranked issues often gain the most media coverage.

In reality, individuals vote for a particular candidate only partially because of issues. And, even when people do vote on issues, it is on a small number of issues. In fact, since 1960 the president who won the popular vote has came from the political party that the public deemed best able to solve the issue that was named the most important problem facing the country. Furthermore, since 1956, with only two exceptions, the president winning the popular vote has come from the party the public deemed better for the nation's prosperity. In the only two exceptions, the 1968 (Nixon) and 1980 (Reagan) elections, the winning party trailed the chosen party by 3 percentage points or less on this measure.[8]

Public opinion on a given issue will matter significantly more when that issue is salient to the American public, and, therefore, the health policy community needs to be well aware of the salience the public ascribes to the health policy issue at hand. For example, in the summer of 2003, 13% of the public named health care as the most important problem for the government to address, while 39% said the economy, and 17% reported war and foreign policy.[9] Ultimately, the potential impact of public opinion can be predicted by the salience that the public or particular segments of the public ascribe to a specific issue.

Who Constitutes the Public?

Political analysts often distinguish among different definitions of the public and each of these groups may have different views on health policy legislation. Here we focus on four political definitions of the "public."

First, at the most general level the term "public" refers to all Americans. The views and opinions of this public can be discerned by national random sample telephone surveys.

Second, "the public" refers to voters or likely voters; that is, the subset of Americans who directly determine the outcomes of elections. During election periods (primary and general elections) the views and opinions of this subset become especially important to legislators and decision makers, particularly on the most salient issues. Note that only rarely does a health care issue make it to the "election agenda," that is, rank high enough on Americans' list of concerns for it to be an issue that candidates fear it will affect the way voters cast their votes. For example, reform of the health care system ranked high enough to become an election issue in the 1991 Pennsylvania Senate race and (as a result) the 1992 presidential election.[10] On the other hand, in 2001 health care costs were rising by double digits, the proportion of Americans without health insurance was rapidly increasing, and 60% of the public reported being dissatisfied with the availability and affordability of health care; yet health care was not a dominant issue in the 2002 congressional election. When likely voters were asked to name the most important issues in deciding their vote, health care generally ranked fourth or fifth (regardless of whether the question was asked open-ended or using a list).[11]

Third, one might be interested in only the views of particular subpopulations of the "public" defined by a specific demographic attribute, such as age, gender, race, religious preferences, or political party identification. When an agenda item pertains to certain groups, their involvement is likely to increase and they are more likely to play a role in an issue's support or opposition, or salience on the agenda. For example, when looking at the Medicare prescription drug debate, the differences in priorities and preferences between younger and older groups are profound. In 2003, adults ages 65 and over were more than twice as likely as adults ages 18 to 64 (32% versus 14%) to say that the cost of prescription drugs was one of the top issues for government to address. Adults ages 18 to 64 are twice as likely as those 65 and older to prefer a prescription drug plan for seniors which offers coverage through private plans (46% versus 23%). Similarly, about half

(51%) of adults ages 18 to 64 favor incentives to join private plans for better prescription drug benefits, compared with a third (33%) of those ages 65 and over.[12]

Fourth, the final "public" includes only those who are politically active. This group is made up of those Americans who communicate directly with their representatives, by either writing or calling, contributing money to politicians or political groups, attending protests or other forums on behalf of a particular interest or candidate, or in other ways make their voices and policy preferences heard. Legislators are most responsive to the views or wishes of these active Americans, particularly when they live in their legislative districts. Political activity is more likely among those who are older, have more years of education, and have strong party identification.[13]

It is important to determine which "public" is most pertinent for the issue at hand. In some cases when political leaders say they are responding to public opinion it is in reality to the opinions of those who are politically active; in others, to the general public as a whole as reflected in opinion surveys. For example, take the controversial issue of abortion. While there exists majority support among the *general* public for the principle of legally available abortion, a review of exit poll data from the 2000 presidential election shows that the majority (58%) of voters who said that abortion was a top issue in their vote indicated that they voted for George W. Bush, the more pro-life candidate.[14] In addition, the 1984, 1988, and 1992 presidential election exit polls showed that the majority of those for whom abortion was important to their presidential vote were those who wanted abortion to be illegal in all circumstances or to see its availability in our society substantially restricted.[15] That is, those who held the pro-life position were more likely to say the abortion issue was important in their vote than those who held the pro-choice position in these elections. Furthermore, more than 50% of the political activity directly related to the abortion issue, including protesting and contacting legislative representatives, came from the 30% of Americans who held pro-life positions.[16] Therefore, these different "groups" of the public—voters versus non-voters, the politically active versus the non-active—hold different policy preferences on the legality of abortion and compose different groups to which political decision makers need to respond.

Americans Often Hold Parallel and Conflicting Values

In addressing public opinion it is important to know that Americans often hold conflicting views. Until these conflicts are resolved we cannot accurately predict where the public actually stands on the specific health policy issues confronting them. For example in 2003, 74% of the public said it is very important for the president and Congress to deal with increasing the number of Americans covered by health insurance.[17] At the same time, however, Americans mistrusted the government and were cynical about the government's ability to do things right. Thus, while the public consistently supports the goal of guaranteeing health insurance to all Americans, it also rejects the idea of the federal government running the health insurance system. Similarly, while the public wants the government to control health care costs, it also believes that the federal government already controls too much of our daily lives.[18]

In each of these cases, the public's conflicting views lead them to support contradictory policies. Only by presenting the specific policy choices in comparison to one another can we see how Americans make trade-offs and resolve their conflicting views and values.

Americans Often Agree on Broad Goals but Disagree on the Means

These differences can be seen clearly only when survey questions are designed that explicitly separate the goals from the various means of achieving them. Public opinion textbooks talk at length about the importance of question wording. The types of questions asked will fundamentally shape the survey results. For example, in 2000, 84% said that health care should be provided equally to everyone, just as public education is; but only 44% said they favored a single (government) plan to provide health insurance for all Americans as a means of guaranteeing universal coverage[19] and 46% said they were willing to pay more in higher taxes or premiums in order to increase the number of Americans who have health insurance.[20]

Furthermore, strong majorities report favoring many approaches to providing health insurance to more people. For example, most support the following proposals: offering businesses tax deductions, tax credits, or other financial assistance to help them provide health insurance to their employees (85%); expanding state government programs for low-income people, such as Medicaid and the Children's Health Insurance Program, to provide coverage for people without health insurance (79%); requiring businesses to offer private health insurance for their employees (74%); offering tax deductions or other financial assistance to help the uninsured pay for private health insurance (72%); and expanding Medicare to cover people under age 65 who do not have health insurance (64%). However, when asked to choose which solution they most preferred, no single solution came close to a majority. In fact, when forced to choose the one option they favor most, none of these options get the support of more than one-fourth of the public.[21] (See Figure 11-1.)

The main point from these examples is that the public often supports goals of public policies, but not the means of achieving them. This suggests an important caveat for public opinion research: do not mix up the goals and the means of achieving those goals in the same questions. Furthermore, an observed increase in support for a particular policy goal does not necessarily mean that there is consensus on the means of achieving that goal. It is often easier to get agreement on general principles and goals than it is to get consensus on the particular

I'm going to read you some different ways to guarantee health insurance for more Americans. As I read each one, please tell me whether you would favor it or oppose it.

When forced to choose…

Of those options you just said you favored, which one do you MOST prefer?*

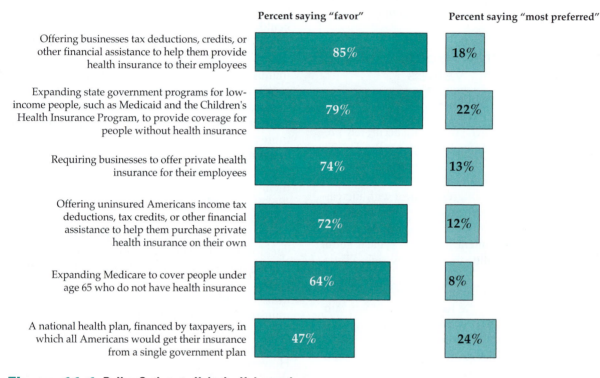

	Percent saying "favor"	Percent saying "most preferred"
Offering businesses tax deductions, credits, or other financial assistance to help them provide health insurance to their employees	85%	18%
Expanding state government programs for low-income people, such as Medicaid and the Children's Health Insurance Program, to provide coverage for people without health insurance	79%	22%
Requiring businesses to offer private health insurance for their employees	74%	13%
Offering uninsured Americans income tax deductions, tax credits, or other financial assistance to help them purchase private health insurance on their own	72%	12%
Expanding Medicare to cover people under age 65 who do not have health insurance	64%	8%
A national health plan, financed by taxpayers, in which all Americans would get their insurance from a single government plan	47%	24%

Figure 11-1 Policy Options to Help the Uninsured

SOURCE: Update to Kaiser Health Poll Report, 2003a.
*Also includes those who said "favor" to only one option

mechanisms and programs that would actually meet those goals.

Potential Consequences of a Policy Affects Its Public Support

Americans' support for a particular policy often shifts when the potential consequences of that policy become more widely known. As a result, measures of public opinion gathered before a large-scale campaign or debate on an issue can be misleading and

are often very different than measures taken at the end of the debate period. As a problem initially emerges on the public agenda, the public wants to see action. This desire to "do something" is often reflected in their answers to public opinion survey questions. However, as the public debate ensues, Americans become more aware of the potential consequences of each policy option, and support for large-scale changes falls. This was seen clearly over the course of the 1993–94 national health care reform debate. Throughout this one-year period, the president went from enjoying strong support for his proposal in its initial phase to seeing public attitudes turn decisively negative toward his plan at the end.[22]

Furthermore, simply providing respondents with more details regarding the potential effects of policies can change their initial support even in the absence of a lengthy public debate. This was seen clearly over the course of the Patient's Bill of Rights debate. Support for this consumer protection law was consistently found to be very high (81% in favor, 12% opposed, and 7% don't know/refused, in 2001).[23] However, after hearing arguments about potential consequences made by opponents of the legislation, support dropped. For example, opposition rises to 31% if they "heard it would increase the cost of health insurance premiums usually shared by employers and workers by about 20 dollars per month for a typical family." Furthermore, 53% report they would oppose such legislation if they "heard it meant that some employers might stop offering health insurance plans to their workers because the employers are afraid they might be sued along with the plan." On the other hand, providing "positive" consequences can increase respondents' public support for a policy. In the case of the Patient's Bill of Rights debate, support for the legislation rose slightly from 81% to 86% if they heard "the law resulted in making health insurance plans less likely to deny coverage for services for people who need them."[24]

A similar pattern can be seen in polling about the uninsured. When Massachusetts residents were given a brief general description of various possible state initiatives to help the uninsured, about three-fourths (76%) favored requiring businesses to offer private health insurance to their employees and pay a fixed amount of the employee's insurance premium. However, when asked if they would still favor this plan if they heard that it would be so expensive that employers would be forced to lay off workers, support dropped to 35%. About half favored a state insurance plan, financed by taxpayers, in which all Massachusetts residents would get their health insurance from a single government plan. But when asked if they would still support such a plan if they heard they would have to wait longer for some hospital and specialty care, support dropped to 30%.[25]

Overall, public support for health care policies can be dramatically affected by whether or not the potential consequences of the policy are either widely understood or explicitly stated in the survey question.

Of course, high-visibility policy proposals often have a large range of potential consequences—some likely, others not. Contemporary policy debates often feature intense campaigns as proponents of a change tout the outstanding (potential) benefits and opponents imagine the terrible (potential) harms. Both sides might exaggerate or dramatize extremely unlikely possibilities. Public opinion surveys measure how the various publics respond to the competing claims and counterclaims.

Public Opinion Changes

Public opinion is not always stable and may shift from support to opposition (or visa versa) as the result of national events, debates, or emerging problems. However, in some public policy areas and for some types of survey questions, researchers have shown that public opinion results can remain quite stable over time.[26] Certain goals, such as covering the uninsured and adding a prescription drug benefit to Medicare, continue to garner support year in and year out. In other cases, particularly during debates over specific policy options, public opinion can change quite rapidly.

Support for national health insurance increases and decreases over time, as does support for fundamental reform of the health care system. "Windows of opportunity"[27] exist when an issue such as health care reform moves to the top of the national agenda and presents an opportunity for mobilizing public support for comprehensive reform. But over time, public interest in the issue is often not sustainable. This can be seen in the results of the debate over health care reform. In September 1993, Americans ranked health care third among the most important problems facing the country—a clear "window of opportunity." By April 1995, it had declined to ninth, behind such issues as high taxes, family values, and the economy.[28]

Unlike some areas of social science research where there are clear findings that remain constant over time, public opinion can vary significantly from one period to another. Debates, advertising, improved public knowledge, or the impact of events can all affect outcomes. Careful analysis of public opinion requires the monitoring of public preferences over time rather than relying on a single observation at any particular point in time.

KEY VALUES AND BELIEFS AMERICANS HOLD[1]

Health policy issues are often complex, involving numerous technical details, yet Americans manage to determine preferences and hold strong views on many of these issues. How does the public draw clear conclusions amid many complex policy choices? Americans consider the health policy proposals within the broader context of their deeply held beliefs and values, and this allows them to reach strong policy preferences across a broad range of issues. Americans organize their responses to surveys and policy questions through a framework of how they generally think about health policy and other social issues. The core beliefs that help make up this framework include beliefs about the relative importance of health care issues, attitudes toward equity, usefulness of new technologies, attitudes toward the role of government, and beliefs about the health care system. In our view there are eleven core beliefs that shape Americans' views on health policy. They are as follows.

Health Is Important but It Is Not Usually the Dominant Issue

To sick people getting well may be the most important priority, but to those who are well it is of lesser

importance. Americans sometimes rate health care issues as a second-level concern, behind issues such as the economy or the war in Iraq. Health care is not the single dominant concern because it is tied to economic factors such as jobs that may include health insurance, or public programs that provide coverage to the poor or elderly based on income contingent guidelines. Only rarely does the general issue of national health care reform attain a level of prominence among all other issues for Americans. What this means is that although polls may show support for increasing health care spending, such preference must be considered within the context of stronger preferences and higher priorities in other areas. For example, Americans have often been more concerned with increasing national defense spending than they with increasing public spending on health care. (See Figure 11-2.)

Health Care, Redistribution, and Self-Interest

Voters often base their political judgments on their evaluation of the nation's overall economic health (sociotropic voting) and not on considerations of their own personal financial situation (pocketbook voting).[29] However, surveys in the health policy area show a somewhat different picture. In its health policy preferences, the public is often more self-interested, either at the individual level or in the perception of being part of a demographic group (e.g., the middle class, seniors, African Americans). Perhaps this is because health care solutions often involve redistribution of resources.

For example, when Congress was debating a Medicare prescription drug benefit, likely voters aged 65 and over (the chief beneficiaries of this issue) overwhelmingly picked prescription drug costs as the most important health care issue in deciding their vote in the upcoming 2002 Congressional elections. Likely voters under age 65 were more likely to cite the uninsured issue and general health care costs (problems experienced more often by non-seniors).[30]

Similarly, the 2000 National Election Survey found that only 28% of upper-income voters supported an

---

[1]Much of this section comes from Blendon et al. 1994c. Adapted with permission from *Health Affairs*.

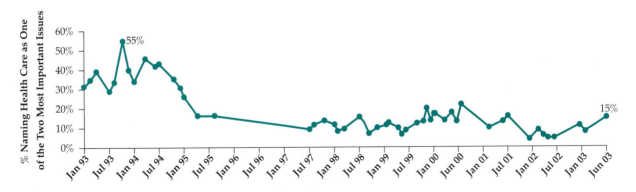

Figure 11-2 **Americans' Perceptions of the Most Important Issues for the Government to Address**

NOTES: "Don't know" responses were included in the base when percentages were calculated.

all-government national health insurance plan (single payer), compared with 51% of lower-income Americans (the group most likely to be helped by such a plan).[31] Likewise, when asked if it was the responsibility of the federal government to make sure that minorities have equality with whites in health care services, even if it means you will have to pay more in taxes, 90% of African Americans said yes, compared with 55% of whites.[32] Taken together, these results suggest that health policy views are often driven by some broad view of individual or group self-interest rather than by more general societal concerns.

A Romance with Technology

While experts are somewhat skeptical of how much new medical technologies contribute to improving health, Americans think they get tremendous benefits out of expensive new medical technologies and procedures. Americans have a greater interest in new medical discoveries and higher expectations for medicine than do people in other industrialized countries.[33] For instance, on surveys Americans rank biomedical research as one of the nation's highest research priorities[34] and do not want to see its fruits "rationed" or unavailable. Polls show that few people (21%) support "rationing" high-cost medical

equipment and procedures.[35] Just how strongly this view is held was revealed in a 1994 poll where 62% of the public agreed "health plans should pay for any treatments which will save lives, even if it costs a million dollars to save one life."[36] In August 1997, 70% of the public said the best thing to do in providing medical care for people who have a serious illness or injury is to provide any treatment that might help, regardless of its cost, even if it means raising health insurance costs for all people.[37] Similarly, in May of 1997, 69% of Americans agreed that if someone is very sick and has almost no chance of survival, all medical treatments, even heroic measures, should be covered by health insurance no matter how costly the care is. Again in 1997, 78% of Americans agreed that insurance companies should be required to cover any medical treatment or test, regardless of cost.[38]

Public Opinion Paradox: Poor System but Good Personal Care

Americans continue to express conflicting views on how they perceive their health care. While they are satisfied with their *personal* health care arrangements and physicians, they believe that there is something wrong with the *national* health care system. For example, in 2003, 56% of the public said that our health care system required fundamental change and 30% said that there is so much wrong with it that we need to completely rebuild it.[39] But, at the same time 91% said they were somewhat or very satisfied with the medical care they received from their doctor during their last visit.[40] Furthermore in 1999, 87% of Americans reported they felt their doctor or provider and other staff members paid attention to their concerns, and 91% said the doctor or provider explained things in a way they could understand.[41] These conflicting beliefs frame the way Americans think about reform debates—change the system, but do not interfere with my personal health care arrangements.

Moral Concern for the Uninsured

Surveys show that moral concern for the uninsured is a strong public value. For example, 86% of Americans say everybody should get the care they need regardless of their ability to pay.[42] Furthermore, in 1995, 65% agreed that the government should do whatever is necessary, whatever the cost in taxes, to see that everyone gets the medical care they need.[43] And in 2003, 74% of the public said it is important to pass a law in the next year to provide health insurance for most uninsured Americans.[44] This fundamental concern for the uninsured remains a powerful factor in shaping public attitudes toward health care reform. Any proposal aimed at assuring universal access is likely to enjoy a great deal of political legitimacy, grounded in the moral convictions of the American people.[45]

Security

Americans are, at least in part, motivated by worries that the problems of the uninsured may one day be their problem. Underlying many survey results is a clear sense of anxiety—the fear that one's own health coverage may at some time prove to be inadequate. To the extent that Americans see their own sense of security threatened, they will be far more likely to endorse significant actions to reform the health care system.[46]

More Americans are personally worried about health care costs than about losing their job, paying their rent or mortgage, losing money in the stock market, or being a victim of a terrorist attack. More than a third of Americans (35%) report they are very worried that the amount they pay for health care services or health insurance will increase. More than three in ten Americans say they are very worried that their income might not keep up with rising prices (33%) and that their health plan will be more concerned about saving money for the company than about what is best for them (31%). Slightly smaller shares are very worried about other health issues (not being able to afford prescription drugs, 24%; declining quality of care, 23%; not getting needed health care, 21%). Far fewer people say they are very worried about other non-health concerns, including not being able to pay their rent or mortgage (15%), losing money in the stock market (12%), losing a job (11%), and being a victim of a terrorist attack (10%) or violent crime (9%).[47]

A Limited Willingness to Sacrifice

One of the most striking features of public opinion surveys is that while Americans frequently state support for a national goal, they are unwilling to make any sacrifice to reach it—whether paying higher taxes, cutting other programs, limiting their choices, or having more government interference in their health care arrangements. The fact that millions of Americans without health insurance may face rationing of health care does not motivate the majority of people who have insurance to share in that rationing or to pay higher taxes so that this situation could be remedied.

As illustrated above, surveys show that a moral concern for the uninsured is a strong public value. For example in 2003, 74% of the public said it is important to pass a law in the next year to provide health insurance for most uninsured Americans. However, less than half are willing to see taxes increased to accomplish this goal. Given three choices, 47% said that the government should make a major effort to provide health insurance for most uninsured Americans, which might require a tax increase to pay for it. Another 37% thought the government should make a limited effort to provide health insurance for some of the uninsured, which would mean more government spending, and 13% preferred to keep things the way they are now.[48] Public reluctance to raise taxes is also illustrated by findings from another 2003 poll. A majority (52%) of respondents disagreed with the statement, "If the only way to make sure that everyone can get health care services they need is to have a substantial increase in taxes, we should do it"; 43% agreed.[49]

Americans' resistance to paying increased taxes needed to fund comprehensive health care reform appears to be embedded in our culture. Americans are less committed than citizens of European industrialized countries to the idea that it is the government's responsibility to even out differences in wealth between people. In 2003, the progressive federal income tax was considered the worst of federal, state, or local taxes.[50] Relatively flat taxes such as state sales taxes, the burden of which often falls disproportionately on the poor, are more widely favored by the public. In addition, they perceive themselves as over-taxed by the federal government. Fifty-one percent of Americans describe their federal income taxes as too high.[51]

Ideology and Party Identification

American views about the role of government in health care are heavily influenced by their ideological orientation and party identification. About 33% of Americans identify themselves as conservative, 26% as liberal, and 36% as moderate.[52] When it comes to political party identification, three in ten Americans consider themselves Republicans, 35% consider themselves Independents, and another 30% consider themselves Democrats.[53]

In thinking about the expansion of the government's role in health care, in almost all cases those who see themselves as being liberal are most receptive

to an enlarged government role, and those who see themselves as more conservative are more resistant to government intervention. The same can be said in most cases when looking by political party. Those who consider themselves Republicans are much more likely to share conservative views of government and resist more government intervention in health care. Conversely, those who identify as Democrats are much more likely to be receptive to a larger government role in dealing with health care. Additionally, conservatives are most likely to see individuals as accountable for their own health care and liberals are more likely to place responsibility on society as a whole.

Distrust of Government

The public's pronounced reluctance to allow the federal government to take a more active role in their lives influences their opinions on almost every issue including health care. Though Americans show strong support for national efforts to improve health, they have a deep suspicion of government.[54] In 2003, only 34% of Americans said they trusted the federal government to do what is right just about always or most of the time.[55] Similarly, 60% told pollsters that the federal government controlled too much of their daily lives, and 63% agreed that when something is run by the government it is usually inefficient or wasteful.[56] Finally, 48% report they would rather have a smaller government with fewer services, while 40% favored a bigger government with more services.[57]

This distrust of "big government" is a long-established American political value, bolstered by the belief that the private sector is inherently more efficient than the government. But this belief is tempered in health care by distrust of the health insurance industry. People suspect that health care providers and insurers are taking financial advantage of them.[58]

Cynicism about "The System"

Americans are cynical about the efficiency and ethical behavior of major institutions and professionals in our society. They believe that the most serious problems facing the health care system are caused by the waste, inefficiency, and greed of the major institutions involved—insurance companies, hospitals, the medical profession, and malpractice lawyers. While there is clearly some truth in the public's perception of a system plagued by inefficiency, this view causes the public to overlook many more significant long-term problems, such as the aging of the population, the frequent use of expensive new technologies, and the cost of using highly trained medical specialists. Because Americans do not see these other factors as important, they are less likely to support proposals to address them, especially if the proposals involve major sacrifices.[59]

This general cynicism becomes more complex when directed toward the medical profession. There is an apparent dichotomy in the way the public views medicine. They see the profession and its leaders in a different light than they do their personal physicians.[60] Over the past four decades, public confidence in the leaders of medicine, as well as other American institutions, has declined. The proportion of Americans expressing a great deal of confidence in the leaders of medicine has declined from 73% in 1966 to 31% in 2002.[61] However, this has not affected the high level of satisfaction most people have with their most recent physician encounter (91%)[62] or their positive feelings toward their own physician (87%).[63] Thus, the public may react differently, depending on how a policy issue is framed— that is, whether the culprit is their own personal physician or the medical profession as a whole.

A Lack of Self-Blame

Americans do not see the problems of the health care system as their own doing. When asked to assess responsibility for the nation's health care ills, only 4% of those surveyed named "patients" as among the one or two most blameworthy groups. While ready to cast blame on the major components of the health care system (including doctors, insurers, and hospitals), the public does not believe that the system's problems may be related to their

own behavior as consumers of health care—or to the lack of incentive for consumers to be price-conscious. As a result, it seems clear that Americans look for reforms that affect primarily the behavior of the major institutions that make up the system, rather than their own behavior.[64]

PUBLIC ATTITUDES IN HEALTH POLICY: A CASE EXAMPLE

When a health issue emerges the public examines it in the light of the broad core beliefs they hold. These, taken together, tend to favor specific incremental changes over more sweeping efforts led by the government. The relationship between our core beliefs and health policy choices, and the subsequent bias toward incrementalism, is illustrated by the case of national health care reform.[2]

These principles and core beliefs can be seen at work when exploring the results of major national debates on health care reform. Since World War II, Congress has had four major debates over reforming the nation's health care system. While each campaign for health care reform centered on a unique policy proposal, there are common features across the contests. Prior to the introduction of each bill, there existed strong public interest in and expectation for reform. After each plan was introduced, opposing interest groups spend millions of dollars to convince the public that enactment of the proposal would result in a health care delivery system even worse than the status quo. Examining these past contests provides important lessons on the role of public opinion and interest group activity in determining the outcome of the national health care reform debates.

[2]Most of this section comes from Blendon et al. 1993b. Adapted from Volume III of the Future of American Health Care series, published by Faulkner & Gray's Healthcare information Center, New York, New York.

Almost 50 years ago, President Truman proposed a comprehensive, prepaid national health insurance plan to be financed through the Social Security tax program. Initially, Truman's proposal had the support of an impressive array of legislators and organizations, prompting political analysts to predict the passage of the plan would proceed smoothly. In response, however, special interests mounted a public relations campaign unprecedented in scope and unparalleled in term of campaign expenditures spent fighting the plan.[65] Unable to match their resources, President Truman ultimately lost out to the interests groups' exaggerated claims regarding the details of his plan, and his proposal failed to attract sufficient public or legislative support. (See Table 11-1.)

National health insurance was again hotly debated after President Johnson's election to office in 1964. As John Oberlander discusses in Chapter 14, Congress considered three competing proposals. House Ways and Means Chairman Wilbur Mills unexpectedly merged all three and created a comprehensive program that resulted in Medicare and Medicaid.[66] While this reform covered only the nation's poor and elderly citizens, proponents of universal national health insurance supported these programs as a necessary first step toward achieving their ultimate goals.[67]

In 1974, the Nixon White House proposed a more extensive national health program called the Comprehensive Health Insurance Program (CHIP). This proposal mandated health insurance coverage for workers through their employers, and provided a separate program to cover the unemployed.[68] Given the similarities between the Nixon bill and the Democratic (Kennedy-Mills) alternative, compromise seemed likely. However, the Watergate scandal significantly reduced the president's influence with Congress and the American public, and dominated the political agenda at a time when health care reform might otherwise have been achieved.[69]

In 1993–94, President Bill Clinton introduced a health care plan and both Democrats and Republicans floated alternative proposals. Once again an administration was proposing comprehensive national health reform, including health insurance coverage for every American citizen. The reasons for the surge of interest in health reform were not immediately apparent to many outside the health field. Some believed that the issue was high on the national agenda because the health care system has reached a state of crisis: a large number of Americans were either uninsured or underinsured, and many were threatened by high health costs. If these conditions were the sole drivers of reform, however, then a national debate over universal health insurance bill would have been enacted in Truman's day, when a far greater percentage of Americans were uninsured and far more were seriously threatened by high medical costs.

The national debate over universal health insurance has never been a reflection of the severity of the aggregate problem. With only 15% of Americans lacking health insurance today,[70] and with Medicare and Medicaid covering many of the nation's poor and elderly citizens, the national health insurance debate was largely driven by something else: *middle-class anxieties over the security of their health insurance coverage.*

Anxiety about health insurance extended far beyond the ranks of the uninsured. The inability of the United States to control sharply rising medical costs was beginning to disintegrate health coverage for working families. Sixty-four percent of Americans said they were worried that their health insurance would become too expensive to afford, 52% feared that very large medical bills would not be covered, 52% were concerned that their health benefits

Table 11-1 Change in Public Support for the Truman Health Reform Plan Over Time

Public Support for Truman Health Plan	March 1949 (%)	November–December 1949 (%)	November 1950 (%)
For	38	33	29
Against	38	47	60
No opinion	25	20	11

SOURCE: Gallup Poll, 1949, 1950.

would be cut, and 31% worried that their family might lose health insurance coverage in the future.[71]

These anxieties were based on real problems. One in four Americans did lose their health insurance during any two-year period.[72] Nearly one-half of the nation's employed workers had had their health benefits cut during the previous two-year period.[73] One in eight households reported someone locked into a job for health insurance reasons,[74] and one in five had had someone denied coverage for a preexisting medical condition.[75] One in five Americans had had a problem paying medical bills in a given year,[76] and 10% reported that there was a time in the past year when they needed medical care, but did not get it for economic reasons.[77]

It is not surprising, therefore, that health care moved to near the top of the national political agenda and became a much more salient issue politically. According to a 1990 survey conducted in ten industrialized countries, Americans were the least likely to say that their own country's health care system works fairly well.[78] Voters in the 1992 presidential election cited health care as the third most important issue, with 19% naming it one of the top two issues in deciding how they voted. Among those who voted for Clinton, health care was the number two issue, second only to the economy.[79]

Given this level of public anxiety and interest, it would seem that enactment of a major health plan was inevitable. But history tells us that public support for health care reform can be fragile. While Americans expressed strong opinions on what they thought was wrong with the health care system, there were four key reasons why the public did not, and still has not, reached consensus on health care reform. Opponents have always appealed to the following uniquely American values in their efforts to defeat national health care reform.

1. Americans want the federal government to solve the health care problem, but don't trust the government to do things right. Americans differ from citizens of most other industrialized countries in their views about the role of government in solving society's problems— the United States has a stronger tradition of reliance on private-sector action. In a multinational survey conducted in 1985, only 36% of Americans said it should definitely be the government's responsibility to care for the sick, compared to 87% in Italy, 86% in Great Britain, and 54% in West Germany.[80]

In addition, Americans' trust in the federal government has never completely recovered from the cynicism of the Vietnam War and the Watergate era. In the late 1950s, three-quarters of Americans said they trusted the government in Washington to do the right thing[81]; in 1993, fewer than one in four (23%) expressed such trust.[82] Between 1972 and 1974, Americans' trust in the federal government dropped from 54% to 37%.[83] Similarly, President Nixon's approval ratings fell from 67% in January 1973[84] to 24% shortly before his resignation in 1974,[85] likely contributing to the defeat of his national health reform plan. Likewise, at the time the Clintons were developing their health plan, less than one in four (23%) Americans expressed generic trust in the government in Washington.[86] This cynicism toward the federal government haunted the Clinton administration throughout its extensive campaign to convince the public that its plan would be good for Americans.

2. There has never been a consensus among the American people regarding an acceptable approach to health care reform. While Americans are willing to applaud the goal of national health reform, they do not agree on the means of achieving that goal. In a 1945 survey, 82% said that something should be done "to make it easier for people to pay for doctor and hospital care." When asked whether each of three different plans (group coverage through an insurance company, a federal government plan as part of Social Security, and a doctors' organization plan) was a good, fair, or poor idea, at least a plurality of Americans rated each plan as good, and at

least two-thirds rated each plan as good or fair. But when asked to choose among the three plans, none came close to achieving majority support and the government option was preferred by only a third (34%) of the public (see Table 11-2).[87]

Similarly, during the debate over the Nixon health reform plan, 66% of Americans agreed that "we need a new nationwide federal health insurance plan." But when asked whether they preferred to receive health insurance from a private insurance company or through the government, the public was almost evenly split.[88]

Again, in the 1993–94 debate, there seemed at first glance to be strong support for a national health insurance program. Fifty-nine percent of Americans said they favored "national health insurance, which would be financed by tax money, paying for most forms of health care."[89] Yet by more than a two to one margin (57% to 26%), they believed that private industry could do a better job managing health care than the government.[90] Similarly, when offered a choice among the three principal reform options (Figure 11-3), the public consistently was divided almost evenly: 32% preferred a plan similar to President Clinton's; 32% opted for a tax credit plan such as the Republican proposal; and 28% preferred a single-payer system like that proposed by Representative

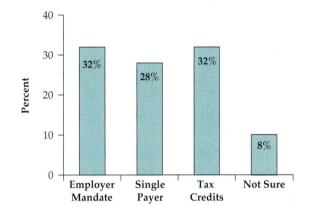

FIGURE 11–3 Americans' Preference for Expanding Health Insurance Coverage

SOURCE: Kaiser Family Foundation/Commonwealth Fund/Harris, 1993.

James McDermott (D-WA) and Senator Paul Wellstone (D-MN).[91] Thus, no matter which of the three options was actually being promoted, two-thirds of the American public believed that there was a better alternative plan proposed.

Each of these examples suggests that caution is necessary in interpreting the public's will. First, agreement on a goal does not necessarily imply agreement on the means of achieving that goal. Additionally, where opinions on the means of achieving a goal are not strongly held, an idea presented alone received higher approval than when it is presented along with alternative proposals that ultimately emerge in the course of the debate.

3. While Americans are willing to spend a lot of money on health care, they have strong reservations about doing it through the tax system. The longest continuous trend measuring public opinion on health care spending in this country shows that the public consistently believes that the United States is spending too little, rather than too much, on health.[92] However, support for such spending does not necessarily translate into support for increased taxes. This pattern is

TABLE 11–2 Level of Support for Three Health Reform Plans, 1945

Type of Plan	Percent Saying "Good or Fair Idea" (%)	Percent Favoring in Forced Three-way Choice (%)
Insurance company plan	88	39
Federal government plan	72	34
Doctor organization plan	69	12

SOURCE: Opinion Research Corporation Poll, 1945, cited in S. Payne.

evident as far back as 1944, when 68% of the public said they thought it would be a good idea for Social Security to cover doctor and hospital care. Support for the idea dropped to 41%, however, when respondents who opposed a payroll tax increase and those who preferred a private-sector plan were removed from the approval ratings.[93]

In the months immediately after the 1992 election, Americans expressed some willingness to pay additional taxes dedicated to a national health reform plan. A March 1993 survey found that 65% of Americans were willing to pay either increased taxes or higher premiums for "a national health care program that would provide every American with access to health care." At the same time, however, only 40% were willing to pay as much as $30 more a month.[94] Moreover, this willingness to pay even a small tax increase was on the decline. By late September 1993, support for higher taxes fell to 48%,[95] and by early October 1993, just 40% supported an increase in taxes to help pay for President Clinton's health reform plan.[96]

4. While Americans are dissatisfied with the health care system overall, they are quite satisfied with the quality of their own health care. Americans have consistently rejected significant health care reform because while they believe there may be problems with the aggregate system, they are highly satisfied with the care they personally receive. In 1993, 71% of Americans reported being satisfied with the quality of their medical care[97]; at the same time, 73% believed that our health care system is fundamentally unsound.[98] This disparity makes it possible for opponents of health care reform to advance the argument that changes made to the aggregate health care system might adversely affect the patient's own health care arrangements.

Even as far back as the 1940s, interest groups have been able to rally Americans against health reform by claiming that the quality of *their own* medical care would be worse under a reformed system. Political

advertisements attacking President Truman's health insurance plan contrasted Norman Rockwell images of the doctor–patient relationship so valued by the public with the threat of government bureaucratic interference. The interest groups' campaign played on public anxieties by questioning whether in the future patients would be able to freely choose their own physicians (which was guaranteed by the Truman plan) with slogans such as, "Your Doctor, or Doctor X?"[99]

Taken together, these four key public attitudes toward health care reform have historically served as constraints on policy makers' ability to restructure the US health care system. The paramount lesson they provide for those interested in promoting health care reform is that early public enthusiasm for health reform ultimately may not translate into continuing public support for major changes in the health care system.

This is in fact what occurred in the case of the Clinton health care plan. The initial public support (in the range of 56% to 59%) for the president's plan declined over time.[100] As of spring 1994, public support stood at 43%, and surveys showed more public opposition than support.[101] Although the Clinton plan contained several elements that had previously been shown to have considerable public support, Americans certainly ended up with a more negative view of the plan as a whole.

The opponents once again left the public fearful of the consequences of major change. A public that earlier had told pollsters of their desire for comprehensive reform later reported concerns that the amount they would have had to pay for health care would increase under the Clinton plan. Moreover, twice as many Americans thought the quality of health care they received would get worse rather than better. The majority (55%) of the public came to believe they would have less choice of physicians, and almost half (46%) believed the president's proposal would entail excessive government involvement in their health care.[102]

Given this level of public anxiety, it is not surprising that by June 1994 only 33% of the public saw the Clinton health plan as good for the country—down from 55% just a few months earlier.[103] This once again illustrates how volatile public opinion can be in the midst of a heated debate and how early support for general principles may not result in majority support for a specific proposal.

This case also illustrate a phenomenon continually found in national public opinion surveys. Knowing that Americans desire health care reform does not necessarily mean that they will favor an all-out government effort to run the health care system. The actors in any given policy debate need to know about the public attitudes not just to the policy option, but, even more important, about their attitudes toward the mechanism by which the policy will be enacted, much less implemented.

CONCLUSION

Public opinion is only one of the many factors that influence the development of health policies in the United States. However, monitoring and responding to public opinion are integral parts of our political system, and have taken on increasing importance with the rise of new communication technologies and the growth of direct democracy. The frequency of major government decisions influenced by direct voter referendum, talk radio, public opinion polling, and communication over the information highway has risen dramatically over the past few years. Increasingly, citizens' views, at a given moment, directly influence decisionmaking that previously was the province of elected representatives and legions of experts and interest groups in Washington. These developments suggest that the role of public opinion in future health policy decisions will be greater than ever.

A sophisticated analysis of polls and surveys is required to understand the nature of public opinion and its influence in health policy debates. In order to draw accurate insights and conclusions, analysts must reach across multiple surveys at multiple times, and should utilize the key principles, core beliefs, and the organizational framework discussed in this chapter.

A peculiar dilemma grows from the fact that the public does not hold the same beliefs and values as many experts in the health care field. Americans think about issues very differently than the experts. The public does not reach the same conclusions using the same type of evidence as health policy experts. As a result, those who seek to influence public opinion on major health policy issues are going to have to develop their case and frame their policy options based on the public's core beliefs, priorities placed on solving health care problems, willingness to live with the consequences of various public policy actions, and level of trust and confidence in both government and interest groups that might be affected by the policy changes.

From the perspective of health policy community, public opinion can be a double-edged sword. On the one hand, the public generally supports the many goals and policies that health care experts have advocated for years. On the other hand, Americans have been much less supportive of the means to achieving the goals. One of the major lessons from past health care reform debate is that, although a "window of opportunity" might exist for major government action, experts tend to overestimate the willingness of Americans to make sacrifices and take risks.

Analysts must also be aware of the major influence actors can have on public opinion in a debate. What Americans believe at the beginning of any reform effort may be totally different from what they believe at the end of the process. In recent years a profession has developed that is focused solely on influencing public opinion in the course of major debates. These political consultants, pollsters, and strategists use the principles we discuss in this chapter to attempt to achieve the policy outcomes they desire. Health policy actors will have to become more skilled in these areas if they are to successfully champion their causes in the future.

STUDY QUESTIONS

1. Why is understanding public opinion important for health policy?
2. How can politicians determine what the most salient issues happen to be at any given time?

3. The authors give multiple answers to the question of "who constitutes the public." What are the answers? Why are they politically significant?

4. The authors note that prevailing American views on health care are contradictory? How? What broader considerations seem to lie behind these contradictions?

5. What evidence exists for general American support behind the expansion of health coverage? What other common attitudes have largely prevented government action on this front?

6. According to the authors, what were the four main political episodes involving health care? What were some of the reasons each presidential effort failed?

7. Why did health care again become a salient issue during the Clinton administration, even though that era saw many more insured than in previous years?

8. How has the erosion of faith in government affected the national health care debate?

9. What are some ways in which would-be health care reformers might overcome the obstacles posed by prevailing American attitudes?

NOTES

1. Page and Shapiro, 1983; Monroe, 1979, 1998; Jacobs and Shapiro, 1994.
2. Columbia Institute, 1995.
3. Schur et al., 1990; American Association for Retired Persons, 1989; Wirthlin, 1989.
4. Jacobs and Shapiro, 2000.
5. Blendon et al., 2001.
6. Kaiser Family Foundation/Harvard School of Public Health/Princeton Survey Research Associates, 1994.
7. Gallup/CNN/*USA Today*, 1994.
8. Gallup/CONUS/*Los Angeles Times*, 1989; Gallup, 1992a, 1992b, 1996, 2000; CBS News/*New York Times*, 2000.
9. Kaiser *Health Poll Report*, 2003b.
10. Blendon et al., 1994a.
11. Blendon et al., 2002.
12. Kaiser Family Foundation/Harvard School of Public Health/Princeton Survey Research Associates, 2003.
13. Verba and Nie, 1972.
14. *Los Angeles Times*, 2000.
15. Blendon et al., 1993a.
16. Verba et al., 1995.
17. Kaiser *Health Poll Report*, 2003b.
18. Blendon et al., 1995b.
19. Kaiser Family Foundation/NewsHour/ICR, 2000.
20. Kaiser Family Foundation/Harvard School of Public Health/Princeton Survey Research Associates, 2000.
21. Kaiser *Health Poll Report*, 2003a.
22. Downs, 1972; Blendon et al., 1995b.
23. Kaiser Family Foundation/Harvard School of Public Health/Princeton Survey Research Associates, 2001.
24. Kaiser Family Foundation/Harvard School of Public Health/Princeton Survey Research Associates, 2001.
25. Harvard School of Public Health/Blue Cross/Blue Shield Foundation of Massachusetts/Cogent Research, 2003.
26. Page and Shapiro, 1992.
27. Kingdon, 1986.
28. Times Mirror Center/Princeton Survey Research Associates, 1995.
29. Markus, 1993; Brewer, 2002.
30. NPR/Kaiser Family Foundation/Kennedy School, 2002.
31. NES, 2000.
32. *Washington Post*/Kaiser Family Foundation/Harvard, 2001.
33. Kim et al., 2001.
34. Harvard School of Public Health/Robert Wood Johnson Foundation/ICR, 2003b.
35. Louis Harris and Associates, 1990.
36. Blendon et al., 1995a.
37. ABC News, 1997.
38. Kaiser Family Foundation/*U.S. News & World Report*/National Opinion Research Center, 1997.
39. CBS News/*New York Times*, 2003.

40. Harvard School of Public Health/Robert Wood Johnson Foundation/ICR, 2003a.
41. Kaiser Family Foundation/Princeton Survey Research Associates, 1999.
42. Blendon et al., 1994a.
43. Harris, 1995.
44. Blendon et al., 2003.
45. Blendon et al., 1994a.
46. Blendon et al., 1994a.
47. Kaiser *Health Poll Report*, 2003c.
48. Blendon et al., 2003.
49. Harris Interactive, 2003b.
50. Gallup, 2003.
51. NPR/Kaiser Family Foundation/Kennedy School, 2003.
52. *Time*/CNN/Harris Interactive Poll, 2003.
53. Princeton Survey Research Associates/*Newsweek*, 2003.
54. Blendon et al., 1995b.
55. NPR/Kaiser Family Foundation/Kennedy School, 2003.
56. Pew Research Center/Princeton Survey Research Associates, 2002.
57. CBS News/*New York Times*, 2003.
58. Blendon et al., 1994a.
59. Blendon et al., 1994c.
60. Blendon, 1988.
61. Harris Interactive, 2003a.
62. Harvard School of Public Health/Robert Wood Johnson Foundation/ICR, 2003a.
63. Princeton Survey Research Associates/*Newsweek*, 2000.
64. Blendon et al., 1994c.
65. Starr, 1982; Quadagno, 2005.
66. Marmor, 1973; Oberlander, 2006.
67. Fein, 1989.
68. Thompson, 1980.
69. Peterson, 1992.
70. Employee Benefits Research Institute, 1995.
71. Kaiser Family Foundation/Commonwealth Fund/Louis Harris & Associates, 1993.
72. US Bureau of the Census, 1992.
73. CBS News/*New York Times*, 1993a.
74. Kaiser Family Foundation/Commonwealth Fund/Louis Harris & Associates, 1993.
75. CBS News/*New York Times*, 1993a.
76. Blendon et al., 1994b.
77. Kaiser Family Foundation/Commonwealth Fund/Louis Harris & Associates, 1993.
78. Blendon et al., 1990.
79. Voter Research and Surveys, 1992.
80. International Social Survey Program, 1985.
81. Opinion Roundup, 1985.
82. CBS News/*New York Times*, 1993b.
83. Opinion Roundup, 1985.
84. Gallup, 1973.
85. Gallup, 1974.
86. Gallup, 1993.
87. Payne, 1946.
88. Opinion Research Corporation, 1972.
89. CBS/*New York Times*, 1993a.
90. Fact Finders/Novalis Corporation, 1993.
91. Kaiser Family Foundation/Commonwealth Fund/Louis Harris & Associates, 1993.
92. Davis and Smith, 1993.
93. Payne, 1946.
94. Blendon et al., 1994c.
95. Princeton Survey Research Associates/*Newsweek*, 1993.
96. ABC News/*Washington Post*, 1993b.
97. CBS News/*New York Times*, 1993a.
98. Gallup/CNN/*USA Today*, 1993.
98. Kelley, 1956.
100. Gallup/CNN/*USA Today*, 1993; ABC News/*Washington Post*, 1993a; *Time*/CNN/Yankelovich Partners, 1993.
101. Gallup/CNN/*USA Today*, 1994.
102. *Time*/CNN/Yankelovich Partners, 1994.
103. Princeton Survey Research Associates/*Newsweek*, 1993, 1994.

REFERENCES

ABC News Poll. (1997). Storrs, CT:Roper Center for Public Opinion Research (August 24).
ABC News/*Washington Post* Poll. (1993a). Storrs, CT:Roper Center for Public Opinion Research (September 22).
ABC News/*Washington Post* Poll. (1993b). Storrs, CT:Roper Center for Public Opinion Research (October).

American Association of Retired Persons Research and Data Resources. (1989). *Opinion of Americans age 45 and over of the Medicare Catastrophic Coverage Act*. Washington DC:American Association of Retired Persons.

Blendon, R.J. (1988). The Public's View of the Future of Health Care. *Journal of the American Medical Association* 259 (24), 3587–93.

Blendon, R.J., J.M. Benson, and C.M. DesRoches. (2003). Americans' views of the uninsured:An era for hybrid proposals. *Health Affairs*, Web Exclusive, W3:405–14; http://www.healthaffairs.org/WebExclusives/Blendon_Web_Excl_082703.htm#18.

Blendon, R.J., J.M. Benson, and K. Donelan. (1993a). The Public and the Controversy Over Abortion. *Journal of the American Medical Association* 270 (23):2871–5.

Blendon, R.J., J.M. Benson, K. Donelan, R. Leitman, H. Taylor, C. Koeck, and D. Gitterman. (1995a). Who has the best health care system?:A second look. *Health Affairs* 14 (4):220–30.

Blendon, R.J., M. Brodie, D.E. Altman, J.M. Benson, S.R. Pelletier, and M.D. Rosenbaum. (2002). Where Was Health Care in the 2002 election? *Health Affairs*, Web Exclusive; http://www.healthaffairs.org/WebExclusives/Blendon_Web_Excl_121102.htm.

Blendon, R.J., M. Brodie, and J.M. Benson. (1995b). What Happened to Americans' Support for the Clinton Health Plan? *Health Affairs* 14 (2):7–23.

Blendon, R.J., M. Brodie, T.S. Hyams, and J.M. Benson. (1994a). The American Public and the Critical Choices for Health System Reform. *Journal of the American Medical Association* 271 (19):1939–44.

Blendon, R.J., K. Donelan, C.A. Hill, W. Carter, D. Beatrice, and D. Altman. (1994b). Paying Medical Bills in the United States:Why Health Insurance isn't Enough. *Journal of the American Medical Association* 271 (12):949–51.

Blendon, R.J., T.S. Hyams, J.M. Benson, and M. Brodie. (1993b). Introduction. In R.M. Sorian (Ed.), *A new deal for American health care*. Washington DC: Faulkner & Gray, pp. 1–14.

Blendon, R.J., M. Kim, and J.M. Benson. (2001). The Public Versus the World Health Organization on Health System Performance. *Health Affairs* 20 (3):10–20.

Blendon, R.J., R. Leitman, I. Morrison, and K. Donelan. (1990). Satisfaction With Health Systems in Ten Nations. *Health Affairs* 9 (2):185–92.

Blendon, R.J., J. Marttila, J. Benson, M. Shelter, F. Connolly, and T. Kiley. (1994c). The beliefs and Values Shaping Today's Health Reform Debate. *Health Affairs* 13 (1):274–84.

Brewer, P.R. (2002). Public Opinion, Economic Issues, and the Vote. In B. Norrander and C. Wilcox (Eds.), *Understanding public opinion*. Washington DC: CQ Press, pp. 243–62.

CBS News/*New York Times* Poll. (1993a). Storrs, CT: Roper Center for Public Opinion Research (January).

CBS News/*New York Times* Poll. (1993b). Storrs, CT:Roper Center for Public Opinion Research (March 28).

CBS News/*New York Times* Poll. (1993c). Storrs, CT:Roper Center for Public Opinion Research (September).

CBS News/*New York Times* Poll. (2000). Storrs, CT: Roper Center for Public Opinion Research (September 27).

CBS News/*New York Times* Poll. (2003). Storrs, CT:Roper Center for Public Opinion Research (July 13).

Columbia Institute. (1995). *What shapes lawmakers' views: A survey of members of Congress and key staff on health care reform*. Menlo Park, CA:Kaiser Family Foundation.

Davis, J.A., and T.W. Smith. (1993). *General social surveys, 1972–1993:Cumulative codebook*. Storrs, CT:Roper Center for Public Opinion Research.

Downs, A. (1972). Up and Down with Ecology—The "issue attention cycle." *The Public Interest* 28:38–50.

Employee Benefits Research Institute. (1995). Sources of Health Insurance and the Characteristics of the Uninsured: Analysis of the March 1994 CPS (Special Report and Issue Brief No. 158). Washington DC:Employee Benefits Research Institution.

Fact Finders/Novalis Corporation Poll. 1993. Storrs, CT:Roper Center for Public Opinion Research (January 14).

Fein, R. 1989. *Medical care, Medical costs:The search for a Health Insurance Policy*. Cambridge, MA:Harvard University Press.

Gallup Organization, CONUS Communication, Inc., & The *Los Angeles Times* Syndicate. 1989. *Election '88*. Princeton, NJ:Gallup Organization.

Gallup Poll. 1949a. Storrs, CT: Roper Center for Public Opinion Research, (March).

Gallup Poll. 1949b. Storrs, CT: Roper Center for Public Opinion Research (November/December).

Gallup Poll. 1950. Storrs, CT: Roper Center for Public Opinion Research (November).

Gallup Poll. 1973. Storrs, CT: Roper Center for Public Opinion Research (January 26).

Gallup Poll. 1974. Storrs, CT: Roper Center for Public Opinion Research (August 2).

Gallup Poll. 1992a. Storrs, CT: Roper Center for Public Opinion Research (March 26).

Gallup Poll. 1992b. Storrs, CT: Roper Center for Public Opinion Research (October 23).

Gallup Poll. 1993. Storrs, CT: Roper Center for Public Opinion Research (March 22).

Gallup Poll. 1996. Storrs, CT: Roper Center for Public Opinion Research. (July 26).

Gallup Poll. 2000. Storrs, CT: Roper Center for Public Opinion Research (October 6).

Gallup Poll. 2003. Storrs, CT: Roper Center for Public Opinion Research (April 7).

Gallup/CNN/*USA Today* Poll. 1993. Storrs, CT: Roper Center for Public Opinion Research (September 24).

Gallup/CNN/*USA Today* Poll. 1994. Storrs, CT: Roper Center for Public Opinion Research (February 26).

Harris Poll. 1995. Storrs, CT: Roper Center for Public Opinion Research (April 14).

Harris Interactive Poll. 2003a. New York: Harris Interactive (January 22).

Harris Interactive Poll. 2003b. New York: Harris Interactive (March 14).

Harvard School of Public Health/Blue Cross/Blue Shield Foundation of Massachusetts/Cogent Research Poll. 2003. Storrs, CT: Roper Center for Public Opinion Research (September 3).

Harvard School of Public Health/Robert Wood Johnson Foundation/International Communications Research Poll. (2003a). Storrs, CT: Roper Center for Public Opinion Research. (February 19).

Harvard School of Public Health/Robert Wood Johnson Foundation/International Communications Research Poll. 2003b. Storrs, CT: Roper Center for Public Opinion Research (May 28).

International Social Survey Program Poll. 1985. Storrs, CT: Roper Center for Public Opinion Research.

Jacobs, L.R., and R.Y. Shapiro. 1994. Public opinion's tilt against private enterprise. *Health Affairs* 13 (1): 285–98.

——2000. Politicians Don't Pander. Chicago: University of Chicago Press.

Kaiser Family Foundation. 2003a. *Kaiser Health Poll Report.* Menlo Park, CA: Kaiser Family Foundation (February 26).

Kaiser Family Foundation. 2003b. *Kaiser Health Poll Report.* Menlo Park, CA: Kaiser Family Foundation (August 7).

Kaiser Family Foundation. 2003c. *Kaiser Health Poll Report.* Menlo Park, CA: Kaiser Family Foundation (October 3).

Kaiser Family Foundation/Commonwealth Fund/Louis Harris & Associates Poll. 1993. Storrs, CT: Roper Center for Public Opinion Research (September).

Kaiser Family Foundation/Harvard School of Public Health/Princeton Survey Research Associates Poll. 1994. Storrs, CT: Roper Center for Public Opinion Research (February 17).

Kaiser Family Foundation/Harvard School of Public Health/Princeton Survey Research Associates Poll. 2000. Storrs, CT: Roper Center for Public Opinion Research (November 13).

Kaiser Family Foundation/Harvard School of Public Health/Princeton Survey Research Associates Poll. (2001). Storrs, CT: Roper Center for Public Opinion Research (July 2).

Kaiser Family Foundation/Harvard School of Public Health/Princeton Survey Research Associates Poll. (2003). Storrs, CT: Roper Center for Public Opinion Research (April 25).

Kaiser Family Foundation/The NewsHour with Jim Lehrer/International Communications Research Poll. (2000). Storrs, CT: Roper Center for Public Opinion Research (January 10).

Kaiser Family Foundation/Princeton Survey Research Associates Poll. (1999). Storrs, CT: Roper Center for Public Opinion Research (July 7).

Kaiser Family Foundation/*U.S. News & World Report*/National Opinion Research Center Poll. 1997. Storrs, CT: Roper Center for Public Opinion Research (May 31).

Kelly, S. (1956). *Professional public relations and political power*. Baltimore, MD: Johns Hopkins University Press.

Kim, M., R.J. Blendon, and J.M. Benson. 2001. How Interested are Americans in New Medical technologies?: A Multicountry Comparison. *Health Affairs* 20 (5):194–201.

Kingdon, J.W. 1986. *Agendas, Alternatives, and Public Policies*. Glenview, IL: Scott Foresman.

Los Angeles Times National Election Day Exit Poll. 2000. Storrs, CT:Roper Center for Public Opinion Research (November 7).

Louis Harris & Associates. 1990. *Survey of Health Care Consumers*. New York: Louis Harris & Associates.

Markus, G. 1993. The Impact of Personal and National Economic Conditions on the Presidential Vote. In R.G. Niemi & H.F. Weisberg (Eds.), *Controversies in voting behavior*. Washington DC: CQ Press, pp 153–66.

Marmor, T.R. 1973. *The politics of Medicare*. Chicago, IL:Aldine Publishing Co.

Monroe, A.D. 1979. Consistency between Public Preferences and National Policy Decisions. *American Politics Quarterly, 7*, 3–19.

Monroe, A.D. 1998. Public Opinion and Public Policy, 1980–1993. *Public Opinion Quarterly* 62 (1): 6–28.

National Election Studies (NES), University of Michigan. The NES Guide to Public Opinion and Electoral Behavior:Government Health Insurance 1970–2000. Accessed at:www.umich.edu/~new/nesguide/2ndtable/t4a_3_1.htm.

National Public Radio/Kaiser Family Foundation/Kennedy School of Government Poll. 2002. (October 23).

National Public Radio/Kaiser Family Foundation/Kennedy School of Government Poll. 2003. (February 5).

Opinion Research Corporation Poll. 1972. Storrs, CT:Roper Center for Public Opinion Research (January).

Opinion roundup:The state of the nation. 1985. *Public Opinion* 8 (4): 21–40.

Page, B.I., and R.Y. Shapiro. 1983. Effects of public opinion on policy. *American Political Science Review* 77:175–90.

Page, B.I., and R.Y. Shapiro. 1992. *The rational public:Fifty years of trends in Americans' policy preference*. Chicago: University of Chicago Press.

Payne, S. 1946. Some opinion research principles developed through studies of social medicine. *Public Opinion Quarterly* 10 (1): 93–8.

Peterson, M.A. 1992. Leading our way to health:Entrepreneurship and leadership in the health care reform debate (Occasional Paper 92–6). Cambridge, MA: Center for American Political Studies.

Pew Research Center/Princeton Survey Research Associates Poll. 2002. Storrs, CT: Roper Center for Public Opinion Research (August 19).

Princeton Survey Research Associates/*Newsweek* Poll. 1993. Storrs, CT: Roper Center for Public Opinion Research (September 23).

Princeton Survey Research Associates/*Newsweek* Poll. 1994. Storrs, CT: Roper Center for Public Opinion Research (June 17).

Princeton Survey Research Associates/*Newsweek* Poll. 2000. Storrs, CT: Roper Center for Public Opinion Research (August 10).

Princeton Survey Research Associates/*Newsweek* Poll. 2003. Storrs, CT: Roper Center for Public Opinion Research (July 24).

Quadagno, J. (2005). *One Nation Uninsured: Why the U.S. Has No National Health Insurance*. New York: Oxford University Press.

Schur, C.L., M.L. Berk, and P. Mohr. 1990. Understanding the cost of a catastrophic drug benefit. *Health Affairs* 9 (3):88–100.

Starr, P. 1982. *The social transformation of American medicine*. New York: Basic Books.

Thompson, M.C. (Ed.). 1980. *Health policy:The legislative agenda*. Washington DC: Congressional Quarterly.

Time/CNN/Harris Interactive Poll. 2003. Storrs, CT: Roper Center for Public Opinion Research (March 27).

Time/CNN/Yankelovich Partners Poll. 1993. Storrs, CT: Roper Center for Public Opinion Research (September 23).

Time/CNN/Yankelovich Partners Poll. 1994. Storrs, CT: Roper Center for Public Opinion Research (March 2).

Times Mirror Center/Princeton Survey Research Associates Poll. 1995. Storrs, CT: Roper Center for Public Opinion Research (April 6).

U.S. Bureau of the Census. 1992. *Current population survey*. Washington DC: Bureau of the Census.

Verba, S., and N. Nie. 1972. *Participation in America:Political democracy and social equality*. Chicago: University of Chicago Press

Verba, S., K. Lehman Schlozman, and H.E. Brady. 1995. *Voice and equality: Civic voluntarism in American politics*. Cambridge, MA: Harvard University Press.

Voter Research and Surveys Election Day Exit Poll. 1992. Storrs, CT: Roper Center for Public Opinion Research (November 3).

Washington Post/Kaiser Family Foundation/Kennedy School of Government Poll. 2001). Storrs, CT: Roper Center for Public Opinion Research (March 8).

Wirthlin Group for the Coalition for Affordable Health Care. 1989. *Medicare Catastrophic Coverage Act Survey* (May 15).

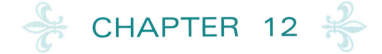

CHAPTER 12

Lobbyists: Ten Myths about Power and Influence

Rogan Kersh

What do health lobbyists actually do? How do they operate? Its not what most people think. Rogan Kersh describes the real world of power and influence in Washington.

INTRODUCTION

A dozen years ago, the authors of the landmark interest-group study *The Hollow Core* could note that "until fairly recently . . . the scope of federal health policy was so small as to attract little attention from interest groups or anyone else."[1] Today no one would dispute the central role of lobbyists in health policymaking. The Clinton health reform battle of 1993–94 was a key catalyst in boosting attention to groups as influential policy actors; most accounts cite the Health Insurance Association of America and other interest groups as central to the Clinton plan's failure.[2] Today a lively, wide-ranging literature on groups and health policymaking continues to expand, within and beyond the academy.

Along with this growing attention have come misconceptions about interest groups and lobbying. This chapter is organized around 10 relatively common claims about health-care lobbying, familiar from academic or journalistic accounts (or both), which deserve careful examination, or perhaps overturning altogether. For slightly exaggerated effect I call them "myths."

Since January 1999, I have followed a group of eleven Washington, DC, health-care lobbyists as they carry out their professional activities. During this time I have also interviewed many other interest-group representatives and their clients, as well as executive branch officials, both career and political appointees, and Members of Congress and their staffers. But direct observations are the heart of my research: of lobbyist discussions with their clients; meetings with Clinton and then Bush executive-branch officials, and with Congressional staff and members; interest-group coalition meetings to strategize and exchange information about administration and Congressional priorities; in-house lobbyist strategy meetings; and so forth.

Most of the lobbyists I follow chiefly represent private (usually corporate) interests. While this fact may skew my findings somewhat, corporate representatives are by far the least studied interest-group actors, compared to lobbyists, for consumer and other public-interest groups, unions, state and local governments, and other membership organizations.[3] Otherwise, the lobbyists make up a diverse group, with respect to type of firm, age, gender, experience, and health policy expertise. A condition of this ethnographic research was anonymity; lobbyists are therefore referred to in this chapter by number ("Lobbyist #1," etc.).

Myth #1: Health Care Is Different

Although the role and influence of interest-group lobbyists in health policy is increasingly well chronicled, health is still often portrayed as a "different" issue realm—attracting more enthusiastic amateur or do-gooder lobbyists than topics like tax policy or financial services. "Health care is not . . . just another line of commerce," goes one typical claim. "It's a matter of life or death for everyone. It should more resemble a religion than a business." Echoed Democratic presidential candidate John Kerry in 2004: "health care is different; it's not as much a matter of the bottom line . . . even in Washington."[4]

Yet to the clients who hire health-care lobbyists, and among corporate and non-profit lobbyists alike, health policy is big business, plain and simple. For example, health policy attracts more lobbyist spending than any other issue. This has been true for several years; interest groups' efforts to influence health policy rose sharply during the Clinton health plan fight of 1993–94, and continued to increase through the tobacco wars of the latter 1990s, the debate over a patients' bill of rights, the clash over Medicare prescription drug benefits, and a whole host of additional health-care issues. Table 12-1 shows total registered lobbyist spending[5] for the 10 most active policy domains over the first half of 2006.

At this rate, health-care lobbyists will report a record (for any issue domain) $400 million in registered spending during 2006; the actual figure will

Table 12-1 Lobbyist Spending by Issue Area, January 1–June 30, 2006

Issue Area	Registered Lobbyist Spending ($)
Health Care	196.5 million
Communication/Technology	178.8 million
Finance, Insurance	154.3 million
Transportation	105.8 million
Energy/Natural Resources	99.4 million
Business (Retail, Services)	87.4 million
Miscellaneous	82.4 million
Defense	60.7 million
Manufacturing	56.3 million
City/County Governments	48.0 million

SOURCE: Lobbyist records filed with US House and Senate, compiled by Political MoneyLine.

be considerably higher, since estimates suggest that as little as half of lobbyist spending to influence Congress is reported in lobbyist filings.[6] "Lobbyist spending," as used here, excludes political action committee (PAC), 527 group, or any other campaign donations. Monies in this category refer to lobbyist salaries, contract payments, research costs, travel, and so forth. Divided by the 535 Members of Congress, reported lobbyist spending on health care in 2006 will be around three-quarters of a million dollars *per member*.

To focus this portrait further: of the 10 top interest-group spenders over the first half of 2005 (the latest full year available), five—the American Medical Association, Philip Morris/Altria, the National Committee to Preserve Social Security and Medicare, the American Hospital Association, and Pharmaceutical Research & Manufacturers of America (PhRMA)—lobby exclusively or primarily on health issues. Two others—the Chamber of Commerce and its legal arm, which are listed as separate entities—devote a significant proportion of their spending to such health policy matters as medical malpractice reform. Any discussion of health-care lobbying must begin with the acknowledgment that, whatever its "special" past, today health is as normalized, professionalized and, yes, corporate as any other realm of US politics and governance.

Myth #2: Here Today, Gone Tomorrow

The classic model of Washington power brokers pictured a closed process dominated by "*iron triangles*"—tight, durable links among powerful interest groups, Congressional committee chairs, and bureaucratic officials. In the past 20 years, this portrait has given way to a very different image, one of loose, open "*issue networks*" comprising experts, specialist staffers in Congress and the executive branch, and stakeholders. *Change* and *fluidity* are now said to dominate lobbying, including on health issues. In the mid-1990s, Mark Peterson charted the "radical change" in health policymaking: the old iron triangles had dissolved into a "far more diverse and open system" that featured "looser, less stable, less predictable, and more diverse patterns of interaction and decision."[7]

Compared to the "iron triangle" model, issue networks appear almost infinitely more open and penetrable—and therefore chaotic. A host of studies apply terms like "bewildering" and "ungovernable" in describing health policy, both as a general domain and with respect to particular topics (Peterson applies the issue network idea to health care as a whole, as well as to the somewhat less sprawling "health care reform policy community").[8]

Despite portraits of constant change verging on chaos, policymaking and lobbying on most health-care issues is much more stable than many current descriptions allow. For accompanying the shift from triangles to networks is another stability-inducing phenomenon, the *issue regime*.

An issue regime is a distinctive constellation of political stakeholders, framing arguments, viable solutions, legislative outcomes, and responses to systemic shocks. Regimes often originate in response to a policy crisis; they thereafter harden into an established set of political practices that help to shape and constrain future policymaking.

Most-health care topics that achieve policy prominence quickly begin to display features of an issue regime. The result is islands of stability within the shifting sea of the health policy network—and a relatively stable set of legislative and administrative outcomes, year in and year out.

One overview of an issue regime may illustrate the general pattern. Medical malpractice burst onto the contemporary political agenda late in 2001, as malpractice insurance premiums spiraled in certain specialties, threatening providers' financial viability and some patients' access to care. Reinsurance costs rose sharply in the wake of 9/11 terrorist attacks, further exacerbating the problem. As bad news mounted, malpractice reform reappeared atop political agendas nationwide. Political responses were swift, even though the 9/11 tragedy was barely three months past. President Bush delivered several major addresses on malpractice policy, Congressional committees organized hearings, and a series of malpractice reform bills were introduced. Media reports breathlessly chronicled a "malpractice crisis," warning of "physician shortages" and "a health-care collapse" in the worst-affected states.[9]

But to those with longer Washington memories, malpractice politics after 2001 was déjà vu all over again. For in two previous crisis episodes—during the mid-1970s and mid-1980s, policy makers had developed standard responses, helping to establish a well organized issue regime.[10] The salient features:

Familiar stakeholders. For three decades, the same leading groups—physicians' representatives led by the American Medical Association, trial lawyers, hospital officials, and insurance executives—have been central players in malpractice policy. All tend to advance arguments first honed in the mid-1970s; employ consistent tactics to mobilize members; and adapt some positions in response to their opponents' views, a process referred to as "issue uptake."[11]

Consistent policy options. Malpractice debates have remained oriented around levels of patient (and attorney) compensation. Policies taken up nationally and in most state capitals—and receiving the bulk of media coverage—are almost all *first-generation* reforms, initially promoted during the 1970s.

Consistent style of legislating. Federal officials are yet to pass a single major malpractice policy since the 1970s crisis, despite repeated efforts. Instead states have been the agents of reform—and most states' malpractice policymaking styles have changed little over 30 years. Some states, like New York or Texas, have passed a series of incremental policies. Others, including Pennsylvania and California, have periodically enacted broad legislation designed to redress the problem of high premiums and to change perceptions of a malpractice "crisis." In Pennsylvania, major reforms were passed in 1975 (Act 111), 1996, and 2002 (Act 13). In the 1970s and current crisis alike, these were only partly successful—laws changed, but not fears of a crisis—and did not result in the usual legislative pause after enactment of a relatively ambitious policy. Act 111, one of the nation's first comprehensive reform packages, was followed by four amendment rounds between 1976–80; Act 13 was supplemented later in 2002 by two additional changes, and reformist pressure remained intense into 2005.

While issue regimes promote stability, they are not iron-clad influences. Changes occur, but the existing regime generally absorbs them. In the malpractice example, the current crisis exhibits at least two significant innovations, compared to the 1970s and 1980s episodes. First, the *context* for policymaking is wider: the malpractice system is more closely integrated with (and affected by) national health policy trends than in the past.[12] Yet despite dramatic changes in US health care since 1970s, the malpractice liability system is little altered. Notable technological advances in medicine have proven to be a double-edged sword: once-miraculous cures are now routine, boosting expectations of success, but the costs of medical errors are far higher now than during the first or second malpractice crises. Yet policy responses have remained steady over time, both at the state and national level.

In a second distinctive change, new *actors* have entered the malpractice policy arena—a key feature of the "issue network" model. Political entrepreneurs, especially tort reform advocates and patient safety groups, have gained prominence in malpractice debates during the present crisis. Yet, in characteristic issue regime fashion, they are swiftly absorbed into existing debates. Groups like the American Tort Reform Association became part of the long-running battle over whether non-economic ("pain and suffering") malpractice damage awards should be capped, usually at the $250,000 level. And patient safety advocates have been "adopted" by trial-lawyer groups seeking to frame malpractice as a problem of incompetent physicians. Safety promoters' aims include frank, open discussions of errors among providers and patients, as well as consistent, swift compensation for medical injuries—reforms that would require broad changes to the malpractice system. And these reforms, under the current malpractice issue regime, receive scant attention in Congress or in most state capitals. Understanding malpractice—and other health topics—in terms of an issue regime helps explain the surprising consistency of health policymaking. Incremental, predictable change generally prevails, despite (or perhaps because of[13]) the forces associated with the modern transformation of triangles into networks.

Myth #3: It's a Man's World

Though no scholarly commentary has singled out health care as dominated by male interest-group advocates, this general view of lobbying has sustained for decades. Jeffrey Berry's comprehensive look in 1996 at the US "interest-group society" termed lobbying a "man's world," though he noted that "barrier[s] to equal employment seem to be eroding." The most recent scholarly study, from 2005, finds that women are still "vastly underrepresented" in the nation's capital, a claim confirmed by the best informal guide to lobbying power in Washington: the annual "Top Lobbyists" listing in the Capitol Hill newspaper *The Hill*. Of the 76 most prominent corporate and independent lobbyists in their latest survey, only six are women.[14]

But in health policy, women lobbyists have achieved a rough numerical parity, and anecdotal evidence suggests that they are also moving up the ladder of influence in private/corporate as well as public interest groups. According to my count of all individuals registered to lobby on health-care issues in 2003–04, 42% were women (46% of non-profit health lobbyists and 37% of corporate interest-group representatives). Although historical evidence is harder to come by, my analysis of 1983–84 health lobbyists finds just 13% women, and a 1990 study put the total proportion of female lobbyists in Washington at 22%.[15]

Women in health policy lobbying are not limited to middle-manager or other positions down the corporate ladder. The president/CEO of AHIP, the chief lobbying association for health plans and insurance companies, is Karen Ignagni; the lead Chamber of Commerce lobbyist on health issues is Kate Sullivan Hare; the head of the peak trade-association group Healthcare Leadership Council is Mary Grealy; and the lobbying shops of two of the largest pharmaceutical companies, Pfizer and SmithKlineGlaxo, are headed by women. Back to *The Hill*'s listing of the capital's most prominent lobbyists: in 2004–05 their assessment was broken out by issue area. In health policy domains, women are well represented among the 10 to 15 top representatives. Fully half of the key health insurance lobbyists are women, for example, and the comparable figure for medical device lobbyists is 56%. In areas like homeland security, oil refining, or business lobbying, by contrast, 91%, 89%, and 100% of the top lobbyists, respectively, named were male.[16] Evidence suggests that state capitals feature more women in prominent lobbying positions as well, in health care and other issue domains, than when the subject was investigated in a 1998 study titled "Female Lobbyists: Women in the World of 'Good ol' Boys.'"[17]

Myth #4: 'K' Is for 'Republican'

George Bush's presidential victory in 2001 marked a transfer of executive branch power from Democratic to Republican. A similar partisan shift within the Washington lobbying community was soon an article of faith both inside and beyond the Beltway, as summarized by journalist Nicholas Confessore: "As Republicans control more and more K Street jobs, they will reap more and more K Street money, which will help them win larger and larger majorities on the Hill. The larger the Republican majority, the less reason K Street has to hire Democratic lobbyists or contribute to the campaigns of Democratic politicians, slowly starving them of the means by which to challenge GOP rule." Confessore's, like many similar accounts, focused on the "K Street Project," a well-publicized effort by Republican strategists and lawmakers to turn lobbyist hiring and contribution practices decisively toward the GOP.[18]

Yet, during and after 2001, despite widespread reports that the advent of a new Republican administration was significantly reshaping the K Street lobbying corridor, surprisingly little change was evident in most lobbyists' regular work, policy emphases, campaign contribution patterns, client base, in-house organization, or hiring practices—at least in the health policy realm. Such continuity suggests increasing stability in federal lobbying.[19]

Two measures buttress this view of interest-group constancy amidst partisan change. If health-care lobbyists shifted sharply toward Republicans, this should show up in patterns of *campaign contributions,* as the GOP received a spiraling share of donations from lobbyists and their clients; and in *organizational practices*—especially new hires—within health care and other sectors of the lobbying community. On neither dimension does the case for Republican dominance hold up fully.

The health industry slightly increased its support for Republican candidates during the 2001–02 cycle following Bush's election, compared to the previous (1997–98) midterm elections. Health-care companies contributed $95 million in the 2002 campaign, 65% to Republicans; in 1998, GOP

Table 12-2 PAC/Soft-Money Contributions, Health-Care Sector, 2002 vs. 1998 (lists all $1 million-plus donors)

Rank	Organization	Amount ($)	Dems (%)	Repubs (%)	Cf. 1998 (Rank, % partisan change)
1	Pharmaceutical Rsrch/Mfrs of Am.	3,505,052	5	95	[not in top 20]
2	American Medical Assn.	2,694,522	40	60	1st, +10D
3	American Hospital Assn.	2,127,495	47	53	2nd, +1D
4	Pfizer, Inc.	1,905,772	19	81	4th, +1R
5	Bristol-Myers Squibb	1,641,813	16	84	8th, +10R
6	Eli Lilly & Co.	1,581,781	25	75	12th, +6R
7	Pharmacia Corp.	1,529,241	21	79	[not in top 20]
8	SmithKlineGlaxo	1,526,938	19	81	11th, +6R
9	American Dental Assn.	1,455,131	42	58	3rd, +2R
10	American Soc. of Anesthesiologists	1,337,227	41	59	7th, no change
11	UnitedHealth Group	1,247,913	22	78	[not in top 20]
12	Wyeth	1,192,129	17	83	[not in top 20]
13	Aventis	1,083,549	20	80	[not in top 20]
14	Johnson & Johnson	1,079,671	39	61	[not in top 20]
15	Schering-Plough Corp.	1,058,528	21	79	17th, +2D
16	American Health Care Assn.	1,058,417	54	46	5th, +1D
17	Amgen, Inc.	1,013,742	21	79	[not in top 20]

SOURCE: Center for Responsive Politics, Federal Election Commission.

candidates garnered 60% of the health sector's $58.3 million. Table 12-2 suggests that this change resulted primarily from a single industry—drug companies, led by their trade association, PhRMA. PhRMA was by far the top health-sector donor in 2001–02, and 95% of their contributions went to Republicans. Table 12-2 displays the 17 health-sector donors that gave more than $1 million during the 2001–02 cycle; 10 of the 17 are drug companies, most of which were not among the top donors in the previous cycle—and they favored Republican candidates by unusually large margins, likely due to GOP legislators' willingness to back the industry's preferred version of the massive prescription drug benefit legislation. Meanwhile, most of the traditional top health contributors maintained existing giving patterns—or, as in the case of the AMA, increased their support for *Democratic* candidates.[20]

During the 2004 election cycle, as "K Street Project" stories continued to spread, the GOP lead retreated to 1998 levels; 61% of total health industry donations were to Republicans. Pharmaceutical giving also shifted slightly toward Democrats in 2004, vis-à-vis 2002; 66% of pharmaceutical industry donations were to Republicans, as opposed to 74% in 2002.

Thus, reports of a decisive move to financing Republican candidates, freezing out Democrats and further cementing the "one-party state" in Washington, appear to have been overstated—at least for the health sector. (Overall corporate donations moved somewhat more toward the GOP in 2002, and fell back in 2004.) What about the *organizational* front: do lobbyists reflect executive branch partisan power shifts within their own trade associations or lobbying firms? The conventional story, again, was that new Republican lobbyists were hired in droves following Bush's victory, and that within the typical organization GOP representatives were given more responsibility. Decrying the "naked effort to make sure that every big lobbyist is a Republican," professor Martin Kaplan noted in 2003 that "the iron [Republican] lock on policy includes the source of big money in Washington"—i.e., lobbyists. Another account portrayed regular meetings of Republican lobbyists and the Project's top Senate ally, Rick Santorum (R-PA): "the lobbyists present pass around a list of the [lobbying] jobs available and discuss whom to support. Santorum's responsibility is to make sure each one is filled by a loyal Republican. . . . After Santorum settles on a candidate, the lobbyists present make sure it is known whom the Republican leadership favors." By 2003 the *Washington Post* concluded that "already in control of the White House and Congress, Republicans are tightening their grip on the largely unseen but vital world of big-time lobbying . . . . The K Street project [is] planting a new crop of Republican lobbyists rich enough to give back to the party in the years ahead." Political scientists Jacob Hacker and Paul Pierson provide a more qualified view, noting in their compelling *Off Center* that Republican "power brokers have an enhanced capacity to induce organized interests to work through them and to do so on their terms."[21]

Definitive studies of the K Street Project's influence, or of Republican inroads in the lobbying community more generally, are yet to come. But they may well show a less potent GOP effect than has been widely asserted since Bush took office. For one, the flow of Republican political talent during the early months of Bush's administration was *away* from K Street, to a substantial degree. Republicans with policy expertise actively sought jobs in the new administration, with nearly 3,500 positions available; conservatives called for expanded political appointments to enable more comprehensive Bush control over the executive branch.[22]

Meanwhile, a set of former Clinton White House staffers was entering the lobbying field. Far from forlornly seeking work, most were snapped up swiftly by lobbying firms—both public interest and corporate—or think tanks.[23] What value could these experienced Democrats supply in an ostensibly "one-party" Washington? Plenty, as it turned out. Public interest and issue groups geared up quickly to stymie Bush policies. As Lobbyist #5, a Democrat, commented in February 2001: "We were worried that [President Bush's policies] *would* turn out to be compassionate conservative policies, but the tax cut—and failure to tackle [a patients' bill of rights or Medicare reform]—took care of that." But corporate and other private interests also hired Democratic veterans of Capitol Hill and Clinton's White House. At Quinn Gillespie, a top lobbying firm co-headed by new GOP chair Ed Gillespie, stories chronicling the firm's four prominent new Republican hires overlooked that at least three former Clinton officials were also brought on board as senior lobbyists following Bush's ascension. Perhaps the highest profile lobbying vacancy during the first Bush term, at the Motion Picture Association of America, was filled by a Democrat, former Congressman and Clinton Agriculture Secretary Dan Glickman. Even pharmaceutical companies—which, as noted earlier, strongly favored GOP candidates in their contributions—were balanced in their new hires. Of the 23 former Members of Congress hired to lobby for the pharmaceutical industry in 2001, 13 were Republicans, and 10 Democrats.[24] My own count of the 47 highest profile health lobbyist hires in 2002–03 found a nearly even split: 25 Republicans, 22 Democrats.

Within individual lobbying firms, a subtle increase in Republicans' influence (compared to their in-house Democratic colleagues) after Bush took office was sometimes apparent. Space permits only a general conclusion here: rather than a wholesale shift toward Republican hiring or influence, most health-lobbying firms appear to have boosted their bona fides with both parties. This again testifies to an established professional lobbying sector, less subject to swings in partisan power than might be expected. Organizational changes were more at the margins, as also seems the case thus far in the wake of the 2004 election.

During that 2004 race, Jeffrey Birnbaum chronicled two "enemies" in the "battlefield of national politics," a Democratic and Republican firm that worked respectively with the Kerry and Bush campaigns. Yet "when it comes to lobbying," Birnbaum notes, "both firms are frequently on the same side. Almost any legislation requires the backing of both Republicans and Democrats to pass in Congress."[25] This captures a basic feature of health (and most Washington) lobbying: the prominent interest-group coalitions forming around most issues include lobbyists associated with both parties, as do the firms housing those representatives.

A host of articles following Congress's return to Democratic control in November 2006 reported a major swing in spending and hiring practices back to Democrats; future versions of this study will examine this transition in detail. Just as rumors of Democratic lobbyists' demise during the halcyon days of the K Street Project were exaggerated, so are tales of their return from the dead.

Myth #5: Lobbying Targets as Rational Choices

How do interest groups decide who to lobby? This topic has been a thorny perennial among interest group scholars at least since 1963.[26] Most relevant research proceeds from a few basic assumptions: that lobbyists divide legislators (or agency officials, but Members of Congress are the usual topics of study here) into supporters, opponents, and fence-sitters, then determine how to allocate lobbying resources among the three.[27] For certain goals, such as securing an earmark (specific allocation) in an appropriations bill, such an analysis is apposite: in such instances, only friendly Members and staffers would be approached. But on most topics, where a majority vote in committee or the full chamber is desired, "choice" and "decision" are less frequently at issue. As Lobbyist #9, a former Member of Congress (MC), told me after exiting an unexpected but "very rewarding" meeting with a top Senate HELP Committee staffer he happened to meet on our ride up in the Hart Senate Office Building elevator, "*this* is how it usually happens. You can draw up a game plan [e.g., listing lobbying "targets"] every day at 9 AM, but by 10 it's fallen apart, and you're nowhere if you can't retreat and regroup—fast." In the swirling Washington policy realm, strategies about where to expend lobbying resources are highly contingent, for several reasons. Two are outlined below.

1. *Uncertain legislative process.* Given the near-constant shifts and reversals characterizing daily events on Capitol Hill, compiling a detailed lobbying list of MC targets on a given bill or during a certain time period is usually a waste of time. "Chaos rules" the legislative calendar, as then-Senate Majority Leader Robert Dole noted in 1995[28]: in a quantum rather than Newtonian universe, few fixed points of reference exist. Predicting timing and all the key legislative and/or executive players on most issues is a talent to which even seasoned Washington hands can only aspire. And since virtually all lobbyists work on several topics simultaneously, determining whom to approach in a multiple-issue legislative arena is less a matter of deliberate choice than of on-the-fly opportunism. Everyone hopes to gain the ear of the relevant committee chair and House/Senate leaders; this being usually impossible, a number of other Members and staffers are worthy targets, a set that shifts repeatedly as the process veers along.

2. *Coalition assignments.* Accompanying, if slightly lagging, the "advocacy explosion" in Washington has been a similar expansion in lobbying coalitions, formed around virtually all issues.[29] Most prominent lobbyists join numerous coalitions: one whom I followed belonged to 54 different health policy groups between 1999–2002, and the average number of coalition memberships among my 11 lobbyists during any given point between 1999–2003 was just under 14 apiece.[30] Among these organizations' many functions is to organize lobbying "opportunities," as the term is delicately put. Setting up meetings for two or more coalition lobbyists with lawmakers or their staffers diminishes the time individual lobbyists must spend angling for a legislator's ear—and

also removes many decisions about 'who to lobby' from direct personal control.

Perhaps the coalition organizer is then the source of painstaking targeting decisions? In some cases, yes. But as an issue is debated in committee markups and floor votes, and hearing rooms and the corridors outside fill with lobbyists eager to register their preferences once more (or, alas, for the first time), the coalition manager's aim is to get the group's message across, with little time for careful pairings based on existing contacts. Most coalitions seek "blanket coverage," as one coalition manager described it to me, of the House or Senate members and key staffers involved in a markup or floor vote, and the managers match lobbyists with legislators in a fashion closer to random than rational.

Take, for example, a Senate vote in June 1999 on a patients' bill of rights (S. 6). A key member from a prominent coalition of corporate health-care interests acted as base organizer, speeding e-mails to each of 38 individual coalition lobbyists on the day of the vote. At 8:13 AM, a list went out of the relevant Senators and staffers, with the request: "Everybody pick at least one, and make sure he knows our view on this!" By 10:09 only 12 responses from coalition lobbyists had been received, heightening the manager's frantic ire. "URGENT THIS REALLY MATTERS," read the next group e-mail header; the message assigned the 26 delinquents their Senator and/or staffer target. "DO YOUR PART," the manager exhorted in conclusion. As the day wore on, e-mail or phone reports poured in: "[Senator X] is on board, I think." "The level of lobbying in [Senator Y]'s office needs to be stepped way up." And, as the floor vote loomed: "We need a better showing of bodies who care on the Senate side!" The takeaway point here: more than two-thirds (26/38) of these lobbyists were *assigned* their contact—and these were experts on the issue, not Washington novices. A survey or interview afterwards asking them whom they "chose" as lobbying targets would likely elicit an answer, but "choice" in this context is so elastic a term as to defy useful analysis.

I tracked all face-to-face meetings between lobbyists and legislators or staffers over various selected periods during the course of my observations. The results of this exercise underscore the problem inherent in analyzing lobbyist "choices." Only between a quarter and a third of a typical set of meetings with a legislative official were actually planned by the lobbyist. At times they went to Capitol Hill *hoping* to encounter one or more of a group of possible targets, but this hardly seems the stuff of strategic choice. I also ask every lobbyist I follow—and most of the 150-plus I have interviewed to date—how they arrive at their mix of legislative targets on an issue, among those officials considered friendly, undecided, and opposed. Beyond the abovementioned earmarks or "rifle shots," however, few can specify targeting practices in any general way, and even fewer saw the question as particularly relevant. "I am a professional opportunist," one senior law-firm lobbyist told me in response. "I take what they [Members and staffers] give me . . . . Sure, if it came down to [my] having to pick Congressman 1, a supporter, or Congressman 2, a [fence-sitter], and that was the only important thing I knew about them, I guess I could make that call. But in 25 years of this [work], it's very, very rarely come down to that [choice], I doubt more than three or four times."[31]

Myth #6: Clients Are King

In most scholarly accounts of policymaking, individual lobbyists are ciphers. They appear as a means for registering the preferences of others, either as an agent for client/corporation principals or as a member of a House or Senate member's "lobbying enterprise."[32] The usual relation is specified as follows:

Client *Interest* → Public official '*Target*' → Policy *Outcome*

Thus, lobbyists are portrayed as vehicles for clients' (or, sometimes, public officials') interests, striving to influence decision makers.

Yet in practice, lobbyists do not always act in faithful obedience to the clients that hire them. Instead, they sometimes advance interests of their own. These include retaining clients and/or signing up new ones; bolstering their own reputation in the Washington policy community for various reasons (status, future employment, a sense of personal worth, and so forth); and promoting what they view as worthy public policy outcomes. These goals are not always best pursued by faithfully striving to match clients' preferences to officials' policy positions. To understand what lobbyists do and why, it is not sufficient to know the interest(s) they represent or the public officials' positions they are seeking to influence.

Of course, interest-group representatives do not actively oppose their clients' preferences, nor do they dominate the public officials they lobby. But ample space for discretionary activity exists, enough that lobbyists must be taken seriously as political actors in their own right. This is an accepted view among Washington officials, who are as likely to ask "Where does Lobbyist Smith stand on this issue?" as they are to wonder "Where does Big Insurance Company stand?"

In practice, client "interests" can be so vague as to amount to little of substance. Many lobbyists spend a great deal of time shaping their clients' preferences, even *creating* interests where none apparently existed before. Where strong client preferences exist, lobbyists often work as hard to alter those as they do the views of their legislative or executive-branch targets. In short, lobbying works in two directions: influencing clients as well as public officials. As for policy makers' hold over lobbyists, this is diminished by the mutual-benefit character of most lobbyist–public official exchanges, and also by the fact that much of what interest-group representatives seek from officials is not terribly costly to obtain. Many lobbyists are better described as independent trustees than as mere delegates of their sponsoring firm, trade association, individual clients, or a Member of Congress.[33]

Again, lobbyists rarely depart radically from their clients' ideological predispositions. But within that broad context ("oppose more government regulation," for example), ample room exists for wielding autonomy—deciding what issues to emphasize, how to do so, when to cut deals, and so forth. As a former Senate committee staffer turned lobbyist put it, "The alliances don't always play out the way you would think. I'm a lot closer to folks on the Hill than I am

my boss in [corporate headquarters]. There's things they know and understand about my issues that my boss doesn't have the faintest idea about; and there's plenty of times when I'm looking after *their* [legislators'] interests instead of sticking hard to the corporate line." This may be a skilled route to long-term lobbying success: favor officials on some issues, positioning oneself to push for client benefits when really necessary. But the fact that even single-firm lobbyists think—and act—independently of their corporate imperatives on a regular basis is telling. Further discussion along these lines arises with our next topic.

Myth #7: The Revolving Door Corrupts Absolutely

Among the most strident complaints about the Washington system of "special interests," inside and outside health care, is that lobbyists move easily and frequently between government and private lobbying firms. This concern is expressed at length in a recent study by the "Revolving Door Working Group" (a watchdog effort sponsored by Public Citizen), which concludes that "The revolving door from the White House and Capitol Hill to well-paid lobbying firms . . . has been spinning out of control in recent years."[34]

In the health-care realm, the Medicare prescription drug benefit is the most recent issue to inspire widespread critiques of "inherent conflicts of interest." Critics adopt similar metaphors: "Authors [of the drug bill] have been streaming in record numbers out of the Capitol and other government buildings and toward K Street . . . people are noticing that the revolving door is spinning out of control."[35] The animating concern is that public officials—Members of Congress and their top staff, executive-branch appointees, even civil servants—quietly favor some interests while in office and then are rewarded with choice lobbying jobs, often changing their political views when they cash in as lobbyists.

Post-government service lobbying restrictions exist, although like many lobbying regulations they carry relatively weak penalties; regulatory standardization and more active enforcement are likely results of the Abramoff lobbying scandal of 2005–06 (more on that later). And the number of elected officials who move into lobbying careers has clearly grown since the 1970s.[36] But is the "revolving door" in fact disgorging corrupt actors with every turn?

This question is difficult to address empirically. The Public Citizen exposé lists a few prominent Members of Congress and Bush administration officials who left public service for lobbying posts, some of whom were directly involved with the issues they later lobbied on, and notes that far more former Members turn lobbyists today than in the mid-1970s. My similarly impressionistic sense is that the raft of outraged commentary serves a valuable watchdog function but far overstates the corruption resulting from the revolving door.

Much as some legislators care deeply about the policy they debate and vote on,[37] most of the lobbyists I followed—and interviewed—had ideological and issue preferences that affected their labors. The distinction between pursuing client interests and advocating policies distinct from (or even opposed to) these is subtle but sometimes apparent in practice. Telling examples concern the evident relish with which lobbyists work on causes about which they care a great deal. I follow one representative (#4) whose background included long service on the staff of a staunchly liberal Democratic Senator; her subsequent work for the Washington office of a multinational company, mostly populated by conservative Republican colleagues, frequently left her discouraged. When an appealing issue arose, she subsequently admitted that "I'll work on this to the exclusion of a lot of things I should be doing instead; then I play catch-up for awhile, [a time] during which I feel like I'm going through withdrawal or something." Another lobbyist represents, for personal reasons, drug and alcohol rehabilitation interests. "This causes me serious problems with my [lobbying] firm," she said. "They represent beer and wine distributors, and other clients who don't much like my advocacy of Betty Ford [Clinic]. But [the firm's director] knows that I'll leave before I give this up."

The reasons that public officials leave office or staff positions are various. Some no doubt conform to the stereotype of "cashing in" with a lucrative lobbying position. But what Washington hands call "priors"—the layers of legislative or executive branch issue wars, professional activities, and colleagues—exert a powerful gravitational pull of their own. Far more lobbyists conform to a portrait of engaged political professionals than to the popular caricature of rank opportunists.

Myth #8: Donations Buy Access (or Even Votes)

What inspires political action committee (PAC) contributions to public officials? In the popular imagination, legislative benefits are the obvious answer. Explains one seasoned journalist: "What [lobbyist-donors] do may be technically legal, but it is nonetheless corrupt, because it's an exchange . . . of campaign contributions and other goodies for special treatment in the legislative process." Scholarly assessments similarly, if more soberly, center on two explanations for donations: influencing policy and affecting election outcomes.[38] Debates among interest-group researchers, as well as outside the academy, continue to percolate about whether PAC funds are intended to "buy" votes (secure Members' support on particular legislative items), win access to members, and/or keep friendly legislators in office, and about the extent of policy influence gained through contributions.

My research suggests that contributions are most often a form of *insurance,* rather than a reflection of the donor's expectation of political gain or even a determined effort to return a particular legislator to office. Rarely do lobbyist-donors have a clear—or even partial—expectation about the return on their investment; rather, they are protecting against unforeseen future dangers as the policymaking process develops. In part this claim is impressionistic, derived from attending numerous fund-raisers and otherwise "following the money." These impressions are augmented by observing hundreds of interactions between lobbyists and the recipients of their contributions.

During the 1999–2000 election cycle (I am now repeating this study for the 2003–04 elections), I asked 80 lobbyists—the 11 I followed regularly, plus

69 of the larger group that I interviewed—to explain the motives for their campaign contributions, both personal and through their organization's PACs.[39] In addition, on the 296 occasions I witnessed or heard about a contribution decision (e.g., one of my 11 lobbyists or their clients giving some amount to a Congress member or political party)[40] I asked what the purpose of that contribution was. For the latter queries, after a lobbyist's initial explanation I asked them to classify their rationale in one of five categories. In 64 cases they refused or were unable to do so; thus I coded 232 total. One example of a coding decision: Lobbyist #10 authorized a $1,000 PAC contribution to a Republican House member. The MC sat on a committee of interest to the lobbyist, but had little seniority. "Why go to this fundraiser?" I asked. "Well, he [the Congressman] asked me to," said the lobbyist. "Sure," I ventured, "but a lot of Members ask you for contributions. Why make this one?" "Ah, well, on the off chance he notices I'm not there [at the fundraiser] . . . best to stay on the safe side," he said. "And [he named a lobbyist for a rival firm] is likely to show up, so I ought to too." After prodding the lobbyist further on what "safe side" entailed, and receiving no concrete response, I coded this as "insurance."

Results appear in Table 12-3 below. The table's four rows represent the different groupings noted just above: first are the general explanations of donation motives given by the 11 lobbyists I followed (the 27 responses reflect multiple answers and/or variations over time; I asked them about the primary purpose of their contributions at three stages in my interactions, between early 1999 and after the 2000 election). The second row aggregates the answers given by 69 other lobbyists in extended interviews, and the third assesses the 232 specific contributions made by "my" 11 lobbyists. The fourth row totals all these. A descriptive summary of the five categories among which I sorted answers:

- *Access/policy influence:* answers here were both retrospective ("He helped us out with [a legislative item] the last session") and prospective ("We have a lot of business before his committee this [session of] Congress").

- *Ideological/partisan:* includes answers like "We only give to Republicans,"[41] "We need more [Democrats] in the Congress," and the like. Though no lobbyist mentioned "influence voters" as a motive, that would also fall into this category.

- *Insurance:* a common formulation was one trade-association lobbyist's account: "I [contribute] to cover all the bases, because you never know." Also frequent in this category were "everybody else does it" claims, as well as variations on a familiar theme, voiced rather convolutedly here by Lobbyist #4: "I doubt [that] my [contributions] rarely if ever help me much, but I'm never sure if it might hurt if I *don't* give."

- *MC status:* includes answers related both to leadership position ("I always give to the Ways &

Table 12-3 Lobbyists' Reported Reasons for PAC Contributions (as % of Row)

	Access/ Influence	Ideological/ Partisan	Insurance	MC Status	Personal	Row TOTAL
Gen'l Resps: my 11 reps. (n = 27)	11	15	41	22	11	100
Gen'l Resps: other 69 reps. (n = 92)	10	26	27	22	15	100
Specific Resps (n =232)	8	19	34	26	13	100
TOTAL (n = 351)	9	21	33	25	13	101 (rounding)

Means chair; it's good politics") and constituency concerns ("We have two plants in that district").

- *Personal:* reasons ranged from "she's a personal friend" to "generally a good guy; I like him, though he's not in any position to help me especially."

As Table 12-3 shows both the general and specific responses of the 11 lobbyists I followed regularly, and the general answers from the 69 other group representatives, rank "insurance" highest among donors' explanations of their contributions, with "MC status" and "ideological/partisan" also mentioned frequently.[42] Compared to my 11 lobbyists, the 69 lobbyists I interviewed listed "ideological/partisan" reasons more often, and "insurance" much less often, but otherwise these differing contexts yielded fairly similar results. Bringing up the rear among all three response groups are contributions designed to win access/influence or on the basis of a personal connection.

I did witness cases where a MC's fund-raising director asked a staffer to meet with a major contributor who otherwise would not have merited an audience; access is a plum sometimes granted. But not all that often, on average. In a separate but related point, the lobbyists I observed and interviewed rank PAC and soft money donations as considerably less important means of affecting policy debates than a host of other activities, such as direct lobbying, researching issues, or media interviews.[43]

Again, most journalistic and many scholarly accounts hold (if often implicitly) that interest groups' campaign contributions are precisely targeted instruments designed to wield maximum political influence. But if lobbyists' own judgment about the purpose of their contributions is both highly uncertain and substantially discounted, perhaps models specifying political clout as a function of campaign spending are flawed in important particulars.

Myth #9: Everybody Does It, Abramoff-Style

In 2005–06, a lobbying scandal rocked Washington. Republican lobbyist Jack Abramoff's catalog of misdeeds inspired a flurry of responses: lawmakers scrambled to rid themselves of tainted campaign monies (over 100 Members of Congress and several state officials returned or donated to charity over $1 million in Abramoff-related funds by mid-January 2006); reformers drew up plans to regulate lobbying; and a host of commentary characterized Abramoff as—in former House Speaker Newt Gingrich's words—"only the tip of the iceberg." As one account of the press coverage summarized, "Abramoff's travesties are the norm in Washington[;] he just got caught giving lawmakers all those meals, drinks, trips and campaign cash in exchange for openly discussed legislative favors."[44] How widespread are practices like Abramoff's—or, more bluntly, how corrupt *is* the world of interest group lobbying?

Abramoff's case will be cited for years to demonstrate the essential corruption of lobbying. Yet it may be more an exception than rule in contemporary American politics. As three political scientists, longtime Washington observers all, note: "Political reforms have reduced the level of corruption in American politics, including the level of bribery, quid pro quo, and special payoffs that involve special interests."[45] Abramoff's case seems exceptional in at least three important respects:

- *Stupendous scale.* Most recent scandals in Washington involve matters of a few thousand or even few hundred dollars. Former Ways & Means Committee Chairman Dan Rostenkowski, for example, lost his seat in 1994 and later was imprisoned, owing to his part in a cash-for-stamps scheme at the House Post Office; the total amount involved was less than $10,000. Abramoff, according to reports in January 2006, admitted to Senate investigators that he bilked clients out of more than $20 *million.* Longtime Washington journalist Jacob Weisberg divides the lobbying world into "swindlers" and "fixers": Abramoff is Exhibit A among the former. But even within the world of flashy caricatures of lobbying power, Abramoff's deeds stand out for their sheer magnitude.

- *Flouting the line.* Concern about lobbyists' unseemly influence over policymaking has exploded since details of Abramoff's actions began to emerge early in 2005. But Abramoff performed at what is widely regarded by lawmakers, journalists, and lobbyists (some enviously, perhaps?) as a different level. Besides defrauding clients, Abramoff has admitted to bribing at least one public official; he also laundered payments to Congressional staff and members through their families and front organizations he created, and paid for lawmakers' trips across the United States and abroad (for example, funding former House Majority Leader Tom DeLay's golf outing to St. Andrews in Scotland), in direct violation of lobbying laws.[46] Trade associations are permitted to pay for Congressional travel, if the trip demonstrably serves some "educational purpose"; individual lobbyists cannot do so.

- *Response.* If "everybody" indeed "does it," no lobbyists in recent years have drawn an official reaction resembling that to the Abramoff scandal. Two indictments have already been handed down, against Abramoff and his lieutenant Michael Scanlon. Powerful House figures like Tom DeLay and former House Administration Committee chair Robert Ney have been driven from office; and—,for a variety of reasons including this and other scandals, the Republicans lost their majority in both houses. Arguably, the system—however maligned and feeble it may be—is working.

So has nothing changed in Washington lobbying practices over the past 10 or 15 years? No, much has. But critics of "corruption" are off the mark; again, Abramoff is not an example of business as usual. Two tectonic shifts have taken place, and they are likely to prove very difficult to disentangle.

One change over recent years is the decline in Washington policymaking of what might be termed "ordinary virtues": tact, civility, restraint, or what the first President Bush used to call prudence. From organizing lavish fund-raisers to rotating from campaign staffer back to lobbying firm to mingling socially with lawmakers as close companions (not to mention spouses), many lobbyists engage in actions that once raised eyebrows but are now routinely accepted. These are all legal—and, indeed, it is difficult if not impossible to formally regulate interactions or

the networks that grow out of them. Clearly a line of reckoning, legally invisible but no less disturbing for that, has been crossed.

Closer associations between lobbyists and lawmakers do not merely represent a shift back to the bad old days of cash-on-the-barrelhead lobbying. Ties between lobbyists and lawmakers have grown tighter in part due to the *professionalization* of lobbying, a second major change in Washington over the past quarter century or so. Instead of an unseemly occupation dominated by, well, fixers and swindlers, "lobbyist" has become a title actively sought by many policy wonks, liberal and conservative activists, top graduates of public administration and law schools, and public officials. Today's lobbyists attend law school, work side by side on Capitol Hill, and socialize daily with the public officials they also seek to influence. In a policymaking environment of increasing size, technical sophistication, and importance to many Americans' daily lives—what political scientist Burdett Loomis aptly describes as the "industry of politics"— replacing ward heelers and hacks with well-trained professionals seems less objectionable.

It is hard to focus reform efforts on these "network" connections; the law cannot reach much of the contemporary intertwining of lobbyists and legislators. This may be where Abramoff's excesses have a long-lasting effect. Not in banning campaign contributions or ending privately financed trips for MCs and staff: these are, perhaps sadly, often the only way policy makers learn something about the rest of the United States and the globe. Instead, the benefit may lie in restoring a sense (which may have to be largely self-generated) of propriety and balance to the complex relationships between lawmakers and the tens of thousands of lobbyists who seek knowledge about and influence over their decisions.

Myth #10: It's All about the Spin

Another widespread view holds that lobbyists provide information that is subtly—or blatantly—repackaged, depending on the audience. "Information is tailored narrowly to spin the target," runs one characteristic claim. "Democratic information for Democrats,

Republican information for Republicans." The notion also makes sense in rational-actor terms: as "cheap speech," lobbyist information is presumably sculpted for maximum appeal to the recipient.[47] This may be true of realms outside health care, but I was dubious about the conventional view after observing lobbyists for several months and reading hundreds of the information packets they prepare for legislators, executive-branch officials, and reporters.

I conducted an experiment to investigate the extent to which information was altered or repackaged. I selected 15 health policy issues high on the Congressional agenda between 2000–03, and collected all the lobbying documents I could for each—making sure to draw from a total of at least five different groups per issue, preferably on multiple sides. The result yielded over 500 discrete pieces of information, ranging from one-page talking points or press releases to bulky studies numbering over 100 pages.

To my surprise, groups almost never altered the information in significant—or even in minor—ways to influence their audience. Republican legislators received the same set of facts and figures as did Democratic staffers and their Members of Congress. Occasionally groups plugged in different information based on an MC's district, but only in 8% of the matched pairings (information provided by a lobbyist to Democratic and Republican lawmakers) did I see arguments shaded toward perceived party affiliation. Rather than an effort to match partisan positions, the information remained constant. I attended more than 90 meetings between lobbyists and staffers or legislators on these 15 issues during the selected time period, and differences of emphasis were certainly present in discussion. But these "leave-behinds"—the research and analysis designed to shift arguments in the lobbyist's preferred direction—remained the same from office to office, audience to audience.

In a longer study of information provision I explore reasons for this constancy.[48] The principal reason was succinctly summed up to me by a senior Senate staffer: the best lobbyists "provide really good information, ideally very quickly, and capitalize on what you already want to do—not something

that's bad for you or your [MC]. If they try to spin you, as opposed to giving good, straightforward information, that's not good . . . and their reputation will decline, *fast*."

CONCLUSION

Myths—and theories—abound about lobbyists in US policymaking. One popular chestnut imagines lobbyists as channeling orders (and cash) from powerful men to pliant members of Congress. A more romantic notion imagines that health care is immune from such crass influence-peddling. And political scientists generally suppose a loose network of experts buzzing around the "hollow core" of each policy issue.

As we have seen, these are all myths, more or less. Health care is not different: quite the contrary. The powerful are increasingly as likely to be women as they are to be men. And most important, lobbyists do not simply "channel" anything. They are permanent, often central, players in a Washington health regime. They have their own political views; they work closely with sympathetic Members of Congress; and they are as likely to shape their clients' views as vice versa.

This fits neatly into contemporary views of power. Political observers frequently note that politicians influence interest groups as often as the interest groups influence the politicians. A close look shows that much the same is true of professional lobbyists and the interests that hire them. The entire Washington establishment—Members of Congress, bureaucrats, and lobbyists—all regularly pressure their constituents, the ostensible "pressure groups."

STUDY QUESTIONS

1. What is an "issue regime"? How does it differ from the previous "iron triangle" model of interest group politics?

2. Many people have suggested that health-care issues are somehow exceptional within the broader scheme of lobbying. Why do they believe this? How is this perception incorrect?

3. How has the role of women changed in health-care lobbying?

4. Why is it important for lobbying firms to have staff culled from both Republican and Democratic circles?

5. How do lobbyists select their "targets"? How much control do they exercise in this process?

6. Myth #6 holds that lobbyists simply represent or channel their clients' views. How does the author challenge this view? How do lobbyists form their views? What do they do about their client's views?

7. Your opinion: The author exposes many familiar myths about lobbyists. Which do you think runs most counter to conventional wisdom? Why?

NOTES

1. Heinz et al., 1993, p 48.
2. Johnson and Broder, 1997; Skocpol, 1996; Hacker, 1997.
3. On the "lack of comprehensive, in-depth studies of individual organized interests" as "a major weakness of the [interest-group] literature," see Cigler, 1994 (quotes); Lowery and Gray, 2004.
4. Dyckman, 2002; Kerry in *Post*, Aug. 14, 2004. A good account of health care's emergence as "big business" is in Barlett and Steele, 2004.
5. All lobbyists seeking to influence members of Congress are required to file quarterly reports with the House and/or Senate, listing amount and sources of lobbying income.
6. Nownes, 2006.
7. Herrnson, Shaiko, and Wilcox, 2005, p. 386 (on the "considerable fluidity in the interest group universe"); Peterson, 1994, pp. 108, 127. Heclo, 1978 pioneered the "issue networks" view.

8. Kendall and Levine, 2000 ("ungovernable"); Franko, 2002 ("bewildering"); Peterson, 1994, p. 108.
9. Kersh 2006.
10. For further details of malpractice politics nationally, see Kersh, 2006; for the Pennsylvania malpractice regime, see Kersh, 2005.
11. Sulkin 2005.
12. Sage 2005.
13. As Peterson, among others, has noted, the policy process's very complexity—especially its multiple veto points—can paradoxically promote stability.
14. Berry, 1997, p. 108; Bath, Nownes, and Gayvert Owen, 2005; "Top Lobbyists—Hired Guns," *The Hill* (April 27, 2005).
15. Schlozman, 1990.
16. See weekly "Lobby League" features in *The Hill*; medical devices ran June 7, 2006; health insurance June 15, 2005; homeland security July 27, 2005; oil refining May 24, 2006; business May 11, 2005.
17. Nownes and Freeman, 1998. See also Nownes, 1999, suggesting that female lobbyists have an "advice advantage" in information provision. Contemporary reports include "State's Female Lobbyists Gaining Power," *Arizona Republic*, April 26, 2004; Ogmundson, 2005; and especially Benoit, 2007.
18. Confessore 2003, p. 7. See also Chaddock, 2003; "List or Blacklist: Democrats Take Aim at Conservative 'K Street Project'," *The Hill*, June 26, 2002; and the rhetorically charged accounts in Continetti, 2006 and Rampton and Stauber, 2004. The K Street Project's (unabashed) self-description was long at http://www.atr.org/kstreet/; the website quietly was taken down in the fall of 2006.
19. This outcome affirms neopluralist accounts of interest representation and influence. See Lowery and Gray, 2004; McFarland, 2004.
20. Bumped out of high-ranking 1998 positions were such groups as the American Nurses Association (6th in 1998); SlimFast Foods

(9th); and the American Academy of Opthalmology (10th); all tended to favor Democratic candidates in both 1998 and 2002.

21. Kaplan, 2003; Confessore, 2003, p. 2; Vande-Hei and Eilperin, 2005; Hacker and Pierson, 2005, p. 145.

22. E.g., Moffit, 2001.

23. Specifics on Clinton Administration veterans who sought lobbying posts is in Salant, 2003.

24. Clemente et al., 2002.

25. Birnbaum, 2004.

26. Beginning with Bauer, de Sola Pool, and Dexter, 1963. A summary of this literature is in Smith, 1995; see also Baumgartner and Leech, 1998.

27. An especially able treatment is Hojnacki and Kimball, 1999.

28. Dole in Ehrenhalt, 1984, p. 819.

29. See, e.g., Hula, 1999; Browne, 1998, p. 146–54; Heaney, 2006.

30. Two points to contextualize these high numbers: first, many coalitions form and disband around *parts* of an issue, as coalition techniques become ever more refined (so that Medicare reform, e.g., spawns mini-coalitions on issues from drug benefits to Part B reimbursement rates). And second, each lobbyist's degree of participation in any one coalition waxes and wanes considerably over time.

31. More detail on these meetings, planned or otherwise, is in Kersh, 2007.

32. Ainsworth 1997, pp. 518 and *passim*. For a succinct statement of principal/agent theory as applied to clients and lobbyists, see Heinz et al., 1993, pp. 373–4. Robert Salisbury describes the "classic model of lobbying" in similar terms: "A group sends its representative to Washington to press its case for or against some policy option, or it hires one of the many would-be agents already located in the nation's capital . . . . The presumption in this model is that the group knows what its policy interest is." Salisbury emphasizes, in contrast, lobbyists' "need and dependence" on government officials. Salisbury, 1990, pp. 224, 229.

33. This claim is defended in greater detail in Kersh, 2002.

34. Holman, 2005, p. 35. For a more cautious but related scholarly assessment, see Piotrowski and Rosenbloom, 2005, 270–1.

35. Sloane, 2004, p. 33.

36. Holman, 2005, p. 44.

37. Fenno, 1973; an interesting recent comment on this theme is Miquel and Snyder, 2006.

38. Weisberg, 2006. The scholarly literature on contributions is voluminous: good recent studies include Primo and Milyo, 2006; Esterling, 2007; and the essays in Corrado et al., eds., 2006.

39. "Lobbyist contributions," as cataloged in this study, were of three types: donations by a lobbyist's *client* (corporation, trade association, or—less often—individual), with the funds directed and often personally delivered by the lobbyist; donations by the lobbyist's *firm;* or donations from the lobbyist's *personal* resources. This chapter does not distinguish between PAC and soft-money contributions, again for reasons of space.

40. About 45% of this total was from three lobbyists, whose organizations made multiple contributions during my observation periods. But 9 of "my" 11 lobbyists are included in the 296 decisions.

41. This from former GOP party chair Haley Barbour (personal interview, October 4, 1999); Barbour's firm's single-party contribution practice is unusual, as Barbour noted. His full explanation, coded as "ideological/partisan": "We try to give to people who need help the most, and who are strong for the [issues] we're for. Rather than who can help us out, if we could even measure that. Our goal is to help Republicans stay in the majority . . . so we only give to Republicans."

42. Esterling, 2007 discusses the propensity of groups to donate to high-status MCs.

43. Fuller details are spelled out in Kersh, 2003.

44. Scherer, 2006; Riskind, Torry, and Nash, 2006.

45. Herrnson, Shaiko, and Wilcox, 2005, p. 389.
46. Revelations were continuing as this chapter was written; details are available in Stone, 2006.
47. Powers, 2003; Lagerlöf and Frisell, 2004. See also Austen-Smith, 1993; Larocca, 2004; Rasmusen, 1993.
48. Kersh, 2007.

REFERENCES

Ainsworth, S.H. 1997. "The Role of Legislators in the Determination of Interest Group Influence." *Legislative Studies Quarterly* 22: 3.

Austen-Smith, D. 1993. "Information and Influence: Lobbying for Agendas and Votes." *American Journal of Political Science* 37: 3.

Barlett, D.L., and J.B. Steele. 2004. *Critical Condition: How Health Care in America Became Big Business—and Bad Medicine.* New York: Random House.

Bath, M.G., A.J. Nownes, and J. Gayvert Owen. 2005. "Female Lobbyists: The Gender Gap and Interest Representation." *Politics and Policy* 33: 5.

Bauer, R.A., I. De Sola Pool, and L.A. Dexter. *American Business and Public Policy: The Politics of Foreign Trade.* New York: Atherton Press.

Baumgartner, F.R., and B.L. Leech. 1998. *Basic Interests: The Importance of Groups in Politics and in Political Science.* Princeton: Princeton University Press.

Benoit, D. 2007. *Women Corporate Lobbyists, Policy, and Power in the United States.* New Brunswick, NJ: Rutgers University Press.

Berry, J.M. 1997. *The Interest Group Society.* New York: Longman.

Birnbaum, J. 2004. "Going Left on K Street." *Washington Post* July 2.

Browne, W.P. 1998. *Groups, Interests, and U.S. Public Policy.* Washington: Georgetown University Press.

Chaddock, G.R. 2003. "Republicans Take Over K Street." *Christian Science Monitor* August 29.

Cigler, A. 1994. "Research Gaps in the Study of Interest Group Representation." In William Crotty et al., eds., *Representing Interests & Interest Group Representation.* Lanham, MD: University Press of America.

Clemente, F., et al. 2002. "The Other Drug War II." Washington DC: Public Citizen.

Confessore, N. 2003. "Welcome to the Machine: How the GOP Disciplined K St. and Made Bush Supreme." *Washington Monthly* (July/Aug.).

Continetti, M. 2006. *The K Street Gang: The Rise and Fall of the Republican Machine.* New York: Doubleday.

Corrado, A., et al., eds. 2006. *The New Campaign Finance Sourcebook.* Washington DC: Brookings Institution.

Dunham, R.S. 2002. "The GOP's Wacky War on Dem [sic] Lobbyists." *Business Week* Online (June 24).

Dyckman, M. 2002. "Health Care is Big-Profit Business." *St. Petersburg (Fla.) Times* December 15.

Ehrenhalt, A. 1984. *Politics in America: Members of Congress in Washington and at Home.* Washington DC: Congressional Quarterly Press.

Esterling, K.M. 2007. "Buying Expertise: Campaign Contributions and Attention to Policy Analysis in Congressional Committees." *American Political Science Review* 101: 1.

Fenno, R. 1973. *Congressmen in Committees.* Boston: Little, Brown.

Franko, F.P. 2002. "The Federal System of Government and Health Policy Priorities." *AORN Journal* 7: 2.

Hacker, J.S. 1997. *The Road to Nowhere: The Genesis of President Clinton's Plan for Health Security.* Princeton: Princeton University Press.

Hacker, J.S., and P. Pierson. 2005. *Off Center: The Republican Revolution and the Erosion of American Democracy.* New Haven: Yale University Press.

Heaney, M.T. 2006. "Brokering Health Policy: Coalitions, Parties, and Interest Group Influence." *Journal of Health Politics, Policy and Law* 31: 4.

Heclo, H. 1978. "Issue Networks and the Executive Establishment." In Anthony King, ed., *The New American Political System.* Washington DC: American Enterprise Institute.

Heinz, J.P., et al. 1993. *The Hollow Core: Private Interests in National Policy Making.* Cambridge: Harvard University Press.

Herrnson, P.S., R.G. Shaiko, and C. Wilcox. 2005. "Interest Groups at the Dawn of a New Millennium." In *idem.,* eds., *The Interest Group Connection,* 2d ed. Washington DC: CQ Press.

Hojnacki, M., and D.C. Kimball. 1999. "The Who and How of Organizations' Lobbying Strategies in Committee." *Journal of Politics* 61: 4.

Holman, C., et al. 2005. *The Revolving Door: A Matter of Trust.* Washington DC: Center for Public Integrity.

Hula, K.W. 1999. *Lobbying Together: Interest Group Coalitions in Legislative Politics.* Washington, DC: Georgetown University Press.

Johnson, H., and D.S. Broder. 1997. *The System: The American Way of Thinking at the Breaking Point.* Boston: Little, Brown.

Kaplan, M. 2003. Interview on 'Marketplace.' Minnesota Public Radio (July 1).

Kendall, D., and S.R. Levine. 2000. "Governing the Ungovernable Health System." *Blueprint* 3: 2.

Kersh, R. 2002. "Corporate Lobbyists as Political Actors." In A.J. Cigler and B.A. Loomis, eds., *Interest Group Politics*. 6th ed. Washington DC: Congressional Quarterly Press.

—— 2003. "To Donate or Not to Donate? Washington Interest Group Representatives' Campaign-Contribution Decisions." Paper presented at the American Political Science Association annual meeting.

—— 2005. "Politics & the New Malpractice Crisis: Pennsylvania." Philadelphia: Pew Trust.

—— 2006. "Medical Malpractice and the New Politics of Health Care." In W.M. Sage and R. Kersh, eds., *Medical Malpractice and the U.S. Health Care System*. New York: Cambridge University Press.

—— 2007. "The Well-Informed Lobbyist: Information & Interest-Group Lobbying," in A.J. Cigler and B.A. Loomis, eds., *Interest Group Politics*. 7th ed. Washington DC: Congressional Quarterly Press.

Lagerlof, J.N.M., and L. Frisell. 2004. "Lobbying, Information Transmission, and Unequal Representation." CIC Working Paper, SP II 2004–02.

Larocca, Roger. 2004. "Strategic Diversion in Political Communication." *Journal of Politics* 66: 2.

Lowery, D., and V. Gray. 2004. "A Neopluralist Perspective on Research on Organized Interests." *Political Research Quarterly* 57: 1.

McFarland, A.S. 2004. *Neopluralism: The Evolution of Political Process Theory*. Lawrence: University of Kansas Press.

Miquel, G., and J. Snyder. 2006. "Legislative Effectiveness and Legislative Careers." *Legislative Studies Quarterly* 31: 3.

Moffit, R.E. 2001. "Personnel is Policy: Why the New President Must Take Control of the Executive Branch." Washington DC: Heritage Foundation.

Nownes, A.J. 1999. "Solicited Advice and Lobbyist Power: Evidence from Three American States." *Legislative Studies Quarterly* 24: 1.

—— 2006. *Total Lobbying: What Lobbyists Want (and How They Try to Get It)*. New York: Cambridge University Press.

Nownes, A.J., and P.D. Freeman. 1998. "Female Lobbyists: Women in the World of 'Good ol' Boys.'" *Journal of Politics* 60: 4.

Ogmundson, R. 2005. "Does it Matter if Women, Minorities and Gays Govern?: New Data

Concerning an Old Question." *Canadian Journal of Sociology* 30: 3.

Peterson, M. 1994. "Congress in the 1990s: From Iron Triangles to Policy Networks." In J.A. Morone and G.S. Belkin, eds., *The Politics of Health Care Reform: Lessons from the Past, Prospects for the Future*. Durham, NC: Duke University Press.

Piotrowski, S.J., and D.H. Rosenbloom. 2005. "The Legal-Institutional Framework for Interest Group Participation in Federal Administrative Policymaking." In P.S. Herrnson, R.G. Shaiko, and C. Wilcox, eds., *The Interest Group Connection*, 2d ed. Washington DC: CQ Press.

Primo, D.M., and J. Milyo. 2006. "Campaign Finance Laws and Political Efficacy: Evidence from the States." *Election Law Journal* 5: 1.

Rampton, S., and J. Stauber. 2004. *Banana Republicans: How the Right Wing is Turning America Into a One-Party State*. Los Angeles: Tarcher Press.

Rasmusen, E. 1993. "Lobbying When the Decisionmaker Can Acquire Independent Information." *Public Choice* 74: 4.

Riskind, J., J. Torry, and J. Nash. 2006. "Senior Aide to Rep. Ney Subpoenaed." *Columbus (Ohio) Dispatch*, June 30.

Sage, W.M., and E.D. Kinney. 2006. "Medicare-Led Malpractice Reform." In W.M. Sage and R. Kersh, eds., *Medical Malpractice and the U.S. Health Care System*. New York: Cambridge University Press.

Salant, J.D. 2003. "Many Clinton Officials Stay Close to Washington." *Washington Post* March 31.

Salisbury, R. 1990. "The Paradox of Interest Groups in Washington—More Groups and Less Clout." In A. King, ed., *The New American Political System*, 2d ed. Washington DC: American Enterprise Foundation.

Scherer, M. 2006. "Newt: I'm Shocked, Shocked by Abramoff Scandal." Available at http://www.salon.com/news/feature/2006/01/05/gingrich/index.html?sid=1422655 (last accessed October 22, 2006).

Schlozman, K.L. 1990. "Representing Women in Washington: Sisterhood and Pressure Politics." In L.A. Tilly and P. Gurin, eds., *Women, Politics, and Change*. New York: Russell Sage.

Skocpol, T. 1996. *Boomerang: Clinton's Health Security Effort and the Turn Against Government in U.S. Politics*. New York: Norton.

Sloane, T. 2004. "As the Revolving Door Spins: Medicare Law." *Modern Healthcare* 17: 3.

Smith, R.A. 1995. "Interest Group Influence in the U.S. Congress." *Legislative Studies Quarterly* 20: 1.

Stone, P.H. 2006. *Superlobbyist Jack Abramoff, His Republican Allies, and the Buying of Washington.* New York: Farrar, Straus, & Giroux.

Sulkin, T. 2005. *Issue Politics in Congress.* New York: Cambridge University Press.

VandeHei, J., and J. Eilperin. 2005. "Targeting Lobbyists Pays Off For GOP." *Washington Post* June 25.

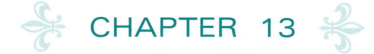

CHAPTER 13

Employers and Health Care: a Sick Business

Cathie Jo Martin

This chapter examines health politics and policy from the business perspective. Martin traces the costs and benefits of placing employers at the center of our health care system and examines the political strengths and weaknesses of the business community.

INTRODUCTION

One of America's great paradoxes lies in expecting business corporations to purvey social welfare benefits.* Capitalism celebrates defeating competitors and eliminating inefficiencies; welfare state norms prescribe equalizing opportunity and guaranteeing security for society's most marginal (and thereby inefficient) members. Business is about survival of the fit, while social policies are about protecting the weak.

Yet in the absence of a government health financing system, American employers have become key actors in both the provision of and policy debates about health care benefits. In this chapter we explain this unlikely scenario—taking up the employers'

roles as health care purchasers, as community activists, and as participants in policy debates. We explore how managers are changing health care markets in their role as health insurance purchasers; we investigate how business leaders engage in local efforts to control health costs and quality; and we reflect on business involvement with national health policy proposals.

This chapter offers five general insights into the uneasy relationship between employers and health care financing. First, the extensive system of firm-based health benefits has been both cause and effect of the absence of a national health financing system. Early corporate liberals (the relatively progressive wing of business) provided some social protections for the usual mixed motives: to enhance worker productivity, to halt unionization, and to meet needs left unfulfilled by the underdeveloped American state. Making the firm a central actor in health care financing, in turn, worked against future development of a public financing system.

Second, private sector financing helped produce a highly inflationary patchwork health care system. Health care costs claim 16% of the GNP and make the United States the highest health spender in the world. Although our health expenditures reflect an extremely sophisticated medical technology—middle class people often receive top-notch medical treatment—the system suffers from administrative inefficiencies, redundancies, and wasted resources that drive costs up without improving health outcomes.

Third, at the firm-level, employers have experimented with many health financing strategies to restrain the rising costs of worker health benefits and in the process have driven major changes in the health financing system. In the 1990s, firms' enthusiasm for managed care led to significant market restructuring. For example, Preferred Provider Organizations (PPOs) offered special discounts to firms when employees sought treatment from the physicians in the network. Health costs flattened out in the mid-1990s, then resumed their rapid rise. The various short-term efforts to save money may have fragmented risk pools and contributed to a longer term escalation in health prices.[1]

Fourth, at a community level corporate health reformers often join forces with labor activists, government bureaucrats and even hospitals to search for solutions to the problems of health quality, costs, and access. Community coalitions have had some success at making better use of existing resources, in eliminating duplication, and increasing coordination in the use of technology. These coalitions also demonstrate a pragmatism that is not evident when the same stakeholders meet at the national level. Still, the regional efforts have had little success in addressing the big issues—health care costs and access. Local coalitions have encountered particular difficulties in expanding access to uninsured people, although they have been somewhat more successful in making the "safety-net" system more efficient and effective.[2]

Finally, some employers have become involved in national legislative efforts to reform the health financing system; however, corporate activists have experienced great difficulty in generating business consensus on policy solutions. In part corporate actors are handicapped by attachments to their own private plans: those with market power to negotiate low prices (as well as the growing number who do not offer health benefits) are especially reluctant to deviate from the current system. The Clinton administration's reform effort exposed many stark divisions among firms: those with large retiree commitments had very different interests from those without them. A government mandate to provide health care coverage to workers—a central feature of the Clinton plan—was not a problem for those firms already paying for health benefits; but those that did not fund their workers' health care bitterly opposed the idea.

Business activism is also hampered by the enormous fragmentation of employer political organization. No unitary peak association exists in the United States to reconcile conflicting corporate interests and to present a united business perspective to legislators. Surprisingly, large firms—the most likely past supporters of comprehensive health reform—are less organized on health issues than the small business and provider interests that generally oppose reform. The Clinton effort painfully demonstrated the weaknesses of large employers in the health care area, and little has changed in the interim.

Business enthusiasm for national policy solutions is further constrained today by the lack of ideas about how to fix the system. Ten years ago managed competition appeared to be the silver bullet that would fire health reform: the concept promised to preserve the perks of the employer-based system while implementing system-wide reform. Although broad support for the concept eventually broke down, the idea had enough power to give reformers considerable political momentum. Today, no new idea has emerged to rally corporate supporters. Instead, managers have become more skeptical about grand solutions to the health crisis.

At the same time, the market-driven solutions that seemed so attractive after health reform's demise in the mid-1990s have also disappointed those searching for a palliative to the problems of cost, quality, and access.

EMPLOYERS AS PURCHASERS OF HEALTH CARE INSURANCE

American employers began providing social benefits in the 1920s, when "welfare capitalists" determined that social benefits (such as pensions, on-site medical services, and group health insurance) could enhance worker productivity and deter unions. Although some social protections were being created at the state level, national health insurance seemed unlikely after the failure of the early efforts of the American Association for Labor Legislation and the later decision not to include national health insurance in the New Deal social security bill. Corporate liberals resolved to fill the gap with company plans. They were encouraged by commercial insurers, who joined with employers to fight national health reform proposals and aggressively marketed the group insurance model to their new-found corporate friends. By 1926 over 400 large firms offered on-site services to their workers and by 1935 over a third of large employers provided some health insurance.[3]

The rudimentary firm-based health benefits created during the inter-war period became a robust system of private social provision after the Second World War. The Taft-Hartley Act of 1947 set up an institutional framework for health and pension trust funds: the funds would be paid for by employer and employee contributions negotiated through the collective bargaining process and usually administered by the unions. Although many within organized labor initially supported the creation of a national health system or community group health plans, political winds (and employer opposition) in the late 1940s and 1950s worked against a public solution.

Trade unions eventually fixed on the Taft-Hartley funds as the best way to secure health coverage for their members. Many of the strikes during this period concerned health care benefits. Thus while employers created the earliest health plans, organized labor collaborated in the expansion of "the shadow welfare state" after World War II.

Taft-Hartley plans addressed the health insurance needs of unionized workers, but the firms' non-union employees—in management and elsewhere—also required health coverage. The passage of the federal Employee Retirement Income Security Act (or ERISA) in 1974 provided an economic incentive and a regulatory framework for companies to create health financing programs for their non-unionized workers. ERISA stipulated that self-insured entities of a certain size—whether they be company or Taft-Hartley funds—were exempted from state regulations, on the grounds that many firms engaged in multi-state operations. This legislation thereby encouraged states to self-insure, or to pool their own workers' risk and to hire outside insurers to administer these company health plans. The long-term consequences of ERISA were profound. Companies seeking to avoid state regulations or constraints on their health packages (for example, mandatory benefits) moved to self-insurance in droves, creating a highly-fragmented health insurance landscape. Because each self-insured group negotiated its own prices, health care fees varied widely among groups. Large companies with the market power bargained for good deals and became attached to their self-insured plans. Even though costs continued to rise, the successful bargainers calculated that they would pay more in a world with evenly distributed health prices.

Firms in the post-war period seemed eager to expand their health benefits. Policy experts convinced managers that good health benefits enhanced job performance and curbed absenteeism. Superior health plans could attract talented workers, increase organizational commitment, and reduce turnover.[4]

Gradually private employment-based health benefits expanded to constitute a major component of the total health financing system. In 1965, households funded 60.5% of the our nation's health care; firms, 17%; and government, 20.7%; by 1989 each sector paid about one-third. In addition, the health benefits that began as a side show in collective bargaining gradually became a major component of total wage costs. Employers spent only 2.2% of salaries and wages on health benefits in 1965; these costs jumped to 8.3% by 1989. Health benefits accounted for 14% of all employer benefits in 1960 and 44% by 2005.[5]

With the corporate share of America's health financing rising, firms have good reason to worry about the seemingly boundless rise in costs. After a lull in the mid-1990s, premiums resumed their steep rise with averages that repeatedly ran into double digits after 2000. Small employers were hit especially hard.[6] Rising corporate costs can be traced to cost shifting in which governments—the most effective health fee bargainers—negotiated ever lower rates, leaving business and commercial insurers to pay more. Hospitals make up Medicare and Medicaid payment shortfalls with whopping bills to private payers.

In response to these pressures, many firms have simply stopped offering health benefits. According to the Bureau of Labor Statistics, 90% of large and medium sized firms offered health benefits by 1988, while only 76% offered benefits in 1998. Today most uninsured people are workers—only 15% are unemployed. Thus while access expanded in the last decade, the recession and the jobless recovery of the early 2000s took a toll. By 2004, one in five Americans (almost 45 million) lacked health insurance coverage. Because uninsured people are three times as likely not to receive necessary medical care, the growing ranks of the uninsured has significant ramifications for the health of the US population.[7]

Brian Klepper (from the Center for Practical Health Reform) reflects on the implications for business:

Cost increases are going so hard and fast that employers are up against the wall . . . All employers should expect a 5–8 percent hit above premium hits in October due to stress-related conditions linked to September 11. Employees are doing a lot of preemptive things because they fear the loss of their health benefits in the future . . . The health care system is going to go into free fall.

FIRM'S EFFORTS TO CONTAIN COSTS

Faced with an alarming rise in health costs, companies have scrambled to contain this seemingly uncontrollable share of their wage package. In the late 1980s, firms began moving their employees into managed care plans. Unlike other markets where price is arrived at by the interplay of supply and demand, the health market is distorted by a third party, the insurer, who traditionally pays for the care at the point of service. Managed care plans sought to restore the natural balance between supply and demand by making patients or their doctors sensitive to prices. In the HMO model, for example, health providers would be paid a fixed fee in advance for each patient; they would have incentives to curtail unnecessary services. The employees would be transformed from patients into wise health consumers; workers would be given a choice of plans, adequate information to choose among them wisely, and—in theory—financial incentives to chose a high quality–low cost plan.

In reality, companies offered few traditional managed care products. Instead, they sought market power through an industrial purchasing model, using their economies of scale to negotiate highly favorable rates with a few loosely managed health care plans. The firms rather than their employees (or the consumers) maintained control; the company negotiated lower costs for employees and greatly limited the choice in health plans.[8] Few firms signed up with traditional HMOs offering a single annual fee for each customer, a focus on prevention, and comprehensive benefits. Instead employers sought services from Preferred Provider Organization (PPO) plans and other soft managed care plans with retrospective, fee-for-service payment, thin benefits, large deductibles, and a wide choice of health care providers.[9]

Managed care worked for about five years, stemming the rising tide of health costs (especially during the mid-1990s during and immediately after the debate over federal legislation). By 2000, however, the savings came to an end and premiums resumed their seemingly inexorable rise. One study found that 92% of people in employment-based plans belonged to a managed care plan by the end of the decade. As the health market for managed care became saturated, insurers began changing their strategies by offering less restrictive plans with more choice, negotiating less adversarial relations with providers, and shifting focus from expanding market share to increasing profitability. In part this may reflect the consolidation that has transformed the group health insurance industry in recent years. With only a few insurance companies to choose from, employers lost much of their leverage to negotiate lower rates.[10]

Hospitals also helped keep rates low in the 1990s by offering significant discounts to their corporate clients. These discounts were not based on new efficiencies or on productivity improvements, but were drawn from the hospitals' stock market investments. When the stock bubble burst, the hospitals' portfolios dropped and providers began negotiating higher premiums. Simultaneously, provider systems merged or went out of business in many areas, creating de facto monopolies over health provision in much of the country. Backlash against managed care hit the news when public opinion surveys ranked these companies beneath oil firms and other popular villains. By 1998 four-fifths of Americans viewed reining in the managed care companies as a top priority issue.[11]

As savings from managed care began to ebb, some employers sought to contain their own share of health costs by shifting the burden onto their employers. Few employers increased premiums to their employees during the last half of the nineties—constrained, no doubt, by the tight labor market: the

employees' share of single-coverage premiums, in fact, dropped from 21% to 14% from 1996 to 2000. But firms created subtle forms of cost-shifting, increasing co-pays and deductibles and decreasing pharmacy benefits. Workers' share in deductibles rose by over 30% in 2002 and fights over health benefits have been at the center of current collective bargaining rounds.[12] Employers also offered options for employees to use pre-tax dollars to defray health costs, including deductibles and co-pays called Flexible Spending Accounts.

Some firms developed defined contribution plans and other "consumer directed" forms of financing health care, seeking to control costs and to limit liability. The defined contribution approach entails employers paying a fixed amount toward premium coverage, offering workers a choice of high and low cost plans (described in detail on the Internet); the approach generally includes a medical spending account, which employees pay into and draw from to fund health needs beyond the employer's major medical insurance. The employees arguably become more cost conscious and choose plans that best fit their individual needs. Still, the transference of liability from the employer to the employee troubles many critics. Employees with high co-pays and deductibles seem to be foregoing necessary primary, preventative, and pharmaceutical care. The transfer of liability falls much harder on individuals and families with chronic, complicated conditions who must use higher levels of health care. In a fully-developed defined contribution plan the firm loses all incentives to restrain the growth of premium costs as well as the responsibility for ensuring that its employees are insured. In addition, defined contribution plans threaten to fragment the risk pool even more than ever.[13]

Some firms have simply given up trying to cope with the soaring costs of health insurance coverage and have ended coverage for their workers, thus contributing to the growing ranks of the uninsured. This trend is most dramatic among small companies; since they have little market leverage and face high rates—the down side of the industrial bargaining model. Low-skilled workers at large companies have also been losing coverage (after all, they don't have much bargaining leverage either). The public holds very different attitudes toward the different kind of employers: there is substantial sympathy for small businesses struggling in the health insurance market; on the other hand, critics have been pummeling the Wal-Marts of the world for dropping dependent coverage, shifting health costs to their workers, and creating other barriers to insurance for low-wage and part-time workers.[14]

BUSINESS AND THE POLITICS OF COMMUNITY HEALTH REFORM

Optimism about employers' capacities to solve health financing problems has perhaps been greatest at the community level, especially in the 1980s when business struggles to control the community health costs resembled nothing less than a social movement. Yet despite this enormous corporate activism, local efforts to expand access and to control costs have ultimately fallen short. The stories of business efforts to change local health care delivery and financing, thus, mirror at the micro-level the disappointments of national endeavors to reform the health care system.

The regional coalition movement represents a high point in employer activism, as employers have been very influential in generating ideas, setting the agenda, and providing political clout for health initiatives in their regions. The community purchasing coalition movement developed in the 1970s: By banding together, reasoned the corporate reformers, firms might gain the market power necessary to leverage lower health costs and the political clout to monitor quality.[15] Cost and quality concerns transcend individual firms, and many benefits managers in Fortune 500 companies determined that their firms' health fortunes were tied to the health care policies of their local areas. In Cleveland, a coalition of

employers called the Health Action Council of Northeast Ohio (HAC) together with a CEO group called Cleveland Tomorrow forced hospitals to generate data on quality. In Minnesota, the Business Health Care Action Group (BHCAG) set out to change the health care market by improving the quality of care through the development of clinical practice guidelines.

Early assessments of the coalition movement tended to be fairly sanguine, and business managers felt enthusiastic joining this win-win effort.[16] Health expert Walter McClure explained that this focus on quality was politically appealing to CEOs, because it suggested that the productivity of health care can be improved and costs can be lowered without sacrificing benefits levels.[17] Foundations played an important role in funding and spurring the development of these community coalitions.[18] The movement also received help from community activists such as Doug Shaller who brought his background in community action to the task of organizing the corporate world.[19]

Ultimately, community initiatives largely faltered, and health costs soared even in regions that appeared to have the greatest initial successes.[20] In Massachusetts, Governor Mike Dukakis developed a comprehensive health plan and convinced both the Business Roundtable and the Associated Industries of Massachusetts to lobby vigorously for cost controls and "pay or play" requirements. This seemingly incongruous corporate position reflected the large employers' desire to be released from the burdens of paying for other employers' uninsured workers; thus, the business supporters of the Dukakis plan sought to impose costs on a group that did not provide benefits.[21] Yet ultimately the heath plan was legislated but never implemented, due to the same zero-sum corporate conflicts that roused initial business support. Participants in the struggle discovered the inevitable bottom line of health care policy: clashing interests are at play and each has something fundamental at stake, every successful cost cut for business is a revenue cut for a hospital, discounts for me lead to cost shifts to you, and firms that do not pay health insurance have radically different interests than those footing the bill.[22]

The California case tells a similar story of great initial optimism and subsequent disappointment. The Californian Pacific Business Group on Health struggled throughout the 1980s and 1990s to improve managed care delivery in the state: business consumers insisted that plans offer standardized packages, base physician compensation on performance measures, and use scientific data to justify purchases of new technology.[23] Yet after successfully restraining health costs throughout the 1990s, the California Employees Retirement System (CALPERS) announced rate increases for 2003 ranging from 19% to 25%.[24]

Finally, the Maine experiment (described in detail by Elizabeth Kilbreth in Part 2) in comprehensive health reform offers at once a cautionary tale about business activism and an ode to governmental leadership. Governor John Baldacci pushed through passage of a universal health care plan called the Dirigo plan after the motto of the plucky state ("I lead"). The initiative aimed to extend access to Maine's 180,000 uninsured residents through private insurers, by providing subsidies to low-income families and an affordable health insurance product to small businesses.[25] The initiative (after some political negotiation) passed in 2003 with bipartisan support and the endorsement of the state Chamber of Commerce and several major employers (such as Bath Iron Works, and Unum). At the point of implementation, however, the business support evaporated in part because the firms were purchased by out-of-state companies with little interest in broader community issues. Governor John Baldacci pushed on with support from a group of small firms, the Maine Small Business Alliance, that can't afford the current market.[26] The Portland Chamber of Commerce (that had opposed the state initiative) developed a private, small business product with Anthem Insurance to forestall the state's effort to pool and share risk and costs across a larger number of firms statewide. Although it is still too early to predict the success of the Maine initiative, the case reinforces a fundamental lesson about corporate leadership: major business players are often

enormously helpful in building political support for reform, yet their support is often ephemeral over the long-term.

EMPLOYERS IN NATIONAL HEALTH REFORM DEBATES

Employers have also become involved in policy debates over remedies to the health care crisis. Yet the large employers—so active in *community* level reform movements—are notably less influential in *national* policy debates. The reasons for this have to do with the diversity of employers interests, the constraints imposed by companies by virtue of their attachment to existing plans, and the organizational limitations of large employers in America.[27]

First, the so-called business community consists, in fact, of quite diverse interests: employers as a group may want cost containment, but as individuals they each want to preserve their market power. Firms deriving profit from the health care industry have different views of cost control than those in other sectors. Firms offering extensive benefits resent surtaxes to pay for the uninsured, but companies without benefits programs (and with a substantial share of uninsured workers) have clear financial incentives to resist such taxes. Many large manufacturing companies that provide benefits want to end cost shifting and to protect the ERISA preemption for their own private plans, yet those with extensive benefits commitments to retired workers have markedly different interests from those without such commitments.

Second, the large employers who are most likely to provide health insurance to their workers (and therefore have the most to gain from health reform) are handicapped by their own legacy of private provision. These large employers have been reluctant to deviate too much from the status quo, as they have deep vested interests in the current system. Thus policy makers have been constrained in the range of solutions acceptable to large firms.[28]

Third, the large employers with the most to gain from health reform are the least organized to act on their collective concerns because US business organization is quite fragmented and large firms lack an organizational forum to consider their collective interests. The big umbrella associations—the Chamber of Commerce, the National Association of Manufacturers, and the Business Roundtable—compete for members and are, consequently, unwilling to alienate minority voices with controversial stands. This organizational weakness makes it difficult for American managers to generate collective positions; and while large firms are quite competent at securing action on their targeted self-interests, they find it hard to take collective action for shared common goals.

Compared with the fragmented large employers, small business groups (representing firms least likely to offer health benefits) have achieved considerable political power through organization. Small employers have an easier task in battles over social regulation because it is easier to oppose than to promote; the small business groups also demonstrate unambiguous organizational advantages over large firms. Small business groups have been better able to play to the media; thus, small firm proprietors were found credible by 71% of journalists in 1982 but only 50% believed CEOs of big corporations.[29] The well-heeled corporate lobbyist wielding power behind closed doors lacks the television charisma of hundreds of restaurateurs storming Congress. Innovations in computer technologies have augmented the advantage of small business groups: grassroots computer mailings first made popular by public interest groups are perfectly suited to their large and varied membership.

Small business groups have also developed organizational decision rules to augment the natural advantages of a broad-based, numerous membership. The major small business groups have enhanced their power with single issue coalitions, which large employers with low-skilled workers (such as Pepsico) sometimes join. Coalitions organize to address a single issue and cannot afford to slip into inaction. Thus the major small business associations have been able partially to overcome the least-common-denominator

politics that handicaps much of the other business sector. These coalitions have also gained power in their close connections to the Republican party; indeed small firms have developed a far tighter alliance with the Republicans—especially in Congress—than large employers.

The dynamics surrounding employers' and health politics became apparent in the early 1990s during the debate over Bill Clinton's national health reform. The Clinton administration tried to devise a health reform proposal that was consistent with employers' preferences for private-sector solutions and with the extant employer-based system. The Clintons proposed to form health alliances to aggregate purchasers, but allowed firms with over 5,000 employees (eventually negotiated down to 500 workers) to opt out of these community pools. Thus, the health alliance concept was consistent with the move toward managed competition already occurring in the private sector and sought to fix the system while leaving large firms alone. The Clintons also proposed the aggregation of health providers into accountable health plans which would move health users away from fee for service arrangements and resembled the point of service plans already serving many corporate clients.[30] The big five insurers (as the primary organizers of managed care networks for corporate purchasers) initially hoped to administer the new Clinton system. Even the employer mandates did not seem to be an especially big change for the large employers, because many already provided health benefits. A defined benefits package with tax caps on employee deductions might help firms to curb their health commitments to unions and could force others in the industry to provide comparable levels of health benefits. Thus, where a single-payer arrangement and the virtual end of the employer-based system would be a very big leap for business, managed competition was a very small step from the status quo.

Due to the policy legacies of the patchwork employer-based system, firms motivated by the collective goal of fixing health financing also had particular (and diverse) interests in preserving their own position in health care markets. Because the Clinton plan deviated so slightly from the status quo, companies could easily calculate the differential impact of the bill on various corporate sectors. For example, firms without significant retiree benefits viewed the bill as inordinately helping companies with such commitments. Thus the very incremental nature of the Clinton plan contributed to its appearance as a zero-sum game. Joined to these concerns were those of single-payer proponents, who believed that the managed competition proposal would do little to achieve cost containment or to reduce administrative costs.[31]

The large employers who were most likely to support the Clinton health reform legislation were also hampered by their lack of an organizational forum. During the agenda-setting stage, large employers helped to make health reform a top political issue, in part working through the Washington Business Group on Health, but by 1990 this group had lost its activist edge with a decision to admit insurers as voting members. Other umbrella associations were unable to develop consensus on a health plan because of divisions within their ranks. The efforts of the National Association of Manufacturers (NAM) to develop a position exemplifies the difficulty. Most NAM members offered health benefits (99% in 1988), a majority supported a Clinton-style plan, and NAM's health care task force endorsed a comprehensive proposal complete with mandates. According to Ira Magaziner, who directed the Clinton reform effort, NAM's president, Jerry Jasoniwski, agreed to ask his board to support the Clinton plan in exchange for five changes in the plan. But before the critical board meeting in February 1994, health providers and fast food companies lobbied hard against the move. NAM staff reported going into the board meeting with "good things to say about the Clinton bill" and watching the board do a 180 degree turn.[32]

A similar story unfolded at the Chamber of Commerce. The Chamber originally testified before Congress in favor of the Clinton reform; in exchange the administration adopted the Chamber's small business discount schedule in the proposal.

Yet, the Chamber's support angered conservative Congressional Republicans, who demanded a meeting with the Chamber leadership and "read them the riot act" according to one participant. John Boehner (R-Ohio) sent letters on Congressional letterhead urging Chamber constituents to cancel their membership in the association and the National Federation of Independent Business initiated a membership drive against the Chamber, effectively forcing the Chamber to reverse its earlier position.[33]

In contrast to large employers, the major small business associations opposing reform were very well-organized and joined forces with small insurers and for-profit providers to battle health reform. Small business groups favored reforms to help small businesses buy group health insurance but opposed employer mandates because many small firms do not offer insurance. The powerful lobbying capabilities of small business were evident through the health reform debate. Thus when the Energy and Commerce Committee attempted to mark up a bill, NFIB mailed action alerts to all its members in the 10 districts with swing legislators, sent faxes to about 10% of its members, and held a press conference the day before Jim Slattery, Democratic Representative from Kansas, was to appear with President Clinton. Pizza Hut, headquartered in Topeka, wrote to all of the local Chambers of Commerce in Kansas. Despite committee chair John Dingell's many concessions to conservative Democrats, legislators ultimately rejected the Dingell compromise effort.

In the years since the failure of the Clinton health plan, large employers have been wary of national policy solutions to problems in health care financing. No clear consensus has emerged as to how to fix the health financing system, and this deficit of ideas creates a major roadblock to national policy efforts. While private firms and employers' coalitions have largely worked to control costs and to improve quality, the national legislative process has focused almost exclusively on quality and access—with little attention to cost control.

For example, the patients' bill of rights—which dominated the Congressional health agenda in the late 1990s—offered neither cost control nor expanded access. The patients' rights legislation had virtually no corporate supporters, because it allowed consumers to sue their health plans (and in some versions their firms). Employers worried that the legislation would expand their liability and drive up costs.[34] The political coalition developed to fight patients' rights legislation, the Health Benefits Coalition, was a direct descendant of the coalition of small business managers and private health care providers that defeated national health reform, the Health Equity Action League (HEAL). But the Health Benefits Coalition had an advantage over the HEAL because the patients' rights legislation achieved a remarkable unity in the business community—everyone was against it. The Health Benefits Coalition mobilized against patients' rights legislation; they were especially adamant about provisions that permitted patients to sue their health plans in federal court. For example, when the bipartisan Dingell-Norwood Patient's Bill of Rights was announced in August 1999, the coalition called the measure "The Health Insurance Elimination Act" and predicted that it would leave millions of additional individuals uninsured. In September 2000, the group announced the initiation of a $1 million ad campaign against the Dingell-Norwood-Kennedy bill.[35]

Large employers have been active at the national level in calling for the improvement of the quality of health services, largely through a coalition called the Leapfrog Group. The group sprang to life after the Institute of Medicine produced an alarming report in November 1999 that pointed to a chasm in the quality of hospitals. According to the report, between 44,000 and 98,000 hospital patients die yearly from preventable medical errors, with these errors costing between $17 and $19 billion a year.[36] The Leapfrog Group was organized by the Business Roundtable and includes the major purchasing coalitions, as well as a number of Fortune 500 companies such as AT&T, Bethlehem Steel, Caterpillar, DaimlerChrysler, Eastman Kodak, Ford, General Electric, Honeywell, IBM, LTV Steel, 3M, Motorola,

Siemens, and Sprint. Many of these firms were active in encouraging Congress to consider a comprehensive overhaul of the health system ten years ago. Now, the group reasons that employers can use their purchasing power to increase consumer knowledge about health care providers and, thereby, improve safety. Leapfrog members are urged to encourage the referral of patients to hospitals that have the best survival odds, that staff intensive care units with doctors having credentials in critical care, and that use error prevention software to prescribe medications. Thus the Leapfrog Group seeks to deal with some of the same issues as patients' rights legislation, but suggests that the prevention of medical mistakes can be achieved through the power of the marketplace rather than with the threat of a law suit.

Recently several groups have formed to work on costs control, although none can claim the title of clear leader in this area. The Wye River Group on Healthcare came together in 1998 to promote patient-driven health care benefits, especially defined contribution plans. The idea behind defined contribution plans is to inject consumer sensitivity back into health spending decisions.[37]

The Center for Practical Health Reform was formed as a non-profit, non-partisan group to brainstorm about and to advocate for national health reform. The group draws members from health care providers and consultants, insurers, and employers. Executive director, Brian Klepper, is a health consultant and the group includes employers such as Southwest Airlines, Dupont-Dowell, Wal-Mart, Microsoft, and Medtronic. Members have agreed upon goals of universal coverage, choice, retaining the private health care system, quality enhancements, and a desire to develop pragmatic changes that will improve the existing private-sector system. The group hopes to conduct roundtable discussions around the country to foster discussions on possible solutions.

Finally, a few recent groups with at least some business representation have formed to think broadly about access issues. The best known of these groups is CoveringTheUninsured.org, a "strange bedfellows group" that was partially funded by the Robert Wood

Johnson Foundation with leadership by Families USA and HIAA to raise public awareness of the problems of the uninsured. But to date the group has generated very little consensus about the appropriate policy directions for reducing the ranks of the uninsured, beyond a few incremental measures. Although all of the groups' 13 members agree that something must be done and most would prefer to retain the employer-based system, they remain deeply divided along predictable lines as to the appropriate solutions and they each have pet peeves. For instance, the Chamber and Health Insurance Association of America (HIAA) continue to oppose mandates and the AFL-CIO wants liability legislation for health plans. One health policy consultant to large employers concludes that although large firms are extremely worried about rising health costs, "they have no clear sense of direction . . . they are flailing but don't have a plan . . . There is no thinking about broader solutions in the business community."[38]

CONCLUSION

The ambivalent relationship between employers and health care has reached a critical juncture. Throughout the 20th century firms expanded the private health financing system to augment worker productivity, to prevent labor militancy, and to preempt public sector initiatives. Yet today the employment-based benefits system is threatening the health of the company and few managers are sanguine about controlling this once-fringe benefit. The very successes of the employer-based system—its diversity of funding arrangements, its individuality in matching health prices to the demographic characteristics of company pools, and its exclusivity in giving better deals to large firms with expansive market power—have worked to the long-term detriment of the system. The multiplicity of options has eliminated economies of scale in administering health plans. Individual actors with some market power have no incentives to risk radical change.

Yet few managers have arrived at an easy way out of the current predicament, especially as business has consistently shown a preference for tax incentives and market solutions, despite the apparent failure of these interventions over the past 2 years. Political realities doom non-incremental reforms and unintended consequences plague marginal adjustments to the health financing system. Employers have worked with other community activists to try and reform regional health systems. But in national policy debates, the large employers who form the bulwark of the employment-based system have had less political input; they have no new ideas, no effective organizations, and no faith that changes will bring them relief.

Perhaps a new idea will galvanize employers. Perhaps the scope of the health problems they face will push them to become engaged again in national policymaking. Alternatively, if the "party of the nonvoters" (about 50% of the potential electorate) ever rejoins the political debate, a national reform movement could radically redraw the contours of American health provision with or without corporate involvement. Under that scenario, Americans might even decide to end their paradoxical, increasingly troubled, employer based health care system.

STUDY QUESTIONS

1. Describe some of the accomplishments of local coalitions comprising organized labor, business interests, government, and medical institutions? Describe some of their failures.
2. Why were American businesses originally motivated to offer health care provisions for their employees?
3. How did the passage of ERISA affect the corporate health care landscape?
4. How did many businesses respond to rising health costs in the 1990's? How are many responding today?

5. What were the governing principles behind anticipated health care savings arising from managed care? Why did these savings prove transitory?

6. Why did the (first) Massachusetts experiment in comprehensive health coverage fail?

7. What part of the business community is best organized for politics?

8. Why has big business been ineffective when it comes to the national health care debate?

9. *Your opinion:* On balance, has the American reliance on employers to provide health benefits been a good thing? Should we strive to maintain this system? Or should we seek to end it.

NOTES

* The author wishes to thank Cathy Dunham and Jim Morone for their enormous knowledge and insights.

1. See, for example, Robinson, 2002.
2. Brown and McLaughlin, 1990.
3. The information in this section is largely drawn from Brandes, 1976; Hacker, 2002, especially p 201; Gottschalk, 2000; Klein, 2004; Gordon, 1991, p 165.
4. See for example, R. Bertera, 1990; Golaszewski, 1992; Tett and Meyer, 1993.
5. Kirk Victor, 1990; Levit, et al., 2002; McDonald, 2007.
6. Abelson, 2002; Fronstin, 2002.
7. Bureau of Labor Statistics home page, "Employee Benefit Survey."
8. *Lawrence Brown. 1983.*
9. Maxwell and Temin, 2002; Robinson, 2003.
10. Prince, 2001; Dutton, 2001.
11. For discussions of the public response see Jacobs and Shapiro; Morone, 1999; Blendon et al., 1998.
12. For discussions of these trends see Trude et al., 2002; Hudman and O'Malley, 2003.
13. Christianson, Parente, and Taylor, 2002; Sullivan, 2001; Stone, 1999.

14. Glied, Lambrew, and Little, 2003.
15. For great discussions of the rise of the coalition movements see Bergthold, 1990; and John, 1985.
16. Fraser et al., 1999.
17. Martin, 2000.
18. The Washington Business Group on Health, the Chamber of Commerce and the Robert Wood Johnson Foundation all helped to fund the coalitions. The Community Care Network Demonstration Program aimed to improve the health of communities with grants to develop public–private partnerships. A program called "Communities in Charge" sought to expand access by helping communities develop "more efficient and effective health care services for low-income, uninsured individuals." Robert Wood Johnson Foundation. 1999. "$16.8-Million Initiative To Help Local Communities." *RWJF Media Release.* Princeton, NJ: Robert Wood Johnson Foundation (January 26).
19. Interview with Dale Shaller.
20. Benko, 2001.
21. Kronick, 1990.
22. See also Morone, 1995; Brown, 1991.
23. Bergthold, Koebler, and Singer, 2000.
24. Interview with Larry Leavitt, Senior Vice-President of the Kaiser Family Foundation.
25. Alan Greenblatt, 2003.
26. Interviews with Trish Riley (Director of the Governor's Office of Health Policy and Finance) and Joseph Ditre (Head of the Maine Consumers for Affordable Health Care).
27. The following section is largely drawn from Cathie Jo Martin, 2000.
28. On this point see Martin, 2000, Hacker, 2002; Gottschalk, 2000.
29. Brown, Hamilton, and Medoff, 1990.
30. A Foster Higgins study found three-fourths of the firms already offering point of service plans. Foster Higgins/NAM, 1992.
31. See, for example, the work of Theodore Marmor.
32. Foster Higgins/NAM, 1992; interview with Ira Magaziner; Interview with NAM staffers.

33. Memo. To Ira Magaziner, from Robert Patricelli, "Follow-up to March 8, 1993 Meeting," (3–18–93); Interview with Chamber Staff.
34. See for example Hewitt Associates, 2001.
35. Information provided by the Health Benefits Coalition, 8–5–1999. Dingell Norwood ultimately passed in the Republican controlled house, 275–151, with President Bush supporting a watered down version.
36. Leapfrog Group. No Date. "About Us" and "Fact Sheet." http://www.leapfroggroup.org; Kohn, Corrigan, and Donaldson, 2000.
37. The group is chaired by John Comola, with additional direction offered by Marcia Comstock (previously at the Chamber of Commerce) and David Kendall of the Progressive Policy Institute.
38. The information in these paragraphs come from interviews with various participants.

REFERENCES

Abelson, R. 2002. Hard Decisions for Employers as Costs Soar in Health Care." *New York Times* April 18: C1.

Altman, S., S. Goldberger, and S. Crane. 1990. "The Need for a National Focus on Health Care Productivity." *Health Affairs* (Spring): 107–16.

Benko, L. 2001. "Coalitions lose mission." *Modern Healthcare* (May 14): 56.

Bergthold, L. 1990. *Purchasing Power in Health.* New Brunswick, New Jersey: Rutgers University Press.

Bergthold, L., S. Olson Koebler, and S. Singer. 2000. "In loco parentis? The purchaser role in managed care." *California Management Review* 43 (1 Fall): 34–49.

Bertera, R. 1990. "The effects of workplace health promotion on absenteeism and employment costs in a large industrial population." *American Journal of Public Health* 80 (9 September): 1101–5.

Brailer D., and L. Van Horn. 1993. "Health and the Welfare of U.S. Business." *Harvard Business Review* 71 (2 March-April): 128.

Brandes, S. 1976. *American Welfare Capitalism.* Chicago: University of Chicago Press.

Brown, C.J.H., and J. Medoff. 1990. *Employers Large and Small.* Cambridge: Harvard University Press.

Brown, L. 1983. *Politics and Health Care Policy: HMOs as Federal Policy.* Washington DC: Brookings Institution.

Brown, L. Shadow Governance: the Political Construction of Health Policy Leadership. *Journal of Health Politics, Policy and Law* 28.2-3 (2003) 517-524.

Business and Health. 1991. "Leaders look at health care." *Business and Health* 9 (2 February): 8–9.

The Center for Population Studies. 2002. "Annual Demographic Survey" (March supplement) Table HI01. "Health Insurance Coverage Status and Type of Coverage by Selected Characteristics." http://ferret.bls.census.gov/macro/032003/health/h01_001.htm.

Chicago Business Group on Health, Health and Medicine Policy Research Group, and Midwest Business Group on Health. 2001. "Business Perspectives on the Uninsured." Conference Report (June 13).

Christianson, J., S. Parente, and R. Taylor. 2002. "Defined-contribution health insurance products: Development and prospects." *Health Affairs* (Jan/Feb).

CoveringTheUninsured.org. 2002. "Two Million Americans Lost Their Health Insurance in 2001" (February 12). Coveringtheuninsured.org/media/docs/release021202.php3.

Craig, J. Jr. 1985. "Private Foundations' Role in Coalitions." J. Jaeger ed., *Private Sector Coalitions.* Durham, NC: Duke University Press.

Draper, D., R. Hurley, C. Lesser, and B. Strunk. 2002. "The Changing Face of Managed Care." *Health Affairs* 21 (1 Jan/Feb): 11–23.

Dutton, G. 2001. "The shrinking pool of plans." *Business and Health* 19 (6): 14–6.

Foster Higgins/NAM. 1992. "Employer Cost-shifting Expenditures." (November).

Fraser, I., P. McNamara, G. Lehman, S. Isaacson, and K. Moler. 1999. "The Pursuit of Quality by Business Coalitions: a National Survey." *Health Affairs* 18 (6 Nov/Dec): 158–65.

Fraser, I., P. McNamara, G. Lehman, S. Isaacson, and K. Moler. 1999. "The Pursuit of Quality By Business Coalitions." *Health Affairs* (November-December).

Freyer, T. 1992. *Regulating Big Business.* New York: Cambridge University Press.

Fronstin, P. 2002. "Trends in health insurance coverage: A look at early 2001 data." *Health Affairs* 21 (1 Jan/Feb): 188–93.

Glascoff, D. 2001. "Corporate Health Care Purchasing Among Fortune 500 Firms." *Marketing Health Services* 21 (3 Fall): 37.

Golaszewski, T. 1992. "A benefit-to-cost analysis of a work-site health promotion program." *Journal of Occupational Medicine* 34 (2 December): 1164–72.

Goldstein, A. 2002. "Budget's Health Care Priorities Detailed." *Washington Post* (January 31), A23.

Gottschalk, M. 2000. *The Shadow Welfare State*. Ithaca, NY: Cornell University Press.

Gugenheim, A.M., and L. Diamond Shapiro. 2001. "Working with employers to increase SCHIP enrollment." *Health Affairs* 20 (1): 287–90.

Hacker, J., and T. Skocpol. 1997. "The New Politics of U.S. Health Policy." *Journal of Health Politics, Policy and Law* 22 (2 April): 315–38.

Hacker, J. 2002. *The Divided Welfare State*. New York: Cambridge University Press.

Health Benefits Coalition. 6–16–1999. "Employers Launch Major Advertising Blitz to Oppose New Health Care Mandates and Lawsuits." Press Release. Washington DC: National Benefits Coalition. http://www.hbcweb.com.

Health Benefits Coalition. 8–5–1999. "The Health Insurance Elimination Act of 1999." Press Release. Washington DC: National Benefits Coalition. http://www.hbcweb.com.

Health Benefits Coalition. 10–28–1999. "Kaiser Survey Misreads Employers' Opposition to the Expanded Right to Sue." Press Release. Washington DC: National Benefits Coalition. http://www.hbcweb.com.

Health Action Council of Northeast Ohio. "Rethinking the Health-Care Marketplace." Obtained from the Council. No date.

Hewitt Associates. 2001. "US Employers Are Frustrated with Health Care Delivery and Looking for New Alternatives." Press release (February 12). http://was.hewitt.com/hewitt/resource/newsroom/ressrel/2001/02-12-01.htm.

Ioma's Report. 2001. "Communications and coalitions help Searsc control HC costs." *Ioma's Report on Managing Benefits Plans* 1 (6 June): 1.

Jacobs, Lawrence and Robert Shapiro. The American Public's Pragmatic Liberalism Meets its Philosophical Conservatism." *Journal of Health Politics, Policy and Law* 24 (5 October): 1021–31.

Judis, J. 1995 "Abandoned Surgery." *The American Prospect*. November 30: 65–73.

Klein, J. "The Politics of Economic Security." *Journal of Policy History* (January 2004): 34–65.

Kohn, L., J.M. Corrigan, and M.S. Donaldson. 2000. *To Err Is Human*. Washington DC: Institute of Medicine.

Kronick, R. 1990. "The Slippery Slope of Health Care Finance: Business Interests and Hospital Reimbursement in Massachusetts." *Journal of Health Politics, Policy and Law* 15: 887–913.

Leapfrog Group. No Date. "About Us" and "Fact Sheet." http://www.leapfroggroup.org.

Levit, K., C. Smith, C. Cowan, H. Lazenby, and A. Martin. 2002. "Inflation spurs health spending in 2002." *Health Affairs* 21 (1 Jan/Feb): 172–81.

Lovern, E. 2002. "Coalition for uninsured renews lobbying efforts." *Modern Healthcare* 32 (8 Feb 25): 10–11.

Martin, C.J. 1993. "Together Again." *Journal of Health Politics, Policy and Law* 18 (2 Summer): 359–93.

——— 2000. *Stuck in Neutral*. Princeton: Princeton University Press.

Maxwell, J., and P. Temin. 2002. "Managed Competition versus Industrial Purchasing of Health Care among the Fortune 500." *Journal of Health Politics, Policy and Law* 22 (1 February): 5–29.

McDonald, J. 2007. "The 7 Trillion Dollar Question." *EBRI Notes.* December, 2006. Employee Benefits Research Institute.

McNerney, W. 1990. "A Macroeconomic Case For Cost Containment." *Health Affairs* (Spring): 172–4.

Morone, J. 1995. "Nativism, Hollow Corporations and Managed Competition." *Journal of Health Politics, Policy and Law* 20 (2 Summer): 391–398.

——— 1999. "Populists in A Global Market: The Backlash Against Managed Care." *Journal of Health Politics, Policy and Law,* 24 (5 November): 887–895..

NFIB. 1995. "NFIB Named 'Most Powerful.'" *Capitol Coverage.* Washington, National Federation of Independent Business (December).

Pacific Business Group on Health. "About the Pacific Business Group on Health." http://www.pbgh.org.

Peterson, M. 1993. "Political Influence in the 1990s: From Iron Triangles to Policy Networks." *Journal of Health Politics, Policy and Law* 18 (2 Summer): 395–438.

Peterson, M. 2001. "From Trust to Political Power." *Journal of Health Politics, Policy and Law* 26 (5 October): 1145–63.

Prince, M., and L. Fletcher. 2000. "Benefit managers fear consequences of patients' rights bill." *Business Insurance* 34 (51 December 18): 3, 6.

Prince, M. 2001. "Employers looking beyond managed care." *Business Insurance* 35 (33 August 13): 1, 25.

Robert Wood Johnson Foundation. 1999. "$16.8-Million Initiative To Help Local Communities." *RWJF Media Release*. Princeton, NJ: Robert Wood Johnson Foundation (January 26).

Robinson, J. 2003. "The Politics of Managed Competition." *Journal of Health Politics, Policy and Law* 28 (2 April): 341–353.

Shortell, S., A. Zukoski, J. Alexander, G. Bazzoli, D. Conrad, R. Hasnain-Wynia, S. Sofaer, B. Chan, E. Casey, and F. Margolin. 2002. "Evaluating Partnerships for Community Health Improvement." *Journal of Health Politics, Policy and Law* 27 (1 February): 49–91.

Stone, D. 1999. "Managed Care and the Second Great Transformation." *Journal of Health Politics, Policy and Law* 24 (5 October): 1213–8.

Strunk, B., and P.J. Cunningham. 2002. "Treading Water: Americans' Access to Needed Medical Care, 1997–2001," Center for Studying Health System Change: Tracking Report No. 1 March.

Sullivan, P. Jr. 2001. "Defined contribution health plans: Future or fad?" *Compensation & Benefits Management* 17 (1 Winter): 11–15.

Tett, R., and J. Meyer. 1993. "Job satisfaction, organizational commitment, turnover intention and turnover." *Personnel Psychology* 46: 259–93.

Trude, S., J. Christianson, C. Lesser, C. Watts, and A. Benoit. 2002. "Employer-sponsored health insurance: Pressing problems, incremental changes." *Health Affairs* 21 (1 Jan/Feb): 66–75.

Uchitelle, L. 2002. "Stagnant wages Pose Added Risks to Weak Economy." *New York Times* (August 11): A1, 18–19.

Wall Street Journal. 1995. "Big Business vs. the GOP?" *Wall Street Journal* (March 13): A14.

Wechsler, J. 2001. "Showdown or slowdown on patients' rights bill?" *Managed Healthcare Executive* 11 (8 September): 11–12.

——— 2002. "Strange-bedfellows coalition seeks to raise awareness of uninsured." *Managed Healthcare Executive* 12 (3 March): 9–10.

Werntz, R. 2002. Phone interview.

Wilson, G. 2003. *Business and Politics*. Washington DC: CQ Press.

Deborah Stone

A report from the real world of patients and medicine. Deborah Stone shows us how impenetrable bureaucracy, overworked staff members, and defensive legalism wipe out our privacy and bury the patient's right to know.

A few years ago, I had a mole removed from my forehead. I'd had a preliminary consultation with the dermatologist—even such simple things are never done on the spot. On the day I returned for the actual excision, the receptionist gave me a form to sign, saying, "We need this form in order to biopsy it."

Of course, I thought to myself, they have to get my consent, if only so my insurer will pay. Nevertheless, I always read forms before signing. The part she was asking me to sign read: "I understand that Medicare will not pay for a pap smear test for one of the following reasons (there were four boxes that could be checked, but none of them was). I agree to be personally responsible for all the charges."

"I don't understand," I said. "I'm not on Medicare and I'm not having a Pap smear."

"You're reading too much into it," the receptionist snapped. "It has nothing to do with Medicare. We need your signature in order to biopsy it," and then, after a pause meant to suggest my impending stupidity, she drawled, "unless you don't *want* it biopsied."

"Well then," I asked, "is this saying that I will have to pay for the biopsy?"

"No," she said, still exasperated. "Your insurance will cover it."

Well-informed patients and strictly regulated consent procedures are the foundations of the medical market place and the supposed guarantees that medicine will treat patients right. In practice, informed consent is a sham. Medical staffs administer these forms as if they are a royal nuisance, and by and large, they brook no questions from patients. "Shut up and sign" is the prevailing attitude.

Most people don't even read medical consent forms before signing, and the clinical staff don't *expect* patients to read them. When someone like me comes along, someone who actually reads forms and asks questions, the staff get flummoxed, annoyed, or both.

Once, on admission to a hospital for a breast lump biopsy (it was benign), the admitting clerk handed me a consent form saying, "This just allows us to bill your insurance company." I read it over. Billing my insurer was only one of about six or seven things for which the form asked my permission. Most notable to me was authorization for the hospital and its physicians to do anything to me they deemed necessary while I was in their custody.

Given that I was going in for a breast biopsy and given the history of breast cancer treatment—namely radical mastectomies performed at the surgeon's discretion without consultation with the woman—I found this consent form horrifying, no matter that I had discussed this very issue with my surgeon and that she had assured me she NEVER did surgical treatment or even lymph node dissections at the same time as the initial biopsy.

I pointed out to the admitting clerk that the form was about more than permission to bill my insurer. "Oh really?" She professed surprise.

Each time I have visited that same hospital for mammograms and follow-up care, the admitting clerk has handed me a consent form with the same cheery line, as if she's offering me a special deal: "This just allows us to bill your insurance company." I practically know the form by heart. It's a HIPAA form, now ubiquitous in the medical world. You can't walk into a clinic or office anymore without being asked to sign that you've received a notice of the institution's "privacy practices." This particular form does indeed say that I authorize the hospital to disclose my health information to my insurer. It also says I've seen the hospital's "notice of privacy practices," which is a separate form—six pages, single spaced—listing myriad ways "we may use or disclose your protected health information."

The form tells me that the hospital may share my health information both inside and outside the conglomerate Boston health system of which it is a part. It may use my information for medical research and for training new health care workers. The health system may use my health information to contact me not only about "patient care issues, treatment choices, and follow-up instructions," but also "with other health related benefits and services that may be of interest to you"—in other words, marketing. And also, "for fundraising to support [the system] and its mission of excellence, provided, however, that such information is limited to demographic information only." Bill my insurance company, indeed.

By signing the HIPAA form, I'm authorizing a mega-hospital system to include me in its research, business operations, marketing, and fundraising databases, not to mention that I'm giving it permission to turn over my "protected health information" to law enforcement, public health, and other government authorities. These HIPAA "notices of privacy" are grossly misnamed. They're notices of publicity. All the paperwork in the name of privacy masks how patient privacy has been gutted. And it's all carried out through the rituals of informed consent—we give you a notice; you read it, understand it, agree to its provisions, and pen your signature to signify your consent.

As if to underline how vacuous and absurd the HIPAA process has become, one diagnostic imaging center I've used keeps a wastebasket by the door with a prominent sign, "Please Discard Unwanted Privacy Notices Here." Both times I've been there, the basket was full. In another doctor's office where I have an annual check-up, the receptionist greets me with something like, "You probably don't want a copy of our privacy notice, but I need you to sign this paper saying you've received it."

Most medical visits now begin with this parody of consent: the patient is asked to sign a piece of paper saying they've received another piece of paper. No one cares whether they've read or understood the piece of paper that provides the important information. This inane ritual inures people to the very idea of consent as a useful and informative procedure.

Okay, maybe the privacy notices aren't so important after all, but surely good information is essential for wise decisionmaking about medical treatment. For another surgery I needed, the consent form warned me of many potential, if unlikely, risks of this procedure, including death. My surgeon had discussed the "one percent" chance of cutting the nerves to my vocal cords, leaving me unable to speak, but he hadn't mentioned death. I raised my eyebrows and uttered some sort of startled exclamation about meeting my maker quite so soon. "Oh, we have to say that for everything," the admitting clerk assured me. "If I were you, I'd just sign it, because you have to in order to have the surgery."

There's something cynical and duplicitous about making patients sign off on every risk, including death, no matter how remote the possibility. Another form I had to sign to have my mole excised, a procedure for which I would be having Novocain, warned me that "all forms of anesthesia involve risk and the possibility of complications, injury, and sometimes death." Crying wolf undermines the credibility of all warnings, to the point that even the people administering informed consent forms tell patients not to believe the information.

A key principle of the law of contract, the principle that underlies informed consent in medicine, is the idea that parties to a contract must give their consent voluntarily. Coerced consent, consent obtained under duress, is not consent and cannot make a valid contract. In practice, there's coercion in every act of medical informed consent. There's subtle coercion in the staff's perfunctory presentation of consent documents, in their impatience with people who actually read them, and in their outright misrepresentation of what these documents say. And there's brute coercion in the situation: as the admitting clerk said to me, unless you sign, we won't treat you.

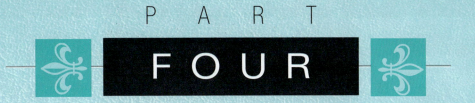

Outcomes: Programs, Politics, Problems

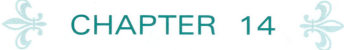

CHAPTER 14

Medicare: The Great Transformation

Jonathan Oberlander

This chapter describes Medicare, the largest federal health care program. The author explains how Medicare has passed through four historical stages. And he points to the great tension that has marked the program's conflicts, past and present: Medicare's original vision reflected liberal ideas which clash with the contemporary conservative vision that emphasizes markets and competition.

Medicare is a major arena of conflict in American health politics. The fault-line in Medicare politics, while not exclusively partisan, primarily divides Democrats from Republicans, liberals from conservatives, advocates of government health insurance from proponents of private insurance. It is a fight that does not lend itself to easy compromises or final resolution because Medicare invokes fundamental debates about the welfare state, health care reform, and generational equity.

Time will not ease this clash. As the baby boomers age into Medicare, the stakes associated with Medicare reform will only grow. Between 2000 and 2030, the share of the American population age 65 and over will increase from 12 to 20% and Medicare enrollment will nearly double, from 40 to 78 million beneficiaries. The fiscal pressures exerted on and by Medicare will be substantial and undoubtedly will intensify debates over program reform. Medicare,

then, figures to be a prominent issue in American politics for years to come.

This chapter explores the dynamics of Medicare politics, identifying major themes and changes in Medicare politics since the program's adoption in 1965. The chapter is organized around four eras in Medicare's history.[1] I begin with the origins of Medicare and the fight over its *enactment*. Next, I describe the politics of *accommodation* that governed Medicare's first 15 years of operation. The third section turns to the *regulation* revolution in Medicare policy that transformed the program's payment systems for hospitals and physicians. The fourth section explores the rise of competition and *markets* as frameworks for Medicare policy. Finally, I conclude by examining how the 2003 Medicare Prescription Drug, Improvement, and Modernization Act is reshaping Medicare and by speculating about Medicare's political future.

THE POLITICS OF ENACTMENT

Medicare's Origins

Medicare's story begins with the failed campaign for national health insurance during the first half of the 20th century.[2] Progressives introduced a model bill for compulsory health insurance to submit to state legislatures in 1915, but it failed due to a combination of political naïveté (advocates assumed "rational argument and statistical persuasion" were sufficient to win legislative passage); mobilization of opposition forces (including employers, the insurance industry, labor leader Samuel Gompers, and after reversing its initial supportive stand, the American Medical Association, which represented US physicians); and bad timing and xenophobia (American entry into World War I enabled opponents to denounce compulsory health insurance as a "German plot," while the 1917 Russian revolution similarly led to charges that reform was "un-American").[3] These same political forces proved to be enduring barriers to establishing national health insurance throughout the 20th century.

The 1935 Social Security bill originally contained a single line authorizing study of health insurance, prompting vigorous protests from the American Medical Association (AMA), which believed government health insurance threatened the organizational, financial, and clinical autonomy of physicians. President Franklin D. Roosevelt, fearing the controversy would jeopardize enactment of his Social Security legislation, refrained from pushing health insurance and ordered the line removed from the Social Security Act. His successor, Harry Truman, became the first American president to formally endorse national health insurance but fared no better in winning its passage. Truman, like FDR, ran into the AMA's unrelenting opposition—they turned debate over national health insurance into a Cold War–era referendum on "socialized medicine"—as well as a conservative coalition of Southern Democrats and Republicans that formed a voting majority in Congress and blocked much of his domestic agenda. Proposals for universal insurance went nowhere in Congress.

Advocates of national health insurance within the Truman administration believed it was time for a new strategy. Wilbur Cohen and I.S. Falk, advisers to Federal Security Agency administrator Oscar Ewing, developed a plan to provide federal health insurance to beneficiaries of Social Security payments for Old Age and Survivors Insurance (OASI). In June 1951, Ewing publicly announced a proposal for 60 days of hospital insurance a year for the 7 million elderly retirees receiving Social Security, saying "it is difficult for me to see how anyone with a heart can oppose this."[4]

The plan reflected a political calculus of incrementalism.[5] By restricting eligibility to the elderly, narrowing benefits to hospital care, and linking federal health insurance to Social Security, the architects of the Medicare strategy hoped to achieve a goal that had eluded the Truman administration and previous reformers: enactment of federal health insurance. In focusing on the elderly, Medicare's architects intended to take advantage of the political sympathy that seniors commanded as a deserving population that was both sicker and more likely to be uninsured than working-age Americans in the 1950s. By omitting benefits for physician services, reformers hoped to tamp down the AMA's opposition to a federal insurance program. And by proposing health insurance through Social Security (which provided the model for Medicare's eligibility rules, financing, and administrative arrangements) they hoped to exploit political associations with America's most popular social program and curry favor with the public.

Ultimately, of course, the Medicare strategy worked—after a half-century of failure, Medicare's enactment in 1965 represented a singular triumph for reformers. But that success came only after a contentious, decade-long debate and an electoral landslide that transformed American politics. Indeed, the carefully calibrated Medicare proposal did not succeed in calming the AMA's opposition to federal health insurance; for organized medicine, 60 days of hospital insurance for the elderly still constituted socialized medicine and set a dangerous precedent for government intervention in the health care system. The AMA saw Medicare as a slippery slope to national health insurance. They consequently campaigned just as hard against Medicare as they had against the Truman plan. Meanwhile, though Medicare attracted substantially more support in Congress than prior national health insurance proposals had (Medicare sponsors came within one vote of winning a majority on the crucial House Ways and Means committee in 1964), it still fell short of garnering enough votes to pass Congress. The 1964 elections—Democrat Lyndon Johnson won the presidency in a landslide and Democrats gained wide majorities in both the House and Senate, thereby breaking the power of the conservative coalition—ended the impasse over Medicare, leading to its enactment in 1965.

1965 Legacies

It is worth highlighting several key features of Medicare as it was enacted in 1965 because they created enduring political legacies and policy dilemmas that continue to influence Medicare today.

First, Medicare provided a limited benefits package focused on protecting beneficiaries against the acute costs of medical care rather than providing comprehensive insurance for all medical costs or covering care for chronic illness. The Medicare legislation enacted in 1965 was significantly broader than the original Medicare proposal—House Ways and Means Chair Wilbur Mills engineered a compromise that added insurance for physicians' services and the Medicaid program for low-income Americans to the bill—but it still omitted coverage of critical services such as outpatient prescription drugs, long-term nursing home care, hearing aids, and dental care. Moreover, Medicare required significant beneficiary cost-sharing without any cap on

catastrophic expenses or limit on how much enrollees could pay in a given year. These limited benefits led directly to the growth in Medigap and employer-sponsored supplemental health insurance policies that many Medicare beneficiaries carry to fill in the program's sizable holes, and set the stage for subsequent fights over expanding Medicare benefits.

Second, Medicare at the start was divided into two programs: Medicare Part A, primarily covering hospitalization, and Medicare Part B, primarily covering physician services. This division was born of political circumstances and divergent histories—Part A, funded by payroll taxes, represented the original 1951 Medicare proposal built on principles of social insurance while Part B, funded by general revenues and beneficiary premiums, reflected the efforts of Wilbur Mills in 1965 to satisfy anticipated beneficiary expectations by extending Medicare benefits without further increasing payroll taxes. Medicare was thus created as a bifurcated program with two different funding mechanisms, two different cost-sharing arrangements, and two separate trust funds. The division, which reflected conventional insurance arrangements at the time of Medicare's enactment, contrasts with contemporary efforts to integrate and coordinate medical services across different settings. It has created distinctive political dynamics—Medicare politics have been driven much more by financial conditions in the Part A trust fund than by Part B—and arguably led to Medicare policymaking that is fragmented by service category rather than focused on more comprehensive approaches to reform.[6]

Third, Medicare borrowed trust fund and payroll tax financing arrangements from Social Security, as well as long-term projections of "actuarial soundness," where they were credited with building that program's public support and political strength. However, predicting pension costs is much easier than forecasting health care spending, so Medicare's actuarial performance proved to be more volatile than Social Security's. The high rate of growth in US health care costs meant that Medicare confronted inflationary pressures from the beginning that pushed program spending upward and often defied prediction. Moreover, as the antitax movement in American politics gained strength in the 1970s and 1980s, increases in the Medicare payroll tax were increasingly difficult to come by in Congress, putting the program in a fiscal straightjacket. As a result, trust fund and payroll tax arrangements did not simply guarantee Medicare's political and fiscal stability, instead they also generated a series of intermittent trust fund crises that fed fears Medicare was "going bankrupt." These funding shortfalls have in turn catalyzed periods of policy activism in Medicare, creating a cycle of crisis and reform that has long defined Medicare politics.

Fourth, Medicare was in key respects a liberal program. Philosophically, Medicare incorporated social insurance principles favored by American liberals. Eligibility was established through payroll tax contributions with compulsory participation for all workers so benefits were earned, rather than provided as welfare only to those recipients poor enough to meet a means test. Medicare provided universal coverage for its intended population (the elderly), regardless of beneficiaries' income, in a single program and that coverage was provided via public health insurance operated by the federal government. Medicare was created, in other words, as a single-payer health insurance program similar to the Canadian system that health care reformers on the Left often hold up as a model. The liberal foundations of Medicare made political sense in 1965 in the midst of the Great Society when liberals were in political ascendance; the program's structure reflected their values and political commitments. However, as American politics turned rightward from the 1970s onward, Medicare's liberal form increasingly clashed with the preferences of conservative politicians who wanted to remake Medicare into a program that reflected their own values and political commitments. That tension between Medicare's original liberal vision and a more conservative vision that favors markets and competition remains the central cleavage in Medicare politics today.

Fifth, Medicare was intended by its advocates as a beginning, not an end.[7] After Medicare demonstrated how effectively government health insurance

could work, its advocates assumed opportunities would soon arise to build on its success, perhaps by covering children next. Medicare would thereby pave the way for a system of universal coverage, the long deferred dream of American health reformers; the strategy was incrementalism, the ultimate goal universalism. But Medicare did not expand as planned, though it did add coverage for end-stage renal disease patients and persons receiving Social Security disability insurance in 1972. Over four decades after its enactment, Medicare remains a standalone program for (mostly) the elderly, and the United States has not achieved universal coverage. Health care reformers today are consequently still deciding whether to build on or around Medicare, whether it is a model to be emulated, ignored, or overcome. And debates over the impact of population aging are shaped crucially by the fact that, unlike most industrial democracies, the United States has isolated the elderly into their own health insurance program that is financed separately from the rest of the health care system, which makes the impact of the baby boomers' retirement seem larger than it really is.[8]

Having outlined the politics of Medicare's enactment and identified attendant legacies, I now turn to the next era in Medicare politics: accommodation.

THE POLITICS OF ACCOMMODATION

Medicare was born in conflict, the debate over its enactment marked by sharp ideological and partisan divisions as well as the AMA's vocal opposition. Medicare's programmatic arrangements were consequently shaped by the desire of program advocates to first win its enactment and then to secure a smooth start for the program. They hoped that a successful start would demonstrate the promise of federal health insurance as a prelude to expanding Medicare into a broader system of national health insurance. Medicare's political sponsors believed the program's enactment and implementation could both be facilitated by the same strategy: accommodation of the medical industry.[9]

The 1965 Medicare law openly announced that the federal government would take a hands-off stance towards medical providers. Section 1801 of the Medicare legislation declared that "Nothing in this title shall be construed to authorize any Federal officer or employee to exercise supervision or control over the practice of medicine or the manner in which medical services are provided . . ."[10] The message was loud and clear: the federal government promised not to disturb the status quo for hospitals and physicians. Medicare would finance medical care for elderly patients, but it would not seek to alter the health care system in any way.

Medicare's accommodation of medical providers shaped its payment policies. Physicians and hospitals were paid generously, retrospectively, and with little oversight. Medicare initially had no predetermined fee schedule set by the federal government. Instead, Medicare paid doctors on a fee-for-service basis according to reasonable charges, which meant that physicians could bill Medicare for amounts equivalent to what they billed other patients as well as what other doctors were charging. That formula was inherently inflationary: the more services physicians provided, the more money they received from Medicare, and paying the prevailing rate encouraged physicians charging below that amount to raise their prices, leading to inexorable increases in the going rate. The formula was also explicitly political; by effectively allowing physicians to charge the government whatever they wanted, program architects aimed to buy doctors' acquiescence to the Medicare legislation and their cooperation in seeing Medicare patients.

The same story unfolded for hospital payment. Medicare paid hospitals on the basis of reasonable costs, essentially reimbursing hospitals retrospectively for whatever costs they submitted on behalf of Medicare patients. Hospital costs were liberally calculated by Medicare and even incorporated a 2% bonus payment that covered capital costs. Medicare was in part following the lead of private insurers; reasonable-cost reimbursement was the industry

norm in the 1960s. Yet Medicare's market power could have enabled Congress or program administrators to enforce tighter limits on hospital payments if they had so chosen. But gaining the cooperation of hospitals in implementing Medicare was the preeminent goal, not cost containment, and once again, Medicare implemented an inherently inflationary payment formula. The more money hospitals spent on Medicare patients, the more money they received. That Medicare was initially administered by Social Security officials who prized political conciliation as a strategy and were more accustomed to sending out checks to beneficiaries than battling medical providers to limit spending only served to reinforce Medicare's permissive posture toward medical providers.[11]

Medicare made one additional concession to providers: day to day program administration (such as claims processing and reimbursement) was delegated to private insurers, largely Blue Cross and Blue Shield plans that enjoyed close relationships with hospitals and doctors and could be expected to maintain the promised hands-off stance. Hospitals and physicians thus could participate in Medicare not only on favorable terms but also by working with private insurers they were comfortable with. This administrative buffer, which preserved a role for private insurers in Medicare, also served to reassure conservative opponents of federal health insurance who disliked centralized administration and to defuse any concern among the public that Medicare would lead to federal bureaucrats running the medical care system.[12]

In sum, Medicare's initial payment and administrative arrangements hardly could have been more accommodating of medical providers. Doctors and hospitals received essentially open-ended payments from the federal government, which foreswore cost control and ceded administrative responsibilities to private insurers. The economic footprints of these policies were predictable. In Medicare's first years spending, unfettered by any federal constraints, accelerated at a rapid rate and concerns about Medicare expenditures and its financial health (particularly the solvency of the hospitalization insurance trust fund) emerged almost immediately after it began operations in 1966. By 1969 Senator Russell Long, chairman of the Senate Finance Committee, had declared Medicare a "runaway program" and opened hearings on its skyrocketing costs and alternative payment mechanisms.[13]

Yet initial efforts to restrain Medicare spending were tepid. In 1972, Congress enacted Professional Standard Review Organizations (PSROs), charged with auditing the care received by Medicare patients to ensure the program did not pay for medically unnecessary services. But in practice PSROs had limited authority and did little to reduce unnecessary care or generate savings for Medicare. Even if PSROs had fettered out fraud and abuse, they left the main sources of Medicare's spending growth untouched: inflationary reimbursement formulas for hospitals and physicians. The truth is that although Medicare costs had become a political issue, the program comprised a relatively small share of the federal budget and the political will did not yet exist to challenge past concessions made to medical providers. Accommodation came at a high price to Medicare's bottomline, but federal health policymakers in the 1970s were unwilling to pay what they perceived as the higher political price of remaking Medicare's payment arrangements by taking on organized medicine.

There was another, unexpected price to be paid for the politics of accommodation. As noted previously, Medicare's architects envisioned the program as a cornerstone for a broader system of national health insurance. Clearly, they did not (and could not) anticipate: the eroding faith in government that followed the Vietnam war and Watergate scandal; the emergence of oil price shocks, stagflation (combining high unemployment and inflation), and sizable federal budgetary deficits; and the rightward shift in American politics during the 1970s and 1980s that halted liberals' expansionary social policy agenda, including plans for national health insurance.

But Medicare's advocates also did not anticipate the impact of the policies they had created for Medicare. Cost overruns in its early years meant that Medicare was viewed more as a fiscal burden and less as a foundation for national health insurance.

A tension existed between short-term goals (ensuring Medicare's successful implementation) and long-term aspirations (expanding Medicare into national health insurance). In order to assure Medicare's implementation, program architects unintentionally compromised their longer-term vision by loading the program with provider-friendly payment policies that inhibited Medicare's expansion. Medicare added coverage for the disabled and end stage renal disease patients in 1972, but otherwise did not expand to new populations. Nor were Medicare's limited benefits liberalized and over time coverage of beneficiaries' medical expenses became increasingly inadequate.

Medicare's accommodation of medical providers had consequences beyond the program. Medicare's inflationary payment policies accelerated medical inflation in the US health care system by enabling hospital charges and physician fees to surge upward for all patients, triggering the nation's first cost crisis and renewing the debate over national health insurance in the early 1970s. But when national health insurance stalled, Medicare remained a standalone federal insurance program. Subsequent efforts to adopt universal coverage were linked to cost control, creating another hurdle for reformers to jump over (the Carter administration argued costs should be controlled before insurance coverage was expanded and having failed to enact system-wide cost controls, never got around to universal coverage). Beset by charges of profligacy and inefficiency, Medicare's allure as a model for national health insurance dimmed.

MEDICARE'S REGULATORY REVOLUTION

Medicare wrote hospitals and physicians a blank check in 1965 that they readily cashed. A program denounced as socialized medicine proved to be a financial boon for the medical industry, and the original Medicare bargain—the federal government would pay generously for seniors' medical care while leaving the status quo in the health care system undisturbed—remained intact for 15 years. Cost containment initiatives in Medicare were half-hearted and broader reforms to restrain national health spending, such as the Carter administration's ill-fated proposal to cap hospital spending, were no more successful. But the era of the blank check in Medicare was bound to end. Once the federal government started paying for medical care through public insurance programs, it could not afford to forever be a bystander to the health care system. Federal policy makers now had their own fiscal reasons to restrain medical inflation, and as the nation's budgetary circumstances changed, those incentives became an imperative.

Prospective Payment Comes to Medicare

Hospitals were the first targets of policy makers' newfound willingness to take on providers.[14] The Carter administration's proposals for system-wide hospital cost containment had failed to pass Congress during 1977–79, giving way to the industry's so-called Voluntary Effort. Rather predictably, the Voluntary Effort failed to work—counting on hospitals to voluntarily give up income wasn't much of a strategy—leaving Medicare to confront medical inflation on its own and leaving members of Congress convinced that federal action was necessary if hospitals costs were to be slowed. Meanwhile, the Reagan administration came to power in 1981 committed to cutting taxes, ramping up military spending, downsizing the federal welfare state, and reducing domestic spending. That policy agenda and the rate of increase in Medicare spending made the program a tempting target for budget cutters. The temptation grew stronger as the federal budget deficit ballooned from $41 billion in 1979 to $208 billion in 1983.

Burgeoning budget deficits in the 1980s transformed Medicare politics by instilling in policy makers the political will to take on hospitals and physicians and cancel 1965's blank check policies.

Coddling medical providers during periods of balanced budgets was one thing; paying them off during an era of widening budget gaps was quite another. In 1983, as part of a larger Social Security reform bill, Congress enacted the Medicare Prospective Payment System (PPS) that established predetermined payments to hospitals on the basis of patients' diagnoses. No longer would Medicare pay hospitals retrospectively on the basis of whatever costs they submitted; from here on out, federal policy makers would set Medicare payments in advance based on a federally-established formula rather than reported costs. And unlike 1965, the formula was not borrowed from the hospital industry, but grew out of state experiments in prospective payment that had been authorized by the federal government in the 1972 Social Security Amendments. Diagnosis-related groups (DRGs), which classified patients by medical diagnoses that then could be linked to a preset payment for each patient a hospital treated with that diagnosis, became the basis for Medicare prospective payment after New Jersey had successfully adopted them for paying their hospitals.

The new mandate to regulate payments to hospitals had a bipartisan constituency. Democrats were comfortable using federal power to limit Medicare costs; cuts in provider payments were preferable from their perspective to raising beneficiary costs. The Reagan administration and Congressional Republicans preferred market-oriented approaches to cost control (such as Health Maintenance Organizations) but believed those approaches would not produce immediate budgetary savings. In order to reduce government's size, the Reagan administration paradoxically ended up supporting policies that expanded federal regulatory powers to contain spending. Moreover, since the prospective payment system moved away from cost reimbursement and instead rewarded hospitals that kept costs down— they could keep any profits from federal payments above what they spent, while hospitals that spent more than the government's payments had to absorb the loss—Medicare's new regulatory powers could be portrayed as promoting market forces and incentives for efficiency, making it more palatable to conservatives.[15]

The Medicare Fee Schedule

Medicare's prospective payment system broke the political stranglehold of medical provides over the program. It also established the precedent of the federal government paying according to prospectively determined prices rather than on the basis of retrospectively determined costs. With Medicare hospital payments under regulatory control, it was just a matter of time before policy makers went after physician payments. Indeed, while the rate of increase in Medicare spending on hospital services fell after the introduction of prospective payment, spending for physician services accelerated, in part because providers were moving care to outpatient settings outside of Medicare's regulatory reach. In 1984 Congress imposed a fee freeze on Medicare physician payments that lasted through 1986. However, Medicare's spending on physician payments kept rising, largely due to increases in the volume of services billed to the program, an increase perceived as physicians' response to the fee freeze. The growing bill for Medicare physician expenditures, limited success of the 1984–86 fee freeze, and continued pressures from the budget deficit fueled Congressional interest in creating a new Medicare physician payment system. As it had been for hospitals, Medicare's original bargain of granting doctors a blank check was abandoned.

In 1989, Congress enacted the Medicare Fee Schedule for physicians based on the resource-based relative value scale (RBRVS). RBRVS created a formula for paying physicians according to the time, skill, and effort associated with different services. The aim was to create a payment system that more accurately reflected the actual costs of delivering services than Medicare's inflationary formula of reimbursing physicians' for their customary, prevailing, and reasonable charges. The assumption was that once those costs were accurately measured, payments for costly specialty care would fall while payments for some primary care services

would rise. By lessening the disparity in payments for specialty and primary care services, RBRVS held out the promise of reducing Medicare spending through financial incentives that favored less expensive care.

Under the Medicare Fee Schedule, which began in 1992, each physician service was assigned a relative value based on RBRVS and then a conversion factor turned that relative value into a dollar amount. The federal government was, in other words, setting prospective prices for what Medicare would pay physicians. Moreover, the 1989 legislation also authorized Volume Performance Standards that empowered Medicare to adjust future physician payments downward in subsequent years if spending targets weren't met, a safeguard against the kind of volume increases triggered by the 1984–86 fee freeze. Like hospitals, physicians were now subject to Medicare cost controls that took away their ability to effectively set their own payment rates, though the reforms proved less successful in reducing the gap between payments to physicians for specialty and primary care.[16]

Medicare's New Regulatory Regime

By the close of the 1980s, Medicare had thus developed a new regulatory regime for paying providers. Both the Medicare Prospective Payment System and the Medicare Fee Schedule were based on technical formulas that ostensibly sought to measure physician and hospital costs on a more objective basis. But stripped of their technocratic imagery and scientific veneer, DRGs and RBRVS were systems of administered pricing and prospective payment that enabled the federal government to impose budgetary controls over Medicare spending. Medicare had entered a new era where federal policy makers asserted power over medical providers. The politics of accommodation, buffeted by the rise of federal budget deficits, gave way to the politics of regulation.

Both the Prospective Payment System and Medicare Fee Schedule were enacted with scant public attention (the debate was too technical to attract a wide audience), bipartisan support (fueled by the impetus to reduce federal deficits), and for the most part, the acquiescence of the medical industry (which managed to win some concessions but could not stop the main thrust of reform). In contrast to Medicare's implementation in 1966, Congress and program administrators (now operating from the independent Health Care Financing Administration rather than from within Social Security) implemented payment formulas with an eye to controlling costs rather than buying cooperation.

In fact, Medicare's new regulatory regime proved effective in slowing down the rate of growth in program spending. As budget deficits persisted throughout the 1980s and 1990s, federal policy makers aggressively used Medicare's prospective payment systems to limit program costs in the name of fiscal discipline. A Congressional Budget Office study found that excess cost growth in Medicare (growth beyond general inflation and demographic changes) declined from 5.5% during 1975–83 to .9% during 1992–2003. Moreover, there was no systematic evidence that the cost controls compromised Medicare patients' access to or quality of care.[17]

The new payment mechanisms did not solve Medicare's spending problems—the program was still subject to broader forces of medical inflation and lacked an overall global budget that could reliably constrain total spending and utilization—but they demonstrated that that the federal government could develop regulatory strategies for cost containment that worked in practice. Indeed, private payers copied Medicare's RVS system for their own payment systems, while DRGs attracted interest from health care systems abroad. Medicare is often derided for lagging behind innovations in American health insurance, but in implementing these payment reforms, at least, Medicare led the way as an innovator.[18] The relative success of Medicare's regulatory policies helped revive the program's reputation and interest in using it in some political quarters as a health reform model.

Finally, just as in 1965, Medicare's payment policies had unintended effects on the health care system. By restraining Medicare spending, the federal government set in motion a chain of events ably described by Rick Mayes.[19] Hospitals shifted costs to private insurers—who lacked Medicare's purchasing power and did not have similarly robust cost control systems in place—to make up lost revenues from declining federal payments after the introduction of Medicare prospective payment in 1983. Insurers who were the targets of cost shifting then responded by raising their premiums for employer-sponsored insurance, resulting in skyrocketing premium increases for health insurance; a sizable increase in the ranks of uninsured Americans; employers' embrace of managed care to stem the tide of rising premiums; and finally, the return of national health insurance to the agenda in the early 1990s. Medicare's regulatory revolution thus unintentionally helped to create, or at least hasten, the revolution in private insurance that managed care unleashed. The cycle, though, was not yet complete: managed care's spread through the private health system in the 1990s would soon boomerang back onto Medicare.

THE RISE OF THE MARKET

Over time, Medicare looked more and more like the national health insurance systems operated by other industrialized democracies. In fact, the regulatory strategies and budgetary controls embraced by Medicare were analogous to (if not as robust or comprehensive as) system-wide cost containment measures used in nations like Canada. We are often told that national health insurance is not a good fit with American political culture, that our affinity for individualism, markets, and liberty precludes the adoption of a national health plan that expands governmental power. And there is little doubt that opponents of national health insurance have successfully exploited Americans' suspicion of centralized government—part of our political DNA—to shake support for health reform. Yet it also appears that once public insurance programs are enacted in the United States and cost containment becomes a fiscal priority, our political culture is flexible enough to permit the adoption of centralized cost controls (even if they are shrouded in technocratic language) that assert government power over the private sector. Pragmatism and fiscal exigency trump ideology and antigovernment bias.

Medicare's trajectory throughout the 1980s and early 1990s thus followed the path of regulation. But Medicare politics was transformed in 1994 and program policy has been driven ever since in a new direction: toward the market. The market era in Medicare policy has not supplanted regulation; indeed, Medicare's regulatory scope has expanded over the past decade. Yet there is no question that Medicare politics have veered right since 1994, with Medicare's policy agenda increasingly populated by proposals to promote private plans, managed care, and competition. The 2003 enactment of the Medicare Modernization Act that created Medicare's Part D program of drug coverage represented the culmination of this trend toward market-driven policy. How this transformation came about and its implications for Medicare is the subject of the remainder of this chapter.

A Political Revolution

As we have seen, Medicare's enactment was highly contested, characterized by deep ideological and partisan divisions. But controversy over federal health insurance for the aged receded after Medicare was adopted in 1965 and attracted broad public support. During the three decades that followed Medicare's enactment, program politics were remarkably stable, more technical than ideological in tone. Major, protracted public debates over Medicare were rare and policy reforms usually reinforced Medicare's existing program structure and philosophy. Absent debate over ideology or programmatic first-principles, Medicare policymaking from 1966–94 was characterized by a striking degree of bipartisanship. To be sure, there were important disagreements between Democrats and Republicans on particular issues, but those differences, as the bipartisan support that emerged for prospective payment reforms demonstrated, were ultimately far less impressive than the similarities between the two parties' positions on Medicare.

Divided government made collaboration across party lines on Medicare reform a political necessity. During Medicare's first 28 years of operation, the program spent 20 years under divided government control, where the party in majority in the House and (or) Senate differed from that of the president. Moreover, because Democrats dominated the House of Representatives, Medicare did not spend any of its first 28 years under unified Republican control of the national government. Medicare lived in a political world ruled by predominantly Democratic Congresses.

That world ended in 1994 and Medicare politics experienced a re-alignment. For the first time in 40 years, the Republican party won majorities in the House and Senate and Medicare's political environment radically changed. The new Congressional leadership at the vanguard of the Republican revolution—led by Speaker of the House Newt Gingrich—believed in conservatism, deregulation, federalism, privatization, and markets. There could hardly have been a greater mismatch with Medicare, which embodied liberalism, federal authority, social insurance, and centralized regulation. After 1994, Medicare was a Great Society program governed by a Republican Congress. It is no surprise that, in the context of efforts to balance the federal budget, Republican Congressional leaders sought to remake Medicare into a program that fit more closely with their ideological vision and political commitments. Put simply, Republican leaders wanted a conservative Medicare program to supplant the liberal Medicare program that had been put into place by Democrats in 1965.

The Rise of Managed Care

The 1994 electoral triumph of the Republican party was not the only element in the transformation of Medicare's political environment. By 1995, the US health system was in the midst of a managed care revolution that reordered the status quo, with dramatic increases in enrollment for HMOs and other health plans that departed from the traditional American insurance model (for instance, by limiting patients' choice of doctors). Medicare had started its own HMO program in 1985 that allowed beneficiaries to enroll in private plans in the hopes of saving the federal government money, but initially enrollment was slow. Meanwhile, various forms of managed care spread through the employer-sponsored insurance market and also gained a foothold in Medicaid. The only bastion of "un-managed" care left in the United States was Medicare. Suddenly, Medicare no longer appeared to be in the mainstream of American medical care and critics attacked the program as a "dinosaur" in dire need of modernization.

The rise of managed care generated pressures on Medicare to conform to the new private insurance standard. For starters, the managed care industry became an increasingly powerful stakeholder in American health politics and Medicare policy, and as they exhausted other markets, they looked to the Medicare population as a growth opportunity. In addition, in the mid-1990s managed care held down spending in the private sector, while Medicare's cost control performance, which had been strong in the prior decade, looked less stellar in comparison. Conservative reformers argued that Medicare was being outperformed and the program had to embrace managed care and competition for it to be sustainable. Managed care consequently provided conservatives with an alternative model to traditional Medicare, a solution to Medicare's problems that offered a ready-made escape from what they saw as the perils of government-run insurance.

The long-term vision was that the traditional Medicare program (and federal government) would give way to private health plans such as HMOs. The government's role increasingly would be to subsidize the purchase of private insurance and oversee a competitive market, rather than operating its own insurance program through Medicare. Private sector managers would replace government bureaucrats in making key decisions about beneficiaries' medical care. Newt Gingrich famously remarked that over time traditional Medicare would "wither on the vine because we think people are going to voluntarily leave it."[20]

A Decade of Market-Driven Policy

The ascendance of a Republican Congressional majority and managed care consequently transformed Medicare politics, opening the door to reforms that sought simultaneously to introduce market forces into Medicare and move Medicare beneficiaries into the market. Yet these proposals often did not achieve political or policy success. The 1995 Republican Medicare reform plan that would have made sizable cuts in Medicare spending and encouraged beneficiaries to move to private plans was enacted by Congress but vetoed by President Clinton. The 1997 Balanced Budget Act (BBA) that created the Medicare+Choice program not only failed to generate the expected advance of managed care plans in Medicare, but came to be widely blamed for triggering the exit of many private plans from Medicare (the BBA did produce sizable savings in Medicare spending, but those savings were the result of extending prospective payment to additional services and of tightening existing formulas for provider payments, not the consequence of the legislation's more market-oriented provisions). The 1999 Bipartisan Commission on the Future of Medicare failed to gain the super-majority necessary to officially submit to Congress its recommendation to move Medicare toward managed competition. And because of favorable selection—plans attracted beneficiaries who were on average healthier than the general Medicare population—and federal payment policies, Medicare actually lost money on beneficiaries who enrolled in private plans, spending more for their HMOs than if they had stayed in traditional Medicare.

In 2003, after nearly a decade of intensive efforts to move beneficiaries out of traditional Medicare, only 5.3 million Medicare enrollees (13% of all beneficiaries) were enrolled in private plans. Conservative reformers could not respond to flagging enrollment by mandating beneficiaries to join managed care plans, a strategy often employed by state Medicaid programs. The Medicare population is too politically influential for that; inducement rather than coercion consequently has been the policy of choice to move them from traditional Medicare into private plans.

THE MEDICARE MODERNIZATION ACT AND POLITICS OF PART D

As of 2003, then, market forces had made only limited gains in Medicare and private plan enrollment of Medicare beneficiaries (which had soared before the BBA) had stalled. But that year Congress enacted the Medicare Prescription Drug, Improvement, and Modernization Act (MMA), giving private plans a new foothold in Medicare and taking market-based reform in Medicare to a whole new level.[21]

The resurgent momentum for market policy ironically was linked to efforts to liberalize Medicare benefits to include prescription drug coverage. Medicare policy has historically been dominated by issues of cost control and provider payment. Medicare did not expand its limited benefit package much after 1965 largely due to affordability concerns, even as it increasingly fell behind private insurance coverage carried by working-age Americans. That many Medicare beneficiaries obtained supplemental insurance coverage through former employers or by purchasing their own Medigap policies also dampened political pressures to liberalize coverage.

Medicare's one foray into large-scale benefit expansion—the 1988 Medicare Catastrophic Coverage Act—ended in disaster.[22] That year the Reagan administration and Congressional Democrats agreed to expand Medicare to limit the out of pocket costs paid by Medicare beneficiaries and add coverage of outpatient prescription drugs. However, only 16 months after its passage, Congress repealed the legislation in response to a backlash by seniors angered by the program's financing arrangements (the costs of the

new benefits were to be paid entirely by the Medicare population without any subsidy from general revenues, and with income-related premiums that imposed a significant new tax on more affluent beneficiaries). It was little consolation that much of the backlash was due to widespread confusion among Medicare beneficiaries (many of whom would have benefited from the program) about who would have to pay the new surtax, confusion largely attributable to misleading mailings sent by interest groups opposed to the program. After the political trauma of catastrophic health insurance, there was little appetite in Congress for expanding Medicare benefits, though the Clinton administration proposed a new Medicare drug benefit as part of its still-born health reform plan in 1993.

Prescription drug coverage re-emerged as an issue in 1999, when President Clinton called for expanding Medicare to cover outpatient medications and Democratic members of the National Bipartisan Commission on the Future of Medicare pushed for the benefit as an essential part of any program reforms. The rising political fortunes of a Medicare drug benefit were closely linked to a critical change in fiscal conditions. In 1998, for the first time in three decades, the Congressional Budget Office announced a federal budget surplus, forecast at $131 billion by 2000 and projected to grow during the ensuing decade. The surplus heralded a new day in Medicare politics, one in which the deficit pressures of the 1980s and 1990s gave way to the politically friendlier contours of surplus politics. Meanwhile, skyrocketing drug costs led Medicare HMOs and supplemental insurance plans to limit or drop their coverage for prescription drugs, or raise premiums. Medicare's omission of drug coverage seemed all the more glaring given the centrality of medications to contemporary medicine.

By 2000, prescription drug coverage for Medicare beneficiaries had become a first-order political issue and figured prominently in that year's presidential campaign. The Bush administration assumed office in 2001 having promised a new drug benefit and having committed to comprehensive reforms that would overhaul Medicare along more market-friendly lines.

But the partisan polarization on Medicare, and the lack of large Republican majorities in Congress, made that agenda difficult to legislate. In fact, neither party could mobilize a majority in Congress for its vision of Medicare reform. Democrats and Republicans remained far apart in how much money should be devoted to a new Medicare drug benefit, how many beneficiaries it should cover, whether drug coverage should be linked to broader program reforms, and whether the federal government or private insurers should offer the benefit. The debate over the design and scope of the drug program was complicated by the fact that by 2002 the federal surplus had disappeared, due to a recession, the economic fallout of the September 11th attacks, and the Bush administration's tax cuts. Without the surplus, Medicare drug coverage could no longer be paid for "for free."

However, the political salience of the Medicare drug issue and the importance both parties attached to seniors' votes meant that there was renewed momentum for enacting the benefit before the 2004 elections. The surplus may have disappeared, but the political dynamics for expansion remained. Neither party wanted to be seen as responsible for blocking a Medicare drug program. There was, in particular, pressure on Republicans to get a bill through since after 2002 they held majorities in both the House and Senate, as well as the White House. Doing nothing risked a backlash among elderly (and perhaps younger) voters and would open the GOP up to Democratic party attacks on not having fulfilled its promise. In contrast, if they got credit for passing a new drug benefit, Republicans believed they could offset Democrats' traditional electoral advantage on Medicare.

The deadlock over the Medicare drug benefit was finally broken at the end of 2003, but just barely, after a dramatic series of events that included: an initial bipartisan deal with Senate Republicans supported by Senator Ted Kennedy, a leading liberal voice on health policy; enactment by a single vote of a more conservative House bill that would have, along with the new drug benefit, converted Medicare into a premium support system (a form of managed competition that would

leave beneficiaries responsible for paying the difference between a federal subsidy and the cost of the health plan they chose); difficulties in the ensuing conference committee's efforts to produce a compromise bill that reconciled the Senate and House approaches; and AARP's late endorsement of the Republican drug plan, an unusual move for a political advocacy group usually aligned with the Democratic party on Medicare issues. The final bill passed the House in November 2003 by 220–215, but only after Republican leaders held open the vote (the longest recorded vote in House history) in order to persuade a few GOP congressmen to reverse their positions and support the bill when it appeared it would be defeated; it later passed the Senate 54–44. Those slim majorities (mainly on party lines) held off opposition from both the right and left. Conservatives objected to the bill as an expensive entitlement that did too little to overhaul Medicare and control costs, thereby adding to growing budget deficits; liberals denounced the bill for inadequate benefits, too much privatization, and as a sellout to drug companies and private insurers.

The drama and controversy did not end with the bill's enactment. In ensuing months, there were allegations of vote buying for one Congressman, admissions that the Bush administration had concealed estimates from the Medicare actuary that projected a substantially higher cost for the program than they had given when the bill was passed, and controversy over the administration's use of advertisements with fake news stories to promote the benefit.

When the dust cleared, the Medicare Prescription Drug, Improvement, and Modernization Act of 2003 (MMA) had created a complicated system of drug coverage and ushered in a series of complex program reforms whose impact was uncertain. Perhaps the most baffling feature of the program was its unusual benefit design. As a result of an agreement that the legislation could cost no more than $400 billion (over 10 years), Medicare's new drug benefit had a peculiar gap that reflected those fiscal limits, a "doughnut hole" in the middle where coverage ended before starting up again after catastrophic expenses (though lower-income program enrollees received more comprehensive coverage). In 2006, the standard Part D plan covered 75% of drug costs through $2,250, then covered nothing for the next $2,850 in expenditures, before picking up coverage again to cover 95% of costs after $5,100 in total spending.

The drug benefit itself is delivered by private companies rather than through the traditional Medicare program.[23] This marks the first time in program history that a benefit is only available through private plans. Beneficiaries can select prescription drug coverage offered as stand alone private policies (so-called Prescription Drug Plans or PDPs) or as part of comprehensive health insurance coverage offered through HMOs and other private plans in Medicare Advantage (the successor to Medicare+Choice). There is no Medicare drug plan directly offered by the federal government; drug coverage in Medicare has effectively been privatized.

It is hard to overstate the importance of this fundamental change in how Medicare works. To be sure, Medicare has always been a mix of public insurance and private delivery, and has always maintained a prominent role for private insurers in administration. And since 1985 private plans have played a growing role in delivering medical care to Medicare beneficiaries. Yet what the MMA has uniquely done is to privatize insurance and cede an entire area of program benefits to private plans that operate instead of, rather than along side, traditional Medicare. For proponents of market-based reform, Part D's exclusive reliance on private plans is a significant political victory, one that provides a testing ground for their belief that competition, consumer choice, and market forces can govern Medicare much better than the federal government. More than that, though, it establishes a precedent for what they would like the rest of the Medicare program to look like. Privatization has gained a beachhead in Medicare that its proponents will undoubtedly look to expand far beyond prescription drug coverage.

The MMA reversed the regulatory era in Medicare politics and the program's embrace of centralized cost control in other important ways. In a repeat of Medicare's 1965 accommodation of hospitals and doctors, the MMA expanded federal insurance but prohibited the government from negotiating prices with drug companies. The prohibition reflected the pharmaceutical industry's political power as well as the ascendance of market ideology (prices were to be controlled instead through plan competition) and marked a sharp departure from the politics of prospective payment that had asserted government power over medical providers. The MMA, which offered an array of expensive concessions to hospitals, employers, and myriad other industry groups, returned interest groups to a dominant position in Medicare policy, in the process subordinating fiscal concerns to political calculations and favoritism.[24]

The MMA also increased payments to private health plans contracting with Medicare, meaning these plans could (because they were being subsidized) potentially offer more generous drug coverage than other insurers, which might induce beneficiaries to leave traditional Medicare for better coverage. By 2006, Medicare payments to private plans were, on average, 12% higher than the average costs of beneficiaries in traditional Medicare; for private fee-for-service plans, which grew rapidly after the MMA, Medicare payments were 19% higher than costs. There was, then, no pretense of cost savings from private plans; privatization was the goal, even if it required enhanced federal subsidies. In addition, the bill established a demonstration project for 2010 in "comparative cost adjustment"—an impenetrable euphemism for a system that would put traditional Medicare in competition with private insurers, with beneficiaries paying more if they enrolled in a more expensive plan (one anticipated effect was that beneficiaries would have to pay more to stay in traditional Medicare).

In the short term, the strategies to enhance private plans' role in Medicare appear to be paying off. In 2007 enrollment in Medicare Advantage plans was estimated at 8.3 million, the highest private plan enrollment in Medicare history. It is unclear how much higher enrollment in private plans will go: this is not the first time analysts have been bullish about private plans in Medicare, only to be disappointed by subsequent results (Medicare+Choice's experience offers cautionary lessons). But the privatization of drug coverage in Medicare, in and of itself a significant advance for private plans, may prove conducive to expanding comprehensive commercial insurance alternatives to traditional Medicare. Industry analysts view Medicare drug plans (PDPs) as loss-leaders that will be used to lure beneficiaries into more profitable Medicare Advantage plans. As a Goldman Sachs report bluntly put it, "Under the most optimistic scenario, Medicare Advantage may represent the end game for Medicare and unprecedented multiyear growth opportunity for managed care."[25]

CONCLUSION

Medicare politics have been profoundly transformed since the program's enactment in 1965. A program that started out accepting the status quo and accommodating medical providers became a source of centralized cost control and innovative payment policies, and that regulatory regime was in turn followed by the rise of market-driven Medicare reform. The character of Medicare politics has also changed. The stable, quiet politics of Medicare's first three decades have given way to an intensely ideological, partisan, and polarizing politics. For the first time since 1965 there is an open political struggle over Medicare's core purpose and philosophy. The original Medicare debate has been reopened.

What's next for Medicare politics? In the short term, the politics of prescription drugs and Part D will dominate Medicare policy. The rollout of Part D during 2006–07 produced decidedly mixed results. Plan premiums were lower than expected, enrollment levels were strong, and beneficiary satisfaction with the new benefit rose over time. However, Medicare beneficiaries were confronted with a dizzying array of choices—beneficiaries typically had to choose from over 50 different standalone drug plans, as well as a host of Medicare Advantage options—that left many profoundly confused. Others are disappointed with the coverage: some Medicare beneficiaries have already fallen into the infamous

"doughnut hole" and that coverage gap, linked to increases in drug spending, will only widen over time. Part D also failed many low-income beneficiaries: some dual eligible beneficiaries (low-income persons on both Medicare and Medicaid) encountered serious problems in switching to new plans and although the program offered generous subsidies and enhanced coverage for low-income beneficiaries, as of 2006 over half of the beneficiaries eligible for the low-income subsidy program were not enrolled.

As Part D's doughnut hole widens, there will undoubtedly be pressures to fill in that gap, though given sizable federal budget deficits there is no guarantee that the Medicare drug benefit will expand substantially anytime soon (it remains to be seen whether more Part D plans will offer gap coverage). At the same time as pressure builds to liberalize the Medicare drug benefit, pressure could also mount to control Medicare spending on outpatient drugs. While the 2003 legislation left cost control in the hands of private plans and prohibited direct federal regulation of drug prices as a sop to the pharmaceutical industry, the political history of Medicare shows that once the government starts paying the bill for a medial services, eventually it imposes its own cost controls. Drug companies may prove a harder target than hospitals or physicians, since they will argue in a way that other medical providers never could that price controls stifle innovation and development of new therapies. But if private plans and competition cannot sustain cost control in Part D and as the federal bill for the program climbs upward, government policy makers may once again step in with more centralized controls.

The ultimate implications of the MMA remain difficult to gauge even four years after its enactment. The law made a number of incremental changes that when added together could catalyze a fundamental change in Medicare that moves the program closer to a framework of market competition run through private insurers. Higher payments to private plans, the privatization of Medicare drug coverage, the premium support demonstration, and other new policies could tilt the balance against the traditional Medicare program, accelerating beneficiary enrollment in private plans and setting the stage for a move to a defined contribution philosophy that transforms the program. But the 2006 elections, which brought Democratic majorities to the House and Senate for the first time since 1994, may signal yet another change in direction for Medicare politics and usher in a policy environment less favorable to privatization (perhaps by cutting federal subsidies to private plans) and more disposed to regulation.

Another issue on Medicare's political horizon is program financing and impending trust fund shortfalls. An obscure provision of the 2003 MMA created a new measure of program solvency that triggers a "Medicare funding warning" whenever program trustees project that general revenue funding will exceed 45% of total Medicare spending within seven years. If such a warning is issued in two consecutive years, the president is directed to propose legislation to Congress (to be considered under expedited rules) that prevents Medicare from reaching the 45% threshold. The political significance of this rather arbitrary benchmark is to create the immediate potential for more Medicare funding crises. Indeed, the new politics of Medicare financing is already playing out and a Medicare funding warning could be issued in 2007; what happens next is unclear, since many believe the law lacks the teeth to compel action.

Even if the general revenue threshold amounts to nothing, a more traditional trust fund crisis is on its way. As the baby boomers age into Medicare, program enrollment will nearly double between 2000 and 2030. Medicare clearly needs substantially more money to cover its growing population and the search for those revenues is likely to dominate program politics for years to come. Yet raising the payroll tax has been essentially off the table in Medicare politics for two decades. When combined with rising medical costs and growing enrollment, the result is that the hospitalization insurance trust fund is projected to be exhausted in another decade. The federal government, of course, will never let Medicare go bankrupt; past funding shortfalls have been resolved by adopting reforms and increasing revenues. But a trust fund crisis, even an artificial or arbitrary one, could reignite wider debates over Medicare reform

and its sustainability. It is hard, then, to escape the conclusion that a major collision lies ahead in Medicare politics, probably sooner rather than later.

Ultimately, Medicare's future will be determined by fundamental political and economic circumstances: the balance of power in Congress, control of the White House, the prospects for national health care reform (which affects the chances for cost control in the health care system as a whole and thus in Medicare as well) and whether Medicare emerges as a foundation for covering the uninsured, and the state of the economy (which crucially affects Medicare's financing). How these circumstances will shape and reshape Medicare is unclear. What is clear is where Medicare is right now. Medicare politics is back to where it started in the 1950s, dominated by a fundamental debate over the role of government and markets in public policy. That debate will not be settled easily and it will not be settled any time soon.

STUDY QUESTIONS

1. What are the four eras of Medicare politics? Briefly describe each.
2. What is the central tension that has run through Medicare's history and that now marks the debates over the policy?
3. Which of the two sides described in the last question—the liberal and the conservative—do you think offers the best answer for Medicare's future? Why?
4. The author describes five political "legacies" that flowed from the original legislation. What were they?
5. The chapter describes how, once the program was passed, Medicare officials accommodated doctors and hospitals with "provider friendly payment policies." What were the consequences?
6. How did Medicare restrain its costs in the 1980s?
7. When Medicare restrained its own costs, it had a series of unintended

effects on the health care system. What were they?

8. "We are often told that national health insurance is not a good fit with American political culture," writes the author. He argues that the Medicare experience challenges this conclusion. What is his argument? Do you agree?

9. How did Newt Gingrich and the new Republican Congressional majority seek to transform Medicare after 1994?

10. What great change did the Medicare Modernization Act of 2003 introduce? Do you think this is a good change in the program?

NOTES

1. I am drawing here on the typology of Lawrence D. Brown in "Technocratic Corporatism and Administrative Reform in American Medicine," 1985.

2. This section of the chapter draws in part on material from Jonathan Oberlander, 2003. The best account of Medicare's enactment, and one that I draw on heavily here, is Theodore R. Marmor, 1973. Other works on the origins of Medicare include: Harris, 1976 and Jacobs, 1993.

3. The "rational argument and statistical persuasion" reference is from Hoffman, 2001: 178. For an historical account of early efforts to enact national health insurance in the United States, see Starr, 1982.

4. Marmor, 2000, pp 14–15.

5. Ibid.

6. Lawlor, 2003, pp 30–2.

7. Ball, 1995, 62–72.

8. White, 2001.

9. Feder, 1977. On the accommodating politics of Medicare's administrators and Medicare's early years, see also Derthick, 1979; Starr, 1982; and Marmor, 2000.

10. Quoted in Oberlander, 2003, p 109.

11. Feder, 1977.

12. Jacobs, 1993.

13. Quoted in Oberlander, p 47.

14. For accounts of Medicare's shift to prospective payment, see Mayes and Berenson, 2006; Smith, 1992; Marmor, 2000; Jost, 1999, pp 39–116; and Brown, 1985.

15. Morone and Dunham, 1985, pp 263–91.

16. Mayes and Berenson, pp 91–2.

17. White, 2006.

18. This argument is made by Moon, 2006.

19. Mayes, 2004.

20. Killian, 1998, pp 169–70.

21. For a comprehensive account of the MMA's origins, see Oliver, Lee, and Lipton, 2004.

22. See Himmelfarb, 1995.

23. This section of the chapter draws in part on Jonathan Oberlander, 2007.

24. On interest group politics in Medicare, Valdeck, 1999.

25. Goldman Sachs Group, 2005, p 29.

REFERENCES

Ball, R. 1995. "What Medicare's Architects Had in Mind." *Health Affairs* 14 (4): 62–72.

Brown, L.D. 1983. *New Policies, New Politics: Government's Response to Government's Growth.* Washington DC: Brookings Institution Press.

—— 1985. "Technocratic Corporatism and Administrative Reform in American Medicine." *Journal of Health Politics, Policy and Law* 10 (3): 579–99.

Derthick, M. 1979. *Policymaking for Social Security.* Washington DC: Brookings Institution Press.

Feder, J.M. 1977. *Medicare: The Politics of Federal Hospital Insurance.* Lexington, MA: D.C. Heath.

Goldman Sachs Group. 2005. *Part D Coming Into Focus.* New York: Goldman Sachs.

Harris, R. 1966. *A Sacred Trust.* New York: New American Library.

Himmelfarb, R. 1995. *Catastrophic Politics: The Rise and Fall of the Medicare Catastrophic Coverage Act of 1988.* University Park: Pennsylvania State Press.

Hoffman, B. 2001. The Wages of Sickness: The Politics of Health Insurance in Progressive America. Chapel Hill: University of North Carolina Press.

Jacobs, L.R. 1993. *The Health of Nations: Public Opinion and the Making of American and British Health Policy*. Ithaca, NY: Cornell University Press.

Jost, T. 1999. Governing Medicare. *Administrative Law Review* 51: 39–116.

Killian, L. 1998. *The Freshmen: What Happened to the Republican Revolution?* Boulder, CO: Westview.

Lawlor, E. 2003. *Redesigning the Medicare Contract: Politics, Markets, and Agency*. Chicago: University of Chicago Press.

Marmor, T.R. 1973. *The Politics of Medicare*. Chicago: Aldine.

—— 2000. *The Politics of Medicare* (2nd ed). New York: Aldine de Gruyter.

Mayes, R. 2004. "Causal Chains and Cost Shifting: How Medicare's Rescue Inadvertently Triggered the Managed Care Revolution." *Journal of Policy History* 16: 144–74.

Mayes, R., and R.A. Berenson. 2006. *Medicare Prospective Payment and the Shaping of U.S. Health Care*. Baltimore: Johns Hopkins University Press.

Moon, M. 2006. *Medicare: A Policy Primer*. Washington: Urban Institute Press.

Morone, J., and A. Dunham. 1985. "Slouching to National Health Insurance." *Yale Journal on Regulation* 2: 263–91.

Oberlander, J. 2003. *The Political Life of Medicare*. Chicago: University of Chicago Press.

—— 2007. "Through the Looking Glass: The Politics of the Medicare Prescription Drug, Improvement, and Modernization Act," *Journal of Health Politics, Policy and Law* 32: 187–219.

Oliver, T.R., P.R. Lee, and H.L. Lipton. 2004. "A Political History of Medicare and Prescription Drug Coverage." *The Milbank Quarterly* 82 (2): 283–354.

Smith, D.G. *Paying for Medicare: The Politics of Reform.* 1992. New York: Aldine de Gruyter.

Starr, P. 1982. *The Social Transformation of American Medicine*. New York: Basic Books.

Valdeck, B. 1999. "The Political Economy of Medicare." *Health Affairs* 18 (1): 22–36.

White, C. 2006. *The Slowdown in Medicare Spending Growth*. Washington: Congressional Budget Office.

White, J. 2001. *False Alarm: Why the Greatest Threat to Social Security and Medicare is the Campaign to "Save Them."* Baltimore: Johns Hopkins University Press.

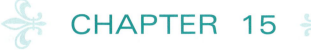

CHAPTER 15

Medicaid: Health Care for You and Me?

Colleen M. Grogan

This chapter provides a broad overview of our largest health care program. Grogan reviews Medicaid's history, its evolving purpose, its many political complications, and the major choice it now confronts: will it continue to evolve into a broad middle class program? Or revert to its origins as program for poor people?

Most people consider Medicaid America's health program for poor people. After all, that's what its architects thought in 1965. However, for a poor person's program, Medicaid gets a lot of attention. In February 2005, the Secretary of Health and Human Services, Mike Leavitt, in office less than a week, chose to make Medicaid the focus of his first formal speech.[1] Leavitt promised to defend the program and forcefully argued that the administration was not simply using Medicaid reforms as a way to make budget cuts. Later in the spring Republican Senators turned Medicaid into one of the major conflicts of the budget process—when they defended the program against most proposed budget cuts.

For the last decade, Medicaid reform has been at the top of the National Governors Association's list of policy priorities. And during the previous administration, President Bill Clinton went to great lengths to defend Medicaid as a core social welfare entitlement. Indeed, Clinton invoked Medicaid alongside Medicare, education and the environment as his sacrosanct programs and commitments—they were mentioned together so often that observers dubbed them Clinton's M(2) E(2). Why does this means- tested, targeted health care program have so many friends—and receive so much political attention?

Even a quick glance at the program explains why. Most people are surprised to learn that Medicaid is our nation's largest health insurance program. By 2002, the number of individuals covered by Medicaid, our health care program for "the poor," surpassed Medicare—our universal program for the elderly. Medicaid has about 51 million enrollees compared to Medicare's 41 million, and it is almost as expensive as Medicare.[2] A few other statistics make its importance crystal clear:

- Medicaid covers 20% of the nation's children;
- pays for more than one in every three childbirths;

- covers two-thirds of the elderly residing in nursing homes;

- helps more than 6 million elderly pay their Medicare premiums and prescription drug costs;

- pays for the bulk of services provided to AIDS patients; and

- finances half of all states' mental health services.[3]

These statistics reveal that we can no longer describe Medicaid as our health care program for "the poor." Rather, it is our health care safety-net for a wide range of people across various illnesses, age-groups, and income levels. Indeed, Medicaid has become an important element of health care security for middle class families. Although not often explicitly stated, it is on this latter point that much of the debate about Medicaid reform hinges. Should it be a program for the poor? Or a stepping stone to assuring that every American has access to some form of health care coverage? This chapter explains how Medicaid came to this crucial crossroads.

FEARS FOR MEDICAID

When Secretary Leavitt gave his Medicaid address he subtly introduced the issue of Medicaid's future—welfare medicine versus mainstream medicine—even while he denied that "reform" meant "cuts."

> Some have predicted that reform would break our commitment to our neediest and most vulnerable citizens: our mandatory populations, such as people with disabilities and children in low-income families or foster care. This is not true.[4]

Leavitt responds to the fear (or myths as he called them) of cost cuts by asserting that the federal government will maintain its commitment to "our mandatory populations." What does he mean by that? "Mandatory," as the term implies, simply

means the states are required under federal mandates to cover certain types of population groups. It is important to understand just *who* these "mandatory populations" are and who they are not. Mandatory populations covered under state Medicaid programs fall into the following four categories:

1. Children up to age 6 under 133% federal poverty level (FPL) and those aged 7–18 under 100% of FPL ($15,670 for a family of three in 2004).

2. Pregnant women and infants up to 133% of FPL.

3. Poor disabled and elderly (65+) persons eligible for cash assistance through the Supplemental Security Income (SSI) program (a federal standard); and

4. Poor families with dependent children eligible for cash assistance through the Temporary Assistance for Needy Families (TANF) program (varies by state, with eligibility levels typically set under the FPL).

The key point to grasp about the mandatory populations is that they represent a very restricted group of people *with very low* income levels relative to families' ability to afford health insurance.[5] This, in short, is Medicaid as welfare medicine.

The Medicaid legislation also specified "optional groups" that states *may* cover (and receive federal funds for) under their Medicaid programs if they so desire. The optional groups include the same populations as above, but at higher income levels, and include other groups as well, such as working parents. For example,

- Pregnant women and infants up to age 1 up to 185% of the FPL (the percentage amount is set by each state).

- Children up to 200% of FPL (State Children's Health Insurance Program [SCHIP]) established by the Balanced Budget Act (BBA) of 1997).

- Working parents up to 250% of FPL.

- Elderly and disabled up to 300% of the SSI Federal benefit rate.

- "Medically needy" persons (can be extended to families, disabled and/or elderly; states set the income level).[6]

These optional groups are important. They are the main way states have been able to expand health insurance coverage through Medicaid[7] in the last decade. The importance of these optional groups for coverage, and therefore Medicaid spending, is enormous: they consume about two-thirds of all Medicaid spending (see Figure 15-1).

Understanding the crucial role optional groups play in expanding Medicaid coverage sheds a different light on Secretary Leavitt's speech. Stating a strong commitment only to the mandatory populations merely reinforces the fear that Medicaid retrenchment will scale back progress in coverage expansions during the last decade since these expansions have happened almost entirely through

the use of optional coverage. In discussing changes and opportunities for Medicaid coverage groups, Leavitt clearly favors distinct treatment for optional populations: either a reduced benefit package or a subsidy to purchase private health insurance.

Leavitt's speech cuts straight to the fundamental question: What can (and should) we expect of Medicaid in the 21st century? Even while promising to protect the program, Leavitt opts for Medicaid as welfare over Medicaid as middle class entitlement. Leavitt is just the latest in a long line of those favoring retrenchment. Every fiscal crisis introduces the same proposal, for it comes from an ambiguity built into the program itself. Yet despite many efforts to retrench, middle class Medicaid survives, expands and flourishes. That's because, like many middle class programs, it has strong (and vocal) constituents.

Understanding Medicaid and its future means understanding the ambiguities that were built into the program from the start—ambiguities about beneficiaries, long term care, and intergovernmental financing. Each has proven a persistent political issue. Each is the source of considerable mythology and confusion. And taken together, they tell us a great deal about where Medicaid will go in the 21st century.

MEDICAID'S POLITICAL HISTORY

Medicaid's adoption in 1965 must be understood in the context of the long struggle to adopt universal health insurance in the United States. By the late 1950s, liberal proponents of health care reform were focusing their attention on senior citizens, a clientele group that was viewed sympathetically and was already tied to the state through the Social Security system. In 1964, most political observers thought Congress would adopt one of three alternative approaches to improve access to health care for the elderly: (1) a universal hospital insurance program based on Social Security (the King-Anderson Bills of 1963 and 1964); (2) a voluntary physician services

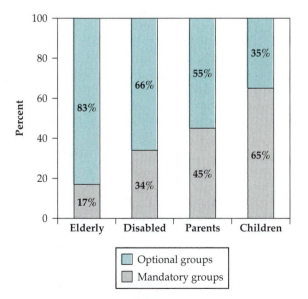

Figure 15-1 **Distribution of Medicaid Mandatory and Optional Spending, 1998**

SOURCE: The Kaiser Commission on Medicaid and the Uninsured, May 2003. "Medicaid: Fiscal Challenges to Coverage." Data obtained from Urban Institute estimates, 2001.

program supported by beneficiary premiums; or (3) an expansion of the means-tested Kerr-Mills program, which offered a wide range of health care benefits to the low-income elderly. Under the influence of Ways and Means Committee chairman Wilbur Mills, the Social Security Amendments of 1965 combined all of these approaches into a single package.

By all accounts, the creation of this massive "three-layer" cake took nearly everyone by surprise.[8] The first layer was Medicare Part A, a hospital insurance program based on the Social Security contributory model. The second layer was Medicare Part B, a voluntary supplementary medical insurance program funded through beneficiary premiums and federal general revenues. The third and final layer was the Medicaid program (originally called Part C), which broadened the protections offered to the poor under Kerr-Mills. The Kerr-Mills means-test was liberalized in order to cover additional elderly citizens, and eligibility among the indigent was broadened to include dependent children, the blind and permanently disabled.

Medicaid's adoption was perceived to be a minor piece of the 1965 Social Security legislation, certainly of far less significance than the creation of Medicare. In President Johnson's speech on the first anniversary of signing the landmark 1965 legislation, he did not even mention the passage of Medicaid.[9] Government estimates of Medicaid's future budgetary costs assumed the program would not lead to a dramatic expansion of health-care coverage.[10] Even assuming that all 50 states would implement the new program, the federal government projected Medicaid expenditures to be no more than $238 million per year above what was currently then being spent on medical welfare programs. As it turned out, this expenditure level was reached after only six states had implemented their Medicaid programs. By 1967, 37 states were implementing Medicaid programs, and spending was rising by 57% per annum.[11]

A key factor that explains Medicaid's early expenditure growth was the establishment of generous eligibility standards under various state "Medically Needy" programs. The Medically Needy programs allowed states to extend Medicaid eligibility to persons with income levels above the regular Medicaid income eligibility established in each state. A number of states initially set a very high Medically Needy eligibility level. For example, New York enrolled families with incomes up to $6,000 per year (for four persons) in 1966. As a point of comparison, by July 1991–25 years later—13 states with Medically Needy programs set income eligibility levels below $6,000 in current dollars. Under New York's generous enrollment standards, almost half of the state's population in 1966 could have potentially qualified for Medicaid's comprehensive medical coverage, including access to prescription drugs and long-term care facilities.[12] In sum, New York state policy makers clearly envisioned Medicaid as the stepping-stone to universal health care for citizens within its borders.

New York state policy makers argued that a liberal definition of the medically needy population was required in order to distinguish the Medicaid program as a whole from welfare. Under the New York program, 70% of the state's Medicaid spending would go to medically needy claimants who did not receive cash assistance. New York was hardly alone in wishing to distinguish Medicaid from welfare. Eighteen other states also devoted more than half of their Medicaid budgets to persons not on welfare. In Wisconsin, for example, 74% of total Medicaid payments were for Medically Needy recipients in 1967.[13]

Not all policy makers agreed with New York's expansionary use of the Medicaid program. To the contrary, many thought the program should be contained for a relatively small number of "truly" needy Americans. In their view, Medicaid costs could and should be controlled exactly because the number of covered person should be strictly contained and narrowly defined.

As a result of these conflicting views, the federal government reached an early impasse with Medicaid: should it embrace an expansive vision of Medicaid, or instead restrict program eligibility to a narrow clientele? It chose the latter course, clamping down hard on New York's attempted liberalization. In 1967, only a year after the New York expansion began, Congress passed legislation lowering the medically-needy eligibility level to 133.33% of a state's AFDC means-tested level.[14] New York's generous $6,000 eligibility level for a family of four was thereby reduced to $3,900. As a result of this federal intervention, about 600,000 potentially eligible persons were denied medical benefits in 1967. The number of potential Medicaid recipients was reduced by 750,000 in 1968 and 900,000 persons in 1969.[15]

In halting New York's attempted liberalization in 1967, federal policy makers made a conscious decision to define Medicaid as a restricted welfare program, off-limits to the employed. "The House is moving toward a program where you provide medical care to those who can't pay, and expect people to pay it if they are working and can earn income," stated one conservative senator in floor debate.[16]

Despite this significant retrenchment in 1967, Medicaid expenditures continued to increase, and the federal government responded yet again in two additional statutory amendments in 1969 and 1972. In 1969, the federal mandate to expand Medically Needy coverage to all groups equally was lifted, and in 1972 the mandate that all states must create Medicaid programs comprehensive in scope and breadth was eliminated. In addition, in 1972, the SSI program was created, which consolidated five separate state-run cash assistance programs for the aged, blind and disabled into a single, federal means-tested program.[17] Because SSI, unlike most means-tested benefits, is run as a *nationally uniform* program, a clear bifurcation among Medicaid beneficiaries was established. The elderly, blind and disabled—who tended to be viewed as highly sympathetic groups—gained Medicaid eligibility based on a *federal* eligibility standard. In contrast, poor mothers and their children gained eligibility according to a (typically much lower) *state* eligibility standard.[18]

As it became clear that Congress was not willing to support significant Medicaid expansions at the state level, states, especially those under fiscal stress, began lowering their eligibility and benefit levels, as well as fees paid to Medicaid providers. As a result many physicians refused to treat Medicaid clients. As early as 1974, Stevens and Stevens described Medicaid as perpetuating a two-class system of medical care, in which middle and upper income people use private hospitals and physicians, and the poor use a fragmented public system.[19]

Yet even these retrenchment amendments had contradictions of their own. While the 1967 measure tightened considerably the definition of "medically indigent," it nonetheless maintained the ability of states to distinguish administratively between welfare recipients and those who needed health care but not cash. The 1967 statute also expanded a series of well-child care benefits for poor children, creating the Early and Periodic Screening, Diagnostic Treatment program (EPSTD). The practical effect was to make the Medicaid benefit package even more comprehensive than it was already.[20] Finally, the 1967 law established the so-called "freedom-of-choice" requirement, which specified that states could no longer create special clinics for welfare clients or require Medicaid recipients to use county hospitals. Thus, while the equal fee requirement was dropped, this statute reaffirmed the mainstreaming goal by requiring that Medicaid administrators had to allow low-income citizens "to use providers of their choice, to enter the mainstream of American health care."[21]

Despite these contradictions, Medicaid's retrenchment stuck in the popular mind, and most analysts describe its early history as pure retrenchment—completely overlooking Medicaid's expansion. Indeed, three myths emerged from this early history and live on to this day: (1) Medicaid was never intended to be our long term care (or LTC) program; (2) Medicaid is a poor peoples' program; and (3) Medicaid reform is predictably partisan.

MYTH 1: MEDICAID WAS NEVER INTENDED TO BE OUR LONG-TERM CARE PROGRAM

Medicaid long term care wasn't just created whole cloth in 1965, but has long historical roots going as far back as the 19th century poorhouses. Don't worry, I'll skip over the details and discuss three historical highlights: (1) the establishment of Old-Age

Assistance under the New Deal in 1935; (2) the creation of medical vendor payments in 1950; and (3) the enactment of Medical Assistance to the Aged under the Kerr-Mills Act in 1960.[22]

Between 1935 and 1965, there was a dramatic increase in the number of nursing homes. This was not an accident, but was clearly encouraged by public policy. These homes, supported largely with public dollars, became the primary American response to problems of chronic disease in an aging population. Thus, the inclusion of long term care (i.e., nursing home coverage) under Medicaid in 1965 was not only intentional, but front and center.

The New Deal in 1935

The history of the modern American nursing home industry begins with a concerted effort by the federal government to close almshouses (also known as poorhouses or poor farms), and thereby abandon institutionalization as a legitimate method for addressing the concerns of poverty. Institutionalization of the poor began with fervor in the 1820s due to a demographic explosion and economic changes which bolstered the view that the causes of poverty could be located squarely within the individual.[23] With this view in hand, the philosophy of almshouse administrators was to change individual behavior through work and punishment.[24]

While these institutions, which housed the poor of all ages, including the sick and mentally ill, grew quite rapidly during the 19th century, social reformers at the turn of the century began designing institutions for certain groups with an effort to reform, rehabilitate and educate. For example, children were sent to orphanages, the insane to mental institutions and the physically disabled to special schools. Not surprisingly, the chronic, non-curable condition of most elderly in almshouses did not fit nicely with the reform and rehabilitation rhetoric of that time.[25] Thus, because there was no "reform movement" for the elderly, they were simply left in the almshouses. As a result, the vast majority of inmates eventually left in the almshouses were sick elderly persons with chronic conditions.[26]

While this shift happened unintentionally, many physicians and social reformers began touting almshouses as the appropriate place not only for poor elderly, but non-poor elderly needing long-term care services as well. The reason physicians and hospital administrators liked almshouses as a solution to "caring" for elderly individuals with chronic care needs was twofold. First, hospitals were growing with a new improved image as places where sicknesses could be cured. The elderly with chronic conditions that could not be cured had no place in these new institutions.[27] Second, they identified old-age with the deterioration of health, and therefore favored a medical institutional model with some type of skilled care to deal with the problems of old age.[28] Despite these "professional" views, the general condition of almshouses continued to deteriorate, and the elderly and their families continued to fear the poorhouse.

In the early 20th century this fear turned into activism, coalescing around the idea of publicly-funded old-age pensions, for two reasons. First, the 1930s depression shifted public opinion about the causes of poverty: from questionable individual behavior to forces over which the individual had no control. As widespread unemployment, sickness, old-age, and death of a spouse thrust hard-working Americans into poverty through no fault of their own, the American public looked to the federal government to help solve the problem of basic economic need.[29]

Second, the horrendous, inhumane conditions of the almshouses became more widely recognized. New Deal activists argued that old-age pensions would allow elderly persons to live with dignity outside of such institutions.[30] When the federal government passed Old-Age Survivors Insurance (OASI, what we commonly call Social Security today) and a federal-state, means-tested program, called Old-Age Assistance (OAA) for poor elderly persons, politicians and Social Security Administrators were quite clear in the statutes that no assistance would be given to almshouse inmates.[31] This clause was inserted in the landmark Social Security Act of 1935 with the clear intent to close the poorhouse.

The poorhouse did, in fact, die out. However, institutional care for the elderly did not. Indeed, to the contrary, institutional care grew.[32] Because many elderly still needed services for chronic conditions, and families either could not or would not care for their elderly relatives, many elderly used their OAA funds to pay for *private* institutional care. Historians Holstein and Cole sum up this irony nicely: "Hatred for the almshouse created a resistance to any public provision of nursing home care; thus, the almshouse . . . led to the now-dominant proprietary nursing home industry."[33]

Medical Vendor Payments in 1950

Although states were allowed to include the cost of medical care in their determinations of need for public assistance payments, few states were actually able to *truly* consider the cost of medical care under the federally defined maximums. States had the discretionary power to define need under their public assistance programs. However, the federal government set funding maximums which meant that above a certain state expenditure level the federal government would cease matching payments. States argued that the maximums were sufficiently low that states could not include the true costs of medical care, and yet they argued further that it was often sickness and medical care expenditures that then caused poverty.[34] In an effort to address this problem in 1950, Congress revised the Social Security Amendments in two important ways. First, the new legislation allowed states, under the federal financial match, to pay medical providers directly for services rendered to public assistance recipients. This revision created the term "medical vendor payments."[35] Second, the bill lifted the prohibition against federally-financed cash payments to elderly persons living in public institutions. This revision reflected the view that it was too restrictive (and perhaps unfair) to finance cash payments to elderly inmates in private institutions, but not public institutions. However, there was also a fear that these dollars would be used, yet again, to finance

poorhouses. Thus, a regulatory clause was included requiring states to establish and maintain standards so that these public institutions "met the definition of a medical institution, not just the old-fashioned poorhouse."[36]

Medical vendor payments were a true "sleeper" issue. When this new concept was presented to the Senate Committee on Finance by President Truman's Commissioner for Social Security, Arthur Altmeyer, many policymakers seemed genuinely perplexed about what the legislation was intended to do, much less its long-term implications. For example, after Commissioner Altmeyer's explanation of medical vendor payments, he stated "I do not know whether I made myself clear," and Chairman Walter George, Democrat from Georgia, said, "I do not quite understand it." After another attempt to clarify, the Chairman and Senators Butler and Johnson (from Nebraska and Colorado respectively) asked a series of questions to determine if this provision would increase federal expenditures. Because medical vendor payments were offered only under the existing individual cash maximums, Commissioner Altmeyer responded that this particular change did not have "much money significance."[37] In fact, as I discuss in more detail below, medical vendor payment expenditures—especially for long term care—rose dramatically after 1950.

The main reason why the significance of medical vendor payments were largely overlooked when enacted in 1950, is that proponents of national health insurance then (and throughout most of Medicaid's history) viewed public assistance as a residual program that could be done away with when national health insurance is enacted. Those in favor of national health insurance did not perceive medical vendor payments as a win to opponents, rather they viewed this provision as a small public assistance expansion that would not harm and might help some vulnerable people a little. For example, when Senator Eugene D. Millikin (Republican, Colorado) wondered about the potential financial and regulatory significance of this then-seemingly small provision, Commissioner Altmeyer quickly assured him that any such significance could not adhere to such meager provisions for public assistance recipients. Part of the reason public assistance programs were discussed as residual is because they were usually viewed in relation to increasing social insurance. Indeed, every state-level public welfare administrator emphasized in their testimony that federally-funded social insurance (i.e., OASI) should be increased and federal-state public assistance (i.e., OAA) would then be allowed to decrease.

As fiscal conservatives feared, public assistance programs continued to increase in the 1950s—in large part due to expansions in medical vendor payments. Although this particular provision did not have much financial significance in the few years following its passage in 1950, the provision allowed for a series of revisions and expansions in 1953, 1956, 1958, and 1960 culminating to the passage of Medicaid in 1965.[38] In 1953, a separate federal-state matching rate for medical vendor payments (apart from cash payments) was established, and the individual medical maximums and federal matching rate for vendor payments subsequently expanded in each of the years listed above. The 1946 Hill-Burton Act also provided funds for nursing home (as well as hospital) construction.[39] Taken cumulatively, these incremental expansions continued, and strengthened, the tie between nursing homes and public assistance that began with the public almshouse. The Kerr-Mills Act, included under the 1960 Social Security amendments, served to solidify that link.

The Kerr-Mills Act of 1960[40]

After President Harry Truman's failure to enact National Health Insurance, and in the wake of medical vendor payments, proponents of national health insurance decided to restrict their goals to expanding hospital benefits only for OASI beneficiaries—in other words, elderly persons over age 65. Following this logic, Aime Forand (Democrat, Rhode Island) introduced the original "Medicare" bill in 1957, proposing universal coverage for the elderly with a restricted hospital-based benefit package administered and financed on a contributory basis by the federal government.[41]

In response to the Forand bill and mounting public pressure to do something for the aged, two crucial provisions were embedded under Kerr-Mills that would profoundly influence Medicaid's subsequent policy evolution: the concept of medical indigency and comprehensive benefits. Kerr-Mills was designed to be distinct from welfare with its continuing stigma of public assistance. The "medically indigent" were older persons who needed assistance when they became sick (but not otherwise), because they had large medical expenses relative to their current income. Proponents emphasized that the "medically indigent should not be equated with the totally indigent"; that is, those who receive cash assistance.[42] Medical indigency was put in place with the idea that sickness should not cause impoverishment.

While it is unclear how much the elderly were helped under Kerr-Mills, the program had a huge impact on the growth and use of nursing homes. From 1960 to 1965, vendor payments for nursing homes increased almost tenfold, consuming about a third of total program expenditures.[43] Even at this time, it was increasingly difficult to view these programs as simply residual entities that would wither away under increases in social insurance. Indeed, when medical vendor payments and Kerr-Mills's medical assistance was folded into a new program called Medicaid and adopted alongside Medicare in 1965, it was in keeping with a by then 30-year historical pattern; that is, adopting a limited social insurance program and "supplementing" it with public assistance. I put "supplement" in quotation marks because, starting with OAA in 1935, these public assistance programs were hardly supplemental. America's social insurance programs (OASI and Medicare) had been sufficiently limited at birth that the adjoining public assistance programs (OAA and Medicaid) were vital—and grew substantially. Nevertheless, as mentioned earlier, Medicaid was perceived as a relatively minor piece of the 1965 Social Security legislation, of much less significance than Medicare. The hope for a small increase in Medicaid given the enactment of Medicare was in keeping with how policy makers, administrators, and advocates had long discussed the hoped-for relationship between public assistance and social insurance.

That this substitution did not occur, however, should not have come as a surprise to anyone looking closely at medical vendor payments and the Kerr-Mills's MAA program. The fastest growing and most expensive component of these two public assistance programs was the cost of nursing homes for chronically ill elderly persons. By 1965, every state had medical vendor payments for public assistance recipients, and forty states had implemented a Kerr-Mills's MAA program for the medically indigent.[44] Because these 40 state programs provided nursing home coverage, while long-term care coverage was essentially ruled out under Medicare, it would have been political suicide to withdraw such benefits from existing Kerr-Mills recipients. Thus, Kerr-Mills and medical vendor payments were consolidated under the new program called Medicaid, and nursing home expenditures continued to increase.

While the increase in nursing home expenditures was perhaps unplanned, three summary points are important to note: first, this increase in nursing home expenditures is part of a larger trajectory that started 15 years before Medicaid; second, Medicaid's enactment in 1965 was not an afterthought, but business as usual; and third, the inclusion of nursing home care coverage under Medicaid was clearly inevitable.

MYTH 2: MEDICAID IS A POOR PEOPLES' PROGRAM

Medicare was knowingly passed with inherited limitations both in depth and breadth. In particular, it left out working adults and their children who are uninsured, and the elderly who need LTC services.[45] While reformers strategically accepted these Medicare limitations as a necessary compromise, others viewed the system as largely "fixed:" Medicare for the elderly and disabled, employer-based health insurance for workers and Medicaid

for the "needy." At the time, most policy makers thought the health care needy were mainly poor, but this was never exactly right and Medicaid quickly became the program to fill in the gaps of this imperfect system.

Middle-Class Reliance on Medicaid for the Elderly

As early as 1970, Medicaid was the dominant governmental purchaser in the nursing home market (see Table 15-1). By 1980, Medicaid spending on nursing home care ($8.8 billion) not only surpassed all other public sources combined ($0.7 billion) but also slightly exceeded out-of-pocket payments ($7.4 billion). Medicaid nursing home expenditures rose rapidly during the 1990s. By 1997, Medicaid nursing home expenditures ($39.4 billion) greatly exceeded out-of-pocket payments for nursing home care ($25.7 billion). In that year, Medicaid picked up almost half (47%) of the $83 billion spent on nursing homes in the United States.

Many seniors in nursing homes are not eligible for Medicaid at the time of their admission. At an average cost of $30,000 per year, however, nursing home care quickly depletes the resources of all but the most affluent of seniors. Between 27% and 45% of elderly nursing home residents become eligible for Medicaid after spending down their resources. A significant proportion of elderly nursing home residents on Medicaid are not poor by typical "welfare" standards.[46] Indeed, some spent their adult lives firmly in the middle class. States cover these "non-poor" persons under either their Medically Needy programs or under a special income rule called the "300% rule."[47] Together, these two sets of programs account for 88% of Medicaid's nursing home spending, and 75% of total Medicaid spending on the elderly.

National nursing home surveys conducted annually during the late 1980s and early 1990s indicate that approximately 60% to 70% of the more than 1.5 million people residing in nursing homes have Medicaid as a payment source on any given day. Somewhere between 33% and 40% of nursing home residents are eligible for Medicaid upon admission.

Table 15-1 Medicaid Myths, Changes, and Opportunities in Elite Discourse: February 1, 2005

Topic 1: Treatment of Mandatory Versus Optional Coverage Groups

Myths	Changes	Opportunities
Some have predicted that reform would break our commitment to our neediest and most vulnerable citizens: our mandatory populations, such as people with disabilities and children in low-income families or foster care. This is not true.	We must find every inefficiency, because waste means covering fewer people. We must stop overpaying for prescription drugs.	We can expand access to more children…We can provide access to more needy people by providing common sense flexibility. Mandatory populations need the help. They must receive the help. The optional populations, on the other hand, may not need such a comprehensive solution. Most of them are healthy people who just need help paying for health insurance.

Topic 2: Middle-Class Medicaid and the Provision of LTC

Some expect that there will be a cut in available resources. NO again.	Medicaid must not become an inheritance protection plan.	We can ensure that seniors and people with disabilities get long-term care where they want it.

Topic 3: Intergovernmental Financing

Some are concerned that we will propose a block grant system, like the one that was discussed in 1995. NOT so. There will be no block grant system for Medicaid.	We must have an uncomfortable, but necessary, conversation with our funding partners, the states.	

SOURCE: Contents of Table are direct quotes taken from Secretary Michael O. Leavitt's "Medicaid: A Time to Act." Speech presented to the World Health Care Congress, Marriott Wardman Park Hotel, Washington, D.C. February 1, 2005. See CMS website: www.cms.hhs.gov for copy of his speech.

NOTE: Secretary Leavitt's quotes are reordered here to fit within the topic headings provided for ease of discussion.

Only about one-third of those who do not have Medicaid as a payment source at admission remain private payers throughout their stay. Two-thirds of such individuals eventually spend down their savings to Medicaid levels.[48] In short, many senior citizens who receive Medicaid do not have a history of poverty before entering a nursing home.

Despite the spending implications of significant elderly reliance on Medicaid for LTC, Congress expanded Medicaid LTC coverage for the elderly in 1988. Congress's main intent was to provide prescription drug coverage for the elderly under Medicare, but to also include two important provisions under Medicaid: protections against spousal impoverishment (when a person resides in a nursing home the community spouse is protected from financial ruin), and the "Medicare buy-in" provision which requires states to pay the Medicare premiums, deductibles, and co-payments of seniors with incomes below the poverty level. Although Medicare's prescription drug bill was repealed in 1989,[49] these Medicaid provisions remained intact solidifying Medicaid's role as America's major long-term care program and signaling that Medicaid would continue to serve a mainstream constituency—the institutionalized elderly—within a means-tested policy design.

Middle-Class Reliance on Medicaid for Children

While Medicaid eligibility for children remained strictly attached to cash assistance welfare throughout the 1970s, this link was increasingly weakened in the 1980s and ultimately severed in 1996 under welfare reform. Today, the majority of children covered by Medicaid have working parents who do not receive cash assistance.[50]

The federal government enacted incremental Medicaid expansions for children and/or pregnant women and infants in every year between 1984 and 1990. By the end of this six-year period, some 5 million children and 500,000 pregnant women had gained Medicaid eligibility in states across the nation.[51] What is most remarkable is that these Medicaid coverage expansions—which helped drive combined state and federal health care spending for the poor from $75 billion in 1986 (measured in 1996 dollars) to almost $180 billion in 1996[52]—is that they occurred when they did (citation). The federal government faced persistent budget deficits throughout the 1980s. Significant cutbacks in Medicaid spending had been made under Ronald Reagan in 1981.[53] In sum, major targeted Medicaid expansions occurred in an era of general fiscal austerity.

Medicaid's traditional constituencies certainly did not fare well at the start of the 1980s. The Omnibus Budget Reconciliation Act of 1981 (OBRA-81), which carried out much of Reagan's budget cutting agenda, reduced Medicaid spending indirectly by imposing severe cutbacks in AFDC. More than 400,000 poor working families lost Medicaid coverage when they were removed from the cash welfare rolls.[54] Given the deep unpopularity of the cash welfare system among both the public and policy elites, it is not too surprising that Medicaid has been damaged historically by its prior linkage to the AFDC program.[55] The Medicaid eligibility restrictions that were enacted in 1981 were actually mild relative to Reagan's original proposal, which would have transformed Medicaid into a block grant program and terminated Medicaid's status as a budgetary entitlement.

Still, OBRA-81 manifested the basic tensions that are endemic in Medicaid policymaking. While the legislation sought to narrow Medicaid eligibility by retrenching AFDC, the measure also mandated that states provide Medicaid coverage to adults who were removed from the welfare rolls for a nine-month transitional period. The aim was to ease welfare recipients' entry into the paid work force. The federal government even offered to share the costs with any state that wished to extend this transition period for an additional six months. Many states eventually opted for the extra six-month option. This little-noticed feature of OBRA-81 illustrates—in this instance simultaneously within the same bill—the multiple and indeed conflicting ways that Medicaid can be portrayed: (1) as assistance for the "totally indigent" (i.e., welfare dependents); (2) as a program to transition welfare dependents into work; and (3) as policy carrot to discourage welfare dependency in the first place.

Expansions in the 1980s fit the latter two portrayals. Most of the Medicaid expansions for pregnant women and children began modestly. They were initially designed as options presented to the respective states for their consideration, with the federal government making available matching funds. Only later were these expansions gradually converted into federal mandates. For example, coverage of pregnant women and infants up to 100% of the poverty rate was a state option in 1986, but became a federal mandate in 1988. Similarly, the Medicare "buy-in" (described below) was optional in 1986 and required in 1988 (see Table 15-2).

Many states responded favorably to the optional expansions. Participating states were, in general, not required to make any changes in their basic Medicaid eligibility definitions when the mandates were imposed. For example, when the 1988 mandate was passed to expand coverage to 100% of the poverty level for pregnant women and infants, 76% of the states were already compliant (see Figure 15-2a). When this mandate was expanded again the following year to 133% of poverty, 40% of states were still compliant (see Figure 15-2b). By at least initially allowing flexibility for state policy makers to shape their

Table 15-2 Nursing Home Care Expenditures in Billions by Source of Funds

| Year | Total | Private | | | Public | |
		Out-of-Pocket	Private Health Insurance	Other Private Funds	Medicaid	All Other Public Sources
1970	4.2	2.3	.0	.2	.9	.8
	(100)	(54)	(0)	(5)	(21)	(19)
1980	17.6	7.4	.2	.5	8.8	.7
	(100)	(42)	(1)	(3)	(50)	(4)
1990	50.9	21.9	2.1	.9	21.1	2.8
	(100)	(43)	(4)	(2)	(45)	(6)
1997	82.8	25.7	4.0	1.6	39.4	12.0
	(100)	(31)	(5)	(2)	(47)	(14)

SOURCE: Health Care Financing Administration, Office of the Actuary.

NOTE: Percentages (shown in parentheses) may not add up to 100 due to rounding.

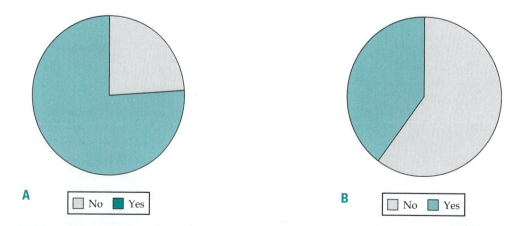

Figure 15-2A State Eligibility Already Above OBRA-88 Mandate of 100% Poverty? **B** State Eligibility Already Above OBRA-89 Mandate of 133% Poverty?

Table 15-3 Major Federal Pregnant Women and Children Expansions for Medicaid Eligibility: 1984–1990

Legislation	Population Affected	Expansion
DEFRA 1984 (Deficit Reduction Act of 1984, P.L. 98-369)	Infants and Children	**Mandate.** Requires coverage of all children up to age 5 born after 9/30/83, who met AFDC financial standards.
	Pregnant women	**Mandate.** Required coverage of first-time pregnant women and pregnant women in two parent families whose principal wage earner was unemployed (AFDC-UP).
COBRA 1985 (Consolidated Omnibus Budget Reconciliation Act of 1985, P.L. 99-272)	Pregnant women	**Mandate.** Requires coverage of all remaining pregnant women meeting AFDC financial standards (that is, those in two-parent families with an employed principal earner).
OBRA 1986 (Omnibus Budget Reconciliation Act of 1986, P.L. 99-509)	Children	**Option.** Allows coverage of all children up to age five born after 9/30/83 with family incomes up to 100% of poverty.
	Pregnant women and Infants	**Option.** Allows coverage of pregnant women and infants under age 1 if income is below a state-established income standard up to 100% of poverty. (Also, allowed states to pay for prenatal care while Medicaid applications are pending.)
OBRA 1986 (Omnibus Budget Reconciliation Act of 1986, P.L. 99-509)	Children	**Option.** Allows coverage of all children up to age 5 born after 9/30/83 with family incomes up to 100% of poverty.
	Pregnant women and Infants	**Option.** Allows coverage of pregnant women and infants under age 1 if income is below a state-established income standard up to 100% of poverty. (Also, allowed states to pay for prenatal care while Medicaid applications are pending.)
OBRA 1987 (Omnibus Budget Reconciliation Act of 1987, P.L. 100-203)	Children	**Mandate.** Requires coverage of all children up to age 7 born after 9/30/83, who meet AFDC income standards (extension of DEFRA 1984 mandate). **Option.** Allows coverage of all children up to age 8 born after 9/30/83 with family incomes up to 100% of poverty.
	Pregnant women and Infants	**Option.** Allows coverage of pregnant women and infants with family incomes up to 185% of poverty.
MCCA 1988 (Medicare Catastrophic Coverage Act of 1988, P.L. 100-360)	Pregnant women and Infants	**Mandate.** Requires coverage of pregnant women and infants under age 1 with incomes under 100% of poverty.

(Continued)

Table 15-3 *(Continued)*

Legislation	Population Affected	Expansion
OBRA 1989 (Omnibus Budget Reconciliation Act of 1989, P.L. 101-239)	Children, Pregnant women and Infants	**Mandate.** Requires coverage of pregnant women and all children (including infants) up to age 6 born after 9/30/83 if family income is below 133% of poverty.
OBRA 1990 (Omnibus Budget Reconciliation Act of 1990, P.L. 101-508)	Children	**Mandate.** Requires coverage of all children up to age 18 born after 9/30/83 with family income under 100% of the poverty level (extends coverage to children age 7 to 18 under 100% of poverty; intent is to phase in coverage of all children in poverty by 2002).

SOURCE: CRS (1993: 36); Coughlin, Ku, and Holahan (1994: 48–51).

respective Medicaid programs, federal politicians - intent on program expansion were able to transform how Medicaid benefits were delivered across the nation.

All told, the targeted Medicaid expansions adopted from 1984 to 1990 increased the number of people receiving Medicaid benefits to 36 million in 1996, up from an average of 20 to 23 million between 1973 and 1989.[56] Then, in 1996, under a larger bill primarily concerned with reforming cash assistance, Congress officially severed the relationship between Medicaid and AFDC (now TANF) eligibility. This meant that children would become eligible for Medicaid based on criteria completely separate from other welfare requirements. In 1997, Congress passed the SCHIP that helped make Medicaid coverage expansions—separate from cash assistance—possible.

When the window of opportunity opened in 1997 for a targeted coverage expansion due to the growing economy, elected officials decided to focus—just as they had in the 1980s—on reducing the number of uninsured *children*. The key administrative question was whether coverage expansion should take place exclusively within Medicaid. While eight major proposals were introduced, the debate quickly narrowed to two major alternatives: a major coverage expansion for children within Medicaid, and a state block grant proposal.[57]

Given Congress's tendency to deal with conflicts between multiple reform proposals not by splitting the difference but rather by accepting them all, it is not surprising that Congress gave its blessing to both the block grant and Medicaid approaches in 1997. This means that under the SCHIP law, with an enhanced federal matching rate, states have the *option* to extend coverage to uninsured children (1) through Medicaid; (2) through the creation of an entirely new, separate program (with a restricted benefit package); or (3) through a combination of both.

While 16 states have opted to use their SCHIP funds for Medicaid expansions, more than half have either implemented new separate (non-Medicaid) SCHIP programs (16 states) or have combination programs (19 states).[58] As mentioned above, a number of states implemented separate (non-Medicaid) programs to expand coverage for low-income children in part to save costs through offering a restricted benefit package, but also because it was feared that working families would not enroll their children in Medicaid due to the welfare stigma associated with the program. Many states wondered whether families with no ties to welfare would be willing to sign up for Medicaid.[59] Enrollment data from the first four years of the SCHIP experience indicate that states can, indeed, successfully repackage Medicaid as a program distinct from welfare.[60]

State policy makers have, in general, responded favorably to the SCHIP option to expand coverage for children and families. While combined Medicaid and SCHIP enrollment declined in the first year after the adoption of SCHIP—due in large part to the effects of welfare reform[61]—there has been a steady increase in enrollment since June of 1998 (see Figure 15-3). Between 1998 and 2001, Medicaid and SCHIP enrollment grew by an average of 30% across the states. Enrollment declined in only three states over this time period.[62] The states with the greatest enrollment increases tended to be those that chose to use SCHIP funds for a Medicaid-expansion program and not to create a new separate program.[63]

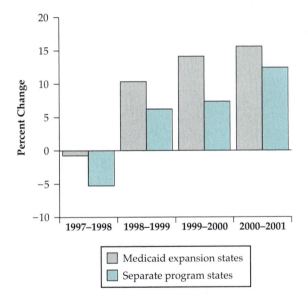

Figure 15-3 Enrollment Expansions in Medicaid and SCHIP by Type of SCHIP Expansion

SOURCE: Mann et al. (2002: 21).

NOTE 1: For this calculation the Rosenback et al. 2001 definition of type of SCHIP program expansion was used. In general, the definition only counts states that adopted relatively broad SCHIP-funded expansions as "Separate Program States."

NOTE 2: Enrollment figures include children, families, and pregnant women.

This suggests that the fear of some progressives that non-poor families would not sign up for Medicaid is baseless, or at least overstated. Indeed, when states devote resources to changing Medicaid's public image and ease of entry (through public relations campaigns highlighting the program's expanded scope and through administrative reforms and simplifications of the enrollment process), they are able to increase enrollment among working, uninsured Americans by significant amounts.[64] As many of the legislative architects of SCHIP hoped, Medicaid coverage increased significantly among children in families who do not receive welfare payments (see Figure 15-4). By 2000, "forty percent of all low-income children were enrolled in Medicaid and SCHIP . . . and two-thirds of these children live in families with one or two full-time workers."[65] By any measure, this is the most significant programmatic shift toward "middle-class" Medicaid since the program was enacted in 1965.

The mid-century strategic notion that Medicare limitations were a necessary, but worthwhile compromise that could eventually take us to universal

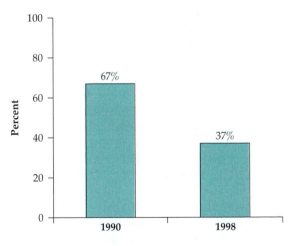

Figure 15-4 Percent of Children Covered by Medicaid Receiving Cash Assistance

SOURCE: This graph is replicated from Mann et al. (2002: 4). They retrieved data from HCFA 2082 and HCFA 64 reports from 1998 to create graph.

coverage was virtually lost by the turn of the 20th century. As of the start of 21st century three facts are clear: Medicare has not expanded as many progressives hoped; employer-based health insurance leaves many workers without health insurance; and Medicaid has tried to plug the holes—not just for the poor, but for middle class families as well.

MYTH 3: MEDICAID REFORM IS PREDICTABLY PARTISAN

Policymakers remain profoundly ambivalent about the reliance of mainstream families on Medicaid for their uninsured children and LTC for their elderly parents. To be sure, politicians recognize the limited long-term care benefits offered by Medicare, eroding employer-based health insurance, and the felt need of middle-class families for governmental assistance. Yet Medicaid, unlike Social Security and Medicare, is not contributory. Program recipients, many policy makers reason, do not have an "earned" right to Medicaid benefits on the basis of payroll tax payments or a lifetime of work.

Indeed, Medicaid policy creates a tricky dilemma for policy makers. On the one hand, the deep reliance of the middle-class families either on nursing home coverage for the elderly or health benefits for children encourages politicians to offer mainstream families ever greater protections and economic security. On the other hand, elected officials are deeply troubled by the offering of such comprehensive benefits to Medicaid-covered families, and the use of Medicaid long term care services as a vehicle for protecting the assets of relatively well-off people.[66]

The central conflict is that most politicians believe means-tested programs should be reserved for the poor who really need the benefits. The problem is that many middle-class families need the benefits Medicaid has to offer. In sum, a fundamental tension has emerged over whether to expand or restrict Medicaid's long-term care role or its efforts to cover the uninsured. The practical result of this dilemma has been to produce a vacillating political dynamic, prone to controversy and uncertainty.

The Middle-Class, Long-Term Care and the Politics of Ambivalence

While there is great disagreement among policymakers about how to reform the Medicaid program, one area where there is bipartisan agreement is that they should discourage middle-class elderly from relying on Medicaid for nursing home care. According to HHS Secretary Leavitt, "many older Americans take advantage of Medicaid loopholes to become eligible for Medicaid by giving away assets to their children. There is a whole industry that actually helps people shift costs to the taxpayer. We must close these loopholes and focus Medicaid's resources on helping those who really need it."

As mentioned above, about 40% of nursing home residents are poor enough to be eligible for Medicaid upon admission, but another 45% begin as private paying residents, spend down their resources, and eventually become Medicaid eligible. Ever since Medicaid was enacted in 1965, middle-class elderly and their families have complained about the spend down process in Medicaid, arguing that it is unfair to elderly, who have worked hard their entire life, to end up having to impoverish themselves and having to die with little (financial) dignity in a nursing home. Over time, policy makers have been sensitive to this argument, and changed the Medicaid program to provide protections to the living spouse so that this person will not lose their home and become poor, and also allowed the elderly to transfer some of their assets to family members, typically their children. It is the transfer of assets on the part of middle-class elderly prior to gaining Medicaid eligibility that has policymakers, like Secretary Leavitt, up-in-arms.

In fact, they've been up-in-arms for a while. Back in 1993, Congress passed a bill making it harder for seniors in nursing homes to gain Medicaid eligibility if they disposed of their assets for less than fair market value during the three years prior to their Medicaid application. An obscure provision, buried in a health reform bill passed in 1996, actually made it a federal crime for a person to "knowingly and willfully" dispose of assets in order to become eligible for Medicaid within the next three years.[67] Despite support among federal leaders, the "Send Grandma to Jail" law (as it was called by the press at the time) was not well-received by the states. Not surprisingly, it just is not popular to demonize our grandparents.[68]

Another way to discourage middle-class people from shedding assets to qualify for Medicaid is to retroactively recoup nursing home expenses incurred by Medicaid recipients from their estates (principally the proceeds of home sales) after death.[69] For many decades states had the option of tapping the estates of the deceased, but, in 1993, Congress actually mandated that every state run estate recovery programs. While a few states implement such programs with vigor, most states simply refuse to follow the law. Again, the idea of taking money from families who just lost a loved-one is not well-received.

Finally, one more approach to rid the Medicaid program of this middle class burden was put forth by Republicans in 1995. Their proposal would have allowed states to make adult children financially liable for their parents' nursing home expenses. It is doubtful Republicans will pursue such a family responsibility initiative today, since it was met with overwhelming popular resistance in 1995. Sixty-eight percent of self-described conservative respondents in a CBS/New York Times poll said they opposed the bill, and it was quickly dropped by Republican lawmakers.

Middle-Class Medicaid to Cover the Uninsured and the Politics of Ambivalence

While several studies have found that party control is related to welfare spending (e.g., a positive relationship between spending and Democratic control), state-level Medicaid policy choices during the 1980s and post-SCHIP enactment appears to be influenced less by differences in political party factors than one might normally expect. Indeed, neither the

partisan composition of state legislatures nor state political ideology correlated with state adoptions of these Medicaid expansions. Ideologically conservative states were just as likely as liberal states to expand Medicaid eligibility to pregnant women and children in the 1980s, though states with heavily Democratic legislators were more willing than other states to expand Medicaid coverage to the highest eligibility level (185% of poverty).[70] In short, Medicaid expansions for poor women and children found a fairly wide base of bipartisan support.[71]

Similarly, there is only a weak relationship between efforts to implement SCHIP expansions and state-level political factors.[72] States led by Republican Governors and/or controlled by Republican state legislatures appear to be just as likely as their Democratic counterparts to take steps to expand Medicaid and SCHIP enrollment. Over three-fourths of the states (78%) set their eligibility levels at or above 200% of the federal poverty line—far above the federal requirement (see Figure 15-5). Again, while Democratic Party control is associated with more generous SCHIP eligibility levels, 20 states led by Republican Governors expanded eligibility to at least 200% of poverty. Moreover, half of these states also had Republican-controlled state legislatures. For example, New Jersey increased SCHIP eligibility levels to 350% of poverty under a Republican-controlled legislature and a Republican Governor. Overall, state experiences with SCHIP suggest that many Republican officeholders are eager to expand coverage to help uninsured working families, with a clear willingness to use Medicaid as the vehicle for promoting this goal.[73]

Beginning in 2001, however, states from California to New York were facing some of their worst budget crises since World War II. Faltering state collections and the weakness of the national economic recovery, together with rapidly increasing Medicaid costs, led many states to consider cutbacks in Medicaid expenditures. While all states have pursued some type of cost-containment strategy within this difficult environment, most states—even those under Republican-control—have been very reluctant to reduce the eligibility gains they achieved over

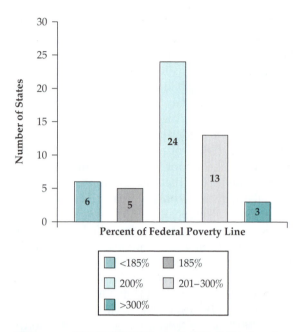

Figure 15-5 SCHIP Financial Eligibility Levels, January 2002

SOURCE: Ross and Cox (2002: 30).

NOTE: Massachusetts and Pennsylvania provide state-financed coverage to children with incomes above SCHIP levels, 235% and 400% respectively. These levels are counted in the graph to show state willingness to expand coverage, however their SCHIP levels are both 200%. Tennessee does not have an upper income limit because its Medicaid waiver is based on the child's lack of insurance.

the last decade. The most popular strategies, regardless of party control, have been to reduce prescription drug prices and payments to providers (see Figure 15-6). Nonetheless, in 2003 over half the states restricted eligibility in some way. The vast majority of states maintained coverage for children, though expansions for working parents have tended to suffer (see Figures 15-7 and 15-8).

Moreover, recent news reports about substantial Medicaid eligibility cuts in Tennessee and Missouri, and potentially Florida, have been alarming.[74] It is important to realize, however, that while the media

has portrayed only the glass half-empty, one can also describe recent state activities as a glass half-full. Some states are chopping Medicaid, but other states, such as Illinois and Kansas are actually increasing eligibility under these extremely fiscally stressed times, and the majority of states are trying to maintain Medicaid coverage.[75] This explains the strong reaction by the National Governor's Association and the National Conference of State Legislatures against President Bush's 2005 proposal to cut $60 billion from projected federal Medicaid spending.[76] Under pressure from their home states, the Republican-led Senate swiftly removed Bush's proposed Medicaid cuts from budget bills under consideration. Although the 109th Congress eventually did pass a $10 billion cut in Medicaid funding to be implemented over the next 10 years, key Republicans in the Senate held up the compromise bill until Medicaid cuts were reduced and a bipartisan Commission to study Medicaid reform was established.

Clearly the Medicaid program can, and has, suffered retrenchment. But, it has not suffered retrenchment as clearly or decisively as other means-tested, targeted programs have (e.g., AFDC in 1996), and its politics does not follow a clear partisan path. While partisan rhetoric around the program exists, Medicaid eligibility policy takes a different turn. As Medicaid takes in more low and middle-income families, politicians—Republican and Democratic—are reluctant to take away Medicaid benefits.

CONCLUSION: WHAT'S HISTORY GOT TO DO WITH IT?

Debunking myths and drawing on history show us where our contemporary policy debates come from—and give us a pretty good idea of where they're going. Three important lessons emerge from this history. First, middle-class reliance on Medicaid for their elderly parents in need of long term care has been with

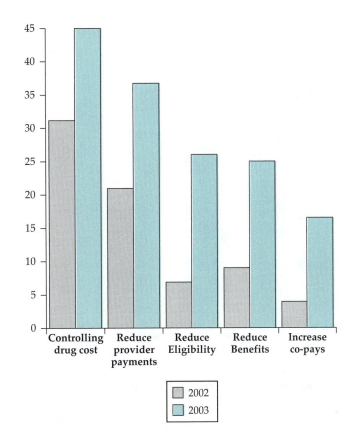

Figure 15-6 States Cost Containment Strategies, 2002 vs. 2003

SOURCE: Kaiser Commission on Medicaid and the Uninsured Survey of Medicaid officials in 50 states and DC conducted by Health Management Associates, 2003. Graph reproduced from KCMU, "Are We Holding the Line on Health Coverage for Low-Income Families? Briefing Charts," July 29, 2003.

us for a long time. Nonetheless, we continue to hear political statements in support of such bills restricting middle-class reliance. For example, besides Secretary Leavitt's recent statement in 2005, New Jersey's Democratic Representative Frank Pallone said the following in 1993: "Clearly the Medicaid program is not intended to be an insurance program for the wealthy."[77] Perhaps. But, Medicaid was intended to fill in the gaps of Medicare. Long-term care services are needed by the majority of elderly at some point in their lives, and when such services are needed—especially expensive nursing home costs—even middle-class elderly find it difficult to pay for care. Because

Medicare, for the most part, does not cover such services, and there is no affordable private market for long-term care insurance, Medicaid has filled in that gap not just for poor elderly, but the middle class as well. It is true that half of all Medicaid applicants transfer some assets prior to submitting their applications. While one in three transfers are for less than $10,000, the remaining are more and sometimes the sum transfer is large.

So, should we "get" these "wealthy" elderly? Are they greedy and taking advantage of taxpayers? Is this the Medicaid "change" we want? If we don't allow the middle class to transfer assets or conduct

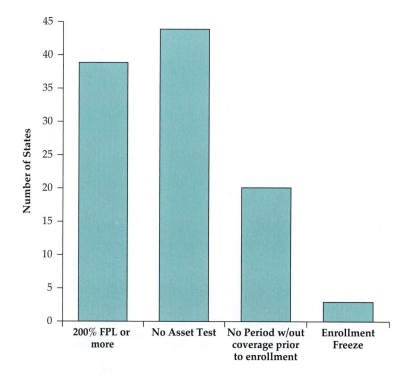

Figure 15-7 **Eligibility for Children's Health Coverage, April 2003**

SOURCE: Graph reproduced from Kaiser Commission on Medicaid and the Uninsured (KCMU), "Are We Holding the Line on Health Coverage for Low-Income Families? Briefing Charts," July 29, 2003. Data based on national survey by the Center for Budget and Policy Priorities for KCMU, 2003.

estate planning, we are essentially saying that middle class elderly must sell their assets and use up their inheritance to pay for long-term care during their last years of life. The problem is most of us think that sounds unfair to the elderly who have worked hard all their lives to build up a nest egg. This is why we created the so-called loopholes in the first place. On the other hand, we also don't like hearing that we—the taxpayers—have to bear the brunt of the greedy elderly who hide their wealth and don't pay for nursing home care. But, that's just it: "We have found the enemy and they is us!" That's the vicious cycle.

But, there is a way out of this cycle, and this is an important Medicaid opportunity. By acknowledging that Medicaid is our universal long-term care

program, we can have a clear earmarked tax fund that we all pay in to. Rather than going after the elderly by trying to take money from their estates when they are the most vulnerable, why not be honest and ask for payment upfront from everyone? Not only are these programs inhumane, they're inefficient. By creating estate recovery programs and transfer of asset policies, we spend sizable amounts trying to prevent innocent elderly from "gaming" Medicaid. Instead, with an explicit tax we could use those administrative resources to implement innovative long-term care models nationwide. Across the political spectrum, Democrats and Republicans alike agree that we should rely more heavily on home and community-based long-term care options, which encourages elderly independence and

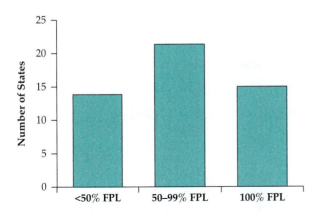

Figure 15-8 **Eligibility for Working Parents, April 2003**

SOURCE: Data obtained from the Kaiser Commission on Medicaid and the Uninsured (KCMU), "Are We Holding the Line on Health Coverage for Low-Income Families? Briefing Charts," July 29, 2003. Data based on national survey by the Center for Budget and Policy Priorities for KCMU, 2003.

are less costly than nursing home use. The states have been remarkably innovative in creating new long-term care delivery models. We should build on this strength that Medicaid already possesses. If we were all in this together, we could have an important, open, and rational discussion about how best to organize long-term care services for our elderly in a humane and, yet, cost-effective way. Finally, this rethinking does not just offer sound policy that is morally superior to the status quo, but that is politically astute as well. While Frank Pallone's rhetoric sounds good out of context, when it is put into practice, middle class children balk, and politicians— Democrats or Republicans—are in trouble.

The second lesson to glean from this history is to realize that we view the problem of "uninsurance" differently today than in the past. When Medicaid was enacted in 1965, policy makers saw the new program as being appropriate for non-workers on cash assistance, whereas workers were supposed to either obtain employer-based coverage or use their earnings to purchase private health insurance. Today, there is

a widespread consensus that Medicaid benefits are necessary for many workers; indeed, to help workers maintain employment. Although policy makers still favor policies that encourage employers to offer health insurance to their employees or encourage workers to purchase private insurance, most of these policy experiments have failed to make any impact on reducing rates of uninsurance.[78] In short, Medicaid and Medicare were designed to fill gaps in the employment based health insurance system. Today, as those gaps are steadily growing, we continue to turn to Medicaid most often as a possible solution.

Indeed, Medicaid expansions for children, when offered, have lowered the rate of uninsured children in working families. Given Medicaid's impact it is not surprising that even conservatives, like Secretary Leavitt, continue to call for Medicaid expansions to cover more uninsured children. Nonetheless, while we can see opportunities for expansion, even in difficult times, the politics of ambivalence shows us that retrenchment is equally likely. The question is whether one should view all restrictions the same way. Are all retrenchments created equal? It is in reference to this question that the third lesson can be helpful.

This third important lesson from Medicaid's history is to realize that the bipartisan connection to Medicaid, and the reason for the politics of ambivalence (instead of a clear partisan path toward retrenchment or expansion), is due to middle-class reliance on the program. The true opportunity that Medicaid provides is to mobilize this middle-class reliance on the program, and thereby transform the politics of Medicaid into a broad-based coalition that views Medicaid as their social entitlement.

In light of this opportunity to transform Medicaid politics, policy reforms that create bifurcations among Medicaid's beneficiaries are particularly damaging. Indeed, a key tension over Medicaid policymaking today is how we offer Medicaid coverage to expansion groups. Secretary Leavitt argues that "mandatory populations need the help, (whereas) the optional populations . . . may not need such a comprehensive solution. Most of them are healthy people who just need help paying for health insurance." In particular,

Leavitt advocates maintaining comprehensive benefits for mandatory populations—those who are tied to cash assistance—but providing a reduced benefit package to optional populations—those whose incomes are higher including people from low and middle-income families. As Leavitt puts it, "Wouldn't it be better to provide health insurance to more people, rather than comprehensive care to a smaller group? Wouldn't it be better to give Chevies to everyone rather than Cadillacs to a few?"

The rhetoric may seem enticing but every generation hears the same call and quickly discovers the flaw in the logic. Medicaid does combine two groups: very low income persons on cash assistance, and many more persons (two-thirds of recipients) not on cash assistance who come from low or middle income families. The latter—working families with political connections—will not give up their benefits without a fierce battle. Neither party has ever shown an appetite for rescinding middle class benefits. Real retrenchment would have to begin—politically—by bifurcating the two beneficiary groups.

In other words, the true opportunity for Medicaid expansions lies in keeping its beneficiaries groups (the so-called mandatory and optional groups) together. Reforms should not allow expansions to create divisions. Rather eligibility expansions should always expand the political base. The vivid lesson for those who fight for universal coverage is to give up on comprehensive benefits for Medicaid's "truly poor." Instead, such persons should fight for the following principle: expansion under the condition that all groups receive equal treatment—even if that means giving less to the "truly needy." Medicaid's history repeatedly illustrates the logic of this strategy. Each time the program expands and the middle class sees Medicaid as their social entitlement (as in the case of long term care), both the quality of care and access to services for the "truly needy" improves. In short, past changes offer reformers a clear road map to future changes. I, too, believe that it would be better to give Chevies to everyone rather than Cadillacs to a few. But, that means changing the benefit package for everyone in Medicaid—not just the so-called optional groups—and making sure

they actually get a Chevy—not half a car but a full one, a car that actually drives.

STUDY QUESTIONS

1. What populations receive coverage under Medicaid?
2. What accounted for the early explosion in Medicaid costs?
3. How did the 1967 'retrenchment' legislation also constitute a broadening of the program's principles?
4. Why was the cost and significance of medical vendor payments underestimated at the time the relevant legislation was passed?
5. How did the Kerr-Mills bill influence the form Medicaid later took?
6. Why must many considered solidly middle class rely on Medicaid after entering a nursing home?
7. The author argues that Medicaid is not a partisan issue. Why?
8. The author argues that there is an endless argument between those who see Medicaid as a middle class program and those who see it as welfare medicine. Explain.

NOTES

1. Leavitt, M. Secretary of Health and Human Services, Speech to World Health Care Congress, Marriott Wardman Park Hotel, Washington DC, Tuesday, February 1, 2005.
2. Hayes, 2003.
3. CMS website: http://www.cms.hhs.gov, February 2003.
4. Leavitt Speech, 2005.
5. Collins and Ho, 2004.
6. Center for Medicare and Medicaid, US Department of Health and Human Services website: www.cms.hhs.gov (as of February 2005).

7. They also use the State Children's Health Insurance Program (SCHIP), which can be structured as part of Medicaid, or as a separate program, or as a combination of these two options. The importance of SCHIP will be discussed in more detail later in this chapter.

8. Stevens and Stevens, 1974; Theodore Marmor, 1970. See Chapter 5.

9. Johnson, 1967.

10. Stevens and Stevens, 1974.

11. Congressional Research Service (CRS), 1993, p 30.

12. Stevens and Stevens, 1974.

13. HEW, 1967, table 15.

14. This bizarre fractional percent to determine eligibility is a testament to Medicaid's complexity.

15. US Senate, 1967, p 1546.

16. Ibid., p 1547.

17. Quadagno, 1988.

18. Waston, 1995. There were some exceptions to the SSI federal standards. Some states were allowed to set lower state-defined SSI eligibility levels.

19. Stevens and Stevens, 1974.

20. Rosenbaum and Sonosky, 1999.

21. Congressional Research Service, 1993, p 1041, appendix H; see also Watson, 1995.

22. See Grogan (forthcoming) for detail about this history.

23. Holstein and Cole, 1996.

24. Ibid.

25. Ibid.

26. Steward, 1925; Katz, 1986.

27. Stevens, 1971; Rosenberg, 1987; Vladeck, 1980.

28. Ibid.; Haber, 1983; Gratton, 1993.

29. Katz, 1986; Stevens and Stevens, 1974.

30. Vladeck, 1980; Stevens and Stevens, 1974.

31. Vladeck, 1980; Holstein and Cole, 1996.

32. US Congress, Senate Hearing, January 23, 1950, p186. The Table on Persons 65 years of age and over living in Institutions was inserted into the record by Wilbur Cohen. *Source:* Special report on institutional population 1940, table 12, Bureau of the Census.

33. Holstein and Cole, 1996, p 29.

34. Altmeyer, 1950; Vladeck, 1980; Stevens and Stevens, 1974.

35. Stevens and Stevens, 1974.

36. Altmeyer testimony, 1950, p 60.

37. Ibid., p 58.

38. Poen, 1982; Stevens and Stevens, 1974.

39. See Holstein and Cole, 1996, for a discussion of how SBA and FHA construction loans encouraged the building of private for-profit nursing homes.

40. Named after its Democratic congressional sponsors, Representative Wilbur Mills and Senator Robert Kerr.

41. Marmor, 1973.

42. Fein, 1998.

43. Vladeck, 1980.

44. Stevens and Stevens, 1974.

45. Of course, it left out more than these two groups mentioned, but these were the groups whose health access limitations became the most concerning to policy makers.

46. Congressional Research Service, 1993.

47. The Medically Needy programs allow states to cover persons who have large medical expenses relative to their incomes. The 300% rule allows states (that so chose) to cover persons needing nursing home care whose income does not exceed 300% of the federally defined SSI level.

48. Cohen, Kumar, and Wallack, 1993.

49. Himelfarb, 1995.

50. Grogan and Patashnik, 2003b.

51. Rosenbaum, 1993.

52. Melnick, 1999.

53. Tanenbaum, 1995.

54. Cohen and Holahan, 1985; Oberg and Polich, 1988.

55. For a provocative argument that the political unpopularity of AFDC reflects racial coding, see Gilens, 1999. AFDC notwithstanding, the political durability of means-tested programs more generally is a matter of debate among welfare state scholars and practitioners. For contrasting views, see Skocpol 1995, and Greenstein, 1991.

56. Melnick, 1999, p 31.

57. Sardell and Johnson, 1998.
58. Mann et al., 2002.
59. Ibid.
60. Ibid.
61. Several studies have documented this decline in Medicaid enrollment due to welfare reform in 1996 (the Personal Responsibility Work Opportunity and Reconciliation Act of 1996). See, for example, Kronenbusch, 2001.
62. Mann et al., 2002.
63. There are many reasons why this might be the case (difficulties coordinating enrollment processes between Medicaid and the new programs for one). See Ross and Cox, 2002, and Mann et al., 2002, for a more detailed discussion.
64. Ross and Cox, 2002.
65. Mann et al., 2002, p 1.
66. Grogan and Patashnik, 2003a.
67. Magnusson, 1996.
68. Joire, 1999.
69. Quinn, 1993.
70. This analysis is based on simple correlation tests. In particular, percent democrat control in state legislature is correlated with percent expansion for pregnant women and infants at .42; percent democrat control and meeting OBRA-88 mandate and OBRA-89 mandate is .18 and .24, respectively. Erickson, Wright, and McIver, 1993, measure of state liberalism (or ideology) is correlated with percent expansion, OBRA-88 and OBRA-89 at .30, .12, and .33, respectively. Obviously, one would need to do a multivariate analysis to test these relationships more rigorously. Kousser, 2002, for example, finds that party control is significantly related to state-level Medicaid expenditures. For our purposes, however, it is of interest to study further whether state responses to certain—more politically favorable—groups are *not* related to party control. A more rigorous extended analysis concerning the effect of party control on specific Medicaid expansions would be useful in a separate chapter. The data source for state level party control is the US

Statistical Abstract for the appropriate year under consideration.
71. Grogan and Patashnik, 2003b.
72. Party in governorship and party control of state legislature is insignificantly correlated with state-level enrollment expansions at −.07 and −.06, respectively. As mentioned in an earlier endnote, these are just simple bivariate correlations. A more rigorous extended analysis concerning the effect of party control on specific Medicaid expansions would be useful in a separate chapter. The data source for state level party control is the US Statistical Abstract for the appropriate year under consideration.
73. Grogan and Patashnik, 2003b.
74. Simon, 2005.
75. Ibid.
76. Pear, 2005.
77. Lynwander, 1993.
78. Collins and Ho, 2004; Commonwealth Fund, 2001; Gabel et al., 2003.

REFERENCES

Cohen, J., and J. Holahan. 1985. *Medicaid Eligibility after the Omnibus Budget Reconciliation Act of 1981.* Medicaid Program Evaluation Working Paper, The Urban Institute. October. Washington DC: Urban Institute.

Cohen, M.A., N. Kumar, and S.S. Wallack. 1993. "Simulating the Fiscal and Distributional Impacts of Medicaid Eligibility Reforms," *Health Care Financing Review* 14 (4): 133–50.

Collins S. and A. Ho, 2004. "From Coast to Coast: The Affordability Crisis in U.S. Health Care." Data from *Commonwealth Fund Biennial Health Insurance Survey* (2001 and 2003).

Congressional Research Service (CRS). 1993. *Medicaid Source Book: Background Data and Analysis (A 1993 Update).* (Washington DC: US Government Printing Office).

Commonwealth Fund 2001 Health Insurance Survey. "Security Matters: How Instability in Health Insurance Puts U.S. Workers at Risk," Charts.

Coughlin, T., L. Ku, and I. Holahan, 1994. *Medicaid Since 1980.* (Washington DC: Urban Institute).

Fein, S. 1998. The Kerr-Mills Act: Medical Care for the Indigent in Michigan, 1960–1965. *Journal of the History of Medicine and Allied Sciences* 53 (3): 285–316.

Gabel J., et al., "Health Benefits in 2003: Premiums Reach Thirteen Year High as Employers Adopt New Forms of Cost Sharing." *Health Affairs* (Sept/Oct 2003): 117–26.

Grogan, C., and E. Patashnik. 2003a. "Between Welfare Medicine and Mainstream Program: Medicaid at the Political Crossroads." *Journal of Health Politics, Policy and Law* 28 (5): 821–58.

—— 2003b. "Universalism within Targeting: Nursing Home Care, the Middle Class, and the Politics of the Medicaid Program." *Social Service Review* 77 (1): 51–71.

Grogan, C. 2005. "The Politics of Aging within Medicaid." In Hudson, R.B., ed., *The New Politics of Old Age Policy.* Baltimore: Johns Hopkins University Press.

Grogan, C. (Forthcoming). "A Marriage of Convenience: The History of Nursing Home Coverage and Medicaid." In R.A. Stevens, C.E. Rosenberg, and L.R. Burns, eds., *History and Health Policy* (tentative title). Berkeley: University of California Press.

Himelfarb, R. 1995. *Catastrophic Politics: The rise and fall of the Medicare Catastrophic Coverage Act of 1988.* University Park: Pennsylvania State University Press.

Holstein, M., and T.R. Cole. 1996. "The Evolution of Long-Term Care in America." In R.H. Binstock, L.E. Cluff, and O. Von Mering, eds., *The Future of Long-Term Care: Social and Policy Issues.* Baltimore: Johns Hopkins University Press, pp 19–48.

Joire, L.S. 1999. "Note: After New York State Bar Association v. Reno: Ethical Problems in Limiting Medicaid Estate Planning." *Georgetown Journal of Legal Ethics* 12 (summer): 789.

Katz, M.B. 1986. *In the Shadow of the Poorhouse: A Social History of Welfare in America.* New York: Basic Books.

Lynwander, L. 1993. "Changes Looming on Medicaid Rules." *The New York Times* July 18, Section 13, p 1.

Magnusson, P. 1996. "Medicaid is Getting Tough with Granny." *Business Week* September 30, p 45.

Mann, C., D. Rousseau, R. Garfield, and M. O'Malley. 2002. *Reaching Uninsured Children through Medicaid: If You Build It Right, They Will Come.* June. Washington DC: Kaiser Commission on Medicaid and the Uninsured.

Marmor, T.R. 1973. *The Politics of Medicare.* New York: Aldine.

Melnick, S.R. 1998. "The Unexpected Resilience of Means-Tested Programs," prepared for delivery at the 1998 annual meeting of the American Political Science Association, Boston, Massachusetts, September 3–6.

Oberg, C.N., and C.L. Polich. 1988. "Medicaid: Entering the Third Decade." *Health Affairs* 7 (4): 83–96.

Pear, R. 2005. "Governors Prepare to Fight Medicaid Cuts." *The New York Times* February 27.

Poen, M.M. 1982. "The Truman Legacy: Retreat to Medicare." In R.L. Numbers, ed., *Compulsory Health Insurance.* Westport, CT: Greenwood Press, pp 97–114.

Quinn, J.B. 1993. "New Law Lets Medicaid Tap Middle-Class Seniors' Estates." *The Washington Post* October 10, p H3.

Rosenbaum, S. 1993. "Medicaid Expansions and Access to Health Care." In D. Rowland, J. Feder, A. Salganicoff, *Medicaid Financing Crisis: Balancing Responsibilities, Priorities, and Dollars.* Washington DC: AAAS Publication, pp 45–82

Rosenberg, C.E. 1987. *The Care of Strangers: The Rise of America's Hospital System.* New York: Basic Books.

Ross, D.C., and L. Cox. 2002. *Enrolling Children and Families in Health Coverage: The Promise of Doing More.* Washington DC: Kaiser Commission on Medicaid and the Uninsured.

Sardell, A., and K. Johnson. 1998. "The Politics of EPSDT Policy in the 1990s: Policy Entrepreneurs, Political Streams, and Children's Health Benefits." *The Milbank Quarterly* 76 (2): 175–205.

Simon, S. 2005. "States Rein In Health Costs: Legislatures are looking to cut Medicaid or add fees. Missouri is poised to end the program, which many of the poor rely upon for care." *Los Angeles Times* April 24.

Stevens, R.B., and R. Stevens. 1974. *Welfare Medicine in America: A Case Study of Medicaid.* New York: Free Press.

Stewart, E.M. 1925. "The Cost of American Almshouses," US Bureau of Labor Statistics, Bulletin No. 386. Washington DC: Government Printing Office.

Tannebaum, S.J. 1995. "Medicaid Eligibility Policy in the 1980s: Medical Utilitarianism and the 'Deserving' Poor." *Journal of Health Politics, Policy, and Law* 20 (4): 933–953.

Thompson, F.J., and J.J. Dilulio. 1998. *Medicaid and Devolution: A view from the state.* Washington DC: Brookings Institution Press.

US Congress. 1950. *Social Security Revision.* Committee on Finance. Hrg., Senate, 81st Congress, Second Session on H.R. 6000, January 23–31, February 1–3, 6–10, 1950. Washington DC: US Government Printing Office.

Vladeck, B.C. 1980. *Unloving Care: The Nursing Home Tragedy.* New York: Basic Books.

CHAPTER 16

AIDS

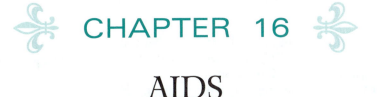

Patricia Siplon

This chapter analyzes the politics of AIDS. Patricia Siplon describes the harrowing early days of epidemic; analyzes the politics of treatment, service provision, and prevention—with special emphasis on the tension between abstinence and harm reduction; summarizes recent policy turns; warns of continuing (even mounting) challenges; and speculates about the future.

AIDS (Acquired Immune Deficiency Syndrome) has had a short history as a policy issue in the United States. Yet, what it lacks in age, it has more than made up for in controversy. It is difficult to think of a disease that has aroused more emotion or spawned more social (and health system) change. Even the recounting of these changes is controversial, with some analysts viewing the response to AIDS as a break-through event that created exciting new models of patient empowerment, scientific innovation, and creative social programming, while others disparage the "AIDS exceptionalism" that they believe has privileged individual human rights above the general welfare.[1]

These wildly differing interpretations of AIDS policy emerged from the politics that created the policy. The politics have their roots in the early days of tracking the epidemic, and in the decisions by affected communities to either actively participate or withdraw from the AIDS policy arena. Like most policy areas, AIDS is constantly changing.

Technological advances cast new light (and new doubts) on some policy approaches; the political landscape has changed significantly over the course of the epidemic. Some activists argue that shifts in ideology and policy have dismantled many of the advances won over the past 20 years. This chapter begins by examining the early days of epidemic. From there I turn to the politics of treatment, prevention, and service provision. Finally, I summarize recent policy shifts and speculate about future trends.

EARLY DAYS AND EARLY DECISIONS

It is impossible to say precisely when the history of AIDS in the United States began. Practically speaking, though, it is useful to start in 1981. On June 5,

1981, the first report identified the health problem. The Centers for Disease Control (CDC) described five cases of *Pneumocysis* pneumonia in previously healthy gay white men in Los Angeles (published in the Center's *Morbidity and Mortality Weekly Report*). A year later, in July 1982, the disease got its acronym—AIDS.

On March 3, 1983, the CDC again stepped up to the plate, and made a critical announcement. It pronounced four groups at increased risk for AIDS: homosexual men with multiple sexual partners; intravenous drugs users (usually heroin); Haitian immigrants in the United States; and hemophiliacs. The groups, quickly dubbed the AIDS 4-H Club, reacted in widely divergent ways that would have tremendous consequences for the future course of the epidemic.

The Haitians reacted most strongly against any attempts to associate them with either risk or infection. In the following two years, Haitian leaders and communities, particularly in New York and Florida, successfully moved to decouple the association of Haitians and HIV (Human Immunodeficiency Virus). They sought both to be removed from the official lists of "at-risk" groups maintained by the CDC and from the list of groups banned by the Food and Drug Administration (FDA) from giving blood. Haitians first convinced the New York City Health Department to remove them from its official risk list in the summer of 1983 then prevailed on the CDC, which also removed Haitians as a category. In April 1985, the battle with the FDA involved major demonstrations in a number of cities, including an April 1990 New York City protest drawing between 50,000 and 100,000 people; the FDA also backed down and rescinded the ban on Haitian blood in December 1990.

The experience of heroin users was very different. In contrast to the other three categories, there was no organized "community" of individuals identified as at risk. Rather, heroin users, who were disproportionately (though by no means exclusively) poor, urban, and members of racial minority groups, had many groups and organizations seeking to speak for them; but these groups had clashing ideas about what constituted advocacy and good policy around HIV prevention and services for injection drug users. Injection drug users became the objects of highly charged emotional battles, particularly regarding prevention efforts.

The hemophilia community's relationship to HIV and AIDS was complicated by delay. As early as 1982, the CDC began identifying hemophiliacs who had no risk factors other than infusion of blood clotting factor; however, this information did not reach hemophiliacs. Instead, physicians and the National Hemophilia Foundation (NHF) told hemophiliacs that their risks of contracting HIV were exceedingly remote, a position maintained into the mid-1980s when approximately half of the US population of hemophiliacs had been infected.[2] Retrospective studies, including an inquiry commissioned by the Congress and conducted by the Institute of Medicine concluded that both the NHF and the Blood Products Advisory Committee of the FDA had been too reliant on information from the private blood products industry and too slow to act in the face of contrary evidence from the CDC.[3] As news of these problems finally began to circulate, it precipitated a split within the hemophiliac community. One side chose an activist orientation that was much like the AIDS activism developing in the gay community; the other side, fearful of losing both confidentiality and decorum, actively resisted the political activism. Thus, although the hemophilia community ultimately produced grassroots organizations working in close alliance with other AIDS activists, it become best known as the "face" of epidemic that fought against any exclusion of individuals living with HIV. This face was epitomized by Ryan White, the boy from Kokomo, Indiana, whose courageous battle against discrimination with his local school district made him a household name.

In contrast to the three other groups, homosexual (mostly urban white) men, came to be clearly and explicitly identified with the epidemic. Indeed the larger gay and lesbian community came to own it. Ownership, in this context means more than association; it also includes the ability to determine the ways in which the disease is socially defined and constructed. In fact, the gay community's struggle against AIDS became profoundly linked to the community's battle for basic rights—particularly privacy, sexual freedom, and freedom from discrimination. The timing of the AIDS epidemic itself was also critical. With Ronald Reagan, a conservative Republican, in the White House, the gay community feared that the administration would react to the disease with disinterest while using the epidemic as an opportunity to eliminate the institutions and freedoms that the gay community had fought for. As a result, the gay community seized ownership of AIDS and began developing its own strategies and policies around treatment, services, and prevention.

PILLS AND PROTEST

Of the many challenges facing people living with the newly-found syndrome, none was more immediate than finding treatment. Initially, of course, none existed. In fact, it wasn't until April 1984 that Health and Human Services (HHS) Secretary Margaret Heckler would be able to announce that the virus that causes AIDS had been discovered. And although she confidently asserted that further rapid advances were in store, including a vaccine ready for testing within two years, her confidence proved ill-founded.[4] For people with AIDS, the goal became staying alive by finding a doctor who was willing to be creative in treating the many illnesses caused by HIV's immune compromising properties.

One such illness, in fact the leading killer of people infected with HIV in the early days of the epidemic, was *Pneumocystis carinii pneumonia* (PCP). Although the first bout of PCP was usually not deadly, subsequent infections left the lungs increasingly damaged and the third or fourth rounds were often fatal. Before the onset of AIDS, other immunocompromised individuals, such as cancer patients on chemotherapy, also suffered from PCP, and known treatments for the condition included an injected drug called pentamidine as well as the sulfa-based drugs Bactrim and Septra.[5] Community doctors be-

gan to treat their patients with these medicines, in some cases, even before they became ill. However, a high number of patients had severe reactions to the sulfa-based drugs leaving pentamidine as one of the only treatment options.

The use of pentamidine soared. By the end of 1983, the CDC had received more than 2,000 orders of what had previously been a rarely requested drug. The CDC ordered pentamidine from England and sent it to requesting physicians on a "compassionate use" (i.e., free) basis. Worried that demand would outstrip supply, the CDC approached several companies and eventually convinced a small company called Lymphomed to supply and eventually distribute the drug.

Lymphomed took advantage of a new law, the Orphan Drug Act, which encouraged drug manufacturers to develop drugs for rare diseases that might not permit them to recoup their research and development costs. The provisions of the Act provided for seven year exclusive marketing rights, research grants, and tax credits. Lymphomed successfully applied for orphan drug status and pentamidine became the first drug targeted to people with AIDS under the orphan drug designation. In what would become a common dynamic, the AIDS community challenged the motivations behind the pharmaceutical company's decision. Although Lymphomed's vice president doggedly defended his company in a Congressional hearing, quoting the National Organization for Rare Disorders' citation of Lymphomed as an "outstanding model for the pharmaceutical industry," Representative Ted Weiss (D-NY), an early ally of the AIDS community, took the company to task for using pentamidine production as a way to grow a small company on the back of a single product "by soaking the clientele."[6]

A still bigger controversy arose when AIDS advocates locked horns with the national public health bureaucracy. Another advance in treatment set off the fight—this time the discovery that pentamidine was more effective when aerolized into a mist and inhaled directly into the lungs. As the information spread, some doctors began to engage in a practice known as "off-label use"—using an FDA-approved drug in a way other than the one listed on the label. Soon, a disparity in care arose. Patients with access to information and private physicians (usually urban gay white men) had access to an effective, often life-saving, treatment that other people with AIDS (including poor and rural people) did not even know about. When one prominent New York City–based gay activist, Michael Callen, found out that his fellow PWA (acronym for "Person with AIDS") Ryan White did not have access to aerolizable pentamidine, he launched a campaign to spread the information. Callen went to the head of the National Institute for Allergies and Infectious Diseases (NIAID), Dr. Anthony Fauci, in May 1987 to request that he release federal guidelines advising doctors with patients at risk for PCP to treat it preventively with aerolizable pentamidine. Fauci—sticking to standard operating procedure—refused because, he claimed, he did not have sufficient evidence on the effectiveness of such treatment to justify issuing the guidelines.

The situation was untenable. The government would not release guidelines because it lacked the clinical trial evidence upon which to base them, but could not enroll volunteers in clinical trials because patients who were informed enough to know about the trials were also informed enough to instruct their physicians to provide off-label treatment. Disgusted with both the government and the private sector, activists and community doctors chose to run their own community-based trials. The first trial was run by the San Francisco Community County Consortium between July 1987 and December 1988. Affected individuals had a heavy influence in the design of the trial. For one thing, there was no attempt to make them "double blind"—the scientific standard in which neither the participants nor the doctors know who was assigned to experimental or control groups. More significantly, there were no control groups—every participant was assigned to one of three experimental groups getting varying levels of medications. In New York City a second community based group, the Community Research Initiative, also launched a trial patterned after San Francisco's, while the National Institutes of Health were called before the Congress in

April 1988 and grilled over why it was that, some nine months after the San Francisco community-based trial had begun, the NIH had failed to enroll even a single person in the three trials they had designed. Lymphomed agreed to sponsor the trials, in part because the company found itself in a race with another drug company, Fisons, over the rights for aerosoluble pentamidine (Lymphomed only had exclusive rights to injections). Based on its collaborative work with the New York and San Francisco groups, Lymphomed received the license for aerolizable pentamidine though the alliance between activist and drug company soon broke again over the recurring issue of pricing.

Lymphomed had already battled with AIDS advocates over prices. Between October 1984, when Lymphomed received orphan drug status for injectable pentamidine, and August 1987, the price skyrocketed from $25.00 a vial to $99.45. In a testimony before the Congress, Lymphomed argued that the price hike was justified by the efforts needed to handle the unexpected demand for the drug.

This answer satisfied neither the Congress nor AIDS activists, who seized on the most effective way to show their displeasure—finding an alternate supply of the drug. The vehicle they used was the PWA Health Group—the largest buyers' club in the country. In September 1989, the PWA Health Group publicly took on Lymphomed in a press conference where it announced it would be begin importing pentamidine from England where it could be had for a fraction of the price. Lymphomed refused to lower its price, and buyers clubs continued to go to England, and, later, Germany, giving savvy people with AIDS a way to openly challenge drug companies on the issue of price.

The pricing battle over aerosoluble pentamidine had a precedent in an even higher profile battle that began on March 24, 1987. On that day, a new organization called ACT UP (AIDS Coalition to Unleash Power)/New York held its first protest. The ACT UP protest targeted the giant pharmaceutical company Burroughs Wellcome (two mergers later, it is now part of the even larger GlaxoSmithKline), which had just announced the release of the first medication licensed as an anti-HIV drug. Although this news was widely hailed as a breakthrough, the company set the price at $10,000 for a year's supply—beyond the reach of many people with AIDS. Some 250 ACT UP protestors took to the streets, and in the process helped define the signature tactics and symbols that would become widely associated with the AIDS activist movement. Employing a powerful combination of visual imagery and information, ACT UP used both props, such as an effigy of FDA Commissioner Frank Young, and information (much of it printed in heavy large lettering against fluorescent backgrounds) including fact sheets and copies of a *New York Times* op-ed piece written by ACT UP co-founder Larry Kramer. In addition to the primary target of Burroughs Wellcome, ACT UP also took on the FDA (for colluding with drug companies and moving too slowly in the drug approval process), NIH (for conducting clinical trials privileging scientific information over the well-being of trial participants), the insurance industry (for denying benefits to people with, or at risk for, AIDS), and the president of the United States (for failing to address the epidemic). By the end of the day, ACT UP had made the national news thanks to large traffic jams and 17 arrests. In time, ACT UP became an organizational model that would spread to cities around the United States and other industrialized democracies. The organization popularized a radical health politics that challenged not only powerful multinational corporations but the whole network of relationships between consumers, government, and the private sector.

The overall impact of the struggles over drug approval and pricing exemplified by these two early treatments was far reaching. AIDS activists helped redefine the paradigms for scientific inquiry, citizen-government, and consumer-corporation relationships. AIDS activists threatened power relationships by challenging well-established rules of science (such as the "gold standard" of placebo testing in clinical trials) and the marketplace (such as the idea of the right of companies to justify their pricing through arguments of the need to recoup (undisclosed) research

and development costs). Such challenges would probably not have been possible without another stream of political activism running through AIDS activist communities—the self-empowerment movement.

SELF-EMPOWERMENT AND NEW TREATMENTS

The AIDS movement did not invent self-empowerment. Rather, it was one consequence of the decision by the larger gay community—gay men *and* lesbians—to take ownership of AIDS as an issue. Many activist lesbians were veterans of the women's health movement which had created new health organizations, service delivery systems (such as birthing centers and women's clinics), and self-help groups. The movement encouraged women to examine their own bodies and experiences, demystifying the medical process. Women reduced the social distance between themselves, the uninformed patients, and their doctors, the highly trained professionals. Rather, women began to see themselves as experts on their own bodies, with experiences and self-knowledge that should be considered in decision making. This concept was transplanted to the AIDS movement, where people infected with HIV began to regard themselves as experienced and knowledgeable for having lived with this unknown virus.

The seminal event within the self-empowerment movement occurred in 1983 at an AIDS conference in Denver, Colorado.[7] About a dozen people with AIDS gathered in a hospitality suite and discussed their experiences of patronizing treatment. Two groups asked two of its members, Michael Callen and Bobbi Callen, to come up with a statement which came to be known as the Denver Principles—a manifesto outlining principles for interaction between health care professionals, the public at large, and people infected with HIV. This last group, they noted, should be known neither as "victims" (which suggests defeat) nor as "patients" (which is only occasionally accurate and implies helplessness), but rather as "people with

AIDS (or PWAs)." The Denver Principles also sought to eliminate discrimination, promote inclusion, and proposed a list of rights that addressed relationships, medical treatment, service provision, and privacy.[8] The activists dramatically announced their principles when they stormed the closing session, unfurled a banner, and took turns reading the points aloud.

The symbiotic interaction between personal and group empowerment allowed PWAs and their allies to challenge medicine and society at all levels. It provided for a consistent approach, privileging, for example, the primacy of PWAs as decision makers in their own medical treatment and as representatives on advisory boards and scientific conferences. The effort to empower PWAs led activists to make medical information free, accessible, and plainly written. In a number of cities, ACT UP chapters wrote and distributed guides to treatment and clinical trials, and in some places new informational organizations were created, such as Project Inform. Still others set up treatment newsletters, like the twice-monthly *AIDS Treatment News* begun by John James in San Francisco and the *Critical Path* newsletter launched by Kiyoshi Kuromiya in Philadelphia. The rise of the internet has further facilitated the spread of this information.

Technological advances led to new treatments. The first AIDS antiretroviral approved in 1987, AZT, belonged to a category of drugs called reverse transcriptase inhibitors that work by keeping the virus from replicating at a specific point in the process. In 1991, a second reverse transcriptase inhibitor was approved, and two more followed in 1994. Then in 1995, the first protease inhibitor, *saquinavir mesylate* (Invirase) was approved, followed by several more protease inhibitors and reverse transcriptase inhibitors in rapid succession. Monotherapy, the practice of using one drug at a time as treatment, quickly gave rise to a new system known as HAART (highly active antiretroviral therapy), or more colloquially, as the "cocktail."

In what the *Washington Post* referred to as "a highly unusual effort by the government to redirect treatment of a specific disease," the Panel on Clinical Practices for the Treatment of HIV Infection within The Department of Health and Human Services

issued a new set of guidelines recommending HAART. This was followed in 1998 with the release of the "living document" entitled "Guidelines for the Use of Antiretroviral Agents in HIV-Infected Adults and Adolescents" which emphasized that all PWAs and many people living with HIV should be on triple therapy (as opposed to single or two-drug combinations).[9] The government's actions had the effect of establishing HAART as the "standard of care," a decision that would have important policy implications. Since 1987, when AZT was first approved, the Congress had provided some funding for states to help purchase antiretroviral drugs. This activity would eventually develop into full-fledged AIDS Drugs Assistance Programs (ADAPs), which would provide funding to states for both antiretrovirals and medications used for the most commonly-occurring infections among people with AIDS.

The Ryan White CARE Act of 1990 introduced the AIDS Drugs Assistance Program. Each state administers and sets eligibility criteria for the program (and decides whether to contribute additional funding to supplement federal contributions); like most state-administered programs, this created widely divergent standards of who qualifies for drug therapy. The cocktail (or HAART) is expensive (between $10,000 and $12,000 per year, sometimes more). North Carolina is the most restrictive state, setting financial eligibility at 125% of the Federal Poverty Line (which was $8,860 for a one-person household in 2002).[10] Delaware, Massachusetts, New Jersey, and New York are the most generous states, and set their eligibility at 500% of the Federal Poverty Line.

In recent years, three factors have converged to create new problems for the Drug Assistance Program. First, ironically, is the "cocktail's" success. Although there are about 40,000 new infections a year in the United States, AIDS deaths have fallen (to 15,000 in 2004). Consequently, the states are supporting a growing number of people living with AIDS on the very expensive HAART medications. Second, combination therapies are becoming more complicated and expensive, both because of resistance to first-line treatment regimens, and because of the introduction of new drugs and boosters for existing drugs. When the FDA approved Fuzeon, the first of a whole new class of antiretrovirals (the fusion inhibitors), hope for the new therapy mixed with concern about the price—$20,000 per year. The third complication is the recent federal and state government budget crisis. During bad economic times, a vicious cycle sets in: the burden on states in the form of increased caseloads for ADAP and other programs goes up at precisely the same time that state revenues and money from the federal government decreases.

The combined effect of these three factors have led states to cut either drugs or people (and, in some cases, both) from their programs. In February 2003, sixteen ADAPs reported that they were restricting their programs in at least one of the following ways: by closing enrollment to new clients, introducing waiting periods, reducing formularies (the lists of drugs covered), restricting eligibility, or otherwise limiting access to treatment.[11] A March 2004 story in the *San Francisco Chronicle* noted that there are currently 1,000 Americans on waiting lists, and this figure does not include the unknown number of people who are not eligible for ADAP but cannot afford the drugs.[12]

As drug prices continue to soar, more and more consumers outside of the AIDS community have challenged drug company research and pricing policies. Like the early AIDS activists who voted with their feet through buyers' clubs for drugs like pentamidine, American consumers are increasingly seeking drugs for lower prices, often outside our borders. What is different now, is that the calls for systemic change are being echoed by Congressional representatives on both sides of the aisle. Although the cause had initially been championed mainly by liberal Democrats, Senator Charles Grassley, an Iowa Republican and (at the time) Chairman of the Senate Finance Committee introduced legislation in April 2004 that would open the way to legalize some drug imports from Canada, Europe, and Australia.

One of the drugs that has been heavily featured in the debate over importation is the AIDS drug ritonavir (sold under the trade name Norvir). The drug has opened new frontiers in the political challenge to pharmaceutical pricing. Norvir was originally developed with federal money—a multimillion dollar grant from the NIH. Abbott Laboratories holds the patent to the drug and markets it, not as it was originally developed (as a protease inhibitor on its own), but as a booster to heighten the effects of other protease inhibitors. Senator Charles E. Schumer (D-NY) described Norvir as "a nexus of all the bad practices that all the drug companies use." Norvir has become an irresistible target for advocates looking to challenge the system.[13] The charges include:

- Thanks to NIH funding, Norvir cost relatively little to develop, but has done very well in sales. The director of the Consumer Project on Technology, James Love, estimates that Abbott's investment in clinical trials was under $15 million, yet Abbott's sales of Norvir totaled $1 billion during its first five years on the market (from 1996 to 2001).[14]

- In December 2003, Abbott quadrupled the price of Norvir bought in the private sector (as opposed to Medicaid or ADAP). The most common booster dose (200 mg) went from $1,600 per year to $7,800.

- Even before the increase, Americans pay twice the price (sometimes more) than citizens in other industrial nations.

- The suspicion that Abbott's was trying to increase market share. This is because Abbott also markets a protease inhibitor called Kaletra, which contains Norvir. When Abbott raised the price of Norvir, it did not raise the price of Kaletra, which means that Kaletra has become cheaper than competitor protease inhibitors boosted by the now more expensive Norvir.

For consumer activists looking to challenge the pharmaceutical industry's pricing policies, it would be hard to find a better test case. Although Norvir is being used to champion the cause of importing cheaper drugs from other countries, it is also being used to demand that the federal government exercise its "march in" authority. This is a never-used power stemming from a piece of legislation known as the Bayh-Dole Act which gives the Secretary of Health and Human Services the power to open competition on a patent that was developed with federal funding (as Norvir was through the NIH grant) but is not sold to the public at "reasonable" prices.

Although HHS is not likely to pursue the "march-in," both the Congress and the NIH have recently held hearings that generated damaging press at a time that the pharmaceutical industry is already on the defensive. The AIDS community—which was once largely alone in the battle over drug prices—now finds itself surrounded by feisty allies.

DUELING IDEOLOGIES IN THE QUEST FOR PREVENTION

Since the mid-1980s we have known that HIV transmission does not occur through casual contact, and in fact, is almost always transmitted through one of three patterns: via unprotected sexual intercourse, through direct contact with contaminated blood or blood products, and from mother to child through the birth process or from breast milk. Given this knowledge, the task of preventing HIV transmission should seem straightforward. Yet nothing could be further from the case. Within the controversy ridden field of HIV/AIDS policy, prevention is arguably the most contentious subject of all. This is because most of the approaches to prevention, whether they involve injection drug users, sexually active gay men, commercial sex workers, experimenting adolescents, or any other risk groups, revolve around a single fundamental goal: convincing people not to engage in behaviors that enable HIV to be transmitted. Yet, there are different ways to view risk behaviors, and a deep cleavage has emerged based on a simple question. Is it better to convince people not to engage in certain behaviors at all or to teach them how to minimize the risk of HIV transmission while engaging in risky behavior? The first option, "abstinence," assumes that

avoiding risky behavior altogether is the only reliable form of prevention. The latter approach, "harm reduction," is predicated on the idea that eliminating the risk behaviors is not desirable or not realistic or both.

The alternatives rest on deeper ideologies. Most abstinence proponents view drug use, homosexuality, and sexual activity outside of heterosexual marriage as morally wrong—in fact, as terrible problems in themselves. The logical conclusion is that HIV transmission is an indication of a deeper evil, and that both problems can be solved only by abstinence. Most harm reduction proponents do not view drug use or various sexual encounters as bad in themselves. Rather, they think that the consequences can be harmful. Thus, unprotected sex can lead to pregnancy, AIDS, and other sexually transmitted infections. Similarly, drug use is problematic, not because it allows people to alter their reality and perceptions (as the abstinence advocates believe), but because it may cause health problems (like AIDS and hepatitis), and social problems (like theft and forced prostitution). One side emphasizes morality, the other health effects.

This struggle is so vociferous because proponents (especially abstinence proponents) view the approaches as mutually exclusive. Abstinence is based on several absolute premises, including the necessity of complete compliance for success. Harm reduction conversely sees a continuum where any modification in behavior that decreases risk is progress (reducing drug use to fewer injections per day, using condoms more often, or completely abstaining from risky behaviors). Harm reductionists regard abstinence as one option. But for supporters of abstinence, harm reduction necessarily undermines the zero tolerance that is crucial to success. There is no relative scale, no continuum beyond just saying "no."

Each of these camps has gathered political allies. Harm reduction was initiated within the gay community by activists and AIDS service organizations that sought to educate and warn at-risk populations without antagonizing or threatening them. As the harm reduction message spread beyond the gay community (which developed the idea), public health professionals, advocates of sexual and reproductive rights (like planned parenthood), and civil libertarians all embraced the idea and its methods.

Abstinence models, on the other hand, were initially supported by conservative politicians, Christian fundamentalist, and Catholic religious leaders. Additional adherents came from the ranks of parents worried about losing control of their children and their children's education and from many churches and abstinence-based drug treatment programs within minority—especially African-American—communities.

Many of the earliest prevention efforts—especially those targeting sexually active gay men and injection drug users—were initiated by private individuals and organizations, often within the gay community. Thus, for example, the whole concept of "safer sex" was invented by gay activists seeking to employ a harm reduction approach that would not demonize gay sex but rather encourage people to minimize their risks during sexual activity. A forty-page document entitled "How to Have Sex in an Epidemic" was an early example.[15] Similarly, (mostly white) volunteers from within the gay community pioneered needle exchange programs inspired by the same harm reduction philosophy that underscored the idea of safer sex.

When activists transplanted these initiatives outside the gay white community they often stirred up fierce controversies. For example, many African-American leaders reacted angrily to the needle exchange strategy as a means of curtailing the spread of HIV among injection drug users. When New York City's Public Health Commissioner Steven Joseph suggested a pilot program, a number of prominent African-American did not mince their words as they denounced the idea: City Councilman Hilton Clark called the plan "Genocide, pure and simple"; the city's special narcotics prosecutor, Sterling Johnson, likened it to "city sponsored shooting galleries"; and police commissioner Ben Ward asked Joseph in a debate why he didn't open a needle exchange program in (white, expensive) Scarsdale instead.

A similar level of outrage over a different form of harm reduction poured out on the Senate floor when North Carolina Senator Jesse Helms discovered a safer sex comic book put out by the Gay Men's Health Crisis (GMHC). Waving the comic book angrily in the air, Helms recounted his confrontation with GMHC, which had assured him that no federal money had been spent on the publication, but which he furiously noted *had* been awarded a federal grant for other risk reduction education. The planned activities included a series of workshops on topics such as gay sexuality and dating, and Helms interspersed his itemization of these (as he saw it, futile) topics with his own appraisal of the disgusting nature of the material.[16]

Such clashes between the communities from which the harm reduction message has come and the conservative partisans within the larger community to which it traveled must be arbitrated by local, state, and federal governments. Sometimes, government agencies promote a harm reduction approach, particularly for sexual education and safe sex; local public health officials, some state health departments, the CDC, and some high visibility officials during the early Clinton administration all took this approach. When the government sides with conservative elements, it has several policy options at its disposal.

The first is simply to refuse funds for harm reduction activities. This was the approach that Senator Helms was advocating on the floor of the Senate, and has been the approach that every presidential administration has taken regarding needle exchanges. Two other options might be called the good cop–bad cop approaches. The good cop uses positive incentives, especially funding, to promote abstinence-based prevention programs. Bad cop strategies include legislation, rules, mandates, and audits that press compliance with abstinence efforts such as mandatory drug testing.

The debate over AIDS education in the public schools illustrates the conflict. Although education is traditionally a state and local issue, the federal government has had a major impact by providing funding (with the inevitable strings). The funding, which now totals more than $100 million, comes from three sources, all dedicated to abstinence-only education: the Adolescent Family Life Act's teen pregnancy prevention component (first passed in

1981); the Welfare Reform Act of 1996 created an annual appropriation (known as "510(b) funds" after the provision in the act); and the Special Projects of Regional and National Significance (SPRANS) Program created in 2000 to provide direct grants to community-based programs (many of them faith based) doing abstinence education.[17] These funding initiatives helped introduce sharp changes in the way that sexuality education is being approached around the country. Today, 86% of public school districts promote abstinence as either the only option (35%) or the preferred option (51%) for unmarried people. From 1988 to 1999, the number of sexuality education teachers who taught abstinence as the *only way* to prevent pregnancy and STDs has gone from 1 in 50 to 1 in 4.[18]

The struggle between harm reduction and abstinence certainly pre-dates AIDS; however, the focus on AIDS as a national (and increasingly international) policy issue has accelerated and accentuated the dispute. Although both sides marshal evidence for their positions, it is the underlying values which shape the substance and fuel the passion of their arguments. The clashing values guarantee that there will be no permanent resolution to the questions of how best to conduct prevention efforts.

SOCIAL SERVICES AND HIV

AIDS activists pressed for social services and spending in unprecedented ways. Their successes are all the more noteworthy when viewed against a larger context of a shrinking national safety net in the United States. An example of such an AIDS-specific gain was the passage of the Housing Opportunities for People with AIDS Act of 1992, which was won in large part because of activist pressure, particularly from Housing Works, a New York City–based AIDS service organization with origins rooted in ACT UP/New York.

The largest pieces of AIDS social spending come from the entitlement programs Medicaid and Medicare, both of which support significant

number of people with AIDS. But the "signature" AIDS social legislation continues to be the Ryan White Comprehensive AIDS Resource Emergency (CARE) Act. The CARE Act was originally passed in 1990 and has been the backbone of AIDS social spending in the United States for nearly 15 years.[19]

The CARE Act illustrates the idiosyncrasies of our legislative process in a number of ways. One important precedent-setting aspect of the bill is that it represents a rare case of social spending based on a specific disease. This made President George H.W. Bush reluctant to sign the act; it would set a "dangerous precedent" for other diseases, he argued. In some other ways, however, the bill absolutely typifies the American political process—after all, it sailed right through what might have been a hostile Congress (with votes of 408 to 14 in the House of Representatives and 95 to 4 in the Senate).

Former Speaker of the House Tip O'Neil famously noted that "all politics are local." The framers of the CARE Act understood this. The Act was written with four titles, each aimed at a different constituency. The first title, which was designed to receive the lion's share of the money, benefited American cities. Of course, this also made sense, because AIDS in the United States has been an urban epidemic, with initial epicenters in Los Angeles, San Francisco, and New York City. But the act also set the standard of an "eligible metropolitan area" as one that had either a minimum case load of 2,000 or at least 0.0025% of its population as of June 3, 1990. Eligible Metropolitan Areas were allowed to define themselves very loosely—Boston became the most infamous example when it qualified by counting most of the state of Massachusetts as well as three counties in Southern New Hampshire. In 1990, there were sixteen qualifying Eligible Metropolitan Areas; by 1999, that number had increased to 51.

In another classic move in Congressional distributive politics, the CARE Act guaranteed that there would be no losers; Title II provided money to the states—with every state included. Even states with few cases were given at least $100,000, and told that it must be spent at least in part on creating "consortia" for HIV care that would address the continuum of care needs of HIV-positive people and their families. States with higher caseloads and less fiscal capacity (determined by average per capita income) could count on larger grants.

Title III bypassed the states and cities, and was used to directly fund projects and organizations that were already dealing with at-risk populations, such as community health centers, migrant health centers, and hemophilia treatment clinics. The funds were to be used for testing, transmission prevention, care, and social services. Finally, Title IV received the smallest funding of all—in fact, it got nothing during fiscal years 1991 to 1993. But it was politically important for it was directed at women, children, and youth living with HIV. As the more sympathetic face of AIDS (together with people with hemophilia and transfusion recipients) they were the "front" behind which many lobbyists and politicians operated. In fact, a study examining the passage of the legislation found that legislators relied heavily on stories of individuals with AIDS to promote the Act. The demographics of their stories are telling: of 19 counted in the study, six were about Ryan White specifically, another five were about infants and children, two were about women, two were about recipients of infected blood, and one gave no demographic description. Only one was about a gay man, who was also an injection drug user.[20]

Just as the original passage of the CARE Act reflects the tilt of the Congressional processes, the later reauthorizations (every five years) demonstrate broad lessons about the distributional politics. As the epidemic has moved across different populations, changes in funding for these groups through the CARE Act have moved much more slowly. This mismatch in need and resources demonstrates one of the truisms of politics: that it is incredibly difficult to take benefits away from one group and give it to another—regardless of relative need. Fighting in this area was particularly fierce in 1995, during the first reauthorization of the Act, when there was sharp debate over which communities *within* a particular city should be recipients of funds, and also *which cities* should get the most money. In the first case, the problem was that in most cities, the organization or

organizations that had initially become involved in AIDS services and care before the Ryan White Act had been passed usually became prominent leaders within the HIV Health Services Planning Councils (HHSPCs) that were set up by the legislation in each Eligible Metropolitan Area to make decisions about the funds they had been allotted. In most cities (with Dallas as a notable exception), these organizations were drawn from the white, gay community. As the epidemic increasingly moved into communities of color, the newer organizations expressed frustration that the older groups continued to control the majority of the Title I money.

While these struggles were raging in cities around the country, a second played out in Washington DC during the first CARE Act reauthorization in 1997. The controversy had its roots in Milwaukee, where the executive director of the AIDS Resource Center of Wisconsin, Douglas Green, made some calculations comparing funding for services provided in Milwaukee to those in San Francisco. He was surprised to find that San Francisco was receiving approximately six times the resources per person living with HIV/AIDS as Milwaukee ($6,000 compared to $1,000). The difference was due mainly to the rules that were set out in the CARE Act for counting AIDS case loads for Ryan White funding. In Title I (the Title providing funding for metropolitan areas), the funding levels were based on *cumulative* caseloads: that is, counting all people who had been diagnosed with AIDS. The two cities most heavily funded by Title I, San Francisco and New York, had the two highest cumulative case loads. But counting cumulatively means that people who have died of AIDS remain in the count—in these two cities that was the case for approximately 60% of the cumulative case load. This geographically based disparity was compounded by a second issue: double counting in Title I and Title II. Both Titles base their funding levels on caseloads. If a state has one or more Eligible Metropolitan Areas that qualify for Title I money, then the people counted in the EMA will be counted again in determining the level of money the state will receive for Title II. But states without any qualifying Eligible Metropolitan

Areas will have their people with AIDS counted only once—for Title II funds.

The battle that ensued in Washington, pitting some cities and their AIDS Service organizations against others, reached an uneasy truce in 1995 with changes in the funding formulas together with a "hold harmless" provision that would limit the amount of funding that a city could lose (no more than 7.5%, with the decrease spread over seven years). But these changes represented not so much a resolution as the first in a long string of struggles that will continue on a predictable five-year schedule—with each reauthorization of the CARE Act legislation. Legislators will always have to juggle three conflicting political desires: they need to win benefits for their own constituents; they know it is difficult to take resources away from those who already have them; and, where it is politically feasible, they seek the fairest way to allot resources in the face of unmet demand.

LOSING GROUND

Despite the important medical advances that have allowed AIDS to become a treatable, chronic condition for thousands of people receiving antiretroviral drugs in the United States, this is a time of frustration for many within the AIDS community. In a number of policy areas—from treatment (where the waiting lists for ADAP are growing) to prevention (where the forces for abstinence are in clear ascendancy over harm reduction) to research (where critics charge that even mentioning certain risk groups and behaviors takes grant applications off the table)—we have entered a period of setbacks for AIDS activists. Many of the policy victories achieved in the 1980s and 1990s are now being rolled back. In addition advocates have been losing ground in another sense. As the epidemic has increasingly been borne by communities marginalized by race, ethnicity, and income, there are fewer activists to forcefully push the AIDS issues important to these communities—issues like expanding addiction treatment programs, the provision of decent

HIV/AIDS care, prevention services in correctional facilities, and the elimination of immigration laws that discriminate against HIV-positive individuals.

Some of these setbacks and stumbling blocks began during the Clinton administration, particularly after Republicans regained the House in 1994. President Clinton's Health and Human Services Department conducted an extensive review of scientific studies done on needle exchange and concluded that such programs were an effective public health strategy that could help reduce HIV transmission without increasing the illegal use of drugs. However, President Clinton rejected this harm reduction strategy and kept his predecessors' ban in place. Similarly, as noted above, one of the enduring legacies of his presidency, the welfare reform enacted in 1996, became a vehicle for abstinence education, requiring states that received money from the federal government for sexual education to promote it above other measures.

But what arguably began under the watch of the Clinton administration has undeniably accelerated with President George W. Bush. The Bush administration submitted a federal budget request for AIDS spending for the fiscal year 2005 of $19.8 billion. This was divided into five categories: care ($11.6 billion, 59% of the total); research ($3.0 billion, 15%); international ($2.3 billion, 12%); cash and housing assistance ($1.8 billion, 9%); and prevention ($0.9 billion, 5%).[21] Yet these seemingly generous numbers mask several deficiencies. First, in the context of state cutbacks, the ADAP around the country face serious challenges. Wait lists are increasing, states are restricting the available drugs, and the costs of the drugs are rising. Despite a recent report by the Institute of Medicine stating that it would be cost effective to provide treatment for everyone who needs antiretrovirals, there has been no government movement in this direction.

On the prevention front, the struggle between abstinence and harm reduction has never been more stark. The United States continues to see approximately 40,000 new infections—and 15,000 deaths a year—yet the prevention budget requested by the president is level funded. More importantly, it is designed to strongly emphasize abstinence-only models and to empower faith-based organizations to carry out prevention activities. Even more ominous from the harm reduction perspective, many advocates report falling under increased surveillance. Organizations that reported never having been audited before (including the Sexuality Information and Education Council of the United States and Advocates for Youth) have come under the scrutiny of both the CDC and the General Accounting Office at the request of conservative members of the Congress apparently looking for fund misuse.

The struggles over treatment and prevention, however, are, in a sense, symptoms of a larger struggle between the AIDS community and the current administration. Similar dynamics to the ones discussed in this chapter are playing out globally—from the Bush administration's near-total emphasis on the "A" in Uganda's successful "ABC–Abstinence, Be Faithful, Condomize" prevention campaigns to its prioritization of faith-based organizations in the awarding of government contracts to do HIV/AIDS work in developing countries. At the 2002 International AIDS Conference in Barcelona, domestic and international outrage within the AIDS community was so strong that it led to a spirited episode of booing that drowned out the attempted speech of US Secretary of Health and Human Services Tommy Thompson. The Bush administration response was equally vociferous: it attempted to find the "ringleaders" of the protest and to prevent them from attending policy meetings; it sought to limit the attendance of government representatives at future International Conferences; and it tried (unsuccessfully) to have organizers of the 2004 International AIDS Conference in Bangkok pass a "gag rule" that would have pledged attendees to refrain from disruptions of the meeting.

AIDS policy is an inherently contentious issue. It involves risk behaviors that hinge on sexuality and drug use. It also involves the challenging of power relationships among and between individuals, health and research professionals, private corporations, moral and religious institutions, and government. Many of these differences are particularly stark today. The AIDS community includes many people steeped in a rights-based tradition that challenges traditional institutions and morally based practices; in contrast, the government is being lead by individuals and groups seeking to restore and reinforce these same institutions and practices. But even if the Republican Party loses its grip on the federal government, AIDS policy will remain among the most contested of policy arenas in the United States.

STUDY QUESTIONS

1. How did the four groups officially classified as at-risk initially respond to the AIDS epidemic? What implications did these divergent responses have for AIDS policymaking?

2. What did the CDC do to ensure increased availability of drugs that treated some of the most common ailments that were, in the end, responsible for the deaths of many people with AIDS?

3. What impact did the early success of ACT UP and similar groups have on the politics of AIDS?

4. How was the concept of medical self-empowerment employed by certain AIDS activists?

5. What policy innovations followed from the passage of the Ryan White CARE Act of 1990?

6. The author describes a fundamental split in AIDS prevention policy. What are the two sides? What are the deeper clashing philosophies that lie beneath the two sides? Where do you stand on this issue?

7. How has the debate over successive reauthorizations of the CARE Act pitted various cities/metropolitan areas against each other?

8. What kinds of policy reversals have AIDS activists suffered in recent years?

NOTES

1. One of the most prominent critics of AIDS exceptionalism is Ronald Bayer. For an early articulation of his argument see Bayer, 1991.
2. Many of these reassuring but false messages were issued in newsletters and advisories sent out by the National Hemophilia Foundation to client members, chapters, and physicians. For examples of the tone and content of these messages see, for instance, the July 14, 1982 *Hemophilia Newsnotes* and Medical Bulletin 10/ Chapter Advisory 13 *Hemophilia Information Exchange/AIDS Update*, January 24, 1984.
3. Institute of Medicine, 1995.
4. The Heckler announcement, together with many other of the other developments of the early days of the US AIDS epidemic are chronicled in Randy Shilt's classic account, *And the Band Played On* p 451.
5. For a fuller accounting of the pentamidine story, on which this summary is based, see Arno and Feiden, 1992.
6. Both Tambi and Weiss's statements are taken from hearings conducted by the Subcommittee of the House Committee on Government Operations, 1988, pp 436, 441.
7. This story is summarized from an account given by Bruce Nussbaum, 1990.
8. The Denver Principles can be found on the websites of many AIDS activist organizations including the one maintained by ACT UP/New York. Available online at http://www.actupny.org/documents/Denver.html (accessed 1 March 2004).
9. The guidelines, which were most recently updated on March 23, 2004, can be accessed, together with older versions, on the AIDSinfo website maintained by the Department of Health and Human Services. Available online at http://www.aidsinfo.nih.gov/guidelines/default_db2.asp?id=50 (accessed 10 May 2004).
10. Both the Kaiser Family Foundation and the National ADAP Monitoring Project (NAMP), to which the Kaiser Family Foundation belongs, together with the National Alliance of State and Territorial AIDS Directors and the AIDS Treatment Data Network, have created an excellent set of reports, fact sheets, and briefing papers on ADAPs. The figures and information listed here come from the Kaiser Family Foundation, "HIV/AIDS Policy Fact Sheet: AIDS Drug Assistance Programs (ADAPs)," April 2003 accessed online at http://www.kff.org (1 March 2004) and the National ADAP Monitoring Project, "Annual Report," April 2003 accessed at http://www.kff.org/hivaids/ADAP.cfm (1 March 2004).
11. National ADAP Monitoring Project, "Annual Report," p 8.
12. Sabin Russell, 2004.
13. Gardiner Harris, 2004, p A1.
14. The Washington-based organization Consumer Project on Technology (CPT) has been an active and vocal participant in the debates over the high prices of patented medication. CPT maintains a webpage on the Norvir issue, from which this information was taken. Accessed online at http://www.cpt.org/ip/health/aids/norvir.html.
15. The collaboration of activists Michael Callen and Richard Berkowitz with medical doctor Joseph Sonnabend in produced the document. See Benjamin Shepard, 2004, p 3.
16. Both the struggle over needle exchange in New York City and Jesse Helm's intervention against a harm reduction approach to risk reduction among gay men are described in greater detail in Patricia Siplon, 2002.
17. An overview of federal funding for abstinence-only educational, as well as an extensive case study of such programs in the state of Texas can be found in a report produced by Human Rights Watch. See Human Rights Watch, 2002.
18. Information is taken from the Alan Guttmacher Institute, 2003.
19. The Ryan White CARE Act is especially significant for being a form of *discretionary spending;*

unlike *entitlement spending*, which is determined by numbers of beneficiaries who are "entitled" to the money by meeting certain criteria, Congress determines how much gets spent each year. The features of and struggles over the Ryan White CARE Act described below are taken from two chapter-length considerations of the topic. For more information on the struggles around this policy area see Burkett, 1995, Chapter 5 and Siplon, Chapter 5.
20. Donovan, 1996, p 81.
21. Taken from the Kaiser Family Foundation, 2004.

REFERENCES

Alan Guttmacher Institute. 2003. "Facts in Brief: Sexuality Education." Accessed online http://www.guttmacher.org/pubs/fb_sex_ed02.html (20 March 2004).

Arno, P., and K. Feiden. 1992. Against the Odds: The Story of AIDS Drug Development, Politics and Profit. New York: Harper Collins.

Bayer, R. 1991. "Public Health Policy and the AIDS Epidemic: An End to HIV Exceptionalism?" *New England Journal of Medicine* 324: 1500–4.

Burkett, E. 1995. The Gravest Show on Earth: America in the Age of AIDS. New York: Houghton Mifflin.

—— "The Denver Principles." 1983. http://www.actupny.org/documents/Denver.html. (1 March 2004).

Donovan, M. 1996. "The Politics of Deservedness: The Ryan White CARE Act and the Social Construction of People with AIDS." In S. Theodoulou, ed. *AIDS: The Politics and Policy of Disease.* Upper Saddle River, NJ: Prentice Hall.

Harris, G. 2004. "Price of AIDS Drug Intensifies Debate on Legal Imports." *New York Times* April 14.

Human Rights Watch. 2002. "Ignorance Only: HIV/AIDS, Human Rights and Federally Funded Abstinence-Only Programs in the United States." 14 (5(G)): September.

Institute of Medicine. 1995. *HIV and the Blood Supply: An Analysis of Crisis Decisionmaking.* Washington DC: National Academy Press.

Kaiser Family Foundation. April 2003. "HIV/AIDS Policy Fact Sheet: AIDS Drug Assistance Programs (ADAPs)." http://www.kff.org (1 March 2004).

Kaiser Family Foundation. February 2004. "HIV/AIDS Policy Fact Sheet: Federal Funding for HIV/AIDS: The FY 2005 Budget Request." http://www.kff.org (1 March 2004).

National ADAP Monitoring Project. April 2003. "Annual Report." http://www.kff.org/hivaids/ADAPs (1 March 2004).

National Hemophilia Foundation. 1982. *Hemophilia Newsnotes.* July 14.

National Hemophilia Foundation. 1984. Medical Bulletin #10/Chapter Advisory #13. *Hemophilia Information Exchange/ AIDS Updates.* January 24.

Nussbaum, B. 1990. Good Intentions: How Big Business and the Medical Profession Are Corrupting the Fight Against AIDS. New York: Penguin Books.

Russell, S. 2004. "State, Federal Budgets Squeeze AIDS Drug Funding; Governor's Plan Would Put Limit on Program for Uninsured Patients." *San Francisco Chronicle* March 7.

Shepard, B. 2004. "From Gay Plague to National Priority to Social Control: HIV/AIDS Policy in the United States." Unpublished manuscript.

Shilts, R. 1987. And the Band Played On: Politics, People and the AIDS Pandemic. New York: Saint Martin's Press.

Siplon, P. 2002. *AIDS and the Policy Struggle in the United States.* Washington DC: Georgetown University Press.

US Congress, House of Representatives, Subcommittee of the Committee on Government Operations. 1988. "Therapeutic Drugs for AIDS: Development, Testing and Availability, Hearing," 100th Congress, 2nd Session. April 28. Washington DC: US Government Printing Office.

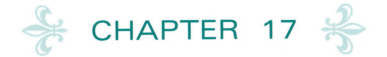

CHAPTER 17

Environmental Policy: A New Focus on Health

Kelly Tzoumis and Leonard Robins

This chapter explains that a traditional focus on public health has slipped out of environmental decision-making. The authors examine the policy response to three problems—Hurricane Katrina, terrorism, and global warming—and show how a public health focus would improve policy making and increase the chances of political success. They call on public health specialists to galvanize a new and more effective environmental movement.

In this chapter we examine how decision making on environmental health issues has gravitated from health to environmental agencies.[1] While the change itself was probably inevitable it has had negative consequences. Critics charge the environmental movement—which like all movements, seizes the rhetoric and symbols that can help win policies[2]—with inadvertently ignoring human health relevant to people "on the ground" at the local level. For example, many Hispanic groups, African-American communities, and low-income populations view the modern environmental movement as being unresponsive to their human health needs.[3]

We illustrate the problem of losing the health dimension by focusing on two major environmental challenges: natural disasters and terrorism and global warming. These are not the only issues of environmental importance we (and the world) will be facing in the immediate future, but they are likely to be at the top of the list of environmental issues that our political leaders will be grappling with in the foreseeable future. Each has an important—often overlooked—health dimension.

The chapter concludes with recommendations for improving environmental policies by bring health—and health professionals—back into the decision-making process. We wish to emphasize, however, that there are no "magic bullet" solutions for any of the issues we raise.

FROM ENVIRONMENTAL HEALTH TO ENVIRONMENT

Environmental health issues have been a major problem since early cities developed living conditions that contaminated water supplies and polluted lakes and rivers which supplied much of the drinking water. One of the famous environmental health problems was the outbreak of cholera in England in 1831. Dr. John Snow made the connection between a water pump and high incidence of the disease.[4] Up until this point cholera had been considered a poor person's disease, something from contaminated air or perhaps divine punishment. Thus medical science and simple statistical observation contributed to the major scientific advances in environmental health as people moved into more urban environments.

American cities experienced similar problems with contamination of drinking water as the country grew. One example is Chicago's very high rates of cholera and typhoid fever in the mid-1800s. State and local governments responded by creating water sanitation districts to manage the supply of drinking water. Several major engineering approaches and technologies were also implemented. Officials raised street-levels several inches to literally pull buildings out of the contaminated soil and water.[5] They also reversed the flow of the Chicago River in 1900, moving the polluted water downstream toward the Mississippi River (and St. Louis) and away from the growing metropolis.[6] These examples illustrate how state and local agencies originally defined the issue of environmental health as more of a "health issue" than an environmental one. Moreover, specific problems were defined and primarily solved by public health officials rather than environmental scientists per se.

Indeed, rarely were health problems considered "environmental" until the modern environmental movement in the 1970s. There were no specialized "environmental protection agencies" dealing with polluted drinking water from urbanization formed prior to the 1970s. Tasks dealing with this problem were performed by public health agencies or other public works departments that handled infrastructure issues. Policy was rarely made in a larger context of ecosystems or environmental protection. This all changed with the environmental movement in the late 1960s and 1970s.

The movement prompted a major shift. Policies implemented by public health agencies primarily at the state and local levels moved to the state and national level; the old problems were defined in a new way. Major pieces of legislation such as the Clean Air Act, Clean Water Act, Safe Drinking Water Act, Endangered Species Act, Resource Conservation and Recovery Act, and Toxic Substance Control Act enacted in the 1970s were viewed primarily as environmental protection policies designed to protect resources such as air, land, water, or species. The provisions, the language and the titles in this legislation were constructed with environment—and not public health—as their central focus. They all granted national government clear leadership in protecting environmental health, emphasized the environment, and largely overlooked health.

New federal organizations were created in the 1970s such as the Council on Environmental Quality and the Environmental Protection Agency (with many parallel state environmental protection agencies) to address environmental problems. These issues have large human health impacts and public health concerns are certainly part of the logic for these organizations and their policies. However, they are regarded primarily as environmental organizations making environmental policies. Thus most of the employees of the Council on Environmental Quality and the Environmental Protection Agency have environmental rather than health expertise, even though their missions importantly include an emphasis on interactions between human health and the environment.

The creation of new environmental-oriented agencies fostered the development of academic disciplines like environmental science and ecology. This redefinition or reframing has had tremendous impact on environmental health policy.

CAUSES AND CONSEQUENCES OF THE CHANGING STRUCTURE AND EMPHASES OF ENVIRONMENTALISM

Policy makers reassigned environmental health concerns from state and local health departments to environmental agencies because they thought the health departments were weak. The causes of this perceived weakness are debatable, but the consequences are not.

To capture this sense of "malaise," we present excerpts from a chapter on public health written for an earlier edition of *Health Politics and Policy* by Camilla Stivers, Associate Study Director of the Task Force of the Institute of Medicine (I.O.M.), which authored the important and influential, *The Future of Public Health*.[7]

The "mission" of public health as seen by public health professionals is to prevent disease and promote health on a community-wide basis. Like most professions, public health professionals believe that practice should be grounded in science. Knowledge about causes of disease, methods of transmission, preventive techniques, and the administration of community-wide programs forms the core of public health expertise, and in the eyes of its members justifies the profession's claims to autonomy and legitimacy. Public health professionals see their skill and dedication as the key to assuring conditions for the health of entire populations, and argue that society should accord them the authority to practice as they think best.

Public health as practiced in state and local health departments in the United States is accorded low status among actors in the policy process and is politically weak. Unlike most other professions, the self-definition of public health is not consistent with its operational definition, that is the actual activities carried on by state and local health departments. Theoretically, the mission of public health can be expanded to encompass a vast range of concerns. From the profession's perspective, almost any aspect of living can be related to the health of society and thus appropriately be considered a potential public health matter. For example, decent jobs and adequate housing contribute to people's good health.

In actual practice, however, the responsibilities of state and local health departments are in tension with the profession's self-image. There is great heterogeneity of duties and functions among the various state and local entities responsible for public health. Thus, there appears to be no consistent societal response to the profession's overall claim to authority.

Finally, many if not most of the people actually doing the work of public health in agencies are not public health professionals by training, a situation at odds with the classic claim of every profession, that outsiders have no right to do its work.

The IOM study concluded that the diversity of organizational arrangements and responsibilities reflected in state and local health agencies suggests that there is no clear organizational focus for state and local public health in the United States, and little agreement among its units of government about what "public health" means operationally. The study uncovered numerous examples of gaps and confusions in the public health system that reflect this lack of focus.

The difficulty of arriving at an operational definition of public health is further complicated by the fact that a great many public health agency personnel have no specific training in public health. The public health profession itself frankly acknowledges, even prides itself on, its multi-disciplinary nature, including within the fold not only physicians, nurses, and sanitarians, but industrial hygienists, statisticians, community health educators, and others. But the tie that binds these different perspectives together, according to the profession, that is, training in a distinctive body of knowledge centering around the "mother science" epidemiology, is not widespread among existing state and local agency staffs. For example, only about one-third of local health department directors have a master's degree in public health, and most public health nurses have little formal public health training beyond what they may have received in nursing school.

The IOM study concluded that, despite obvious expertise, dedication, hard work, and some success on the part of many professionals, on the whole public health agencies are ill-equipped to cope with the functions they perform, let alone fulfill the broader vision of the profession. The study traced the current difficulties of public health to fragmented authority, antiquated laws, frequently inadequate fiscal resources, and lack of public understanding and support.

Problems with Contemporary Public Health Practice

Fragmented authority for carrying out public health functions began in the 1960s as the leadership role in protecting the environment was gradually removed from public health departments and lodged in newly created departments of environmental services or ecology. This development appears to have been a response to the proliferation of environmental programs and permit requirements

that took place as environmental hazards worsened. In a climate of growing concern over pollution, the traditional "health department model" for handling environmental problems "appeared increasingly outdated." Such fragmentation concerns public health professionals not only because of growing confusion about who has the power to act to solve health problems, but also because they fear neglect—due to lack of knowledge—of the health dimensions of issues removed from their control. The tendency to remove environmental health and other responsibilities from health departments has led to a generalized "conventional wisdom" that public health agencies are incapable of solving complex, important problems.

Perhaps the most striking of all the difficulties facing public health today is a lack of public knowledge and support. State and local health departments not only have no apparent constituency, a serious handicap in a political system where organized interest groups play a key role in policy decisions, but in addition the general public has little knowledge of what health departments actually do. The IOM study found during a series of site visits that while many people who are not trained or employed in public health generally understand and favor the public health mission, they have little awareness of specific activities or programs carried on by public health agencies in their communities and the benefits they produce. When asked, respondents could furnish definitions of public health such as, "It's things that benefit everybody . . . Promoting health on a general level . . . What the private sector can't or won't do"; but when queried about what the local or state health department does specifically, most were able to make only vague suggestions, such as, "They take care of poor people . . . You can go there to get a shot . . . Don't they inspect restaurants?"[8]

While environmental functions are unlikely to be returned to state and local health departments, it is vitally important that *those dedicated to the environment* begin to re-emphasize the health aspect of the field. Otherwise, the current political weakness of the environmental movement is likely to continue.

In a recent poll by Peter Hart and Bill McInturff, "seventy-nine percent of voters said they supported stronger national standards to protect our land, air, and water. Yet only 22 percent said environmental concerns were major factors in how they voted in any recent election . . . They view the threats posed by environmental problems as distant and diffuse, and unlikely to harm them personally."[9]

Environmental policies must be *demonstrably* beneficial to humans over time if they are to be enacted and sustained. Intrinsic value arguments cannot be presented as having the same importance as those for improving human health and well-being. While the dominating role of state and local health departments is unlikely to return, the health concerns of environmental health professionals must assume a more prominent role in the environmental movement if it is to succeed.

A NEW ROLE FOR ENVIRONMENTAL HEALTH: NATURAL CATASTROPHES AND TERRORISM

Two major new challenges requiring the attention of environmental health professionals are acts of terrorism and natural catastrophes. Both types of events are similar in that they have limited or no warning for environmental health responders. Certainly, natural events like hurricanes, tornadoes, and even volcanic eruptions, have some lead time in predictability, but it is not always clear when the event will occur or what its impact will be. There is at best usually only modest lead time with natural events. With terrorist acts, there is no lead time. However, the impact from these events can be somewhat

mitigated by preparation and planning—particularly by environmental health responders. It requires environmental health professionals to predict what the probable health risks will be for various populations caused by these disaster events and to inform emergency responders as well as the general public as to potential exposures.

Hurricane Katrina

One example of this new role for environmental health policy was illustrated in the aftermath of Hurricane Katrina in the Gulf of Mexico, particularly in the New Orleans area. Katrina hit New Orleans on Monday, August 29, 2005, as a category 3 hurricane and passed within 10 to 15 miles of New Orleans, Louisiana. The storm brought heavy winds and rain to the city, and the damage breached several levees protecting New Orleans from the water of Lake Pontchartrain. The levee breaches flooded up to 80% of the city with water, reaching a depth of 25 feet in some places. Hurricane Katrina caused significant loss of life and disrupted power, natural gas, water and sewage treatment, road safety, and other essential services to the city.

More than $37 million immediately went to workers involved in emergency response and hazardous waste clean-up from awards made by the National Institute of Environmental Health Sciences (NIEHS), one of the National Institutes of Health within the US Department of Health and Human Services.[10] The grants were to provide training designed to protect workers and their communities from exposure to toxic materials encountered during hazardous waste operations and chemical emergency response.

Environmental health played a significant role in the immediate post-hurricane rebuilding of New Orleans. The National Center for Environmental Health (NCEH) identified 13 environmental health issues and supporting infrastructure that needed to be addressed. The initial assessment included environmental issues of drinking water, waste water, solid waste/debris, sediments/soil contamination (toxic chemicals), power, natural gas, housing, unwatering/flood water, occupational safety and health/public security, vector/rodent/animal control, road conditions, underground storage tanks (e.g., gasoline), and food safety.[11]

It was also generally recognized that hurricane preparation—particularly for prevention on environmental health issues—was not well coordinated within the various government and non-governmental agencies involved. At the same time, environmental health risks were being assessed, the mayor of New Orleans was prematurely inviting people to return, before Hurricane Rita hit the city with a second flooding.

Supplies shipped by Center for Disease Control's (CDC's) Strategic National Stockpile provided pharmaceuticals, technical assistance teams, and treatment capacity due to the hurricane's catastrophic effect on the hospital infrastructure in Louisiana and Mississippi. CDC's supplies served an estimated 30 acute care hospitals south of Interstate Highway 10, and volunteers organized around its "contingency stations" to become temporary stand-ins for hospitals, warehouses, and distribution facilities damaged by the storm. Alongside strong responses from state and local medical teams, CDC support remained crucial until normal infrastructure support began to return a week and a half later.

Within days after landfall, medical authorities established contingency treatment facilities for over 10,000 people, and ultimately treated many, many thousands more. Partnerships with commercial medical suppliers, shipping companies, and support services companies insured that evolving medical needs could be met within days or even hours.

In sum, one major message from the hurricane disaster was the need for greater coordination between environmental health professionals, the Federal Emergency Management Agency (FEMA), and the other agencies involved with the evacuation and repopulation of the city.

Terrorism

Another challenge that environmental health professionals have recently had to face is the threat of terrorism. Terrorism in the United States is a relatively new arena for environmental health providers. Terrorism can almost never be predicted. Moreover, when infrastructure facilities like drinking water plants, nuclear plants, waste water treatment centers, and other large facilities were built, the thought of terrorism rarely entered the minds of the designers. Today we know that essential environmental health facilities like large drinking water plants are at risk to terrorists. A new challenge for environmental health is how to plan for terrorism events which could threaten the lives of millions of people.

On September 11, 2001, with the fall of the World Trade Towers, the entire nation—*the entire world*—confronted terrorism first-hand on live television broadcasts. This event posed a challenge for environmental health officials no one predicted. Moreover, subsequent anthrax attacks through the nation's postal service "popularized" the term bioterrorism.

When the World Trade Center and sections of the Pentagon came crashing down, the rubble left for rescuers and cleanup crews was laced with asbestos, heavy metals, diesel fuel, PCBs, and dozens of other toxins. New York City was enveloped in a cloud of smoke, soot, and toxic ash. The pivotal role of environmental health in terrorism preparedness became clear for the first time. Environmental health providers are now on the frontlines in defending public safety in this age of terrorism.[12]

At the World Trade Center, 450 emergency responders—fully one-sixth of the victims of that attack—perished while doing their jobs, while environmental and medical officials, as well as volunteers, stood helpless to save them. In addition, many workers who cleaned debris from the site in the aftermath were harmed because they did not understand the environmental health risks. On the eve of the two-year anniversary of the terror attacks, the Environmental Protection Agency (EPA) released an evaluation of its response to the incidents that gave credence to critics who said the government downplayed risks and returned people to their homes and offices prematurely.[13]

As a result of the terrorist attacks, Congress passed the Public Health Security and Bio-terrorism Response Act (in 2002), which provided money through the CDC for counterterrorism planning and funding to states for counterterrorism planning. The money has generally been dispensed and much of the focus has been on local police and fire responders rather than environmental health responders.[14]

The 2002 Public Health Security and Bio-terrorism Response Act raised federal spending on public health infrastructure from $67 million in fiscal year 2001 to $940 million in fiscal year 2002. The money generally is being dispensed through CDC in the form of cooperative agreements with the states. Within certain guidelines, each state decides how to spend the money. For environmental health agencies, this trickle-down system has worked unevenly. In some localities, environmental health has received significant new funding. In others, little money has made it from the state level down to local health departments or, within health departments, down to environmental health. And at about the same time this money was appearing, many states were experiencing budget crises that resulted in cuts to funding for public health. Thus, many environmental health budgets are declining, despite the infusion of federal money.[15]

The Lesson

Both events, Hurricane Katrina in August 2005 and the terrorism attacks associated with September 11, 2001, as well as afterwards with anthrax scares, present a consistent and clear message for the United States, if not the world. Environmental health providers need to be more central to the team of emergency response providers both in providing protection immediately after the event as well as preparing for the possible event.

Natural catastrophes and terrorist attacks will continue to occur in the United States. The challenge is to implement the lessons we learned through the large and cumbersome complex of organizations that deal with environmental health policy.

CHALLENGES FOR THE FUTURE: GLOBAL WARMING AND ENVIRONMENTAL HEALTH POLICY

Another large challenge on the agenda for environmental health policy makers is global warming. This is one of the most complex political and scientific issues confronting the world and in particular the United States. Unlike terrorism or natural catastrophic, global warming is gradual and predictable. However, global warming's impacts are likely to have an even greater impact unless we start taking action now.

Generally, American policy makers have been slow to join international policy makers and organizations who see global warming as a serious, major environmental health threat; the international consensus calls for immediate reductions in the gases that contribute to warming. Part of the explanation for the American reluctance stems from the perceived economic cost to limiting the emissions associated with global warming. Additionally, many in the United States challenge the scientific evidence, suggesting the evidence of man-made global warming is weak. This is a unique situation for environmental health officials because science has generally identified such problems and suggested solutions; however, in the United States, by far the largest emitter of global gases, weak scientific arguments have been used to delay working with the international community to address global warming.

This section gives a brief overview on the subject of global warming and then focuses on how political actors have used the rhetoric of science to argue for delay when issues of economic cost are key. Effective participation in the global warming debate in the United States is, in our judgment, the most serious task of environmental health professionals in the foreseeable future. They must become expert in its substance and politics.

Background on Global Warming[16]

Levels of carbon dioxide and other "greenhouse gases" in the atmosphere have risen steeply during the industrial era as economic and population growth have spurred activities like deforestation and heavy fossil fuel use. Like a blanket round the planet, greenhouse gases trap heat energy in the Earth's lower atmosphere. If levels rise too high, the resulting overall rise in air temperatures—global warming—is liable to disrupt natural climate patterns which result in major ecosystem changes.

Carbon dioxide produced by human activity enters the natural carbon cycle. Many billions of tons of carbon are exchanged naturally each year between the atmosphere, the oceans, and land vegetation. The exchanges in this massive and complex natural system are precisely balanced; carbon dioxide levels appear to have varied by less than 10% during the 10,000 years before industrialization. In the 200 years since 1800, however, their levels have risen by over 30%. Even with half of humanity's carbon dioxide emissions being absorbed by the oceans and land vegetation, atmospheric levels continue to rise by over 10% every 20 years.

The Intergovernmental Panel on Climate Change (IPCC) concluded that "new and stronger evidence [demonstrates] that most of the warming observed over the last 50 years is attributable to human activities." Uncertainties in the process of projecting future trends lead to a wide range of estimates, but the IPCC predicted a rise of 1.4–5.8°C in global mean surface temperatures over the next 100 years. Even at the lower end of this range the impact of warming is likely to be dramatic. These impacts on human lives will be unavoidable and in places extreme. People in some areas may benefit from climate change, but most will suffer—in many cases extremely.

Developing countries will suffer more than others, both because their lack of resources makes them especially vulnerable to adversity or emergencies on any major scale and because most are near the equator and other areas likely to receive the most negative consequences of global warming. Yet people in developing countries have created only a small proportion of greenhouse gas emissions.

At the global level, climate scientists have attributed the majority of warming in the past 50 years to the human-caused increase in greenhouse gases such as carbon dioxide (CO_2), methane (CH_4), nitrous oxide (N_2O), and certain industrial gases. This environmental health issue is not new because scientific evidence of human interference with the climate first emerged in the international public arena in 1979 at the First World Climate Conference. As public awareness of environmental issues continued to increase in the 1980s, governments grew even more concerned about climate issues. In 1988, the United Nations General Assembly adopted a resolution urging: ". . . protection of global climate for present and future generations of mankind." In the same year, the governing bodies of the World Meteorological Organization and of the United Nations Environment Program created a new body, the IPCC, to marshal and assess scientific information on the subject. In 1990, the IPCC issued its First Assessment Report, which confirmed that the threat of climate change was real. The Second World Climate Conference, held in Geneva later that year, called for the creation of a global treaty. The General Assembly Responded by passing a resolution formally launching negotiations on a convention on climate change, to be conducted by an Intergovernmental Negotiating Committee (INC). The INC first met in February 1991 and its government representatives adopted the United Nations Framework Convention on Climate Change, after just 15 months of negotiations in May 1992. At the Rio de Janeiro United Nations Conference on Environment and Development (more commonly known as the Earth Summit) of June 1992, the new Convention was opened for signature. It entered into force in March 1994. Ten years later, the Convention had been joined by 188 countries. This almost worldwide membership makes the Convention one of the most universally supported of all international environmental agreements.

The major global warming international agreement to reduce emissions that contribute to warming the planet is commonly referred to as the Kyoto Protocol. The Kyoto Protocol to the United National Framework on Climate Change treaty was adopted in Kyoto, Japan, in December 1997. It was open for signature from March 1998 to March 1999 at the United Nations Headquarters in New York. Immediately, 84 countries signed the protocol and subsequently enough countries have signed so that it is now in effect. Those parties that have not yet signed the Kyoto Protocol may do so at any time. Most countries have already signed.

The United States has not signed the Kyoto protocol and there is little chance of that happening anytime soon. In fact, major industrial sectors of the United States, such as automobile manufacturers and the energy industry, have been openly hostile to the Protocol—they have taken out advertisements linking the signing of the protocol to economic disaster. More recently the debate in the United States may have begun to shift. Former Vice President Al Gore has won considerable attention (and an Oscar) for his documentary about global warming, *An Inconvenient Truth*. After the Democrats recaptured Congress in 2006, some (though hardly all) formerly hostile industrial companies began to soften their opposition to addressing the issue. Even so, significant action—much less signing the Kyoto Protocol or helping draft a new international agreement—remains unlikely.

The stakes are huge on all sides: the economic impact of either action or inaction on climate change will be high. However, taking measures to reduce emissions will be essential to maintaining high levels of health and quality of life on this planet.

The United States Delay: Uncertain Science as the Reason?

In the United States, where the best science on global warming has been conducted, the scientific evidence compiled to date on the observed ecological effects of climate change in the United States and their consequences, and the relationships between observed biological changes and human activities is strong, according to a review of the scholarly literature contained in a recent Pew Center report on global climate change.[17]

That report reviews more than 40 studies that associate climate change with observed ecological impacts in the United States. Using objective evaluation criteria, it found that more than half the studies provide strong evidence of a direct link. These studies span a broad range of plant and animal species from various regions of the United States.

Despite the diversity among studies, the observed ecological responses are consistent with one another, as well as with the changes that one would expect based on the nature of US climate change observed to date. Although many species and ecological systems have yet to be studied (often due to inherent limitations of available data) and it is difficult to attribute ecological changes to a particular cause, a number of robust findings emerge from this report. Sufficient studies now exist to conclude that the consequences of climate change are detectable within US ecosystems.

The key issue is simple: inevitable scientific uncertainty is used to delay action because of the perceived economic costs. The environmental health community has struggled to respond. It is hard to refute the claim that the planet has undergone many natural, large-scale, lifecycle changes over time. The earth's climate has always varied—from ice ages, volcanic activities, or even the reversal of the poles.

Nonetheless, the EPA states there is compelling evidence from around the world demonstrating that a new kind of climate change is now under way, foreshadowing drastic impacts on people, economies, and ecosystems.[18] According to the EPA, the heat-trapping property of gases released by human activity is undisputed—although uncertainties exist about exactly how the Earth's climate responds to them. The EPA further states that it is not easy to calculate the extent to which human-induced accumulation of greenhouse gases since pre-industrial times is responsible for the global warming trend. This is because other factors, both natural and human, affect our planet's temperature. Furthermore, the EPA claims that scientific understanding of these other factors—most notably natural climatic variations, changes in the sun's energy, and the cooling effects of pollutant aerosols—remains incomplete. In short, scientists think rising levels of greenhouse gases in the atmosphere *are* contributing to global warming, but to what extent is difficult to determine. We are certain that human activities are rapidly adding greenhouse gases to the atmosphere, and that these gases tend to warm our planet. This is the basis for concern about global warming. According to those who want to delay action, the fundamental scientific uncertainties are these: How much more warming will occur? How fast will this warming occur? How much is caused directly by human action, how much by natural causes? And what are the potential adverse and beneficial effects? These uncertainties will be with us for some time, perhaps for decades.

In sum, the inevitable uncertainty of science has been utilized as a rationale by some interests in the United States to ignore and even criticize the global warming prevention efforts by the rest of the international community. The scientific community has not adequately responded to this strategy by demonstrating the problems with this delay—including the obvious points that uncertainty also means the problem could be *much more* than assumed and that delay can have the same negative results as a delay in treating serious disease; nor has the scientific community successfully demonstrated what we already know with certainty.

The Kyoto treaty expires in 2012 and international efforts are underway to plan for new policies to combat global warming. There is widespread agreement, even among supporters, that Kyoto contains flaws. World leaders would enthusiastically welcome our participation in developing a new and improved approach to combating global warming. Tragically, the United States continues to use the flaws of Kyoto to say no; other countries use American opposition (after all, we are the greatest human creator of global warming) to resist making sacrifices themselves.[19]

One final point. Most of the protest against the United States' delay has come from environmental protection interest groups, not environmental health agencies and experts at the local or national levels.

This reflects badly on those in environmental health. More importantly, it hurts the effort to combat global warming, for it is concerns with environmental *health* and quality of life that most move the public.

CONCLUSIONS

We have outlined some current and future challenges for environmental health providers. Both events like Hurricane Katrina and terrorist acts like those that occurred on September 11, 2001 are likely to occur again in different forms that demand policy responses from environmental health professionals. It is not clear that the environmental health movement is moving effectively toward implementing the hard lessons we learned from these events. Nor has the movement met the challenge posed by the even larger dangers of global warming.

What is to be done? A first "process" proposal we would like to present is that a national summit on environmental health be convened that encompasses both public health and environmental protection experts as well as grassroots communities. This recommendation may seem platitudinous, but was demonstrably effective at the international level during the Earth Summit conducted by the United Nations in 1992 where major work resulted in developing global warming policies.

Out of such a summit we hope a better alignment of the organizational components of environmental health policymaking would emerge, particularly at the national level. This does not necessarily mean creating duplicative agencies to deal with environmental health, but better organization of the agencies already in existence. This is actually a much smaller task than the recent bureaucratic redesign for homeland security, but one of equal or even greater importance.

A second recommendation concerns the education and training of environmental health experts. More emphasis should be placed from early education all the way to upper levels university studies on a multidisciplinary approach to environmental health fields. Again, this may seem like stating the obvious, but it speaks to a serious gap in training. The Institute of Medicine analysis of public health (discussed above) emphasized improved training in the politics of the policymaking process; political intelligence is essential to the increased effectiveness of public health agencies and professionals.

The essential precondition for improving the effectiveness of the environmental health field, however, is to increase the visibility and importance of environmental health concerns within the environmental movement. This would be of benefit to both environmental health specifically and the environmental movement generally, but achieving it will be difficult.

Today, the environmental movement is undergoing a searching and sometimes searing self-evaluation. Set off by a provocative paper by Michael Shellenberger and Ted Nordhause entitled "The Death of Environmentalism," its purpose is to develop a strategy for repairing a perceived loss of influence in the political arena. Many environmental activists believe that this has sadly resulted in both effective resistance to new recommendations from environmentalists and selectively repealing environmental regulations put in place during the 1960s and 1970s—"the Golden Age of Environmentalism."

We believe that we need a "New Politics of Environmentalism."[20] The environmental movement will need more than a message "reframing" if it is to obtain and retain a long-term increase in influence. Instead, it will have to emphasize the value of its recommendations for the betterment of human health and an improved quality of life rather than subtly and sometimes not so subtly implying that we must all sacrifice for the good of the environment.

In conclusion, we turn the argument around and end by urging environmental health specialists to work harder at integrating themselves and their concerns into the overall environmental movement. They can and will be the most effective advocates for an emphasized role of environmental health in environmentalism.

Just as increased emphasis on the health dimension would work to the advantage of the environmental movement, so a rigorous and popular environmental movement would be the essential driving force behind the enactment and successful implementation of effective environmental health policies. In the eloquent words used by Ben Franklin during the founding of our Republic, "United We Stand, Divided We Fall."

STUDY QUESTIONS

1. How were health issues relating to the environment 'reframed' during the 1970's?
2. What were some of the results of the reframing of environmental health? What were the effects experienced by the public health profession?
3. How would the environmental movement as a whole be strengthened by a renewed focus on health?
4. What were some of the environmental health concerns facing emergency responders in the New Orleans area following the landfall of Hurricane Katrina?
5. Even with an increase in federal funding for public health in the wake of 9/11, why are some state and local environmental health programs still faced with resource shortages?
6. Why are some developing countries expected to suffer disproportionately from global warming?
7. What are some of the points relating to global warming on which scientists broadly agree? What are some of the points of uncertainty?

NOTES

1. For an excellent treatment of environmental health politics, see Barry Rabe, 1997.
2. Baumgartner and Jones, 1993.
3. See Novotny, 2000.
4. Vinten-Johansen, Brody, Rachman, and Rip, 2003.

5. Hill, Libby. *The Chicago River: A Natural and Unnatural History*. Chicago: Lake Claremont Press.
6. Theriot and Tzoumis, 2005.
7. National Academy of Medicine, Institute of Medicine, 1988.
8. Stivers, 1991.
9. Results are available from the Nicholas Institute for Environmental Policy Solutions, Duke University.
10. Joint Task Force of Centers for Disease Control and Prevention and US Environmental Protection Agency, 2005, p 5.
11. Ibid.
12. Lyman, 2003.
13. Berg, 2004.
14. Ibid.
15. Ibid.
16. United Nations, 2005.
17. Parmesan and Galbraith, 2004.
18. EPA, 2005.
19. Revkin, 2005, Sec 4, p 3.
20. Tzoumis and Robins, 2005.

REFERENCES

Baumgartner, F., and B. Jones. 1993. *Agendas and Instability in American Politics*. Chicago: The University of Chicago Press.

Berg, R. 2004. "Terrorism Response and the Environmental Health Role." *Journal of Environmental Health* 67 (2): p 29.

Environmental Protection Agency. 2005. "Uncertainties." Global Climate Change website. http://yosemite.epa.gov/oar/globalwarming.nsf/content/ClimateUncertaintie.html.

Hill, L. 2000. *The Chicago River: A Natural and Unnatural History*. Chicago: Lake Claremont Press.

Joint Task Force of Centers for Disease Control and Prevention and US Environmental Protection Agency. 2005. Hurricane Katrina Response – Initial Assessment. September 17.

Lyman, F. 2003. "Messages in the Dust: What are the Lessons of the Environmental Health Response to the Terrorist Attack on September 11th." September. National Environmental Health Association.

National Academy of Sciences, Institute of Medicine. 1988. The Future of Public Health. Washington DC: National Academy Press.

Novotny, P 2000. Where We Live, Work and Play. Westport, CT: Praeger Press.

Parmesan, C., and H. Galbraith. 2004. Observed Impacts of Global Climate Change in the U.S. Pew Center on Global Climate Change. November.

Rabe, B. 1997. "The Politics of Environmental Health," Chapter 18 in T.J. Litman and L.S. Robins, *Health Politics and Policy*, 3rd ed. Albany, NY: Delmar.

Revkin, A.C. 2005. "A Climate Change, A Change of Thinking." *New York Times* December 4, Section 4, p 3.

Stivers, C. 1991. "The Politics of Public Health: The Dilemma of a Public Profession," Chapter 19 in T.J. Litman and L.S. Robins, eds., *Health Politics and Policy*, 2nd ed., Albany, NY: Delmar.

Theriot, C., and K. Tzoumis. 2005. "The Chicago River: An Experiment in Innovative and Technological Approaches." *Golden Gate University Law Review* 35 (April): 377–90.

Tzoumis, K., and L.S. Robins. 2005. "The New Politics of Environmentalism." June 28. Unpublished manuscript, available upon request.

United Nations. UNFCC. 2005. *Caring for Climate: A guide to the Climate Change Convention and the Kyoto Protocol*. Bonn, Germany: Climate Change Secretariat.

Vinten-Johansen P., H. Brody, N. Paneth, S. Rachman, and M. Rip. 2003. *Cholera, Chloroform, and the Science of Medicine: A Life of John Snow*. Oxford University Press.

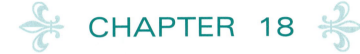

CHAPTER 18

The Elderly: Health Politics Beyond Aging?

William P. Brandon and Patricia Maloney Alt

This chapter explains what is happening in the politics and policies toward senior citizens. The authors suggest how we should think about aging, offer us an inventory of the political landscape and review the major programs (and clashes). Underlying their description runs a fundamental philosophic debate between the politics of community or "solidarity" (espoused by liberals) and the politics of individualism and "the opportunity society" (promoted by conservatives).

Health care for the elderly resists narrow definition and contrasts to other areas of American health politics where the focus has been on the provision of acute medical services.[1] What we call the "aging-support" system incorporates both health care and social welfare systems and focuses on issues such as the turmoil in Medicare and Social Security. The aging-support system includes many social services that are not usually regarded as health considerations.

The principal legislation in the field, the Older Americans Act of 1965, makes coordination of services a primary goal. Particularly given the graying of the "Baby Boom" generation (born from 1946–64), concern over the future of health policy for elders has been increasing. Despite many political changes in recent years, the aging-support system's emphasis on integration and coordination in all sectors of care, particularly at the local level, is unlikely to change.

It is a mistake to conceive of the aging-support system chiefly as a set of formal programs established by government—particularly given the increasing pressure to use non-governmental care resources. The elderly rely on family and on the institutions with which they interact. Over the course of the 1990s, the burden grew on families, particularly on women, to take up the slack for an ever more dependent group of oldest-old. Increasingly, it is the baby boomer near-elderly who are providing this unpaid care. Their involvement in caregiving might prove to be the "hook" that gets them interested in aging policies.

The scope of services and other support for the elderly has had to shift to reflect the heterogeneity of those who are sixty-five and older. Simple stereotypes regarding all of the elderly as poor or near-poor, frail, and bordering on mental incompetence are increasingly inappropriate. Many in this age group still work for wages or as volunteers. Life expectancy continues to rise, which increases the number of frail elderly, but the average health status at every age is also improving. Gerontologists generally deal with this new diversity by dividing the elderly into the young-old (65–74), the old (75–84), and the old-old (85 and over), and emphasize the need for services that recognize the diversity of the target population.[2] The picture of elders as frail and poor may have been accurate when Medicare and the Older Americans Act were passed in 1965; today, it is not accurate overall, but many poor, minority, and/or female elders still face disadvantages when dealing with their health and social service needs. In the debate over whether to increase reliance on the private provision of services it is important to make sure that those citizens who lack private funds have adequate access to the publicly-provided or subsidized services that they need.

The aging-support system only emerged in the 20th century. There were no nursing homes, no public pension systems (aside from veterans' benefits), few private pensions, and little formal retirement as recently as 90 years ago.[3] Over the course of the 20th century, care for our elders was often an easier political "sell," than programs like universal health insurance. Today, a sea-change seems to lie ahead. The United States has a large group of baby boomer near-elders who are not facing up to their own future needs. There is also a growing political effort to slow or reverse the increase in public spending for programs such as Medicare and Medicaid. The year 2005 saw the beginning of a major debate over fundamental reform of Social Security and the convening of the latest White House Conference on Aging; Congressional reauthorization of the Older Americans Act by Congress loomed just ahead. The Medicare prescription drug legislation passed in 2003 and introduced confusing structural changes in a program that will not be fully implemented until 2007.

As Deborah Stone points out, "government seems to be pulling back from the little authority it once exerted over providers to its Medicare and Medicaid beneficiaries . . . converting its two financing programs from a 'defined benefit' model to a 'defined contribution' model." In the latter years of the 20th century, the model emerged of government "restricting its role to something like paying a voucher on behalf of beneficiaries, letting each monitor his or her own benefits as an informed consumer in the managed care market."[4] The proposed (though unsuccessful) changes in Social Security and the emphasis on an "ownership society" in President Bush's second term continued this trend, with significant implications for aging policy. The battles over these changes—reorganization, restrictions, roll backs, privatization—are in their early phases for each is fiercely contested.

The goal of this chapter is to provide a framework for understanding these current and future policy debates. The politics of aging involves three dimensions: *societal understanding, institutional structures*, and *policy issues*.

SOCIETAL UNDERSTANDING

Nothing in biology determines the way that we think of life or its phases. At most, physical constraints provide limits for the societal understandings that develop in each culture. These societal understandings define and structure meaning for both the individual and the community. For example, Social Security, private pensions, Medicare, nursing homes, and retirement communities all emerged from our society's ways of thinking about aging; each reflects our convictions regarding appropriate activities and environments for the elderly. Over time, these structures have become widely accepted and guide the next steps in the evolution of our societal understandings; our empirical arrangements, and the values embedded in them, develop a sense of inevitability—it becomes difficult to imagine our society without Social Security or nursing homes. At this level of analysis it is difficult to disentangle "subjective" from "objective," because one reinforces the other and changes in objective social institutions (like nursing homes) lead or follow changes in subjective understandings (what it means to be "old").[5]

Several brief examples will help clarify the thesis that how we think of aging is a social creation.[6] Perhaps the clearest example is the understanding of retirement as a natural life phase. The idea of reaching an age at which one stopped productive work was largely unknown in North America and England during much of the 19th century—although elderly people might change what they did as their physical powers waned.[7] Formal retirement depended upon the availability of pension schemes. Private pensions, in turn, could become common only with the concentration of capital produced by large-scale industry. Industrialization reduced the heterogeneity of work that had allowed responsibilities in agriculture or traditional hand manufacturing to be altered to accommodate failing physical strength, eyesight, or mental ability.[8] As late as 1940, when Social Security began paying benefits, only about 40% of those 65 and over were "retired." By 1984, about 90% of the same group were "retired."[9] However, by the middle 1990s the trend toward ever-earlier retirement for men had slowed, and the average age of retirement for women had begun to rise. With the age of Social Security eligibility rising for future retirees, this trend is likely to continue.[10] In 2002, 18% of men and 9.8% of women over 65 were in the labor force.[11] Considering that many women in that age range had never been gainfully employed, this is a significant percentage of both genders still working past what is now the "normal" retirement age. As life expectancy continues to grow—and elderly health improves—some argue that people should stay in the workforce longer, thereby easing the pressure on Social Security, making better use of the individual's "age dividend," and increasing the supply of labor.[12]

Another example of the relation between social meanings and institutional structures is the nursing home, a dwelling associated with a way of life. It is easy to forget that the Kerr-Mills Act of 1960 and Medicaid (1965) virtually created the nursing home industry in this country.[13] In contrast, some social welfare states like Sweden and the United Kingdom strive to keep elderly persons living in their own homes by providing home care and other services and by deemphasizing skilled nursing facilities.[14]

Others, like the Netherlands, have more recently moved from an emphasis on nursing homes to home care.[15] Consequently, individuals in those societies may not experience the same difficulties—guilt, feelings of failure, the risks of financial ruin—that often surround decisions regarding entry into long-term care institutions in the United States.

In recent years, advocates for the elderly and policymakers in the United States have increased the scope, quality, and accessibility of community-based long-term care services to enhance the quality of life of the non-institutionalized elderly and to help them continue living in the community. For example, funds were added to the Older Americans Act specifically for community-based care, including the National Family Caregiver Support Program. Medicaid waivers have also allowed states to establish an array of community programs. After 25 years of successful operation, however, it was clear that those programs could not solve all the problems which families faced in dealing with caregiving.

Another increasingly important issue in the move to community-based care has been the potential for cooperation or competition for funding between services for the aging and those for groups with lifelong disabilities. As Rosalie Kane points out, the movement at the state level has been toward encouraging coalitions and overlapping programming. Yet the worldviews of aging and disability advocates have been quite separate, with the younger physically disabled claiming services as a civil rights issue while senior advocates have emphasized services as a health care issue. There has been substantial concern that reducing nursing home use and allowing the money to follow the person into Home and Community Based Services will result in a battle for funds between seniors and the younger disabled.[16] The Supreme Court's 1999 *Olmstead v. LC* decision mandated that publicly funded services be provided to disabled individuals in the most community-based setting possible. What that means for aging services has yet to be fully explored, but at a time of increasing emphasis on private choices in health care, the decision certainly places a premium on movement away from nursing home care.[17]

The plasticity that makes it possible for different societies to evolve different patterns of living for their elderly is also illustrated by the formation of powerful groups that articulate the political interests of the elderly. The United States began its universal social health insurance program, Medicare, by covering the elderly who receive Social Security. In contrast, other industrial nations began government health coverage for workers and expanded it to the rest of society. During the 15 years that it took to enact Medicare, proponents had to conceptualize retirees as a group who were uniquely needy.[18] As we shall see, the effort to enact Medicare generated or strengthened many of the interest groups that subsequently shaped a view of politics based on age cohorts. In many European countries the elderly are incorporated into broad-based and socially active labor and political coalitions.

The fact of social plasticity makes us collectively responsible for the condition of the elderly in our society. This consideration is especially important in regard to the future of aging in America. The baby boomers focused attention on, and often altered, social values when they were young. Many also have a history of resisting the notion of aging, seeking "antiaging" medicine and supporting new slogans such as the Alzheimer's Association's "maintain your brain" campaign.[19] We should not expect them to fall passively into accepted patterns when they become old. There will be more elderly after 2015 than at any other time in American history. And the boomers may be history's healthiest[20] and wealthiest elderly cohort. On the other hand, many lack sufficient savings for retirements that will last longer and involve more expensive health care. Moreover, many who retire in the next 20 years will face confusing changes in Medicare and proposed shifts in Social Security.[21]

INSTITUTIONAL STRUCTURES

Many of the federal policies that affect the elderly originate in institutions that are not organized specifically to deal with aging. In these arenas, advocates of the aging clash, bargain, or cooperate with groups representing other interests. Here, for example, aging interest groups encounter the lobbying efforts of the American Medical Association, hospital interests, employers concerned about the cost of retirement benefits, and labor unions. Over the long term the relative power of the elderly and their advocates will depend on their ability to mobilize and to work together. That may become problematic if boomers continue to resist definition as "elders," preferring to consider themselves as "shoppers" for personalized health care rather than as "citizens" entitled to benefits.[22]

Yet a policy system that is focused on the elderly still exists. In part, the system's components serve symbolic purposes; in part, they constitute administrative routines that are capable of reaching the elderly. The government structures established by Congress to respond to the needs of the elderly are a creation of the 1960s and early 1970s. The first Commissioner of Aging was not appointed until 1965. The first White House Conference on Aging (WHCOA) was convened by the Kennedy administration in 1961. These conferences put issues relating to the elderly and aging in the media limelight and advance the political agenda of the elderly.

Interest groups representing the elderly were relatively weak until the late 1970s.[23] By 1980, however, critics began expressing concern that the elderly might become an organized political force of staggering proportions.[24] Their power was demonstrated first by the passage, then by the repeal of the Medicare Catastrophic Coverage Act of 1988. This was the first rollback of a major social welfare program in American history and featured the startling image of angry elders attacking powerful Representative Dan Rostenkowski's (D-Ill) limousine.[25] Some voices from younger generations suggested that chronological age might become a major division in US politics.[26] Certainly the initial pressure for Medicare drug coverage was an example of an age-centered cohort. However age was not a principal factor determining the interest group alignment around the Medicare Prescription Drug, Improvement, and

Modernization Act of 2003 or the proposed major changes in Social Security.

The chief institutional features of the political landscape can usefully be divided into four categories: government, interest groups, private service institutions, and the communications media.

Government

In the executive branch responsibility for government programs to aid the elderly is diffuse. Using 1978 data Carroll Estes counted at least eighty different federal programs benefiting the elderly directly through cash assistance, in-kind transfers, and direct provision of goods and services.[27] Those programs were scattered among six cabinet departments and seven independent agencies. Tax, regulatory, or employment policies would add to the number of programs benefiting the elderly. These programs affect caregivers as well beneficiaries. In the past two decades, many governmental supports for aging policy have been weakened, with the House Select Committee on Aging gone (it lasted from 1974 to 1993) and the Assistant Secretary for Aging in DHHS "little more than a figurehead."[28]

Federal aid to the elderly is largely administered through agencies that serve a wide range of beneficiaries rather than by bureaucracies dedicated to a single beneficiary or "clientele" group.[29] Thus, the Social Security Administration handles old age, survivor, and disability insurance (OASDI) and the Supplemental Security Income program (SSI), which is a national means-tested income-support program for low-income elderly, blind, and the totally disabled. The Centers for Medicare and Medicaid Services (CMS) is responsible for Medicare and for Medicaid.[30] Though Medicaid was passed primarily as a program for low income groups, it has become particularly important for the elderly, their families, and their advocates, because it functions as the nation's largest payer for nursing home care (see Chapter 15 for the details).[31]

The Administration on Aging (AoA), which was established under the Older Americans Act (OAA) of 1965 (PL 89–73), is more important as a symbol of national commitment than for its power as measured in money or staff. It is the apex of a decentralized network of agencies. Amendments to the OAA in 1973 helped codify an existing informal aging services delivery network by requiring states to establish planning and services areas to ensure that OAA funding would be funneled to strengthen local providers.[32] The 1973 legislation also expanded the scope of activities that can be undertaken by the aging network, which is composed of the AoA, State Agencies on Aging, the Area Agencies on Aging (AAAs), and other local agencies that receive OAA funding. Thus, OAA legislation involved "devolution" to the states and to the local levels before that word was widely used to describe administrative arrangements in the United States.[33]

Over the past decade expenditures have risen slowly, matching inflation, while the proportion of the population over 65 has climbed much more rapidly. When the "baby boom" generation becomes eligible for OAA programs, the gap between resources appropriated and the number of eligible recipients will be even more striking (Figure 18-1).

OAA and its amendments have created a somewhat unusual intergovernmental network of agencies, which are supported through a hybrid type of funding. It can be characterized as a prototypical New Federalism program in which the federal government provides funds in broadly defined block grants. It also resembles a categorical grant program, due to the large number of detailed requirements that restrict the actions of both state and area agencies on aging. The agencies are primarily designed to promote and coordinate services delivered by private institutions and other government entities. Overall, the increases in authorized funding for programs administered by the AoA have been modest and have never kept pace with the growth in responsibilities for the state and area agencies on aging.[34] In fact, during the 1990s funding for AoA programs was flat, although it showed a slight increase at the beginning of the 21st century (Figure 18-2).

Interest Groups

As late as 1969, Theodore Lowi could characterize the elderly as unorganized and apathetic and

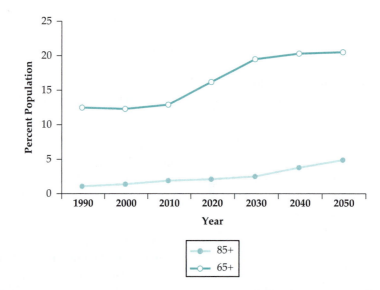

Figure 18-1 Percentage of the Population Ages 65+ and 85+, Selected Years 1990 & 2000 and Projected 2010-2050

SOURCE: U.S. Census Bureau

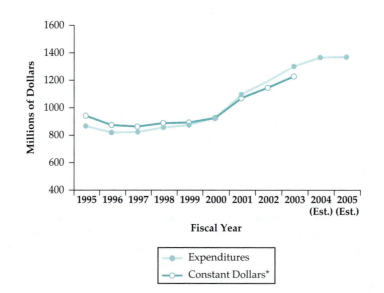

Figure 18-2 Administration on Aging Expenditures.

SOURCE: U.S. Office of Management and Budget, Budget Appendices
*Adjusted to 2000 Dollars Using Implicit Price Deflator

powerless in the struggle to achieve Medicare.[35] For most of the time since then, no one would describe the elderly in these terms. They successfully opposed administration proposals to cut Social Security benefits early in the Reagan presidency, influenced the great Social Security compromise of 1983, and forced the repeal of the 1988 expansion of Medicare that would have covered beneficiaries' catastrophic medical and drug expenses. More recently, elders' concern about prescription drug prices provided the leverage for the passage in 2003 of the Medicare Prescription Drug Improvement and Modernization Act, although many of them found the actual law confusing and disappointing.[36]

The existence of a large array of groups organized around some issue does not mean that they control policy relevant to the issue. Many interest groups may cancel each other out, thereby leaving space for the legislator or executive policy maker to exercise some autonomy.[37] There is also the possibility of a political backlash against the perceived success of interest groups in frustrating legislative reform. The Republicans wrested control of both House and Senate from the Democrats in 1994 by challenging "business as usual" in Washington. The Republican campaign emphasized interest groups influence over congressional Democrats. The Democrats took the legislature back in 2006, in part, by campaigning against indicted lobbyists and industry influence.

In 21st century political whirlwind, attacks on "special interest" groups like the AARP became unusual—perhaps because the relative strength of aging interest groups had waned. Even AARP, the largest and most visible group during the fight over Medicare prescription drug legislation in 2003, suffered a backlash primarily from its own members rather than from politicians or opponents. Critics attacked the AARP, which threw its support behind the legislation, for putting its own business interests ahead of the elderly.[38]

Today, relatively even partisan strength at the national level has led to serious reconsideration of all of the major programs for the elderly. Republicans in Congress have sought, with some success, to reform national policy on aging to make it conform more closely to the budgetary and ideological priorities of the dominant conservative wing of their party. Policy makers no longer see the problems of funding entitlement programs for the elderly as separate from such national economic issues as balancing the budget and reducing the federal deficit (under Clinton) or cutting taxes and encouraging capital investment (under Bush). Traditional aging-related interest groups have played a less-decisive role in policymaking during this time, with the striking exception of the AARP's involvement in the 2003 Medicare Modernization Act.[39]

Mass Membership and Ideological Organizations

Three membership organizations with more than a million members focus on advancing the interests of the elderly: the American Association of Retired Persons (now called just AARP) with 35 million members; the National Committee to Preserve Social Security and Medicare (NCPSSM) with 3.2 million members; and the Alliance for Retired Americans (ARA) with 3 million members. Some organizations are more known for their ideas than for the size of their membership. An example is USA/Next, which used to be known as United Seniors Association (USA).

The American Association of Retired Persons (AARP). Founded as a retired teachers' association in 1947, this organization prospered from the sale of life and health insurance to the elderly. It only began to exert political influence in 1970 over the issue of control of the 1971 White House Conference on Aging.[40] Because it is the largest organization and is well funded from the sale of insurance and other services and government grants, it now sponsors a great deal of policy research and employs many lobbyists and policy analysts. It tends to work with Washington insiders in support of programs for the elderly. Although the membership is still slanted toward the middle and upper middle classes, many of its policy positions would benefit low-income elderly if enacted.[41] Consequently, AARP was the chief target of the insurgent NCPSSM when

AARP supported the Medicare catastrophic health insurance proposal in 1988. Unlike the other organizations described below, AARP is officially nonpartisan and therefore does not make political contributions.

Moreover, AARP incorporated the AARP Andrus Foundation, a 401(c)3 foundation that accepts gifts and bequests, using them to fund research in aging policy and gerontology. In 2003, it committed 7.4 million dollars to academic research and "action demonstration projects."[42]

AARP has been changing its focus over time. Changing its official name to an acronym, for example, deemphasized "retired persons" in order to reach out to younger people and build a base of support among baby boomers. It has also recently moderated its public policy positions in ways that one informed observer interprets as "membership marketing strategies through which AARP's staff and national volunteer leaders could be 'players' in the Washington national scene . . . (and) establish a record that is 'fighting the good fight' with respect to policy proposals affecting old-age programs. But the fight, win or lose, should *not* . . . threaten to jeopardize the stability of the organization's membership, which generates AARP's financial resources through dues and purchases."[43]

Between 1994 and 2003 the AARP was noticeably restrained in its positions. However, with the Medicare Modernization Act of 2003, it found itself in the midst of controversy once again. In contrast with NCPSSM and ARA, which actively opposed the legislation, AARP sought to build grassroots support for the prescription drug benefit by sponsoring rallies in five major cities that featured televised speeches by President Bush. High-ranking administration health officials were present in person to answer questions and elicit support. After these rallies, AARP announced that it would spend 7 million dollars in advertising in one week to support the bill.[44] Iglehart, among others, points out that without AARP's endorsement the bill would not have passed the Senate. Specifically, Democrats feared that AARP would punish them in the next election if they opposed its power on the Medicare drug legislation.[45] Since enactment,

the AARP has committed itself to working to improve the obviously flawed Medicare drug plan. AARP also continued to be staunchly opposed to the privatization of Social Security.[46] Interestingly, while there was a strong backlash among liberals and Democrats against the AARP's support for the Medicare drug plan, including many membership cancellations, its strong opposition to the Personal Retirement Accounts approach to Social Security has also earned it deep hostility from conservative groups such as USA/Next.[47]

The National Committee to Preserve Social Security and Medicare (NCPSSM).
The NCPSSM was founded in 1982 by James Roosevelt (1907–91), former Congressman (D-CA) and son of President Franklin Delano Roosevelt. It originally seemed to be little more than a fundraising effort that used misleading letters about threats to Social Security and Medicare to attract members and donations. The organization became a major irritant to AARP and the congressional elites responsible for passing the Medicare catastrophic legislation in 1988, when NCPSSM became the principal vehicle for mobilizing well-off seniors' discontent against the act.[48] Since the Act's repeal, the Committee's leadership and fundraising practices have changed in ways that make it less threatening to Washington insiders and more effective at lobbying. Its professional staff have become part of the issues networks that determine aging policy in Washington, as shown by its admission in 1995 to membership in the Leadership Council of Aging Organizations, an umbrella group of 51 centrist and liberal advocacy groups.[49] The National Committee to Preserve Social Security and Medicare opposed the Medicare Modernization Act of 2003 and Republican efforts to reform Social Security in 2005 by providing arenas for experts to discuss the "pitfalls of privatization."[50]

The National Council of Senior Citizens (NCSC)/Alliance of Retired Americans (ARA).
This organization began as Senior Citizens for Kennedy in 1960 under union aegis. With aid

from the Democratic National Committee, the organization grew by developing local senior citizens clubs across the country. After it became the NCSC in 1961, it focused almost entirely on Medicare until that legislation was enacted.[51] Subsequently, it concentrated on income security and health issues.

The National Council of Senior Citizens disbanded at the end of 2000; its members were absorbed into a new organization, the ARA. ARA, which was founded in May 2001, proclaims its mission to "ensure social and economic justice and full civil rights for all citizens, so that they may enjoy lives of dignity, personal and family fulfillment and security . . . [aiming] to influence government through action on retiree legislative and political issues at the federal, state, and local levels." It is allied with a number of unions, including the AFL-CIO, and openly supportive of the Democratic Party.[52] However, neither the National Council nor its ARA successor have been very visible in recent debates over aging policy.

United Seniors Association (USA/USANext)

Founded by the late Hollywood actor and former conservative Senator George Murphy (1902–92, R-CA) and conservative direct-mail guru Richard Viguerie, this organization claimed to have four hundred thousand members and revenues of $5.1 million in 1993. In light of the large cost of direct-mail fundraising, some dismissed the organization as another vehicle to enrich Viguerie's for-profit corporations.[53] Under the leadership of former Reagan administration official Charles Jarvis, who took over in 2001, it changed its name to USA/Next and deemphasized its focus on seniors. USA/Next began operating an impressive web site, including links to numerous conservative groups.[54] Jarvis stated that USA/Next had $28 million in annual revenues and explained that he had dropped individual membership subscriptions and aggressively sought contributions from industry—"health care companies, energy companies, the food industry, just about everybody except for financial investment companies."[55] In 2005, USA/Next ferociously attacked the AARP's

stand against Bush's proposed Personal Retirement Accounts, claiming that its polls were skewed and implying in ads that AARP was anti-military and pro-gay. Calling AARP "the boulder in the middle of the highway to personal savings accounts" Jarvis promised that "we will be the dynamite that removes them."[56] The political orientation of both membership and ideological organizations is often affected by their origins. Retirees from the professions, who often held conservative views, made up the bulk of AARP membership in its early years. It now has a broader membership and is more middle-of-the-road. Yet it must be careful about offending members, many of whom are more attracted to the services and information that it offers than to its ideological commitment. Thus, when its policy analysts at the center of the issues networks in Washington get too far in front of its membership—as happened with the Medicare catastrophic health insurance act in 1988 and the Medicare Modernization Act in 2003—the organization will suffer. In contrast to AARP, the National Committee to Preserve Social Security and Medicare and the Alliance of Retired Americans both reflect the very liberal outlook of their leaders and members, who mainly come from organized labor.

Professional Associations and Resources

In addition to elderly mass membership groups and ideological advocacy groups, three other organizations provide the professional infrastructure that helps define aging and gerontology as a distinctive field. The Gerontological Society of America (GSA), the American Society on Aging (ASA), and the National Council on Aging (NCOA), the major professional organizations in the United States, reflect the liberal mainstream views of engaged professional social services and health workers. Each was founded between 1945 and 1954 and now has between 5,000 and 10,000 members.

Interest in aging issues has grown in other professional societies as well. For example, the American Public Health Association's (APHA) Gerontological Health Section grew from a Task Force on Aging in the 1970s into a full-fledged section that sponsors its own panels and works with the Archstone Foundation to recognize excellence in aging services.[57] Similarly, organization-membership groups such as the National Association of Area Agencies on Aging continue to thrive as they seek to represent their members and elders as a whole.[58]

Media and the Internet

Both the "issues network" and "hexagonal lobbying" models of policymaking emphasize the importance of communication among interested parties.[59] The role of public media and newer technologies such as the Internet is central in all modern attempts to understand policymaking. Newspapers, magazines, and television have always paid attention to "worthy" news about the elderly, but they like to concentrate on controversies. Hence, they focus on the fights over the Medicare Modernization Act or proposed reforms in Social Security as political battles, but also make a serious effort to explain these extremely complicated policy issues to the general public. For example, in January 2005 both the *New York Times* and the *Washington Post* and most major newsmagazines and broadcast channels ran numerous stories on the Social Security debate.

Another increasingly influential source of information is the Internet. Each of the major advocacy organizations and the key government agencies that deal with issues of interest to the elderly now have their own websites. In addition, many sites provide listings of other websites of interest to seniors; the subjects range from the Administration on Aging to senior dating services. One major concern for many advocates is the "digital divide" separating seniors, especially low-income and minority seniors, from other generations in their ability to access health and health policy information on the Web.[60] Even those with Internet access can have difficulty in discerning organizational focus, political biases and which net sites are simply marketing fronts.

Summary

The emergence of an increasingly distinct aging-support system began with the development of

government civil service pensions and Social Security. It became more differentiated from other medical and social service programs during the 15-year campaign that followed the decision in 1951 to pursue social health insurance only for the elderly.[61] Nonetheless, federal agencies and congressional committees charged with the most important substantive decision making generally combine responsibility for aging-support issues with other domestic policy issues.

From the 1994 congressional elections onward, the generalist structures of the federal government were especially important, because they had to sort out the fundamental issues of what programs and beneficiaries would suffer the largest funding cuts and who benefited when new resources were parceled out. The interest groups that focused on the elderly became stronger in the last quarter of the 20th century, spanning a wide range of political outlooks and using diverse methods. However, their strength was by no means ensured as the 21st century dawned. Indeed, early indications in the struggle to reform Social Security suggest that organizations based on age cohorts may be eclipsed by broader-based political cleavages.

As the numbers of elderly increased, writers such as Phillip Longman[62] expressed fear that they would become politically invincible.[63] More recently, Third Millennium,[64] an advocacy and educational association representing Americans born after 1960, published a manifesto that, while explicitly eschewing generational war, called for an end to shortsighted political decisions that mortgage their constituents' futures and the futures of *their* children. Increasing government debt and the growing costs of Social Security and Medicare were the principal issues that Third Millennium targeted in the early 1990s.

It is not clear how effective the elderly will be in protecting the entitlements that they have gained and in achieving further advantages from the political system. The elderly have tended to vote in much greater percentages than other age groups. Yet gerontologist Robert Binstock argued that the very diversity of the elderly keeps them from forming an effective voting bloc. "A person who celebrates an older birthday does not suddenly change a lifetime of political attachment, self- and group-identities and specific economic and social interests."[65] He and others argue that the political attitudes of the elderly are not noticeably different from those of other age groups and that the baby boomers will, if anything, be an even less cohesive political force than was the preceding generation.[66]

Others have made persuasive arguments that the boomers will be driven primarily by their own self-interest and might well be more conservative on some policy issues than their parents.[67] In a 2004 opinion poll, the AARP found that boomers are "less likely than [older generations] to favor welfare programs for lower income people, and far more likely to support privatizing Social Security and Medicare."[68] The ongoing battle over Social Security may well be the place where this new dynamic between age cohorts plays out.

The diversity of views is increasingly registered by the proliferation of interest groups that purport to represent the elderly and the increasing ideological disagreement among them. Robyn Stone[69] has identified the causes for the dwindling visibility of aging advocates:

- The loss of "champions": individuals strongly identified with championing programs for elders.

- The failure of successes: the fact that far fewer elders live in poverty leads to the suspicion that advocates for "greedy geezers" take resources away from the needy young.

- Too many organizations fighting for a slice of a limited pie: rapid expansion of programs generate warfare among them for the right to serve particular groups of people.

- Special interests discover aging: biomedical research groups and voluntary health associations such as the Alzheimer's Association join the competition for limited resources with compelling new promises;

- The persistence of ageism in US society: the ongoing cult of youth and widespread baby boomer denial of aging's reality create pressure

to divert funds away from care for elders to "anti-aging," longevity-enhancing visions.

This view of interest groups, which questions their power as organizations to determine the outcome of political issues, is consonant with an emphasis on issues networks in understanding American political phenomena. Position papers, websites, and analytic studies sponsored by interest groups, along with the more important government reports and congressional hearings, are ways to introduce and legitimate ideas. Thus, explanatory models based on bargaining from positions of political power, which characterized the iron triangle as a relatively definable and stable structure (built on interest group, government bureaucrats, and congressional committee) are less useful for understanding contemporary policymaking than the modern information model. Information models, however, are notoriously slippery, because they tend to dissolve distinctions between structure and process and to make each very context-dependent.

With this background we move to an examination of several important aging issues drawing on the four features—government, interest groups, private institutions, and the media—described in this section.

POLICY ISSUES

The outcome of the presidential and congressional elections in 2004 seemed to provid a strong foundation for Republican initiatives in domestic policy during the second George W. Bush administration. With control of the presidency and majorities in both houses of Congress after the November 2004 elections, Republicans at the federal level were well positioned to shape future domestic arrangements in the United States. By the close of that campaign the notion of "the ownership society" appeared to serve as the organizing concept for domestic policy for at least the next four years.[70]

At least in the short run, it did not turn out that way and—bedeviled by an unpopular war and entangled in scandal—the Republicans lost their majority in both Congress and in state legislatures. However, it would be a mistake to dismiss the Bush administration's ownership society. We explore what this perspective means and how it bears on aging policy. The remainder of this chapter looks at policies regarding prescription drugs, Medicare restructuring and income security as they affect the elderly.

In contrast to the notion of "the ownership society," the theme of "compassionate conservatism," was prominent in the disputed election that initially brought George W. Bush to power in January 2001. Although compassionate conservatism was often mentioned in the 2004 campaign, it was not as prominent as it had been four years earlier. After four years, compassionate conservatism seemed a little vague despite administration legislative successes in the domestic areas of education ("No Child Left Behind"), two rounds of significant tax cuts and considerable rhetorical emphasis on "faith-based initiatives." Partially, this vagueness is because the administration, which came to power intending to make its mark on domestic policy, had to focus on foreign affairs after the terrorists' attack on the United States on September 11, 2001.

Even so, the first George W. Bush administration achieved what is generally regarded—but not universally hailed—as the most significant structural changes in Medicare since it was enacted in 1965.[71] This legislation, "The Medicare Prescription Drug, Improvement and Modernization Act of 2003" (PL 108–173), built on important changes in Medicare and federal programs for low income persons in the Balanced Budget Act of 1997 (PL 105–33). These two recent Acts of Congress are important for understanding federal health policy both in the details of how it affects the elderly and in its stakes for the underlying direction of health and aging policymaking.

Medicare

The "ownership society" in Medicare is most visible in provisions favoring the development of private managed care plans that will attract seniors away from the federally run, fee-for-service, social insurance model that has marked Medicare since it was founded. The conservative idea also espouses private, tax-free accounts that will permit individuals who do not yet qualify for Medicare to keep dollars that now go into a common insurance pool for first-dollar health care and investment. (If not spent for health care, the funds and any profits from their investment carry over from year to year and at death can pass to one's heirs.)

Republican policymakers have long desired to achieve these two goals. One involves the strategy of having the US Centers for Medicare and Medicaid Services (CMS) paying for beneficiary premiums in *private health plans* rather than simply enrolling them in traditional, government sponsored Medicare. The other moves health care dollars into a personal account which the individual "owner" would use to self-insure for medical bills up to a large threshold beyond which catastrophic insurance would provide coverage. Both of these policy goals were advanced by the Medicare Modernization Act of 2003, which introduced many changes in Medicare beyond providing the new coverage for prescription drugs used outside the hospital (called "outpatient prescription drugs").

Because the Medicare Modernization Act of 2003 built on important changes initiated by the Balanced Budget Act of 1997, the discussion of contemporary Medicare policy must begin with that law.

Balanced Budget Act of 1997

The Balanced Budget Act explicitly attempted to shift Medicare beneficiaries out of the government-run fee-for-service indemnity plan that allowed them to see any physician who accepted Medicare patients. The Act's proponents wanted to induce Medicare beneficiaries to enroll in managed care plans. Medicare would pay a set monthly amount or premium to the managed care plan which would, in turn, provide all needed services to their Medicare enrollees. Managed care plans claim to provide more efficient care by requiring patients to use the plan's physicians and facilities. In return for a higher volume of patients provided by the managed care plan, health providers typically accept lower payment than they charge patients outside of the plan.

The Move Toward Managed Care

Part of the attraction of managed care is the hope that it reduces costs. Conservative policy makers also favor the growth of managed care because it inserts a for-profit or non-profit intermediary between the government and the provider chosen by a patient, thereby shifting the responsibility for the costs of care to the managed care plan or health provider. In time, many conservatives would like to further emphasize individual responsibility and choice by converting the government's promise of access to a range of medical care services—a "defined benefit"—to a promise to provide money in a "defined contribution" to help the individual purchase whatever level or type of care he or she seeks to have. The latter arrangement, where the beneficiary receives money for a health insurance policy (or pension fund) rather than a definite health service or retirement benefit in the future, is an important concept in understanding the Republican reforms of both pensions and health care benefits.

Liberals, including many Democrats, welcome any cost-saving resulting from managed care, but they generally distrust efforts that increase private variation in previously uniform government social insurance programs, especially those that may work to the disadvantage of minorities and low-income populations. They also desire to avoid preparing the groundwork that would allow benefits to vary according to the income of the recipients. Such "means-" or income-testing is a mark of welfare. The liberals' view is often summarized: "programs aimed at the poor soon become poor programs."

The effort to move senior citizens into managed care plans began during the Ronald Reagan Administration (1981–89) although it was disrupted when health maintenance organizations in Florida were caught using scandalous marketing to attract healthy elderly while avoiding those in poor health (precisely what liberals had predicted). During the Bill Clinton administration (1993–2001), however, the number of elderly enrolled in managed care greatly increased. By that time there were a number of checks on abuses by managed care plans, such as the requirement that plans must contain a mixture of government Medicare or Medicaid beneficiaries and individuals with insurance provided by employers. (Those with commercial insurance could move to other plans if they perceived that quality was falling, which would force management to address problems.)

The federal government's complex payment formula, experts agreed, overpaid health care plans in areas where medical costs were high.[72] Many experts also believed that managed care plans attracted Medicare beneficiaries who were healthier than the average Medicare patient. Better health among Medicare beneficiaries who enrolled in managed care plans would mean that that those plans had lower expenses than the government experienced from its much larger fee-for-service indemnity population.[73] The cost of treating those in fee-for-service Medicare determined the premiums paid to plans. High earnings—whether from healthier enrollees, greater efficiency, or reduced services—allowed plans to provide extra benefits that fee-for-service beneficiaries did not receive from the government-run program. A very common added benefit to entice increased enrollment in managed care plans was coverage of outpatient prescription drugs.

However, generous extra benefits and even the existence of managed care plans open to Medicare beneficiaries were concentrated in geographical areas where Medicare payments were high and in urban areas. In other areas, senior citizens and the disabled had no choice aside from the traditional fee-for-service indemnity Medicare.

Seeking to foster managed care plans and make them available throughout the United States, and especially in rural areas, Republican Congressional leaders created a more complex reimbursement formula in the Balanced Budget Act of 1997, with special provisions to insure that managed care would develop in rural and low-cost areas. It also reduced the earnings of plans in the high-cost areas where they were flourishing. Public information campaigns marketing the new "Medicare+Choice" program created by the Balanced Budget Act of 1997 were developed to inform seniors of their "choices" among traditional fee-for-service Medicare and the several competing plans that were expected to emerge in most areas of the country.[74]

However, in a startling lesson of the importance of "unanticipated consequences," the law's actual effect was the opposite of what was intended. It seems that the managed care plans were motivated to seek the enrollment of Medicare beneficiaries *because* the business was very profitable. Under the new financial structure, managed care plans began leaving many counties in the United States where they had provided health care to seniors. Little expansion to new areas occurred. In 1999, 6.3 million persons or 16% of all beneficiaries were enrolled in managed care plans under Medicare, but by 2003 that number had fallen to 4.6 million and 11%.[75]

The Balanced Budget Act repealed the requirement that plans enrolling government-sponsored beneficiaries must also enroll significant numbers of commercially insured workers (who were presumed to have choices among plans that they would exercise by avoiding inferior plans). Repealing this effort to enforce quality allowed some plans to become Medicaid-only plans, but it did nothing to enhance the appeal of managed care to Medicare beneficiaries.

Moreover, to live up to its billing as a "balanced budget act" in its much larger indemnity program, the Balanced Budget Act cut reimbursements for a wide range of health care providers and required that many ancillary services be paid a flat fee—a "prospective payment"—for delivering a specific service or treating a specific kind of patient.

The broader purpose of the Act which most truly represented the shared goals of the Democratic President and the Republican House of Representatives, was to strengthen the financial basis of the Medicare Trust Fund and to reduce federal government deficits. In this regard, the Act was an outstanding success. The year when the Medicare Trust Fund was projected to pay out more than it received in payroll taxes changed from 2001 to 2029.[76] Overall federal budgets, which had been in deficit since before the presidency of Ronald Reagan, began to post a surplus. These fiscal developments were crucial for the passage of a Medicare drug benefit in 2003, because they created a pot of some 400 billion dollars that legislators were told they could allocate for outpatient prescription drugs without cutting other programs.

The cuts in health care reimbursements imposed by the Balanced Budget Act were severe enough to generate an outcry from health care providers of all types. Several subsequent pieces of legislation attempted to mitigate the negative impacts on health providers of some of the harsher provisions, but none reversed the decline in interest by managed care plans in enrolling Medicare beneficiaries.[77]

Medicare Savings Accounts

In contrast to the major policy initiative of Medicare+Choice, the Balanced Budget Act also established a modest pilot program that allowed up to 390,000 Medicare beneficiaries to set up "medical savings accounts" (MSAs). These accounts received Medicare dollars calculated on what the government would pay for a health plan premium for the individual. No taxes were owed on the money put into the account or on any interest that accrued. The Medicare beneficiary with a MSA was to use it for medical expenses and to purchase a high deductible or "catastrophic" health insurance policy. The deductible before the policy began paying could be no greater than $6,000 in 1999. Funds that were not used to provide health care or buy the catastrophic health insurance policy in the year that they were deposited were retained to cover care in future years.[78]

The drive to establish individual accounts was in part a response to the rise in unregulated managed care in the 1990s after Congress rejected President Clinton's health care reform. The seemingly successful methods used by managed care to constrain the increase in premiums paid by employers generated a public relations and policy backlash from the public, physicians and hospitals.[79] By the end of the 1990s some health policy analysts and many conference panels called for "consumer-driven health care" as an alternative cost-containment strategy to managed care. This strategy for cost-containment involved replacing managed care by a consumer/patient who would have incentives to make cost-conscious spending decisions in purchasing health care for his or her family. Individuals faced with a choice of spending money for health care or keeping it for future health care consumption and short-term investment would make their own decisions about health care instead of surrendering decisionmaking power to distant insurance companies.

The new solution for rising health care costs was based on the assumption that if individuals paid for health care with their own money, optimum levels of consumer satisfaction would be achieved and (probably) rising health care costs would be constrained. It reflects the views of economists and policy analysts who want to see health care conform as closely as possible to the economist's model of the competitive market. According to this model of consumer sovereignty, consumers with adequate incomes will purchase the amount of health care that yields them the optimum satisfaction relative to the entire mix of goods that they wish to consume.[80] This view contrasts with the more traditional view that health care should be provided to individuals on the basis of their objective need for it.[81] Proponents of consumer-driven health care usually neglect to explain how to persuade newly empowered health care consumers to invest more heavily in preventive care than did the insurance companies and health maintenance organizations when they were the acknowledged decision makers.

The inclusion of Medical Savings Accounts in the Balanced Budget Act pleased conservative legislators and those policy analysts who desire to expand competitive markets in health care; some insurance interests also worked for its passage. The limited MSA program attracted little attention after enactment. However, the Balanced Budget Act was the first legislation that allowed a defined contribution to replace what had previously been a defined benefit in a public program. Thus, Medical Savings Accounts established a precedent that the Medicare Prescription Drug, Improvement and Modernization Act of 2003 would build on.

The Balanced Budget Act of 1997 further encouraged the defined contribution approach in Medicare by expanding the alternatives to traditional fee-for-service indemnity Medicare beyond

health maintenance organizations. In addition to opening Medicare up to preferred provider organizations and other kinds of medical plans, one provision allowed the development of a fee-for-service plan that could reimburse doctors and hospitals at higher rates than Medicare. To remain solvent, such plans would have to charge a stiff premium on top of the Medicare dollars that they received. They were designed for the affluent to buy the very best medical care and amenities. Although the implementation of these plans has received little attention, the concept parallels the development of so-called "boutique medicine" at the end of the 1990s. In boutique medicine, physicians decide to serve a very small number of patients who pay much higher fees and an annual premium. Patients who are willing to pay for such "Cadillac" care appear to enjoy the higher levels of service without waiting that this kind of practice allows.[82]

Medicare Prescription Drug, Improvement and Modernization Act of 2003

The Medicare reform of 2003 added a Part D to Medicare that provides outpatient prescription drugs in 2006 for all who enroll. It also reformed Part C by changing Medicare+Choice to "Medicare Advantage," requiring managed care plans to provide drug coverage and providing a number of incentives (including $10 billion over seven years) for them to serve Medicare beneficiaries, especially in geographical areas where they had failed to thrive in the past. A full account of this policy change—the ideas, the politics, and the early experience—can be found in Chapter 13, "*Medicare*." Here we emphasize the enduring implications for politics of the elderly.

Dividing Beneficiaries

The most unusual feature of this effort to protect Medicare beneficiaries against the high cost of drugs is the absence of protection between $2,250 and $5,100 in an individual's annual expenditures for outpatient prescription drugs. In this so-called "donut hole" between $2,250 and $5,100 beneficiaries with the stand-alone drug plans who do not qualify as low income must pay 100% of all outpatient drug costs. Proponents of the legislation felt compelled to accept this gap as the least damaging strategy to keep the 10-year cost under the 400 billion dollars—a ceiling that had been negotiated to win over reluctant Congressional votes. After a $250 deductible, the drug plan pays 75% up to the $2,250. The plan then pays nothing more until a beneficiary crosses the $5,100 threshold, when the plan starts paying 95% of the cost. In 2006, premiums for this plan were originally estimated to be about $35 each month.[83] Counting the cost of a year's premiums, beneficiaries enrolling in the stand-alone plans need to spend $1,590 out of pocket before the drug plan pays an equivalent amount (i.e., breakeven is achieved). All told, the enrollee will have paid $4,020 in one year before reaching the $5,100 threshold, after which the plan pays 95% of outpatient prescription drugs purchased during the rest of that year.[84]

Thus, the new Medicare benefit will be especially attractive to those who are relatively affluent and have high annual drug bills; for them the 95% reimbursement above $5,100 is useful catastrophic protection. Up to that level, the Act is at best marginal in the help that it provides. It is these "first dollars" that proponents of consumer-driven health care want consumers to consider carefully before spending. While the price of a drug is important, the growth in the volume of drugs is causing much of the increase in drug costs. By forcing consumers to pay a $250 deductible plus $420 in premiums, the drug plans and the health care system generally guard themselves against the cost of drugs for self-limiting acute conditions. These financial arrangements and the 25% copayment may lead seniors with chronic conditions and modest incomes to take less than the prescribed doses of medications. For example, it will be tempting for a senior who feels OK to take his or her cholesterol-lowering medication every other day instead of every day.

The point we would underscore is that for the first time in its 40-year history both Medicare benefits and payments will vary by income.[85] Previously, low-income Medicare beneficiaries could qualify for Medicaid, which paid Medicare Part B premiums, deductibles and outpatient prescription drugs along with the other benefits of Medicaid.[86] Under the Medicare Modernization Act, low-income elderly and disabled beneficiaries who meet both income and asset (i.e., wealth) tests do not have to pay premiums or deductibles and are covered through the "donut hole." States have to pay the federal government most of what they save by not having to provide drugs for Medicare beneficiaries who also receive Medicaid. This income-based differential marks the first example of Medicare providing more care for poor beneficiaries than for others with the same medical needs.

In paying for the program all Medicare beneficiaries with high incomes are required to pay higher Part B premiums even if an individual does not sign up for any drug benefit. Heretofore, social insurance programs in the United States have been financed by equal payment, in order to avoid the stigma associated with low-income means-tested programs and to reinforce the principle of social solidarity. Now, a surtax on the Medicare Part B premium starts with individuals with incomes of $80,000 or couples with incomes of $160,000, who have to pay 35% of Part B costs. There are five Part B premium rates in all.[87] And the 2005 increase in the basic Medicare Part B premium was the steepest one-year increase in Medicare history.[88]

Bruising Politics

The politics surrounding the passage of Medicare reform may be as important for future efforts to legislate the administration's conception of the ownership society. Three noteworthy episodes received widespread media attention during the enactment of the legislation. First, almost all Democrats who were appointed to the conference committee that resolves differences in bills passed by the House and Senate were excluded from the conference committee deliberations. The second peculiarity occurred when the bill came up for a final vote by the entire membership of the House of Representatives at 3 A.M. on a Saturday. Instead of stopping Congressional voting after the usual 15 minutes, which would have led to defeat of prescription drug legislation 216–218, the voting was kept open for just under 3 hours. During that time the House Republican leadership and President Bush pressured representatives to change their vote. The third incident was the claim made in an op-ed column by a Republican Congressman that someone offered to donate $100,000 to his son's campaign fund if the Congressman would change his vote from "no" to "yes." (The obviously outraged Congressman continued to vote "no.") Later the Congressman recanted his claim, saying that it was "technically incorrect."[89]

These three episodes suggest that the bill to cover outpatient prescription drugs under Medicare as finally enacted was very much a piece of Republican legislation. Democratic Senate Minority Leader Daschle and Senator Kennedy had strongly supported the original Senate bill. Coverage of outpatient prescription drugs has long been a benefit that liberal Democrats wanted to provide. After seeing the version developed in the House, however, they disavowed the legislation. Thus, the Medicare Modernization Act was essentially Republican legislation in contrast to Balanced Budget Act of 1997. The 1997 legislation involved hard bargaining, but its enactment required that it advance both Republican congressional goals and the aims of a Democratic President who had successfully stood up to the previous highly partisan Congress.

Turning to the politics of interest groups, a key ingredient in the narrow vote in favor of the Medicare Prescription Drug Act was almost certainly the support of AARP. The endorsement by this giant organization of seniors served as protection for Republican legislators in the next election and increased the likelihood of picking up a few critical votes from nervous moderate Democrats. AARP, reasoning that some outpatient prescription drug benefit even if flawed was better than none, broke with its liberal Democratic allies after canny House leaders sweetened the bill enough to get AARP to swallow it. AARP had been a major opponent of medical savings accounts and of efforts to introduce means testing into the Balanced Budget Act of 1997.[90]

The other liberal interest groups continued to vigorously oppose the prescription drug bill as did the liberal Democratic Senators who had supported the initial Senate bill. On the right, conservative legislators and several interest groups including the Heritage Foundation and the National Taxpayers Union opposed Medicare reforms as a fiscally irresponsible expansion of government programs, which in the long term threatened the existing practice of employer-sponsored insurance for retirees.[91] These objections to the Medicare Modernization Act by fiscally conservative Republicans and some of the conservative think tanks that have worked with them may augur future difficulties for the Republican health policy network.[92]

Moreover, the cost-estimates for Medicare Reform damaged Congress's trust in the administration. Many in Congress recognized that the initial 400 billion dollars which was "set aside" to finance the reform for a decade was largely a polite artificial fiction in light of predictable decreases in general federal revenues. A desire finally to provide outpatient prescription drugs led legislators in both parties to accept the 400 billion expense so long as the 10-year costs did not greatly exceed that amount. Indeed, their recognition of the need for fiscal discipline forced Congress to create the infamous "donut hole."

What legislators did not know is that in mid-2003, well before final passage of the Medicare Modernization Act, the Chief Actuary of the Centers for Medicare and Medicaid Services had projected that actual costs would be much higher than the 400 billion dollar limit that Congress and the president had set. The political appointees above him let him know that sharing this knowledge with Congress would cost *him* his job, so he misled Congressional staffers. When it discovered that the administration had suppressed this critical information, Congress was furious.[93] By February 2005, the administration calculated 10-year costs at $720 billion.

This sorry record of hidden cost increases, highly partisan politics, and damaged administration credibility had a vivid impact on the skepticism that met the Bush Administration's proposals to reform Social Security. We now turn to that issue.

Social Security Reform

For most Americans, a comfortable retirement depends on a "three-legged stool"—income from employer-sponsor retirement plans, personal savings, and Social Security.

The second leg of the stool, private savings amassed during prime working years, has long concerned economists, who point out that the average American has a very low rate of personal savings when compared to citizens of other advanced industrial states.[94] Despite rhetoric about the importance of personal rather than social responsibility and the development of such instruments as 401(k) plans that reward savings with tax benefits, Americans have not shifted their discretionary incomes from consumption to savings. On the contrary, personal savings have plummeted in the last few decades, with the average household saving dropping from 11% of disposable income in 1985 to about 1.5% today.[95] In light of this remarkable decrease, carving out part of the employee contribution to Social Security for personal accounts may encourage individuals to be even more negligent about saving.[96]

Social Security, the third leg of the stool, is the largest domestic government program in the United States and covers 90% of those 65 and over. It represents a stable national social insurance commitment to provide a "safety net" for the elderly, the disabled, and the surviving children of workers.

Ball and Bethell describe its five key elements.[97]

- Coverage: equitable protection for the entire population with no one forced into poverty in retirement.

- Earned benefit: all beneficiaries or their families contribute to the program, hence there is a right to benefits.

- Equality: everyone is in the same boat, with broad support for the program and uniform defined benefits.

- Dedicated financing: covered through the payroll tax, with inflation protection. Able to cover low income workers affordably. Cost containment and administrative efficiencies are realized.

- Responsibility for program purpose and content: a clear designation of congressional and federal administrative responsibility; transparency; and public accountability.

For most beneficiaries, Social Security is their single largest source of income. Unlike most company pensions and personal savings, Social Security has been indexed since 1972 so that payments have increased as the cost of living rises, meaning that elders are *not* on a "fixed income." The large reduction in poverty rates among older Americans (from 35% in 1960 to 10% today) is mainly due to increases in Social Security. The Congressional Budget Office estimated that without Social Security almost half of elderly Americans would have been in poverty in 2000.[98] Thus, the long-term economic stability of Social Security is crucial, because it is the principal financial source of well-being for seniors and their families.

One of the major achievements of the 1980s was the eleventh-hour cooperation among Congress, the president, and major private interests that corrected a significant imbalance between revenues and expenditures in the Social Security trust funds. The agreement was reached by an important process. It involved establishing a bipartisan National Commission on Social Security Reform (which was also known as the Greenspan Commission after its chairman, Alan Greenspan). Like other commissions organized during the Reagan administration, this bipartisan commission allowed the President to back away from his public opposition to the Democratic Congress without angering supporters on the political right. The political cover also shielded members of Congress from Social Security beneficiaries who were upset about the one-time postponement of a cost-of-living allowance (COLA), from federal employees and retirees who were angry that new civil servants would have to enroll in Social Security which had exempted government workers with their advantageous pension plans, from taxpayers who would have to pay more in payroll taxes, and from other disgruntled interests such as AARP.[99] Although the National Commission on Social Security

Reform (1983) played a prominent role, it was behind-the-scenes negotiations between David Stockman (President Reagan's director of the Office of Management and Budget) and Robert M. Ball (a liberal who had served as commissioner of Social Security from 1962 to 1973) that forged the final bipartisan compromise.[100]

The compromise was designed to create a 5.5 trillion dollar reserve fund by the year 2025 that was meant to make Social Security financially sound for years to come. However, the existence of burgeoning reserves in the Social Security trust funds since 1983 (instead of the rapid decline experienced in the earlier decade) generated its own political controversy. The issue was whether the growing Social Security trust funds should be regarded as part of the annual federal budget or kept separate.[101]

If the budget included the revenue of the Social Security trust funds, the federal deficit appeared smaller; excluding this major revenue source, on the other hand, masked the proportion of the national wealth that was going to government and made the deficit appear worse.[102] By the time of the 2005 debate over Social Security, the confusion over the role of the Social Security and Medicare trust funds in the federal budget had, if anything, worsened. Dueling forecasts from a wide variety of sources made the situation almost incomprehensible for the average citizen.

When the baby boomers retire (from about 2012 to 2030) their Social Security benefits will be supported by a relatively smaller workforce paying payroll taxes. That appeared to create a crisis—fewer workers supporting more retired people. However intergenerational transfers as a whole will not change much because there are also projected to be fewer children for the workforce to support, and more women in the workforce will help to keep up the payroll contribution. The key question is not the worker/retiree ratio but the worker/non-worker ratio. The latter is projected to rise only 6% over the first half of the 21st century—far less than the 50% projected jump in the worker/retiree ratio.[103]

A prefunded surplus was developed by the 1983 compromise to allow the Social Security system to shift some of the retirement burden from future workers to the current generation of workers.[104] Analysis in the mid-1990s indicated that the OASI could pay benefits until 2030 without expenditures exceeding revenues, whereas the Disability Insurance (DI) fund would be in deficit by about 2016.[105] Of the 47 million Americans collecting payments from Social Security, almost 18 million are not retired workers; they are spouses and children of disabled, retired, and deceased workers, and some six million disabled workers. These non-retirees receive 38% of all Social Security benefit dollars. A very real question persists about whether disabled workers, dependents, or survivors should have the ability to invest in "personal accounts" or whether they would need the funds for everyday living and would wind up in much worse shape as they age.[106]

Over time, enormous disagreement developed about the actual facts regarding Social Security. The result of presumed experts on both sides of the liberal–conservative divide talking past each other was increasing levels of political rancor among insiders and confusion among ordinary citizens. With the facts in dispute, it is no wonder that there was even more disagreement over the appropriate remedies. As pointed out above, some of this confusion stemmed from a recurring debate dating back to the origins of Social Security in 1935 over the relative value of "defined benefits" programs versus "defined contributions" and from partisan and ideological disagreement about the respective roles of government and individuals in such key areas as protecting citizens' health and ability to care for themselves and their families.[107] Even the language used in such discussions was politically charged. After polls and focus groups showed that voters, especially older ones, distrusted changes in Social Security that included the word "private," the Bush administration changed its terminology to speak about the importance of allowing "personal accounts" as a part of Social Security. Similarly, Democrats sought to substitute the word "challenge" for "crisis," which President Bush continually used in discussing Social Security funding.[108]

From the perspective of the libertarian Cato Institute, the prospect of Social Security reform could lead to "changing fundamentally the relationship of people to their government . . . [in] the biggest shift since the New Deal." Similarly, Peter Wehner, a White House aide, sent out a memo arguing that "We consider our Social Security reform not simply an economic challenge, but a moral goal and a moral good . . . one of the most significant conservative governing achievements ever."[109]

Thus, ideological disagreements about fundamental values played a central part in the discussion (in contrast to the more pragmatic concerns that could ultimately be bridged to achieve the 1983 compromise on Social Security). The urge to take a government social insurance program and make it subject to private decisions (and available to for-profit investment firms) came not just from a desire to maximize economic returns to the individual but also from deep-seated beliefs about the need to downsize government and to get it out of the business of guaranteeing collective economic security.

Even the conservative columnist George Will agreed that there was no "crisis" in Social Security, when compared with the impending solvency issues in Medicare and Medicaid. However, he saw an "opportunity" to reform Social Security, stating that "the philosophic reasons for reforming Social Security are more compelling than the fiscal reasons."[110]

Underlying the Social Security and Medicare discussions and the "ownership society" theme was a rethinking of the role of social insurance in modern countries. From the conservative perspective, social insurance and social solidarity were ideas whose time had come and gone. Advocates of the current system, on the other hand, firmly believed in the original vision of collective responsibility for social need. Both sides, in short, took a principled (even moral) perspective and wrapped it in complex cost benefit analyses.

Amid the cacophony of claims and counterclaims, some fairly basic threads can be discerned. There was agreement, for instance, that under current funding methods Social Security will not be able to meet its obligations at some point in the future.

There was, however, great disagreement about exactly when that problem will occur and how serious it will be. Like any other forecasting discussion, this one hinges on what numbers are entered into the formula, and what factors the forecast takes into account. Even the politically neutral Congressional Budget Office and the Social Security Trustees disagreed on the exact point at which the shortfall will occur, although both placed the gap between outlays and revenue at 1.7% to 2% of GDP in 2080, given no change in the current program.[111]

One simple way to strengthen the trust fund balances would be to very gradually raise the age at which retirees will receive full Social Security benefits (as the Social Security Improvement Act of 1983 did). Increasing the accepted retirement age would encourage people to work and keep contributing payroll taxes longer and reduce the period during which they will receive benefits. However, raising the normal retirement age might generate greater alienation among younger workers, many of whom were already skeptical about ever receiving any return from the Social Security contributions that they are forced to pay.[112] A logical variant on this proposal would include counting average earnings for 40 years of highest earnings, rather than 35. This would not mean individuals would have to work longer, but that their benefits would be lowered by factoring in five additional lower-earning years. Given that average life expectancy has increased more than five years since 1935, such a change seemed reasonable to many.[113]

The Social Security Advisory Council also unanimously recommended bringing all new state and local hires under Social Security (as the 1983 compromise enacted for Federal employees). The consequence would be to bring new payments into the system. Many would qualify for Social Security benefits from work for other employers, so the increased payroll taxes might not create many new beneficiaries. Another key change would be to reexamine the price index which is used to adjust benefits, which overstates inflation according to many analysts.[114]

Two other widely recommended changes affect the trust fund revenues: a small, gradual increase in the payroll tax and lifting the $90,000 maximum "cap" on earnings subject to that tax. The $90,000 limit represented 90% of wages when it was imposed. Now it includes only 85% of wages.[115]

Among the many thoughtful but complex "fixes" that were considered, the most controversial was the concept of "privatizing" some portion of the worker's contribution to Social Security. This approach would involve giving younger workers a part of their contribution to Social Security to invest. It fits with the "ownership society" notion that individuals should be able to determine their own lives as much as possible, including the level of risk they take in ensuring their retirement income. Such a perspective parallels the emphasis on "choice" in Medicare plans and in Medicaid waiver programs for community-based long term care. Its supporters foster skepticism about the ability of government to protect its citizens, but their real charge is against the appropriateness of government doing so. As George Will pointed out, this argument is not over whether government should be involved in its citizens' lives, but how that involvement should be shaped. He sees the "crux of modern conservatism" as "government taking strong measures to foster in the citizenry the attitudes and aptitudes necessary for increased individual independence."[116]

Two quite different questions should be asked about Will's view. Is there a public obligation to support through social insurance—not means-tested and stigmatized charity—those who are unable to reach full "individual independence?" And does this collective obligation require provision for the elderly as an age cohort, in light of the fact that almost all of them used to experience this independence when younger but in old age a substantial number are unable to assert that independence?

The second major question is whether those of us who are still able to exercise full independence might make the best use of the choices open to us when secure social insurance programs guard one against extreme poverty or overwhelming health care costs. Moral development and life choices will vary according to the nature of the safety net provided—or not provided—by society. In the context of a reluctant and minimal provision of services only for the poor, realistic "moral" individuals will be risk averse and will feel forced to maximize wealth to seek protection for themselves and their families. In contrast, a broad entitlement that provides for the minimal material needs of individuals or families allows an individual to accept as rational risks that may not be crowned with success or great wealth. For example, an individual living in such a society will find it much easier to choose a career in art, public service or teaching that may fulfill deep needs but generate few financial rewards. A compelling argument can even be made that the economic risk of starting one's own business is easier to undertake in the knowledge that an underlying safety net will not allow those whom the entrepreneur loves to go hungry or homeless if the venture fails.

In short, debates about Social Security (and Medicare) are, ultimately, debates about what kind of society the United States ought to be. This conflict among specific sets of values by which to guide America in the 21st century exemplifies "societal understanding" as we titled the general discussion of the social creation of reality that began this chapter. The debates have grown so heated because, as John Oberlander points out in Chapter 14, Democrats and Republicans now stand for very different visions of the good society.

SUMMARY

We have traced the emergence of a definable aging-support system providing income, social services, and health care. In keeping with the political focus of this book, the chapter provided considerable detail about the relevant public structures and those private interests that have developed to support and influence them. It has also illustrated the contemporary movement toward fundamental political change, the impact of such change on an aging population and the support system which helps the elderly and their families cope with infirmity, difficult living situations, and income insecurity.

From 1981–93, the conservative Republican administrations of Ronald Reagan and George H.W. Bush were committed to helping citizens cope with the health and social problems within a traditional framework. Their administrations strengthened Medicare and Medicaid by developing new ways to control health care costs.[117] At the same time efforts to encourage elders to enroll in managed care programs were relatively unsuccessful.

However, since the Congressional elections of 1994, and particularly since the election and reelection of President George W. Bush in 2000 and 2004, the notion of downsizing the federal government's role in protecting its citizens' health and income security has been increasingly emphasized. The "ownership society" focus of the 2004 election reflects ongoing complicated political maneuverings over Medicare and Social Security. The effort to "privatize" at least a part of both programs has been part of the Republican agenda since at least the middle 1990s. The understandable but perhaps exaggerated concern over the solvency of these programs as the baby boomers become eligible for benefits has been used as an opening for an ideological effort to rethink and restructure the overall role of government. While the Democrats have had some electoral success—on national, state and local level—they face a social policy agenda framed by conservative visions of social reform. One of the great questions for the future is whether Democrats and proponents of social solidarity will be able to reframe the political debate in a way the speaks to the contemporary, global political economy. [118]

At the same time, the aging advocacy groups which were so significant in the evolution of Medicare and the Administration on Aging have become less unified and focused. Complicated economic arguments which seem to pit benefits for elders against the future financial well-being of their children and grandchildren proved to be more difficult to address than the old 20th century issues surrounding "ageism" or prejudice against the old. To some extent the very success of Social Security and Medicare in reducing the level of impoverishment of older Americans and in extending their lives has made their need-based claims less compelling.[119] As needs become more equally distributed across age cohorts in the United States, it is quite possible that the 21st century will see a rise in intergenerational struggles for limited resources. With the first wave of baby boomers turning 65 in 2011, the current generation of Americans urgently needs to engage in an extended dialogue about these issues. As Judith Feder argues, we are challenged to "prevent the unraveling of community" and must "decide whether we are a society in which it is every man, woman, or child for him/herself or one in which we are all in it together."[120]

STUDY QUESTIONS

1. In what ways has the American Association of Retired People (AARP) changed since its inception, particularly with regard to its political advocacy role?

2. How have the interests of the disabled (of any age) and the elderly clashed?

3. What are some ways in which societal understandings about the aged affects aging?

4. Why might many younger workers resist efforts to raise the retirement age for the sake of strengthening the financial health of Social Security?

5. How did the 2003 Medicare reform legislation attempted to keep new expenditures to a minimum?

6. What is a health Savings Account? What are the pros and cons of health savings accounts? Why do they particularly appeal to conservatives?

7. The authors contrasts the ration between retirees and non-retirees (on the one hand) and the ratio between workers and non-workers on the other. What is the difference between the two ratios? Why is this important for the future of social security?

8. The authors point to a great philosophical (even a moral) difference between conservatives

and liberals in the field. On the hand, a belief in social solidarity. On the other, an emphasis on what George Bush has called an "opportunity society." Describe these differences between the two positions. Illustrate with examples taken from Medicare and social security.

9. Which of the underlying visions —social solidarity or individual opportunity— do you personally find more appealing? Which do you think should guide policy towards the aged?

NOTES

1. This chapter draws on a similar chapter by Dr. Brandon and Dr. Dana B. Bradley that was published in the third edition of *Health Politics and Policy* (1997). The authors of this chapter acknowledge that source and wish to express their appreciation to Dr. Bradley for her contribution to the 1997 publication.
2. Moody, 1986.
3. In 1910, only 49 private companies had pension plans; by 1925, the number had risen to 370. Military pensions, which only became common after the civil war, were awarded to alleviate particular hardship and were not intended to be a general entitlement. President Theodore Roosevelt promulgated an executive order that defined age as a disability in 1904, thereby automatically making 62-year-olds eligible for half disability; those 65, for two-thirds disability; and those 70, for full benefits. Haber, 1983, pp 108–15; Haber, 1983; Quadagno, 1988.
4. Deborah Stone, 2000, p 957.
5. Winch, 1958; Winch, 1970; Brandon, 1982.
6. Estes, 1983.
7. Quadagno, 1984.
8. Kreps, 1971; Quadagno, 1988.
9. US Bureau of the Census, 1942; US Bureau of the Census, 1986.
10. Alt, 1998; Manchester, 1997; US Congressional Budget Office, 2004b.
11. US Bureau of the Census, 2003; It should be noted that Social Security was changed in 2000 to permit older workers to collect Social Security pensions without paying a stiff financial penalty. Until this change in the law, Social Security was structured to encourage the elderly to cease more than minimal paid work upon reaching the age of eligibility.
12. Gomperts, 2005; Aaron and Schwartz, 2004.
13. Brasfield, 1987; Colleen Grogan, this volume.
14. Zappolo and Sundstrom, 1989; Johnson, 1989; Jazwiecki and Schwab, 1989.
15. Van Praag and Uitterhoeve, 1999.
16. Kane, 2004.
17. Putnam, 2004.
18. Marmor, 2000.
19. Alzheimer's Association, 2005.
20. Fries, 1980; Fries, 1983; Manton, 1982.
21. US Congressional Budget Office, 2004c.
22. Morone, 2000.
23. Pratt, 1976.
24. Samuelson, 1978a; Samuelson, 1978b; Ossofsky, 1978.
25. Brandon, 1991; Himmelfarb, 1995.
26. Third Millennium, 1993.
27. Estes, 1983.
28. Robyn Stone, 2004.
29. The Departments of Agriculture, Commerce, Labor and Veterans Affairs constitute exceptions to the generalization that federal programs are organized with reference to function rather than client group.
30. For details about Medicare and Medicaid, see Chapters 14 and 15 respectively.
31. Levit et al., 2004; Smith et al., 2005.
32. Bradley, 1994.
33. Morone, 2001.
34. Chemlimsky, 1991.
35. Lowi, 1969.
36. Kaiser Family Foundation, 2005b.
37. Salisbury, 1990.
38. Binstock, 2004.
39. Callahan, 2004.
40. Pratt, 1976.
41. Day, 1990.

42. AARP, 2005.
43. Binstock, 2004.
44. Ibid.
45. Ibid; Iglehart, 2004.
46. Barry, 2004; Goozner, 2005.
47. Justice, 2005.
48. Oberlander, 1995; Oberlander, 2003.
49. Day, 1995; Binstock, 2004.
50. National Committee to Preserve Social Security and Medicare, 2005.
51. Pratt, 1976.
52. Alliance for Retired Americans, 2005.
53. Hutcheson, 1995; Nielson, 1985.
54. USA/Next, 2005.
55. Andrews, 2004.
56. Justice, 2005.
57. American Public Health Association, 2005.
58. Ibid.
59. Heclo, 1978; McConnell, 2004.
60. Kaiser Family Foundation, 2005a.
61. Marmor, 2000.
62. Longman, 1987.
63. See also Feldstein, 1988 and Day, 1990;
64. Third Millennium, 1993.
65. Binstock, 1989.
66. Binstock, 2004.
67. Alwin, 1998; Williamson, 1998.
68. Love, 2004.
69. Robyn Stone, 2004.
70. Rosenbaum, 2005; Kessler, 2004.
71. Congressional Quarterly Almanac, 2004, 11–3; Oliver, Lee, and Lipton, 2004.
72. Before the Balanced Budget Act of 1997 the federal government had for years set premiums for health maintenance organizations at 90% of the average cost of fee-for-service Medicare patients in the same area, thereby claiming for the government some of the savings generated by managed care. If managed care plans were very profitable, earnings beyond a threshold had to be returned to enrollees in added benefits not provided by Medicare or to the government. Plans universally chose to avoid sharing excess income with the government.
73. Weissert and Weissert, 2002, pp 288–9; *Congressional Quarterly Almanac,* 1998.
74. Oberlander, 2003, pp 178–81.
75. Harris, 2004.
76. Oliver, Lee, and Lipton, 2004.
77. Harris, 2004.
78. *Congressional Quarterly Almanac,* 1998.
79. Rochefort, 2001; Declercq and Simmes, 1997; Weissert and Weissert, 2002, 305–6, 308.
80. Rice, 1997; Rice, 1998.
81. Donabedian, 1976, 31–2.
82. Romano and Benko, 2001.
83. *Congressional Quarterly Almanac,* 2004.
84. Oliver, Lee, and Lipton, 2004.
85. Income-tested differentials in both benefits and payment were considered as part of the Balanced Budget Act of 1997, but Democrats and liberal interest groups, especially AARP, succeeded in keeping them out of the final bill. Many conservative Republicans even felt that in 1997 it was premature to push for means-testing (Weissert and Weissert, 2002; *Congressional Quarterly Almanac,* 1998).
86. Medicare beneficiaries who also receive Medicaid are often referred to as "dual eligibles." A large proportion of them are chronically ill or disabled; many are in nursing homes. It is, therefore, a group that consumes large amounts of health care resources.
87. *Congressional Quarterly Almanac,* 2004.
88. Harris, 2004; Pear, 2004b.
89. *Congressional Quarterly Almanac,* 2004.
90. *Congressional Quarterly Almanac,* 1998; Oliver, Lee, and Lipton, 2004.
91. Oliver, Lee, and Lipton, 2004; Kesler, 2004.
92. Pear, 2005b.
93. Oliver, Lee, and Lipton, 2004.
94. Moynihan, 1988.
95. *Washington Post,* 2005.
96. Smitherman, 2005.
97. Ball and Bethell, 1989.
98. *Washington Post,* 2005.
99. Light, 1985.
100. Achenbaum, 1986; Moynihan, 1988.
101. Datallo, 1992.

102. Moynihan, 1990.
103. Aaron, 1997.
104. National Academy on Aging, 1995.
105. Federal Old Age and Survivor Insurance Trust Fund and Disability Insurance Trust Fund Board of Trustees, 1995.
106. National Committee to Preserve Social Security and Medicare, 2004.
107. Aaron, 2005.
108. Allen, 2005.
109. Rauch, 2005.
110. Will, 2005b.
111. US Congressional Budget Office, 2004a.
112. Bernstein, 1995; Third Millennium, 1993.
113. Aaron, 1997.
114. Ibid.
115. *Washington Post,* 2005.
116. Will, 2005a.
117. Brandon, 1991.
118. White, 2003; Oberlander, this volume.
119. Binstock, 1997.
120. Feder, 2004.

REFERENCES

Aaron, H.J. 1997. "Privatizing Social Security: a bad idea whose time will never come." *Brookings Review* 15 (3): 17–21.

—— 2005. *The big picture risks of privatization.* Talk at Conference on "Pitfalls of Privatization: Is it Worth the Risk?" National Commission to Preserve Social Security and Medicare, January 14.

Aaron, H.J., and W.B. Schwartz, eds. 2004. *Coping with Methuselah: The impact of molecular biology on medicine and society.* Washington DC: Brookings.

AARP. 2005. Website retrieved at http://www.aarp.org on January 10, 2005.

Achenbaum, W.A. 1986. *Social Security: Visions and revisions.* Cambridge: Cambridge University Press.

Allen, M. 2005. "War on words shapes debate." *Washington Post* January 23, p B03.

Allen, M., and J. Weisman. 2005. "New doubts on plan for Social Security." *Washington Post* January 19, p A01.

Alliance of Retired Americans. 2005. Website retrieved January 15, 2005 at http://www.retiredamericans.org.

Alt, P. 1998. "Future directions for public senior services: meeting diverging needs." *Generations* 22 (1): 29–33.

Alt, P., and A. Baker. 1987. *Aggressive use of medicaiding to increase federal funds.* Paper presented at the American Society for Public Administration annual meeting, April 1.

Alwin, D. 1998. "The political impact of the baby boom: are there persistent generational differences in political beliefs and behavior." *Generations* 22 (1): 46–54.

Alzheimer's Association. 2005. Website retrieved January 10, 2005 at http://www.alz.org.

American Association of Homes and Services for the Aging. 2005. Website retrieved January 17, 2005 at http://www.aahsa.org.

American Public Health Association. 2005. Website retrieved January 16, 2005 at http://www.apha.org.

American Society on Aging. 2005. Website retrieved January 16, 2005 at http://www.asaging.org.

Andrews, E.L. 2004. "Clamor grows in the privatization debate." *New York Times* December 17, p A26.

Apfel, K. 2005. *Is there a crisis?* Talk at Conference on "Pitfalls of Privatization: Is it Worth the Risk?" National Commission to Preserve Social Security and Medicare, January 14.

Ball, R., and T.N. Bethell. 1989. *Because we're all in this together.* Washington DC: Families USA Foundation.

Barry, P. 2004. The new law and you. *AARP Bulletin.* January, pp 16–18, 20.

Bernstein, R. 2005. *Price indexing.* Talk at Conference on Pitfalls of Privatization: Is it Worth the Risk? National Commission to Preserve Social Security and Medicare, January 14.

Binstock, R.H. 1989. "The phantom old age vote." *New York Times* (January 2), p 23.

—— 1997. The old-age lobby in a new political era. In R.B. Hudson, *The future of age-based public policy.* Baltimore, MD: Johns Hopkins University Press.

—— 2004. "Advocacy in an era of neoconservatism: responses of national aging organizations." *Generations* 28 (1): 49–54.

Blancato, R.B. 2004. *Aging in America: 1995 to today.* Center for American Progress: August 8. Retrieved January 17, 2005 from http://www.americanprogress.org.

Bloksberg, L.M. 1989. "Intergovernmental relations: Change and continuity." *Journal of Aging and Social Policy* 1 (3/4): 1–36.

Board of Trustees, Federal Old-Age and Survivors Insurance and Disability Insurance Trust Fund. 1995. *The 1995 annual report.* H.R. Doc 104–57. 104th. Congress 1st session. Washington DC: Government Printing Office.

Board of Trustees, Federal Old-Age and Survivors Insurance and Disability Insurance Trust Funds 2004. *2004 Annual report of the Federal Old-Age and Survivors Insurance and Disability Insurance Trust Funds.* Washington DC: US Government Printing Office.

Bradley, D.B. 1994. *Constructing state old-age policy: A Pennsylvania perspective.* Unpublished PhD dissertation, Carnegie-Mellon University, Pittsburgh, PA.

Brandon, W.P. 1982. "Fact" and "value" in the thought of Peter Winch: Linguistic analysis broaches metaphysical questions. *Political Theory* 10 (2): 215–44.

—— 1991. Politics, health and the elderly: Inventing the next century—the age of aging. In T.J. Litman and L.S. Robins, eds., *Health politics and policy* (2nd ed.): 335–55. Albany, NY: Delmar.

Brasfield, James M. 1987. *The management of invisible policies: Medicaid and long term care.* Paper presented at the meeting of the Southwestern Social Science Association. Dallas, TX: March 18–21.

Callahan, J.J. 2004. "The world of interest-group advocacy: an 'insider's' view." *Generations* 28 (1): 36–40.

Chelimsky, E. 1991. *The administration on aging: Harmonizing growing demands and shrinking resources* (GAO/T-PEM D-91–9). Washington DC: US General Accounting Office.

Congressional Quarterly Almanac. 1998. Big Medicare, Medicaid changes enacted in budget bills.

Congressional Quarterly Almanac. 1999. Vol. LIII: 6–3–6–12. Washington DC: Congressional Quarterly Inc.

Congressional Quarterly Almanac. 2004. Medicare Revamp Cuts It Close. 108th Congress, 1st Session.

Congressional Quarterly Almanac. 2003. Vol. LIX (pp 11–3–11–13). Washington DC: Congressional Quarterly Inc.

Dattalo, P. 1992. Social Security's surpluses. *Social Work* 37 (July): 377–9.

Day, C.L. 1990. *What older Americans think: Interest groups and aging policy.* Princeton, NJ: Princeton University Press.

Day, C.L. 1995. *Old-age interest groups in the 1990s: Coalition, competition, and strategy.* Paper presented at the annual meeting of the American Political Science Association, Chicago, IL: August 30–September 3.

Declercq, E., and D. Simmes. 1997. "The Politics of 'drive-through deliveries': putting early postpartum discharge on the legislative agenda." *Milbank Quarterly* 75 (2): 175–202.

Donabedian, A. 1976. *Benefits in medical care programs.* Cambridge, MA: Harvard University Press.

Estes, C.L. 1983. *The aging enterprise: A critical examination of social policies and services for the aged.* San Francisco: Jossey-Bass.

—— 2004. Social Security privatization and older women: a feminist political economy perspective. *Journal of Aging Studies* 18: 9–26.

Feder, J. 2004. Crowd *out* and the politics of health reform. *Journal of Law, Medicine and Ethics* 32 (3): 461–5.

Feldstein, P.J. 1988. *The politics of health legislation: An economic perspective.* Ann Arbor, MI: Health Administration Press.

Freudenheim, M. 2005. "Health savings accounts off to slow start." *New York Times* January 11, p C17.

Fries, J.F. 1980. Aging, natural death, and the compression of morbidity. *New England Journal of Medicine* 303: 130–5.

—— 1983. The compression of morbidity. *The Milbank Quarterly* 61 (Summer): 397–419.

Gerontological Society of America. 1987. *To meet the challenge of aging: Annual report 1987.* Washington DC: Gerontological Society of America.

Gerontological Society of America. 2005. Website retrieved on January 12 at http://www.geron.org.

Gomperts, J. 2005. "The age dividend." *Washington Post* January 23, p B3.

Goozner, M. 2005. Don't mess with success. *AARP Bulletin.* January: 12–15.

Haber, C. 1983. *Beyond sixty-five: The dilemma of old age in Americas past.* Cambridge: Cambridge University Press.

Harris, G. 2004. A record increase of 17 percent is set for premiums in Medicare. *New York Times* September 4, pp A1, A13.

Heclo, H. 1978. Issue networks and the executive establishment. In Anthony King (Ed.), *The new American political system* (1st ed.). Washington DC: American Enterprise Institute, pp 87–124.

Himmelfarb, R. 1995. *Catastrophic politics: The rise and fall of the Medicare catastrophic coverage act of 1988.* University Park, PA: Pennsylvania State University Press.

Hodge, P. 2005. *US: 2005 White House Conference on Aging.* January 4. Retrieved on January 17 from http://www.thematuremarket.com.

Hudson, R.B. 2004. Advocacy and policy success in aging. *Generations* 28 (1): 17–24.

Hutchinson, R. 1995. "There's a new kid on the senior's block (op-ed.)." *Charlotte Observer* March 1.

Iglehart, J.K. 2004. The new Medicare prescription-drug-benefit—a pure power play. *New England Journal of Medicine* 350 (8): 826–33.

Jazwiecki, T., and T. Schwab. 1989. Conclusion. In Teresa Schwab, ed., *Caring for an aging world: International models for long term care, financing, and delivery.* New York: McGraw-Hill, pp 366–76.

Johnson, M. 1989. Long-term care for the elderly in England. In Teresa Schwab, ed., *Caring for an aging world: International models for long term care, financing, and delivery.* New York: McGraw-Hill, pp 162–92

Justice, G. 2005. A New Target for Advisers to Swift Vets. *New York Times* (February 21). http://www.nytimes.com/2005/02/01/politics/21 social.html. Retrieved October 27, 2005.

Kaiser Family Foundation. 2005a. *Online health information poised to become important resource for seniors, but not there yet.* January 12. Retrieved on January 16 from http://www.kff.org.

Kaiser Family Foundation. 2005b. *Americans favor malpractice reform and drug importation, but rank them low on health priority list for the Congress and President*, January 11. Retrieved January 16 from www.kff.org.

Kane, R. 2004. "Coalitions between aging and disability interests: Potential effects on choice and Control for Older People." *Public Policy and Aging Report* 14 (4): 15–18.

Kesler, C.R. 2004. Four more years. *Imprimis: The national speech digest of Hillsdale College* 33 (12): 1–3, 6, 7.

Kingdon, J.W. 2003. *Agendas, alternatives and public policies* (2nd ed.). New York: Longman.

Kofman, M. 2004. "Health savings accounts: Issues and implementation decisions for states." *State Coverage Initiatives*, Issue Brief, 5 (No. 3, September). Washington DC: Academy Health.

Kranish, M. 2005. Bush argues his Social Security plan aids blacks. *Boston Globe* January 14. Retrieved from http://www.boston.com on January 30, 2005.

Kreps, J.M. 1971. *Lifetime allocation of work and income: Essays in the economics of aging.* Durham, NC: Duke University Press.

Lammers, W.W., and P.S. Liebig. 1990. State health policies, federalism and the elderly. *Publius* 20 (3): 1331–48.

Levit, K.R., et al. 1994. "National health expenditures, 1993." *Health Care Financing Review* 10 (Fall): 247–94.

Liebig, P.S. 1992. "Federalism and aging policy in the 1980s: Implications for changing interest group roles in the 1990s." *Journal of Aging & Social Policy* 4 (1/2): 17–33.

Light, P. 1985. *Artful work: The politics of Social Security reform.* New York: Random House.

Longman, P. 1987. *Born to pay: The new politics of aging in America.* Boston: Houghton Mifflin.

Love, J. 2004. Political behavior and values across the generations: A summary of selected findings. Washington DC: AARP.

Lowi, T.J. 1969. *The end of liberalism: Ideology, policy, and the crisis of public authority.* New York: W.W. Norton.

Lyman, R. 2005. Florida offers a bold new stroke to fight Medicaid cost. *New York Times* January 23. http://www.nytimes.com/2005/01/23/national/23 medicaid.html. Retrieved January 22, 2005.

Manchester, J. 1997. "Aging boomers & retirement: who is at risk?" *Generations* 21 (2): 19–22.

Manton, K.G. 1982. Changing concepts of morbidity and mortality in the elder population. *The Milbank Quarterly* 60 (2): 183–244.

Marmor, T.R. 2000. *Politics of Medicare* (2nd ed.). New York: Aldine de Gruyter.

McConnell, S. 2004. "Advocacy in organizations: the elements of success." *Generations* 28 (1): 25–30.

Moody, H.R. 1986. The meaning of life and the meaning of old age. In T.R. Cole and S.A. Gadow, eds., *What does it mean to grow old?: Reflections from the humanities.* Durham, NC: Duke University Press, pp 9–40.

Morone, J.A. 2000. "Citizens or shoppers? Solidarity under siege." *Journal of Health Politics, Policy and Law* 25 (5): 959–68.

Morone, J.A. 2001. Introduction. In R.B. Hackey and D.A. Rochefort, eds., *The new politics of state health policy*. Lawrence, KS: University Press of Kansas, pp 1–7.

Moynihan, D.P. 1988. "Conspirators, trillions, limos in the night." *New York Times* May 23, p A19.

Moynihan, D.P. 1990. "Surplus value." *The New Republic* 202 (June 4): 13–16.

Munnell, A. 2005. "Keep it simple." *Washington Post.* January 23: B03.

National Academy on Aging. 1995. Pacts on Social Security: The old age and survivor's trust fund.

National Alliance of Senior Citizens. 1994. *Annual report 1994.* Photocopy.

National Association for Home Care and Hospice. 2005. Website retrieved January 17 at http://www.nahc.org.

National Committee to Preserve Social Security and Medicare. *1994 annual report (1993–4).* Washington DC: National Committee to Preserve Social Security and Medicare.

National Committee to Preserve Social Security and Medicare. 2004. *Disability insurance and survivors' benefits.* Washington DC: October.

National Committee to Preserve Social Security and Medicare. 2005. Website retrieved at http://www.ncpssm.org on January 16, 2005.

National Council on Aging. 1994. *Annual report 1994.* Washington DC: National Council on Aging, Inc.

National Council on Aging. 2005. Website retrieved at http://www.ncoa.org on January 15, 2005.

Nielsen, W.A. 1985. *The golden donors.* New York: E. P. Dutton.

Oberlander, J. 1995. National Committee to Preserve Social Security and Medicare (NCPSSM). In Craig Ramsay, ed., *U.S. health policy groups: Institutional profiles.* Westport, CT: Greenwood Press.

Oberlander, J. 2003. *The political life of Medicare.* Chicago, IL: University of Chicago Press.

Oliver, T.R., P.R. Lee, and H.L. Lipton. 2004. A political history of Medicare and prescription drug coverage. *The Milbank Quarterly* 82 (2): 283–354.

Ossofsky, J. 1978. "Correspondence." *National Journal* 18 (March 1): 408–9.

Pear, R. 2004a. "AARP, eye on drug costs, urges change in new law." *New York Times* January 17, p A12.

Pear, R. 2004b. "Social Security payment will increase, as will Medicare bite." *New York Times* October 20, p A17.

—— 2005a. "Applying brakes to benefits gets wide GOP backing." *New York Times* January 9.

http://www.nytimes.com/2005/01/09/politics/09budget1.html. Accessed January 14, 2005.

—— 2005b. "Bush vows veto of any cutback in drug benefit: Stands by Medicare Law: Threat comes amid furor at Capital over rise in estimated costs." *New York Times* February 12, pp A1, A12.

—— 2005c. "Agency running Social Security to push change: Some workers object." *New York Times* January 16, pp A1, A21.

Pear, R., and R. Toner. 2004. "Partisan arguing and fine print seen as hindering Medicare law." *New York Times.* October 11, pp A1, A18.

Pratt, H.J. 1976. *The gray lobby.* Chicago: University of Chicago Press.

Putnam, M. 2004. "Issues in the further integration of aging and disability services." *Public Policy and Aging Report* 14 (4): 1, 19–23.

Quadagno, J. 1984. "From poor laws to pensions: The evolution of economic support for the aged in England and America." *The Milbank Quarterly* 62 (Summer): 417–46.

Quadagno, J.S. 1988. *The transformation of old age security; Class and politics in the American welfare state.* Chicago: University of Chicago Press.

Rauch, J. 2005. "The No. 1 moral issue is—abortion? No, Social Security." *National Journal* 37 (3): 92–3.

Rice, T. 1997. "Can markets give us the health system we want?" *Journal of Health Politics, Policy and Law* 22 (April): 383–426.

—— 1998. *The economics of health reconsidered.* Chicago, IL: Health Administration Press.

Riggs, J.A. 2004. "A family caregiver policy agenda for the twenty-first century." *Generations* 27 (4): 68–73.

Rochefort, D.A. 2001. The backlash against managed care. In R.B. Hackey and D.A. Rochefort, eds., *The new politics of state health policy.* Lawrence, KS: University Press of Kansas, pp 113–41

Romano, M., and L.B. Benko. 2001. "Members only." *Modern Healthcare* 22 (October): 38–44.

Rosenbaum, D.E. 2005. "Bush to return to 'ownership society' theme in push for Social Security changes." *New York Times* January 16, A17.

Salisbury, R.H. 1990. The paradox of interest groups: Washington—more groups, less clout. In Anthony King, ed. *The new American political system* (2nd ed.,). Washington DC: AEI Press, pp 203–29, 327–30.

Samuelson, R.J. 1978a. "Another look at those figures on the aged." *National Journal* 18 (March): 399.

Samuelson, R.J. 1978b. "Busting the U.S. budget—the costs of an aging America." *National Journal* 18 (February): 256–60.

Smith, C., C. Cowan, A. Sensening, A. Catlin, and the Health Accounts Team. 2005. "Health spending growth slows in 2003." *Health Affairs* 24 (1): 185–94.

Smitherman, L. 2005. "Social insecurity." *Baltimore Sun* January 23, C1–2.

Stone, D. 2000. United States. [In symposium "Reconsidering the Role of Competition in Health Care Markets"]. *Journal of Health Politics, Policy and Law* 25 (5): 953–8.

Stone, R. 2004. Where have all the advocates gone? *Generations* 28 (1): 59–64.

Third Millennium. 1993. *Third millennium declaration.* New York: Third Millennium.

USA/Next. 2005. Website retrieved at http://www.usanext.org on January 29, 2005.

US Bureau of the Census. 1942. *Statistical abstract of the United States 1941* (No. 63). Washington DC: US Government Printing Office.

US Bureau of the Census. 1986. *Economic characteristics of households in the United States: Fourth quarter 1984* (Current Population Reports, Series P 70, No. 6). Household Economic Studies. Washington DC: US Government Printing Office.

US Bureau of the Census. 2003. *The Older population in the United States: March 2002* (Current Populations Reports, Series P20–546). Washington DC: US Government Printing Office.

US Congressional Budget Office. 2004a. *The outlook for Social Security* (June).

US Congressional Budget Office. 2004b. *Retirement age and the need for saving* (May 12).

US Congressional Budget Office. 2004c. *The retirement prospects of the baby boomers* (March 18).

Van Praag, C., and W. Uitterhoeve. 1999. *25 Years of social change in the Netherlands: Key data from the Social & Cultural Report 1998.* Nijmegen, Netherlands: Uitgeverij SUN Publishers.

Washington Post. 2005. Social Security (Editorial), January 17, p A16.

Weissert, C.S. and W.G. Weissert. 2002. *Governing health: The politics of health policy* (2nd ed.). Baltimore: Johns Hopkins University Press.

White, J. 2003. "The Social Security and Medicare debate three years after the 2000 election." *Public Policy and Aging Report* 13 (4): 15–19.

White House Conference on Aging. 2005. Website retrieved on January 16 at http://www.whcoa.org.

Will, G.F. 2005a. "Acts of character building." *Washington Post* January 30, p B07.

—— 2005b. Social Security: Opportunity, not a crisis. *Washington Post* January 20, p A25.

Williamson, J.B. 1998. "Political activism and the aging of the baby boom." *Generations* 22 (1): 55–9.

Williamson, J.B. 2004. "What is the central goal for Social Security reform? Adding individual accounts or preserving the Social Security mission?" *Gerontologist* 44 (6): 851–5.

Winch, P. 1958. The idea of a social science and its relation to philosophy. London: Routledge & Kegan Paul.

Winch, P. 1970. Understanding a primitive society. In B.R. Wilson, ed., *Rationality.* New York: Harper & Row, pp 78–111.

Zappolo, A.A., & G. Sundstrom. 1989. Long-term care for the elderly in Sweden. In Teresa Schwab, ed., *Caring for an aging world: International models for long-term care, financing, and delivery.* New York: McGraw-Hill, pp 22–57

20 Classic Observations about Health Politics and Policy

Theodor J. Litman

It is always useful to try and summarize what we have learned from experience. Here is one editor's list of 20 classic conclusions from the health politics and policy literature. See if you can find each of these in other chapters.

1. Every nation's health care system is unique, based on its own social, political, cultural, and economic history.

2. There is no health care magic bullet, no single program or technique that will "solve" health care policy once and for all. All health systems require constant decisions— and wise policy makers.

3. A striking feature of the international experience is the association between universal coverage and lower costs.

4. All modern health care systems, built as they are around sophisticated medical technology, are inherently costly.

5. Regardless of spending levels, all governments (state, federal, international) feel that health care spending is crowding out other forms of spending.

6. Efforts to attain health care reform are more likely to succeed when couched in terms of cost containment, rather than improved access to health care.

7. Politics will always dominate policy analysis in the legislative process.

8. Health policy is dominated by the tyranny of the budget.

9. A system of competing health care payers leads to cost shifting, with each source of payment (public and private) seeking to protect itself at the expense of others by shifting costs to someone else.

10. A system of multiple competing payers can avoid cost shifting, gaps in coverage, and a high inflation rate only through a strong, central public authority which sets and maintains firm ground rules.

11. Any major domestic reform, especially one that imposes buyer costs, must enjoy a broad base of public support.

12. States vary in their fiscal ability and political willingness to underwrite care. Some of the most needy states are also the least able or willing.

13. Despite 25 years of trying, no state government has succeeded in assuring universal access to affordable health care for all its citizens.

14. Even very well designed programs must be effectively administered. All health programs must change with the times, with developments in the health care, and with the beneficiaries themselves.

15. Be wary of generalizing from successful local experiments. Promising ideas face all kinds of unexpected problems when policy makers try to implement them on a larger scale. Small pilot programs rarely look as good on the state level; state level experiments rarely look as good on a national scale.

16. Programs for poor people are usually poor programs.

17. Pinning one's hopes on an employment based health care system is increasingly risky in a dynamic, global economy.

18. Universal coverage alone will not alter the wide gaps in housing, living conditions, the morbidity rates, and the mortality rates between the poor and middle classes.

19. The demise of health and welfare systems has been greatly exaggerated. Even in an austere fiscal environment, health care programs are more likely to win expansions than to face elimination. This is because elected governments are eager to create and distribute benefits and reluctant to reduce or eliminate services to the middle class.

20. No nation has ever enacted a comprehensive health insurance program over the opposition of its medical profession without negotiating concessions and winning over some important health care factions.

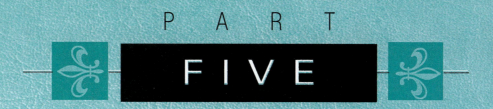

P A R T

FIVE

The United States in International Context

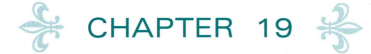

CHAPTER 19

American Health Care in International Perspective

Joe White °

This chapter places American health care politics and policy in an international perspective—highlighting how our own system is unusual. The article describes the "international standard" for organizing and financing care by showing what most other health systems have in common. The international perspective illuminates the underlying causes of our problems (like high costs); it highlights the kind of health policies that often succeed—and those that are more likely to fail.

Artists know that the appearance of a figure depends in part on the painting's background, or setting. Within this book's analysis of American health policies, the purpose of this chapter is to provide some background, or contrast, that can highlight important aspects of the subject.

The proper background for this picture consists of other "Rich Democracies:" countries that have large enough per capita incomes and responsive enough political arrangements so that underlying economics and sociology enable similar policies, if the political systems so choose.[1]

While I will fill in some details below, the basic outline of the international backdrop to American medical care is clear enough. Other countries have national health care or insurance systems that provide much more equitable access at lower cost than in the United States. Hence the international background highlights how differently the United States collects the money for health care (finance) and pays the providers of care (payment). To a lesser extent, the background may provide some contrasts to how Americans organize care (delivery) and to health system politics.

WHAT CAN WE LEARN FROM COMPARISON?

From a social scientific perspective, comparing countries is a way of increasing the number of cases for analysis. Just as we can learn more about

416

welfare-to-work policies by looking at actions and results in 50 states, we might learn about health policies by adding to American experience the experience of the 20 or so countries at comparable levels of development.[2] In making such comparisons we have to be careful because nations may vary from each other in ways that states do not. Yet that should not scare us away. After all, Texas is very different from Maine; indeed, Maine may be more similar to parts of Canada than to Texas.

International comparisons can provide three kinds of information: about possibilities, about cause-and-effect relationships, and about preferences.

Possibilities

The more cases we look at, the more phenomena we might see, so the more alternatives we might consider for changing our own system. For example, if Americans wanted to insure all citizens, would expanding Medicare to everyone be the obvious choice? Apparently not. Canada has something similar, but organized by the provinces instead of the national government. France has a dominant national insurer that covers most people but a series of smaller funds for particular populations. Japan has thousands of insurers, defined by employment and location. In those countries insurance is compulsory for all; in the Netherlands and Germany membership in the multiple "sickness funds" is compulsory for most citizens but optional for a minority (some of whom choose private insurance). In the United Kingdom, instead of having insurance, citizens are given the right to use a state bureaucracy, the National Health Service (though general practitioners (GPs) are not exactly employees of the organization). Sweden also provides health services, but at the county rather than the national level. Australia has a version of Medicare nationwide for ambulatory care, but hospital care is provided by state public hospitals. "National Health Insurance (NHI)" turns out to include a very wide range of possible arrangements.[3]

Looking abroad can expand our sense of possibilities in other policy areas as well. For example, in the United States care within hospitals is basically

supervised by admitting physicians, who have practices outside the hospital as well. The full-time hospital staff consists mostly of trainees, the interns and residents. In Germany, physicians with ambulatory care practices generally do not have hospital privileges; once a patient is admitted, their care is managed by full-time, fully trained, hospital doctors. Each system has its own advantages and disadvantages.[4]

By expanding our knowledge of possibilities, looking at other countries can increase the menu of possible "solutions" to policy problems. That does not mean approaches can be adopted exactly from other countries, but it does help with generating ideas for reforms in the United States.

Yet studying other countries can and should also have the opposite effect. If a supposed "problem" has not been significantly ameliorated (never mind solved) in any of 20 or more countries, maybe American failures are not due to American institutions. Maybe the problem is really, really hard. As my mentor, Aaron Wildavsky, commented to me, "even Stalin and Beria couldn't get doctors to move to the countryside." Thus we might gain more realism about what's possible, not just a wider range of options to consider.

Cause and Effect

Analysis of how systems work in other countries can also provide evidence about cause-and-effect relationships. For example, observation of the same relationship in multiple settings may make it more credible. American evidence suggests that an aging population per se is not nearly the most important cause of increases in health care costs. Since conventional wisdom often exaggerates the importance of aging, the fact that evidence from other countries supports exactly the same conclusion could make the finding more convincing.[5]

Yet it is more difficult to use comparison to analyze causation than to survey possibilities, for a series of reasons. It can be very hard to measure some effects in the first place. The controversies over assessment of any new technology or drug make that clear enough, as do the controversies over rating the performance of individual hospitals or health plans. This problem is particularly severe if the goal is to compare the quality of national health care systems.[6] Measurement of the dependent variable is less of a problem if the variable is health care costs or the extent of insurance coverage. There can be some disagreement about what costs count or what benefits matter, but there is very little doubt that costs are much higher, and insurance less extensive, in the United States than in all comparable countries.

Even when outputs can be measured, and causes identified, doubts can be raised about the implication of that finding for American policy choices, in three ways. Perhaps the association between seeming cause and effect in other countries is spurious because the better performance is due to some other, unmeasured cause. For instance, lower Canadian health care costs could be due not to superior cost control methods, but to Canadians being healthier because of lower levels of poverty, crime, and other problems. Perhaps changing the policy (cause) will have negative effects on some other valued output. Hence the policies that lower Canadian costs may be claimed to have unacceptable effects on quality. Perhaps also a policy would work differently in the United States than in other countries, due to a difference on some mediating variable. For example, maybe the kinds of payment restrictions that work in Canada won't work in the United States because Canadians are much more law abiding and we'll cheat more.[7] None of these objections are in fact compelling, but an analyst who argues that the United States would benefit from adopting Canadian-style insurance needs to be able to address them all.

Preferences

Each nation has not only health care policies but health care politics. Within that politics, groups define their interests and fight for them. Analysts also identify "problems." To most people, each of these processes may seem natural; but for political scientists, they all require explanation.

Why are some conditions put onto the political agenda as "problems" and others not?[8] For example,

how did "quality" become an issue in the United States in the late 1990s?[9]

Why do some groups take stands that would seem contrary to their economic interests? For example, why do American businesses that pay lots of money for health insurance not turn to the government, which seems to have more power to control costs, and ask it to take over?

Do we decide which problems are most pressing based on some objective measurement of their level? Or, do problems get prioritized based on the self-interested perspectives of groups that try to sell those definitions in order to win changes that serve their own purposes? Here an instance would be the frequent claim in the United States that there should be a greater emphasis on "primary care" and less on "specialty care."[10] Is this claim clearly justifiable from data? Or is it just the result of the social position of its advocates?

Comparison to other countries can help us answer such questions because we can see how similar groups take similar or different positions under similar or different circumstances.

In the rest of this chapter I will identify some conclusions about possibilities, cause and effect, and preferences that I have drawn from my comparative studies of health policy.

POSSIBILITIES

The most obvious possibility, as mentioned above, is to provide health insurance to all citizens. The fact that all other rich democracies do it strongly suggests it is possible!

The second and equally obvious background fact is that other countries spend much less money on health care than the United States does. Table 19-1 shows that in 2002, the United States paid 14.6% of GDP on health care. The second highest spender in these terms, Switzerland, spent 11.2%. Germany spent 10.9% and all other countries were under 10%.[11] The gap could only have widened afterwards, as US health spending reached 15.3% of GDP in 2003 and 16% by 2005.[12]

Table 19-1 Health Spending Per Capita and as Share of GDP, 2002

Country	Per Capita Spending ($PPP)	Percent of GDP	Change in % Share of GDP, 1992–2002
Australia	2,504	9.1	1.0
Austria	2,220	7.1	0.2
Belgium	2,515	9.1	1.1
Canada	2,931	9.6	−0.4
Denmark	2,583	8.8	0.3
Finland	1,943	7.3	−1.8
France	2,736	9.7	0.7
Germany	2,817	10.9	1.0
Iceland	2,807	9.9	1.6
Ireland	2,367	7.3	0.2
Italy	2,166	8.5	0.1
Japan[a]	2,077	7.8	1.6[b]
Luxembourg	3,065	6.2	0.0
Netherlands	2,643	9.1	0.7
New Zealand	1,857	8.5	1.0
Norway	3,083	9.6	1.4
Spain	1,646	7.6	0.4
Sweden	2,517	9.2	0.9
Switzerland	3,446	11.2	1.9
United Kingdom	2,160	7.7	0.8
United States	**5,267**	**14.6**	**1.6**

[a] 2001 data
[b] 1992–2001

SOURCE: Adapted from Anderson et al. 2005: 905; data available from OECD 2004. Data is limited to the countries with national per capita incomes over $20,000 per year.

NOTES: PPP is purchasing power parity, a metric that attempts to relate national currencies to convert other national currencies into dollars by comparing what the currencies can purchase at national price levels. It is an imprecise adjustment, but generally considered more appropriate (and stable) for this kind of analysis than translating other currencies into dollars using exchange rates. GDP is gross domestic product, a standard measure of the size of an economy. It is a better measure of the overall "burden" of health care costs.

Looking more closely at other rich democracies, we can see that there is both an *international standard* of financing and payment arrangement, and room for a lot of variation within that standard.

Outside of the United States, every advanced industrial country has some system that guarantees a decent standard of health care to virtually all citizens. But they DO NOT provide complete equity of access to health services; nor do they all cover the same set of services.

All provide virtually universal coverage—a minimum of 99% of the legal population. But, in order to do that, the power of government is used to force people—at least a majority of the nation—to contribute to earn membership in a system. Switzerland is a bit of an exception: a majority is not compelled.

But Switzerland has laws that give individuals strong financial incentives to voluntarily purchase insurance, in a context where few people are poor, and there are strong group pressures for conformity. So universal coverage is possible, but entirely voluntary universal insurance appears not to be.

Each country covers all "medically necessary" hospital and physician services and at a minimum provides pharmaceutical benefits for the poor and the elderly. In all cases the definition of "medically necessary" excludes extras such as cosmetic surgery and private rooms. Yet all systems have populations with somewhat worse and somewhat better access than the norm. The difference between the United States and other countries is not the existence of inequality per se. The difference is, in other countries everyone is guaranteed decent standard coverage, and a few have more. In the United States hardly anyone is guaranteed anything; most people have decent coverage but a large segment has much less. In other countries there is an "escape valve" for the well-to-do. In the United States there is a ragged "safety net" for the poor.

There are inequalities in other systems in part due to factors such as geography and patients' knowledge. Rural areas can never have the same access to services as urban areas, and immigrants who don't speak the national language will always be at some disadvantage. And, in all systems, some portion of more privileged people can buy extra services or better access or amenities. Hence universal insurance of a decent standard appears to be possible; equal access does not.

In other countries, most people do not "buy" insurance on a market. Instead, people contribute to a system. Whether people pay a payroll contribution (so a proportion of wages, like with Social Security), or spending is financed from government revenues, payments are in rough proportion to ability to pay. They are not related to need for care. Thus larger families don't pay more than smaller families or single people—same income, same payment. Sicker people don't pay more than healthy people. The basic principle, then, is that contributions should be a fairly steady share of income through your life, regardless of how much health care you or those on whose behalf you contribute actually need.

As mentioned above, there are many ways to organize the compulsory insurance. This means, for example, that believers in a "single payer" system for the United States should realize that other systems can work pretty well. For example, in Germany and the Netherlands, only people with incomes below a certain level are compelled to join particular "sickness funds," the term for public law insurers. Others can purchase private insurance. In Germany about 10% of the population is privately insured; in the Netherlands it is more like a third. While perceived inequities can be controversial in those systems, the basic guarantee remains solid. There are lots of ways to set up safety valves. The Japanese system is a total hodgepodge, with varied flows of funds from individuals, employers, general taxation, and local taxation. It somewhat resembles what would happen if the United States expanded the parts of its hodgepodge (employer-based insurance, Medicare, Medicaid) to cover its citizens in a messy but universal manner.

Yet all other rich democracies have arrangements that differ greatly from those in the United States, where private insurers charge according to the perceived risks of individuals or groups, so charge more to those who need more, regardless of their income. In principle also, in the United States, sellers and buyers of insurance can choose each other in market transactions. In contrast, most people in most systems have very little choice about which insurance funds they can be in. This means there is a lot less entrepreneurship (for better or worse) about insurance per se. Insurers in other countries are much more like old-fashioned non-competitive public utilities in the United States than like American health insurers. Other countries' experiences show that universal insurance can include private, for-profit or private, non-profit insurers. What isn't possible, if you want to cover everybody, is insurers who can pursue profit without being very heavily regulated as to their rates and marketing practices.

Cost control also is different in other countries. While most hospitals and physicians in the United States collect revenues from many payers on many different terms, in all other countries the terms and sources of income are more limited. Most have some degree of budgeting for individual hospitals, rather than paying hospitals fees for whatever services they provide. There is something resembling a standard fee schedule for physicians, unless they are paid a form of capitation in the case of GPs. There are some limits on capital investment, so providers of care cannot just go out and buy new equipment or expand their facilities in ways that increase costs. For example access to capital is restricted so hospitals or doctors can't get the money to build unapproved facilities. Conversely, cost control in other countries generally does not rely on each payer trying to negotiate better prices by threatening to take its business to other caregivers. In short, they rely much more on *coordinated payment*, and much less on *selective contracting*.[13] Hence they illustrate a very different approach from the cost control methods of the American private market.

American advocates may argue that some benefit or other is absolutely crucial to the decency of any universal system. This is, ultimately, a personal choice. But by looking at other countries one can see that there are many possible benefit structures. Canada's version of "Medicare" is much like ours in terms of the covered services. Germany and Japan, in contrast, have substantial drug benefits for all. Some countries cover abortion, some don't. In Japan, normal pregnancy is not covered by sickness insurance, because it is not considered an illness. (It is financed by other arrangements.)

In short, there are many possible variations in the structure of a national health care guarantee, the benefits it covers, and the details of its cost controls. Yet, outside the United States, all share limitations on choice by both insurers and beneficiaries, compulsory contributions related much more to income than to projected expenses, coverage of medically necessary physician and hospital services, and cost controls based on some coordination of payers to maximize their power vis-à-vis providers.

Experience in other countries is less useful for discovering new possibilities in the organization of health care delivery, because the United States has such a wide range of systems internally. The role of GPs as gatekeepers in the British NHS or in the Netherlands is mirrored in some American HMOs. Yet I have mentioned the use of "hospitalists" in many countries, and one can also see extensive roles for midwives in some (Netherlands, New Zealand). There are also wide ranges in both the proportions of various specialties within the physician population, and to some extent how specialties are defined.

These and other examples of health policies in other countries can provide ideas for readers about what goals are reasonable (insuring virtually everybody is; total equality is not) and the range of "solutions" to problems. In judging possibilities, however, people are likely to look for evidence of causes and effects. That will always be more controversial.

CAUSES AND EFFECTS

Assessments of cause and effect are difficult for all the reasons stated earlier. Yet I have already slipped in some judgments as statements about what seems not to be possible. For example, the fact that no system has ever achieved universal coverage without compulsion suggests that compulsion is a necessary cause for universal coverage.

For an analyst, some of the most interesting evidence from a country other than one's own may involve unusual policies. Such extreme cases may raise doubts about simplistic theories of cause and effect. For example, Japanese experience shows that regulation of fees can be used to manage medical care systems quite thoroughly. Campbell and Ikegami recount how high fees were used to encourage adoption of imaging technology and then, when the Japanese imaging industry had been encouraged and costs for the health care system seemed too high, low fees were used to discourage adoption.[14] This Japanese policy flexibility happened to depend on some unique political conditions, but it still should give pause to economists and health services researchers who believe price regulation is an entirely blunt instrument. Analysts in other countries could also learn a great deal from looking at American experience, which provides unmatched evidence of how market forces, allowed pretty free rein, work in health care.[15]

As background for understanding American health policy conundrums, the following statements of cause and effect seem particularly relevant. I will put them in order from what I think should be least controversial to most—though all are, I think, reasonable conclusions.

First, it does not appear possible to have universal health insurance without both making insurance compulsory for the lower income two-thirds or more of the population, and making payments proportional to income.

Second, aging per se does not appear to be nearly as important a cause of increased health care costs as are policies about payment for care. Within payment I'm including both what is paid for and how payment is made.[16] Cross-national evidence helps to make this clear, first, because there is hardly any correlation between the age distribution in countries and their levels of health care costs. But a wide range of evidence also shows that aging per se is not a key driver much of anywhere.[17]

Third, the major explanation of America's high costs is the prices we pay for services. That, of course, does not tell anyone WHY Americans pay so much per service. But comparisons to other countries show that most of the cost difference cannot be explained by the volume of services.[18] Nor are high American costs explained by the availability of high technology. When regression lines are calculated to relate availability of cardiac care facilities, cardiac catheterization labs, radiotherapy machines and other equipment to per capita health care costs, the United States is a consistent outlier, with far higher costs than the supply of facilities would project.[19] This is an especially important finding because so much of American policy debate seems to presume that cost control requires management of utilization, or even

tough ethical decisions about who should and should not get care.[20] In contrast, from an international perspective the key question is why American prices are so high and how to get them down. That directs attention to factors such as staffing in health care institutions (which in turn is highly related to administrative overhead caused by the insurance system) and pay levels for caregivers and various hangers-on (the whole business side of the health care enterprise).

Fourth, the degree of inequality created by cost-sharing depends on the price of care. Many analysts believe that cost-sharing can create an unacceptably two-tiered system, in which richer people go to the "better" doctors who can charge extra for their services, while poorer are stuck with the lower-quality providers. In the extreme case, sick people may go without care because, even though they have insurance, they can't pay the copayment or coinsurance required to pass through the gate at the doctor's office or hospital. This is a serious concern, but needs to be modified. It seems an obvious point, but whether 10% or 20% cost-sharing is a major barrier depends on what it is 10% or 20% of. Since prices are so much lower in Australia or France or Japan than they are in the United States, the same percentage might reduce equity much less in those countries than here.

Fifth, it appears that coordinated payment (fees set by government or a cartel of payers negotiating with all providers) normally works better for cost control than does selective contracting (letting many different payers negotiate with different groups of providers). This is harder to judge, because other countries use selective contracting so sparingly. Moreover, there can be times—the mid-1990s in the United States are the example—where selective contracting controls prices as well as most coordinated payment systems. Nevertheless, American costs are higher than those in other countries by a nearly ridiculous margin, and that contrast, plus the logical argument that coordination of any sort concentrates payer power in a way that gives payers the advantage, suggest strongly that coordinated payment, if seriously pursued, is a more reliable cost control method.

The conclusions here reflect my basic earlier point that it is easier to judge cause and effect when the effect—in these cases level of insurance or costs—is easier to measure. Nevertheless, it seems fair to make one last background judgment: the much higher costs in the United States do not appear to be justified by higher quality of care.

The United States likely buys some extra amenities for its patients, such as more privacy in hospital rooms and fancier hospital lobbies. It clearly does not buy better overall health results. Among the 21 higher-income countries within the OECD database, the United States has the highest level of potential life-years lost to health problems for individuals under age 70. This figure partially reflects the high infant mortality levels in the United States, which are more closely related to social ills than to quality of medical care (save for the uninsured!). We can control for infant mortality and some other social ills (such as homicide against black males) by looking at life expectancy at age 40. Even at age 40, however, the data in Table 19-2 shows that United States was tied for 16th in life expectancy for both males and females in 2000.[21]

A few studies have looked at performance in treating specific diseases. One compared US performance on twenty-one quality indicators to the performance of the Australian, Canadian, United Kingdom, and New Zealand health systems. Eighteen of these indicators were clearly related to medical treatment.

Table 19-2 Life Expectancies at Birth and at Age 40, 2000

Country	At Birth, Total Population	At Age 40, Males	At Age 40, Females
Australia	79.0	38.4	43.0
Austria	78.1	37.0	42.1
Belgium	77.7	36.6	42.0
Canada	79.4	38.8	43.1
Denmark	76.9	36.2	40.3
Finland	77.6	36.1	42.0
France	79.0	37.3	43.9
Germany	78.0	36.7	42.0
Iceland	79.7	40.0	42.1
Ireland	76.5	36.0	40.3
Italy	79.6	38.2	43.4
Japan	81.2	39.1	45.5
Luxembourg	77.9	36.6	42.1
Netherlands	77.9	36.8	41.6
New Zealand	78.5	38.2	42.2
Norway	78.7	37.8	42.4
Spain	79.1	37.6	43.6
Sweden	79.7	38.7	42.8
Switzerland	79.7	38.6	43.6
United Kingdom	77.4	36.7	40.9
United States	**76.7**	**36.5**	**41.0**

SOURCE: OECD 2004. Data is limited to the countries with national per capita incomes over $20,000 per year.

US performance was somewhat better than average, but clearly not the best by this measure among these countries.[22] We can try to isolate the quality of medical care per se by looking at outcomes for particular medical events, such as heart attacks, strokes, and breast cancer. Another study made such comparisons, but although the United States did better than average, it did not have the best results.[23]

There is some reason to believe the extra United States spending provides some higher quality of life. Americans are getting something for their money in cases where patients would wait longer for elective surgery in some other countries (e.g., for hip replacements), or where less surgery is done and the lower level may result in greater discomfort (e.g., lower levels of cardiac surgery so somewhat higher levels of uncomfortable angina in Canada than the United States). Yet many countries do not have significant waiting list problems. Moreover, "the amount of U.S. health spending accounted for by the fifteen procedures that account for most of the waiting lists in Australia, Canada, and the United Kingdom," would be only 3% of total US health care costs.[24] Hence it is highly unlikely that the much higher American spending is justified by convenience of access to surgery.

Hence the best one can say for the US health care system, in terms of value, is that we might buy a small amount of extra value for a portion of our population for a huge amount of extra money—meanwhile providing worse value to our uninsured. Anyone who says the United States has the "best healthcare system in the world" has not looked at the rest of the world.

PREFERENCES, OR THE PECULIAR POLITICS OF HEALTH CARE

Health care is a world unto itself. It shares with some policies, such as pensions, controversies such as who will pay for whom. It shares with other policies, such as administration of the law and efforts to ensure that good information is available in markets, the need to rely on professionals (attorneys, accountants, physicians) to implement policies. It is nearly unique in the range of professions and perspectives it involves (not just physicians but many other caregivers, plus the managers of a wide range of institutions, plus the public health side of health policy, plus all the institutional commentators such as economists and health service researchers). The combination of redistribution, professionals, and overall complexity makes health care a peculiar subsystem in any country's politics and sociology.

Within any country, one might be tempted to conclude that where people stand depends on where they sit, in two senses. First, people in different positions may have different material interests. Second, their jobs involve processes of socialization—both in formal training and through their work—which shape their ideals about policy. A comparative perspective makes this conclusion seem particularly obvious.

This is the hardest subject on which to meet social scientific standards. So I will speak mainly from anecdotal observation, and we can begin with a simple example. In a number of different countries, I have heard orthopedic surgeons described as very different from pediatricians. The former are described as jocks, super-confident, super aggressive, not very cooperative (to put it lightly). The latter are supposedly much more cooperative, communicative, gentle, touchy-feely. These are stereotypes and do not predict any individual's behavior. Yet they are common enough that one cannot help figuring that some self-selection and some of the basic nature of the work shape the personalities involved.[25] The nature of the work is common across countries, so the behaviors also tend to be similar across countries.

The medical world has villages and tribes and maybe rival nations. Physicians are divided into the many specialties and the broad division between generalists and specialists. Nurses and physicians have versions of the same conflicts and issues—status, control of the hospital, pay, etc—virtually everywhere. The public health profession virtually always feels that it does not get enough credit (or pay) for improving peoples' health, compared to the medical profession.

Consider cost control politics and policy. Any system has cost controllers. To the Treasury, or the corporate VP for human resources, spending on health care is not, per se, a good thing. It is a cost to be limited. Even if costs are not growing quickly, it will be a large cost, and money could be used for other purposes (other spending, tax cuts, dividends, buying a competitor). So, except in the very rare conditions where earnings are booming and costs are stagnant, there will always be pressures to control costs, coming from organizational actors who will only care about the consequences if they are forced to care about them (e.g., cutting costs may threaten the government's popularity, or provoke a strike). This is one reason why cost control is a big issue regardless of nations' relative success at the task.

When they search for policy options, cost controllers tend to think in similar ways, and so they tend to come up with similar ideas. In virtually all countries, budgeters think something like, "we have to control costs; so we should focus on where the biggest costs are; the biggest costs are in hospitals; so we should try to get people out of hospitals, which are expensive places." In addition, new technology (particularly forms of anesthesia) make it easier to do procedures outside of the hospital. For both these reasons—what's possible and what's believed—levels of hospitalization and length of stay have declined virtually everywhere. Unfortunately, as Uwe Reinhardt has shown, that policy may not actually reduce costs.[26] Yet it is so entrenched in both the core perspectives of payers, and the interests of those physicians who can make more money outside of the hospital than in it, that we can expect getting people out of the hospital to remain a common policy virtually everywhere, regardless of the merits.

Physicians are another example of fairly predictable preferences based on training and role. Physicians' attitudes about practice can be shaped by the conditions of practice and general attributes of national culture. In Great Britain the constraints on supply may have been so severe for so long, and the

national emphasis on keeping a stiff upper lip provide a convenient enough justification, that British physicians could rationalize a less aggressive practice style more easily than in the United States, with its very different culture and supply conditions.[27] Nevertheless, the profession as a whole tends to share a set of values across countries. Giorgio Freddi gives a nice summary:

1. The remuneration of physicians according to the fee-for-service formula, whereby fees are paid directly by patients to doctors and are freely determined by the latter.

2. The right to independent practice, that is clinical autonomy, connoted by the sanctity of a highly individualized doctor-patient relationship, which ensures that diagnostic and therapeutic decisions are subject to no external control.

3. The responsibility to lead and coordinate other health professionals.

4. The processing of professional issues according to a social consensus model of behavior which excludes the conflict-based processes inherent in unionization.[28]

These attitudes appear to have led to, for example, resistance against being pushed to practice in clinics in any country in which physicians had any choice in the matter.[29] Inasmuch as these values derive from the fundamental training and work orientation of physicians, we should expect doctors to be at best skeptical about all policies that try to force them to work in teams controlled by anyone else, or to "integrate" care at the expense of personal discretion, or to favor "health promotion" over the "medical model." If behavioral change is desired, policies should recognize the underlying attitude of physicians and adapt accordingly. For example, paying physicians extra money as fees for service may indeed get them to do more screening tests. Conversely, it would be a shock if physicians anywhere, not just in the United States, endorsed health care reforms that called for them to move into large, "integrated" group practices.[30]

More generally, citizens and policy makers should expect to see continual claims that primary care is undervalued relative to specialty care, simply because there is a primary care community to make those claims. They should expect to see advocacy for health promotion, accompanied by arguments that spending more on health promotion and prevention would reduce spending on hospitals, because people trained in public health believe that. In a more recent development, the rise of a health services research profession naturally leads to claims that it is not getting enough money.[31] This call for more spending on data and research is hardly limited to the United States.[32] Similarly, believers in research and information technology professionals can be expected to promote the idea that better information systems (integrated medical records, etc.) would save lots of money and improve quality.

None of this makes all countries' health politics the same. Far from it. Attitudes depend in part on what people think they can get: British physicians might want the high incomes available from American fee-for-service practice, but that would be so politically implausible that they do not appear to lust for those incomes very passionately. Participants in systems become accustomed to how they are organized. Politics is path dependent—past decisions profoundly shape future possibilities.

Because private health insurance is a larger part of American health care, private health insurers are more politically important: they have more political resources and more to lose. Hence the similarities of medical sociology are not a strong predictor of the prospects for NHI in the United States. Instead, the comparative background highlights differences in partisan values (e.g., the conservative party in the United States is much more opposed to measures like NHI than the conservative parties in much of Europe have been),[33] mobilization of interest groups to oppose redistribution (e.g., the small business lobbies and insurers in the United States), and the fact that our costs have become so high that the redistribution to cover our uninsured (and maintain coverage for much of the currently insured population) must be much larger than the redistribution in

countries where income is more equal and health care costs a lot less.

Similarities in the sociology of the health care arena are better predictors of the politics of non-insurance issues. Controversies over how to improve quality, or the balance of medical professions, or methods of cost control, or relative emphasis on prevention and cure, will create cleavages on predictable lines. Supposedly neutral experts, such as economists and health services researchers, have predictable interests and biases.

CONCLUSION

This chapter provides an introduction to the perspectives on American health policy that can be gained by looking at policies in other countries.

As with any social science research, it is difficult to totally prove any hypothesis. Arguments about possibilities are easier to demonstrate than claims about cause and effect, because all one has to do is show an example of the first. Some comparisons are simply very clear from the data: the United States has much less extensive health insurance and far higher costs. Others are much more obscure, such as any differences in quality of care. Nevertheless, the arguments about cause and effect presented here are, I believe, on very firm ground.

It is important for citizens and policy makers to know that the United States could do a much better job of controlling costs, with universal insurance coverage, and little if any decline in quality. That evidence does not predict that change could be easy or its benefits automatic. The measures that control costs might best be imposed over long periods of time, as restraint on cost growth rather than quick rollback of expenses. Cost control that eliminates functions (such as most of what insurers in the United States do, or the extra jobs involved in billing all those insurers by all their different rules), would be economically wrenching for those whose jobs are eliminated. Other countries give little evidence of how to manage such a transition, because no country has had to transform such a large, ragged, and entrepreneurial system of health care finance.[34]

My arguments about how health care policy perspectives tend to be driven by an underlying sociology based on training, social roles, and material interests suggest fewer specific policy options. Yet they do suggest that the kinds of reforms that are particularly popular among health policy elites now, such as efforts to improve quality by reorganizing medical practice, or to somehow integrate public health and population health policies, must be more difficult than their seeming popularity in elite conversation suggests.[35] The obstacles appear to be extremely common properties of the practice of medicine.

There is less evidence that other countries improve on American health care quality than that they provide better access to care at lower costs. Hence the comparative backdrop highlights most clearly what is most unacceptable and inexcusable in our health care system. It costs too much and insures too few.

STUDY QUESTIONS

1. What is the "international standard" in health care finance and management? Describe some of the variations within the general standard.
2. Name the five "causes and effects" that can be discerned through comparative analysis of national health care systems.
3. In what way is the American health care system really a "hodgepodge"?
4. What indicators show that the American health care system is not, in fact, the "best in the world"?
5. What might some of the political obstacles be to instituting some version of national health insurance (NHI) in the United States?
6. How/why do the medical profession and public health officials often clash? What are the implications of such friction?

NOTES

1. For explanation of why similar levels of economic development tend to be accompanied by some convergence in sociology and politics, see Wilensky, 2002, which is also the source of the term "rich democracies."
2. The basic set of countries for reference would be the members of the OECD, which constitutes kind of a developed nations "club." Of the 30 OECD member nations, 21 had per capita GDP in 2001 of $20,000 or above, with national currency translated into US dollars according to purchasing power parity. These countries were Australia, Austria, Belgium, Canada, Denmark, Finland, France, Germany, Iceland, Ireland, Italy, Japan, Luxembourg, the Netherlands, New Zealand, Norway, Spain, Sweden, Switzerland, the United Kingdom, and the United States. Some other countries approach that level and have versions of NHI that actually seem to work somewhat; they include Korea, Portugal, and Taiwan (which does not get to be an OECD member). My own research has focused on Australia, Canada, France, Germany, Japan, the Netherlands, and the United Kingdom.
3. White, 2001.
4. The United States' difficulty is coordination of care within the hospital, given that the physician supposedly in charge of the patient is rarely there. The German difficulty is coordination between sectors; for instance, the hospital may run tests that the ambulatory care physician already ran, and once the patient is released, her outside physician may not be so well informed about the course of care inside the hospital.
5. White, 2004; Gray, 2005. Of course, having better evidence does not in fact mean people will recognize it, and in this case the conventional wisdom is so conventional, though wrong, that I do not expect the average American policymaker or editorial writer to notice the error.
6. A state of the art example is OECD, 2003; for a good example of the measurement difficulties see chapter 3, on Stroke Treatment and Care.

7. The third objection comes not from the usual right-wingers, but from my friend David Rose. I have argued at length that none of these objections are true (White, 1995), but they all are raised.

8. The classic analysis of this question is Kingdon, 2003.

9. For a discussion see Leape, 2005.

10. Stevens, 2005.

11. Both Switzerland and Germany may be so high because of unusual reasons. In the case of Switzerland, it, next to the United States, is the country in which private insurance plays the biggest role. In the case of Germany, after unification the Germans chose to provide a West-Germany level of health spending to East Germany, which unfortunately did not and does not have a comparable economy. So that significantly increased spending as a share of the overall German economy.

12. Heffler et al., 2005. See, also, the Introduction in this volume.

13. White, 1999.

14. Campbell and Ikegami, 1998.

15. Light, 1998; Robinson, 2005.

16. I am aware that most economists and health services researchers believe "technology" is the major cause of increasing costs. Yet this seems unrealistic in two ways. First, technology does not have a natural cost; the cost depends on policies about how much will be paid for any new procedures or equipment. Second, whether a technology is even implemented depends on whether payment policies make it profitable for either the sellers or the buyers (who have to in turn sell the services that they would use the technology to provide). Hence the effect of "technology" is subsumed by payment policies.

17. White, 2004; Gray, 2005; OECD, 2003.

18. Anderson et al., 2003.

19. OECD, 2003, 201–4.

20. For a typical example see Daniels, 2005.

21. The data in the OECD database is only complete for all 19 countries through 2000. Where later data is available, it does not change the pattern.

22. Hussey et al., 2004. The items that I have excluded as non-medical were three indicators of suicide rates. Four indicators involved screening and vaccination rates; nine were survival rates from acute diseases; the others were rates of smoking, pertussis, measles and hepatitis B, and asthma mortality for ages 5–39. The United States had the best rating on three items and tied for first on another. It had four seconds, three thirds, three fourths, and a fifth. Australia had the best overall performance in this set of measures.

23. For example, in 1996 the US had the third lowest one-year case fatality rate for men and fourth-lowest for women ages 40–64, among seven countries (OECD, 2003, p 37). One-year case fatality rates for ischemic stroke victims age 65 and over were higher in the United States than in Denmark or the Canadian provinces of Alberta and Ontario; similar to the rates in Sweden; and lower than in the United Kingdom (OECD, 2003, p 63). The United States' five-year breast cancer survival rate was second best out of eight countries (OECD, 2003, p 85), though that result might be due to earlier diagnosis in the United States rather than better treatment.

24. Anderson et al., 2005, p 908.

25. Orthopedic surgeons may have gotten interested in the work from experience with sports injuries. It at least used to help if one was large and strong to manipulate bodies and bones. They hope not to have long-term relationships with patients. When bones are already broken, there's a limit on the opportunities to be gentle. Pediatricians are dealing with frightened children, usually in the presence of a parent, expect long-term relationships, and so on. It would be interesting to see if this informal sociology holds true as a larger and larger part of orthopedic surgeons' practice consists of frail elderly people getting hips and knees replaced.

26. Reinhardt, 1996.

27. Payer, 1996.

28. Freddi, 1989, p 5.

29. Glaser, 1994.

30. Individual economic incentives matter a lot. So more and more American physicians can be expected to participate in group practices, simply because that may allow them to work saner hours (because their colleagues rotate taking call) and share huge capital investment costs. Those incentives, however, are more likely to cause physicians to join single-specialty than multi-specialty groups.
31. Readers can consult any issue of the Academy Health newsletter to confirm this observation.
32. See OECD, 2003 for an example.
33. This is a major theme in the comparative public policy literature, though framed differently by different analysts; see e.g., Wilensky, 2001.
34. The closest example would be Australia in 1984, where adoption of Medicare involved extending insurance to about the same proportion of the population as would be involved in creating universal coverage in the United States. But Australia already had systems of public hospital care for citizens of all states, and its overall health care costs were much lower than in the current United States.
35. For a particularly trendy example, from those who pay to create trends, see Mechanic, 2005.

REFERENCES

Anderson, G.F., P.S. Hussey, B.K. Frogner, and H.R. Waters. 2005. "Health Spending in the United States and the Rest of the Industrialized World." *Health Affairs* 22 (4): 903–14.

Anderson, G.F., U.E. Reinhardt, P.S. Hussey, and V. Petrosyan. 2003. "It's the Prices, Stupid: Why the United States Is So Different From Other Countries." *Health Affairs* 22 (3): 89–105.

Campbell, J.C. and N. Ikegami. 1998. The Art of Balance in Health Policy: Maintaining Japan's Low-Cost, Egalitarian System. Cambridge: Cambridge University Press.

Daniels, N. 2005. Accountability for Reasonable Limits to Care: Can We Meet the Challenges? In D. Mechanic, L.B. Rogut and D.C. Colby, eds., *Policy Challenges in Modern Health Care*. New Brunswick: Rutgers University Press, pp 238–48.

Freddi, G. 1989. Problems of Organizational Rationality in Health Systems: Political Controls and Policy Options. In G. Freddi and J.W. Bjorkman, eds., *Controlling Medical Professionals: The Comparative Politics of Health Governance*. London: Sage Publications, pp 3–27.

Glaser, W.A. 1994. "Doctors and Public Authorities: The Trend Toward Collaboration." *Journal of Health Politics, Policy and Law* 19 (4): 705–727.

Gray, A. 2005. "Population Ageing and Health Care Expenditure." *Ageing Horizons* 2: 15–20.

Heffler, S., S. Smith, S. Keehan, C. Borger, M.K. Clemens, and C. Truffer. 2005. "U.S. Health Spending Projections for 2004-2014." *Health Affairs* Web Supplement (23 February) W5-74–W5-85.

Hussey, P.S., G.F. Anderson, R. Osborn, C. Feek, V. McLaughlin, J. Millar, and A. Epstein. 2004. "How Does the Quality of Care Compare in Five Countries?" *Health Affairs* 23 (3): 89–99.

Kingdon, J. 2003. *Agendas, Alternatives, and Public Policies*, 2nd ed. New York: Longman.

Leape, L. 2005. Preventing Medical Errors. In D. Mechanic, L.B. Rogut and D.C. Colby, eds., *Policy Challenges in Modern Health Care*. New Brunswick: Rutgers University Press, pp 162–76.

Light, D. 1998. *Effective Commissioning*. London: Office of Health Economics.

Mechanic, D., L.B. Rogut, and D.C. Colby, eds. 2005. *Policy Challenges in Modern Health Care*. New Brunswick: Rutgers University Press.

Organisation for Economic Co-Operation and Development. 2003. A Disease-Based Comparison of Health Systems: What is Best and at What Cost? Paris: OECD.

—— 2004. Health Data/Eco-Sante (database).

Payer, L. 1996. Medicine & Culture: Varieties of Treatments in the United States, England, West Germany, and France. New York: Henry Holt and Company.

Reinhardt, U. 1996. "Perspective: Our Obsessive Quest to Gut the Hospital." *Health Affairs* 15 (2): 145–54.

Robinson, J.C. 2005. Entrepreneurial Challenges to Integrated Care. In D. Mechanic, L.B. Rogut, and D.C. Colby, eds., *Policy Challenges in Modern Health Care*. New Brunswick: Rutgers University Press, pp 53–68.

Stevens, R. 2005. Specialization, Specialty Organizations, and the Quality of Health Care. In D. Mechanic, L.B. Rogut, and D.C. Colby, eds.,

Policy Challenges in Modern Health Care. New Brunswick: Rutgers University Press, pp 206–20.

White, J. 1995. Competing Solutions: American Health Care Proposals and International Experience. Washington DC: The Brookings Institution.

—— 1998. Health Care Reform: What is the Problem? In T.R. Marmor and P.R. DeJong, eds., *Ageing, Social Security and Affordability.* Aldershot UK: Ashgate, pp 246–70.

—— 1999. "Targets and Systems of Health Care Cost Control." *Journal of Health Politics, Policy and Law* 24 (4): 653–96.

—— 2001. National Health Care/Insurance Systems. In N.J. Smelser and P.B. Baltes, eds., *International Encyclopedia of the Social & Behavioral Sciences.* New York: Elsevier, pp 10301–5.

—— 2004. "(How) Is Aging a Health Policy Problem?" *Yale Journal of Health Policy, Law, and Ethics* 4 (1): 47–68.

Wilensky, H. 2002. Rich Democracies: Political Economy, Public Policy, and Performance. Berkeley: University of California Press.

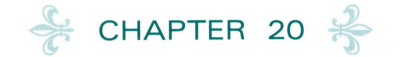

CHAPTER 20

Taking Medicine To Market: Competition in Britain and the United States

Daniel Ehlke

This chapter examines the rise of the British National Health Service. It explains how British health reformers turned to market competition and placed in the middle of a government run system. Finally, the chapter compares the idea of market competition in health care as it has played out in Britain and in the United States.

Health care challenges every effort to introduce free market forces but as costs keep rising, policy makers around the world keep trying. This chapter looks at British efforts to inject market forces into their national health service. Americans might feel a bit dizzy when they first encounter the British experience. After all, we often imagine that markets are the opposite of government; while many chapters in this book challenge that idea, the English case completely explodes it. In Britain, market reforms operate entirely *within* the centralized, government run, British National Health Service (the NHS). Indeed the reforms are known as "internal markets"—internal to a vast, bureaucratic, public health service.

While injecting markets into a governmental program may sound unusual to American ears, in many ways, the British results parallel our own reform experience: the British internal market was intended to alter the power relations within the medical profession, transform the relations between payer and provider, and to empower consumers, while delivering greater "value for money." As in the American case, results have been mixed—the only constant in recent years has been change.

BRITISH HEALTH CARE BEFORE 1948: ANTECEDENTS OF THE NHS

By the end of the 19th century, two kinds of hospitals had developed in Britain. Wealthier people received care at the so-called voluntary hospitals.[1] These were private institutions financed by members of the nobility and others who could afford to cover the costs of such institutions.[2] Municipal hospitals treated the poor and, to some extent, the middle classes. Overseen and funded by local governments, municipal hospitals varied widely in quality, reflecting the uneven distribution of wealth among the different communities. Care of any quality was often hard to come by in rural areas, which suffered from a shortage of medical professionals and facilities.[3]

Physician services also divided into two categories. As in many nations, the British drew a sharp distinction between office-based general practitioners (or GPs) and hospital-based specialists. A rivalry soon developed between the GPs and the hospital specialists. For the most part, the latter enjoyed greater prestige, viewing GPs and their patients as being beholden to them.[4] Government programs would perpetuate this bifurcation among British medical professionals.

The State established a role in medicine by 1911 with the passage of national health insurance for workers. The Liberal Party under the leadership of Prime Minister David Lloyd George championed the legislation. Lloyd George, who became best known for guiding the nation through World War I, was a legendary political survivor, changing positions frequently across a range of issues in order to preserve his position at or near the apex of the national power structure.[5] Though a decidedly dynamic figure himself, he led a Liberal Party that was even then heading into a state of long-term decline. Already competing with a fledgling Labour Party for votes, Lloyd George hit upon the construction of a limited welfare state as a means of improving the fortunes of the laboring class and, with it, those of his own party.[6]

The national health insurance established by the Liberal government in 1911 was quite narrow. Under the plan, the government financed a portion of basic health care costs with employers and, to a far lesser extent, the workers themselves paying the rest. Dependents of workers were not covered. Nor were hospital costs.[7] The legislation was partly inspired by the German health care system, in which the provision and finance of health care was (and is) closely related to employment sectors; the Germans also limited coverage to the "workingmen" within society.

This early experiment with national health insurance established a working relationship between the GPs and the State. Initially the GPs feared State intervention in the affairs of the profession and physicians represented by the British Medical Association (BMA) opposed the plan.[8] After threatening to refuse care under national health insurance, most doctors chose to participate in the new scheme and quickly grew fond of the steady flow of income it provided. Hospital-based physicians remained excluded from the national health insurance system and would continue to operate independent of significant government intervention for nearly another three decades.

The interwar period would feature a lengthy debate concerning ways to improve British health care generally, and the proper role of the government in health care. By the 1920s and 1930s, the British health care system was in a state of crisis. During the great depression, many hospitals, municipal and voluntary alike, were under funded with some forced to close. Voluntary hospitals increasingly found themselves in the unfamiliar position of actually lagging in quality behind many municipal hospitals.[9] This trend accelerated once legislation allowed local authorities to take over the ancient poor law medical institutions, thereby encouraging local government to construct a more unified system of health care provision. Voluntary hospitals soon followed suit, banding together to centralize care under their collective auspices. By the 1930s, the hospital sector was marked by ever-greater centralization of operations.[10]

The partial and haphazard centralization did not solve the problems of the health care system. Inequities developed, particularly between rural and urban areas. Poor conditions and low quality of care marked hospitals serving every class. By the late 1930s, there was a growing consensus that something had to be done to improve the state of British health care. There was little agreement, however, as to just what might constitute the proper prescription.

As World War II descended on continental Europe and threatened the British Isles, government officials prepared for the possibility of massive military and civilian casualties by enlisting a large proportion of the medical community in the service of the state. The general practitioners extended their tradition of cooperation with the state; and now that tradition expanded as hospital-based specialists were enlisted into this Emergency Medical Service.[11] This system had its share of weaknesses and hiccups, particularly in its early phases. Many doctors were forced to abandon lucrative practices to provide care where the state expected need could be greatest, with significant reductions in revenue the result. These kinks were, in good measure, ironed out once government and medical personnel agreed on a fair (and, in some cases, generous) rate of compensation.

Like GPs before them, many hospital-based physicians learned to work with public officials. Ironically, the Emergency Medical Service would prove largely unnecessary. Though a fair swath of England, and London particularly, suffered under the depredations of Hitler's Luftwaffe, resultant casualties were far lower than the government had predicted in the immediate run-up to war. The episode was nonetheless significant within the context of the State's role in the national health care system. Along with the National Health Insurance Act of 1911, the Emergency Medical Service of the late 1930s and early 1940s, a set a precedent of substantial government intervention in British health care. Indeed, the effectiveness of the Service led to calls for a postwar National Hospital Service, one which the government swiftly promised its citizenry.[12]

In addition to providing hospital-based physicians with experience in working with government, World War II also had broader significance for the development of the British health care system. England had been a heavily stratified society. Now, groups who had been thoroughly segregated from one another found themselves thrown together under considerable adversity. The same fears of widespread (mainly urban) casualties that led the government to establish the Emergency Medical Service also led to mass evacuations of women and children from London and other urban centers, into (an often more genteel) countryside. Well-off rural residents were, for the first time, brought into contact with some of the poorest within society.[13]

For the most part, this experience and the shared common peril of daily (and nightly) bombing raids had the effect of blurring class boundaries. The national solidarity contributed to postwar acceptance of measures aimed at the further leveling of British society. This spirit found voice in the work of social reformer and sometimes-government advisor William Beveridge.

At the request of Labour leaders in the wartime coalition government, Beveridge prepared a report in which he outlined measures for improving the well-being of the British populace after the war. Unveiled at the height of World War II in November 1942, his report was a tour de force, enlisting government to put its authority to bear in slaying what he called the "five giants": illness, ignorance, disease, squalor, and want.[14] The report created national excitement. A Gallup poll taken in 1943 discovered that 95% of the public had heard about the report and overwhelmingly supported its three major goals: a health service, a children's program, and a full employment plan.[15]

In the area of health care, many (though certainly not all) of Beveridge's recommendations would be swept into law by a very rare political event: "a landslide upset." Winston Churchill's conservatives, anxious about "the follies of socialism," called for "pragmatic reform." Labour, which more enthusiastically embraced the popular Beveridge report, won its first majority in the House of Commons by a stunning 146 seat margin. Labour's Minister of Health, Aneurin Bevan, touted Beveridge's vision, beginning with the establishment in 1948 of the NHS.[16]

THE NHS SUCCESS STORY

As we have seen, the period from approximately 1911–41 had witnessed two trends in the field of British medical organization: an ever-increasing proportion of the medical community was brought into contact with the State and the hospital sector underwent considerable centralization, with many previously stand-alone facilities combining with other facilities. Though the system remained rather haphazard, power increasingly resided in three sectors: medical professionals, local authorities, and the national government. By 1945, many could agree on the need for a unified health service. What remained open to (fierce) debate was just how such a system would look and—more specifically—who would hold the reins of power.

Local authorities initially appeared the best candidates to lead the health service. Their role in the hospital sector had, after all, been steadily increasing prior to the war, and such an approach would be a good bit less politically ambitious than outright nationalization of health care.[17] In the end, however, Aneurin Bevan settled upon nationalization. Under Bevan's NHS, all hospitals would be state run.

Bevan divided England and Wales into a total of 14 health service regions, each focused around a prominent teaching hospital. In order to avoid a London-centered region from lording over (and draining resources) from outlying districts, Bevan drew regional boundaries that met in a point within the city. This way the various neighborhoods of the capital would be divided between four regions, preventing the rise of a preponderantly powerful London-based bloc.

Operations within health regions were to be overseen by a new administrative construct: the Regional Health Board, or RHB. RHB members were appointed by Bevan himself though, insofar as possible, the government worked to keep leaders within health care's *ancien regime* in positions of power. Their responsibilities were broad, and included capital planning, and the formation of Hospital Maintenance Committees, or HMCs. These latter committees would form a unified control structure of the diverse hospital facilities to be found within the various regions—effectively turning, a number of different institutions into a single organism.[18]

At least that was how it was to work in theory—in practice, there was a large loophole in the form of teaching hospitals. Though the health regions had been partly determined on the basis of their geographical distribution across the country, teaching hospitals were only brought into the fledgling NHS on the condition that they would retain a considerable degree of independence. Though a representative from their respective RHBs were added to the governing boards of these institutions, they largely retained freedom of action under the new system.[19]

Anticipating and, indeed, encountering resistance from organized medicine, Bevan ensured that the system incorporated key compromises to the important groups comprising the medical community. When it came to physician compensation, for instance, GPs were to receive capitation (that is, set fees per patient examined), rather than an outright state salary, thus preserving their nominal independence from State control. Similarly, specialists were granted the privilege of retaining private practices, and seeing (private) patients in NHS facilities. Ironically, specialists accepted the very state salary scheme opposed by GPs.

Even after these significant compromises were struck, professional opposition remained and the BMA threatened a strike.[20] At the very last minute, however, the BMA leadership recommended its members accept and serve the new regime. Parliament passed the law in November 1946, a little more than a year after the unexpected rise to power of Attlee's Labour government. The NHS went into effect on July 5, 1948.

Beveridge and his allies had, from the start, envisioned a national health service that would improve the well-being of society, while actually lowering health care costs. In the event (and perhaps unsurprisingly), this did not occur. Indeed, NHS resource needs were consistently underestimated by Attlee's government.[21] While absolute costs rose considerably, much of these early increases could be chalked up to inflation; as a proportion of GDP, health care spending remained stable, and at a decidedly low level—rising from roughly 3% to 4% of GDP over the next 15 years.[22]

Despite the relatively low investment required to maintain the NHS, the Service would continue to face cost-cutting pressures from the Treasury ministry, or Exchequer. The initial cost overruns shifted the power over the NHS from the Health Ministry (the political guardian of the NHS) to the budget hawks at the Chancellor of the Exchequer. From very early on, Treasury officials dominated the NHS, constantly laboring to control health spending, at one point establishing a maximum level of government investment.[23] For this, and numerous other reasons, health expenditure would remain very low throughout the postwar period, particularly relative to that of the United States.

The NHS was, from the start, a hugely popular program. Large proportions of the British populace have and, indeed, continue to express support for the NHS. Indeed, a 2002 poll showed a full 80% of citizens surveyed to believe the NHS was critical to British society.[24]

Ironically, the very popularity of the NHS leads politicians to portray the NHS as being endangered and vulnerable to the whims of the government of the day. The party in opposition, Conservative and Labour alike, often finds health policy a convenient means by which to focus criticism on the government. That this has proven a consistent theme in British politics is, in turn, the result of health care having been thoroughly politicized. This is not to say that health care somehow falls outside the realm of politics in the United States. However, the British system is very much a command-and-control entity—the government is responsible for the smooth operation of the health care system. And the opposition always seeks to score political points by blasting the stewardship of the Party in power.

The historical circumstances surrounding the establishment of the NHS also ensure that it remains central to British political conflict. Having served generations of citizens over nearly six decades, the NHS stands as one of the crown jewels of Labour's postwar political legacy. Since it had been skeptical

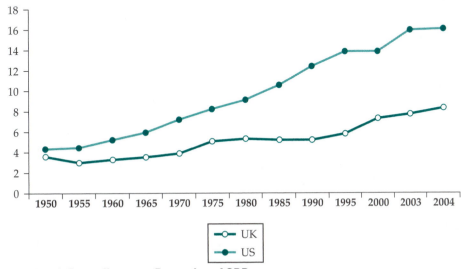

Figure 20-1 Health Expenditures as Proportion of GDP

SOURCE: (UK data) Department of Health Statistics; (US data) Health Care Financing Administration.

about the organization up to the moment of its passage, the Conservative Party has spent decades proving its worth as a custodian—even enhancer—of the Service. In more recent years, the Conservatives (or Tories) have presented themselves as a big-tent party, genuinely concerned with the well-being of all citizens, particularly the most vulnerable. In Britain, health policy has been central to this effort at party transformation.

Today, both parties joust over how to reform the NHS. Unleashed in the early 1970s, the forces of change have been going strong for the last 25 years.

THE NHS IN FLUX: 1974–PRESENT

The NHS forged an alliance between three groups: the general practioners, specialists in the hospitals, and local government. The three acted with considerable independence within the NHS structure. By the late 1960s, policy makers, academics, and some (though by no means all) elements within the medical profession were pushing for management and structural reform aimed at unifying the three components of health care delivery.[25]

The first important reforms, passed in 1974, did not engage general public, perhaps because of their highly technical nature. The new program established local health authorities (LHAs) under the supervision of slightly reconstituted Regional Health Boards, now dubbed RHA[authorities]. Reformers aimed to better delineate the roles of managers—and generally improve management—within the system. The changes had few practical consequences for patients and were most significant for presaging more radical efforts to alter the structure and management of the NHS under future governments.

The press for change came partially from the shortcomings of the NHS. By 1970, Britain was spending less on health care (as proportion of the economy) than France (which spent 20% more), Germany (37% more), and the United States (53% more). The strains were beginning to show. However,

the trouble in the NHS reflected a larger crisis that seemed to enmesh the entire British political economy in the mid-1970s. Just when Watergate and the Vietnam War shook Americans' faith in the efficacy (and, indeed, good intentions) of political leaders and governing institutions, the British underwent a period when their nation also seemed ungovernable.

The roots of this political crisis lay in an economic malaise that spread across much of the world (with the possible exception of the major oil-producing countries) during the 1970s. Pervasive and prolonged economic torpor called into question basic assumptions that had driven domestic and, indeed, global policy for the past three decades. At the international level, the establishment of a fixed exchange rate mechanism under the postwar Bretton Woods regime protected nations from the treacherous currency markets, ensured financial stability and, for many, facilitated rapid economic improvement. In the British case, stability was further enhanced by successive governments' close control of the economy and, more specifically, their policy of preserving something approaching full employment.[26]

Demand was largely regulated through cyclical injections of money in the form of government spending, which would, in turn, be followed by periods of spending restraint. Also concerned about the problem of inflation, governments from the 1940s through the 1970s chose to respond by attempting to cooperate with trade unions to control income across the economy during particularly inflationary periods.[27] By the mid-1970s, the effects of oil and energy shocks were creating the phenomenon of stagflation on both sides of the Atlantic—that is, economic stagnation paired with high inflation.

British attempts to rein in industrial income in this environment were met with mass strikes across the economy. This came to a fearful head during the so-called Winter of Discontent of 1978–79 when even the dead went unburied in parts of the country on account of striking gravediggers.[28] The Labour government seemed powerless in the face of political chaos. Armed with the convincing slogan "Labour isn't Working," and buoyed by promises to regain control over events, the Conservative Party under Margaret Thatcher coasted to election victory in 1979.[29]

Thatcher prescribed the bracing discipline of economic markets for the ills of the British economy. But how to apply that idea to the troubled, underfunded, yet ever popular NHS? The government called on Sir Roy Griffiths, a supermarket executive. Initially charged with examining staffing issues within the NHS, Griffiths went beyond his remit (or charge) by evaluating the entire operational structure of the organization. Griffiths found a glaring lack of accountability across the NHS, and called for the increased use (imposition really) of nonmedical general managers who could call doctors to account and push efficiencies on the system; the Griffiths Report also called for tighter national government budget controls. The idea was to inject private managerial practices in the NHS.[30] Griffiths' suggestions were, for the most part, implemented in the mid-1980s. By strengthening management and accountability, his reforms would make it easier for Thatcher to enact more radical changes in the years to come.

The conservatives did not take more forceful action until they had won a third successive election in 1987. Then, after considerable study, the government enacted the *National Health Service and Community Health Act of 1990* which revolutionized the way the NHS did business. In the past those who provided care and those who financed it were, if not the same people, then at least a part of the same entity—the State. Now the reformers split these functions—the purchaser and the provider. District Health Authorities and a new breed of GP, the GP "fundholder," would be entrusted with a limited budget; they were charged with negotiating favorable deals with health care providers (hospitals, for the most part) on behalf of their patient clients.[31]

This purchaser–provider split, it was thought, would increase efficiency by forcing the providers to compete for business from the purchasers. Competing hospitals would contract with as many purchasers (the District Health Authorities or the GP "fundholders") as they could manage. Three assumptions guided the reforms: First, since the hospital's income would be based on how many blocks of patients they could win contracts for, hospitals would streamline their operations, and build up reputations for good quality patient care. Second, the contracts between purchasers and providers would effectively "lock in" higher standards of care. Finally, the reformer's thought that the scheme would ensure the empowerment of GPs at the cost of specialists (since GPs would guide their patients into the hospital system), thus establishing a better balance between the two key sectors of the medical profession and righting imbalances that had stretched all the way back to the 19th century.[32]

While the internal market was designed to break the monopoly of the providers and inject market forces into the NHS, the entire construct played out within the State (and thus remaining "internal"). Public health authorities would, under the Thatcher reforms, remain the driving force among the "purchasing" class of actors. The state would have to authorize the formation of trusts and, indeed, the assignation of GP fundholding privileges. The postreform NHS was an example of what some, including the very academics that inspired system change, a quasi-market, representing a halfway point between public enterprise and private corporation.[33]

Where did the 1990 reforms come from? As we have seen, there was a clear political trajectory that seemed to point toward fundamental change of the NHS, beginning in the 1970s. The election and re-election of the Conservatives under Thatcher accelerated reform efforts that had been percolating for a considerable period. Perceived "crisis" within the system (and the British State as whole) seemed to justify a veritable revolution in the way the NHS functioned.

At the same time, however, the 1990 reforms drew their inspiration from more distant, or external, sources. While it was a British executive who got the ball rolling when it came to management reforms of the NHS, it was an American scholar and sometime government official, Alain Enthoven, who provided much of the theoretical backing and practical advice on just what form any reforms should take.[34] Enthoven was the chief originator of the concept of the internal market, even though such an idea had little relevance, on the face of it, for an American health care system that looked very different (and was substantially already a creature of "the market"). His consultation with the Thatcher government was crucial in the formulation of the 1990 package of reforms.

The Thatcher reforms worked their way through the NHS between 1990 and 1997. John Major, Thatcher's successor as Tory leader, continued the changes she introduced. At the end of this seven-year period, reviews of the new system were mixed. This was inevitable, as it has long proven difficult to measure outcomes of any sort associated with a given health care system. Bound up, as it is, in political conflict, health care systems are altered more as a result of perception and political imperative, than objective measurement of system outcomes. Market reforms often generate charges of inequity; and Conservatives had always been politically vulnerable to charges of not enthusiastically supporting the NHS. Predictably, the Labour party—moving steadily back toward the center under the leadership of Tony Blair—opposed every Conservative change.

Blair entered office in 1997 seemingly dedicated to the eradication of the internal market. His stated goal was more than a bit vaguely expressed as the substitution of competitive principles, with those of "collaboration."[35]

Such broad goals could have been put into practice through a variety of further reforms and this is, in fact, just what occurred. Whereas the Thatcher reform package remained operative for a span of seven years, the chapters in Blair's health care reform agenda would each last a few years, before being succeeded by the next change. These chapters roughly corresponded with the various health secretaries who held the post following the 1997 election.[36] Frank Dobson (1997–99), was followed by Alan Milburn, who served until 2003. Milburn, in turn, was replaced by John Reid (2003–05) who was, in turn, displaced by Patricia Hewitt during a cabinet reshuffle in 2005.

The late 1990s and first several years of the 21st century were thus turbulent times for an NHS in a continuous state of flux. Blair's "new Labour" team

was first intent on formally abolishing the internal market, though it was still unclear what they would replace it with. Indeed, the government left little mark of its own on the NHS during its first two years in office.[37] The momentum of market reform appeared to have ebbed. Surveying the wreckage of the internal market experiment, the normally optimistic Alain Enthoven remarked that, "The government couldn't shake its identity as a provider and make the transition to becoming primarily the purchaser of health services."[38]

Appearances aside, however, further change was afoot. During 1998 and into 1999, the Health Ministry developed plans to establish a National Institute of Clinical Excellence, or NICE. This body was charged with establishing the suitability and effectiveness of various drugs and treatments.[39] Along with a host of other such regulatory bodies, it was designed to improve the quality of care within the NHS. Though new within the context of the United Kingdom, the new policies received some inspiration from American private insurers that often set down just which course of treatments they would authorize, and finance.[40]

A more (outwardly) energetic approach to reform commenced shortly after Alan Milburn took the helm at the Department of Health in 1999. The winter of 1999–2000 witnessed a flu epidemic that appeared to swamp NHS resources, and furthered an impression of 'crisis' within the institution. The government set forth a new package of reforms the following year. These echoed the 1990 reforms, with the reorganization of NHS hospitals [into (more) autonomous foundation trusts chief among them].[41] Quietly, the Blair government began to refine pro-market reforms that had been conceived during the Thatcher era.

At the same time that he was injecting market thinking, Tony Blair pledged to break the long fiscal austerity that had marked the NHS since its inception. By 1997, the United Kingdom's health spending as percentage of GDP stood at 6.7%—far behind France (9.4%), Germany (10.7%), the United States (13%), and even Portugal (8.5%) or Greece (9.4%). Blair promised increases in health spending through 2008, a pledge designed to place British health care spending in line with that the expenditure rates found in other EU nations.[42] Critics questioned whether the rapid increases would be accompanied by greater complacency and inefficiency within the NHS. All the same, from an American perspective this was, in itself, an enviable position in which to find oneself—seeking to increase the size of the health sector. After all (and as previous chapters have demonstrated), detractors of the American system constantly pointed to the proportion of GDP dedicated to health care—already past 16%—on the other side of the Atlantic.

Toward the end of Alan Milburn's tenure as health minister and the start of John Reid's, the NHS continued to undergo radical transformation. In particular, the private sector was invited to take a far more active role in the provision of health care. Private corporations for instance, were allowed to present bids for primary care under NHS auspices. This had the practical effect of changing the role of the organization from a direct provider of care, to a purchaser of care on behalf of the British citizenry.[43] Labour was thus the party to achieve the veritable apotheosis of the internal market envisioned by Thatcher and her team.

Recent developments have perpetuated the pro-market changes. The role of the private sector within the NHS continues to increase. In January 2006 the local authorities in Yorkshire, England made headlines by "hiring" a subsidiary of US health firm UnitedHealth to run several GP practices in the region.[44] By incorporating more "alternative providers" into the system at the community level, the government hopes to counteract the traditional bias patients have shown toward seeking hospital care.

While citizens have, in the main, taken the reforms in stride, the same cannot be said for some members of the medical profession. Polling shows that members of the public were generally agnostic when it came to whether it was the private or public sector that provided care—as long as they received the care they required.[45] Ahead of a recent meeting of the BMA, however, some doctors appeared fearful that the NHS would effectively cease to be public.

Indeed, the gathering debated whether members should join a campaign to ensure that the NHS did not fall into the private sector.[46] Sixty years after members of the profession voiced opposition to the idea of a NHS, doctors have now become among its most ardent defenders.

AMERICAN MEDICAL MARKETIZATION

Around the time the NHS internal market was established (1990), one of its creators, Alain Enthoven, convened a meeting in the resort town of Jackson, Wyoming. His Jackson Hole Group drew on business leaders and policy makers and worked to bring managed competition to the American health care system.[47] Managing competition within the context of the NHS involved injecting market principles into an overwhelmingly public, tax supported enterprise (through the operation of an internal market). This process needed to be reversed in the American system since much of American health care was, after all, already provided by way of a market (of sorts), with direct State involvement being limited largely to Medicare and Medicaid. Whereas the emphasis would thus be on "competition" in the United Kingdom, "management" was stressed in the United States. For all the problems of the British system, reformers began with more or less universal access to health care; American reformers faced the dual problems of rising costs and shrinking coverage.

Of course, there are multiple ways in which attempts might be made to "manage" the health care marketplace. Members of the Jackson Hole Group decided to push the formation of insurer networks, which would then bargain for the best care at the lowest price.[48] They also promoted Health Maintenance Organizations (HMOs) which (theoretically, at least) unified care of individual patients. Such organizations had grown popular with health policy analysts in the 1970s but the organizations themselves had failed to capture large segments of the health care market.[49] This was, however, about to change.

Reformers had been pressing pro-competition reforms since the Nixon administration had promoted HMOs in February 1971: "An HMO cannot afford to waste resources that costs more money in the short run," enthused Nixon. "But neither can it afford to economize in ways which hurt patients for that increases long-run expense." Assistant secretary of health, Lewis Butler, had expressed the hope that 90% of all Americans would be covered through HMOs by 1980.[50]

Each generation of pro-competition reformers in the United States offered the same diagnosis of the American system as the Tories had offered of the British: not enough accountability to the patient. Though nonmarket tendencies in the American system could be traced to private actors rather public enterprise, they existed nonetheless. In the United States, it was (medical) professional prerogative, insurance coverage, employer lassitude, government tax expenditures, government regulations, and government programs that all conspired to block a genuine market in American health care.[51]

Reformers on both sides of the Atlantic, however, saw providers as the greatest obstacle to achieving efficiency in health care. This was particularly the case in the United States, in which money largely went wherever physicians decided it should go.[52] Even in the tightly budgeted NHS, however, would-be reformers starting with Griffiths pointed to inefficiency and a lack of accountability arising from provider autonomy—in the NHS case, the panacea was first thought to be the insertion of professional managers, and then the establishment of an internal market. Each attempted to "discipline" the medical profession.

The American health care system, by contrast, appeared to require the construction of a true market, an external market, in effect. But the upshot was almost exactly the same. Market forces would break the traditional prerogatives of the medical profession and bend providers to the consumers' desires.

Among the converts to the market model of health reform were Bill and Hillary Clinton. Early in his first term, President Clinton entrusted the task of health care reform to his wife and several close advisors. The package they produced was heavily influenced by Enthoven and other reformers seeking to meld market discipline to universal coverage. In the Clinton plan, insurance networks or alliances (recall the British District Health Authorities and GP fundholders) would be empowered to bargain for the best price of services among health care providers. The reforms also sought to expand and formalize the responsibility of businesses to collectively finance health care for their respective employees.

Of course, the Clinton health reform plan went down to defeat. As it turned out, a version of managed competition emerged independent of comprehensive government action. Faced with continuing increases in health expenditure, business corporations took direct action. Many required their workers to enroll in HMOs or other forms of managed care. The managed care organizations competed for contracts by promising to cut health care premiums. They would do this, in turn, by forcing efficiencies on medical providers.

For a brief time, they appeared to succeed. National health spending flattened out—and even dipped—between 1995 and 1999. Then the bottom fell out—or more accurately, the top blew off. Managed care organizations had held prices untenably low to attract enrollees. Now, they began to make up the lost ground and raise prices. More importantly, health care consumers (and their physicians) rebelled at the limits imposed on providers. Horror stories of managed care companies denying needed care turned into a major political story—the Democrats touted "a patient's bill of rights" and took to the floor of Congress to read the name's of constituents who had been cruelly (sometimes fatally) denied insurance coverage for needed care.

Amid the political furor, health care costs resumed their inexorable march—from 13.1% of GDP in 2001 to 16.% by 2005. And, as other chapters in this volume document, with rising costs comes shrinking coverage. The great difference today, is that the market solution—an American reformer's grail for 35 years—no longer holds the same allure thanks to the consumer uprising against managed care.

LEGACIES OF THE MEDICAL MARKETPLACE

What lessons are to be learned by the divergent, yet eerily similar experiences with markets in health care on both sides of the Atlantic? Certainly they reveal the extent to which changes in one system can be, and sometimes are, transferred to one that is very different. This story echoes a familiar generalization repeated in every chapter of this section on international systems: it may be impossible to limit health care expenditure without direct government control of the system as a whole—in fact, the monopsonistic NHS proved too austere at cost control while the pluralistic American health care has, of course, had the opposite problem.

The experience of both countries also yields a more subtle lesson: it takes time, patience, and political commitment, to introduce large-scale change into any health care system. Moreover, big changes generally flow out of past experience. The British medical system, for example, slowly came under state control—from Lloyd George's worker's program in 1911 to the medical emergency measures during World War II—long before anyone proposed a NHS.

Many of the themes that run through contemporary conceptions of health reform can appeal to elements on both the political right and left. While Margaret Thatcher, a Conservative, first championed market reforms, Labour's Tony Blair pushed the idea further and more successfully (though with many fits and starts). Likewise, in the United States, Republican Richard Nixon first championed pre-paid group practice but it was the Clinton administration that gave managed care its great push forward. Despite the political overlaps, however, the practical dynamics of the reform process—and of markets themselves—are every bit as likely to sow (indeed, exacerbate) political divisions, as they are to bring disparate forces together.

Where will the NHS go next—further into markets or back away from them? When health care reform makes it back to the top of the national political agenda in the United States, what will it look like? Will it swing toward markets or rebel against them? Only time will provide the answers to these questions. A veritable certainty, however, is that health care will continue to surprise and, at times, confound, policy makers, providers, and patients on both sides of the Atlantic.

STUDY QUESTIONS

1. What political developments led to the establishment of the NHS?
2. How was World War II a catalyst for increased state intervention in British health care?
3. What are some of the ways in which the British health care system differs from the American system?
4. What led the Thatcher government to fundamentally change an ever-popular NHS?
5. How does 'managed competition', as conceived in the United States, differ from that applied in the United Kingdom?
6. How has the application of market-based principles to health care fared on both sides of the Atlantic?

NOTES

1. Parry and Parry, 1976, p 204.
2. Rivett, "NHS Inheritance," in *A Short History of the NHS*, accessed July 14, 2006.
3. Ibid.
4. Personal interview, Dr. Nicholas Mays, London School of Hygiene and Tropical Medicine Health Services Research Unit. Conducted in London (LSHTM), September 25, 2005.
5. Fromkin, 1989, p 124.
6. Sykes, 1997, pp 156–7.
7. Rivett.

8. Eckstein, 1960, 94.
9. Rivett.
10. Ibid.
11. Parry and Parry, 200–1.
12. Webster, 2002, p 7.
13. Timmins, 1995, pp 31–3.
14. Ibid., p 42.
15. Jacobs, 1993, p 113.
16. Jacobs, 1993, p 117 [socialism], p 168 [most unusual].
17. See Geoffrey Rivett's comprehensive (online) history of the NHS.
18. See Rivett.
19. Rivett; Parry and Parry, pp 209–10.
20. Parry and Parry, pp 205–7.
21. Webster, 2002, p 30.
22. Rivett.
23. Webster, 2002, 31–2.
24. Lowe. 2002 "Financing Health Care in Britain Since 1939," *History & Policy* (May) [available online: http://www.historyandpolicy.org/archive/policy-paper-08.html].
25. Rivett, "1968-1977: Rethinking the National Health Service."
26. Hall, 1986, p 76.
27. Ibid., pp 80–3.
28. Timmins, p 352.
29. Ibid., p 351.
30. Timmins, pp 406–8.
31. See, for instance, "The NHS: The Conservative Legacy," 1999.
32. Baggott, 1997, pp 283–306.
33. Enthoven, 1999, p 14.
34. Timmins, pp 455–6, 460.
35. Webster, 1998, p 5.
36. Rivett, "Introduction."
37. Glennerster, 2001, pp 399–400.
38. Enthoven, 1999, p 39.
39. "NICE Opens for Business," 1999, p 962.
40. Timmins, 577.
41. "NHS Reforms: The Issue Explained," 2003.
42. Sussex and Towse, 2000.
43. Rivett, "Introduction."
44. "U.S. Giant Takes Over GP Practices," 2006.
45. 83% answered thus, in a poll cited in Dreaper, 2006.
46. Ibid.
47. Quadagno, 2005, pp 187–8.
48. Ibid., p 188.
49. Hollingsworth, 1986, p 159.
50. See Blumenthal and Morone, Chapter 5.
51. Enthoven, 1993, pp 26–7.
52. Mahar, 2006.

REFERENCES

Baggott, R. 1997. "Evaluating Health Care Reform: The Case of the NHS Internal Market," *Public Administration* 75 (Summer).

Dreaper, J. 2006. "NHS Reforms Split Medical Opinion," *BBC News*, June 26. Available at: http://news.bbc.co.uk/2/hi/health/5110478.stm. Retrieved July 23, 2006.

Eckstein, H. 1960. *Pressure Group Politics: The Case of the British Medical Association*. Palo Alto, CA: Stanford University Press.

Enthoven, A.C. 1993. "The History and Principles of Managed Competition," *HealthAffairs* Supplement, pp 26–7. Available at:http://content.healthaffairs.org/cgi/reprint/12/suppl_1/24.pdf. Retrieved July 23, 2006.

—— In Pursuit of an Improving National Health Service. London: The Nuffield Trust, 1999. Evans, R. "Sharing the Burden, Containing the Cost" (this volume).

Fromkin, D. 1989. *A Peace to End All Peace*. New York: Henry Holt. Glennerster, H. 2001. "Social Policy." In Anthony Seldon, ed., *The Blair Effect: The Blair Government 1997-2001*. London: Little, Brown and Company.

Hacker, J. 1997. *The Road to Nowhere: The Genesis of President Clinton's Plan for Health Security*. Princeton, NJ: Princeton University Press.

Hall, P. 1986. *Governing the Economy: The Politics of State Intervention in Britain and France*. New York: Oxford University Press.

Hollingsworth, J.R. 1986. *A Political Economy of Medicine: Great Britain and the United States*. Baltimore: Johns Hopkins University Press.

Lowe, R. 2002. "Financing Health Care in Britain Since 1939," *History & Policy* (May). [available online:

http://www.historyandpolicy.org/archive/
policy-paper-08.html].

Mahar, M. 2006. *Money-Driven Medicine: the Real
Reason Health Care Costs So Much*. New York:
HarperCollins.

Mays, N., London School of Hygiene and Tropical
Medicine Research Unit. 2005. Personal Interview
conducted by the author, London School of
Hygiene and Tropical Medicine, September 25.

"NHS Reforms: The Issue Explained," *Guardian* May 7,
2003. Available at: http://society.guardian.co.
uk/nhsplan/story/0,,459310,00.html. Retrieved
July 24, 2006.

"NICE Opens for Business," *British Medical Journal*
April 10, 1999. Available at: http://www.
pubmedcentral.gov/articlerender.fcgi?artid=
1174696. Retrieved July 23, 2006.

Parry, J., and N. Parry. 1976. *The Rise of the Medical
Profession: A Study of Collective Social Mobility*.
London: Croom Helm.

Quadagno, J. 2005. *One Nation Uninsured: Why the
U.S. has No National Health Insurance*. Oxford:
Oxford University Press.

Rivett, G. *A Short History of the NHS*. Available at:
http://www.nhshistory.net/nhs_inheritance.
htm. Retrieved July 14, 2006.

Sussex, J., and A. Towse. 2000. "'Getting UK Health
Care Expenditure Up to the European Union
Mean'—What Does That Mean?," *British Medical
Journal*. March 4. Available at: http://www.
findarticles.com/p/articles/mi_m0999/is_7235_320/
ai_61025585. Retrieved July 24, 2005.

Sykes, A. 1997. *A History of the Liberal Party*. London:
Longman.

Timmins, N. 1995. *The Five Giants*. London:
HarperCollins.

"U.S. Giant Takes Over GP Practices," *BBC News*
January 13, 2006. Available at: http://news.bbc.co.
uk/2/hi/health/4608782.stm]. Retrieved July 24,
2006.

Webster, C. 1998. "Blair and Bevan: More Than Fifty
Years Apart," *Healthmatters*. 33 (Spring. Available at:
http://www.healthmatters.org.uk/issue33/blairandbevan.
Retrieved July 24, 2006.

—— 2002. *National Health Service: A Political History*.
Oxford: Oxford University Press.

CHAPTER 21

Devil Take the Hindmost? Private Health Insurance and the Rising Costs of American "Exceptionalism"

Robert G. Evans

An economist draws on the international experience to analyze American health care—and its high costs. He boils down the international experience into three universal debates or planes of conflict: provider versus payer, payer versus payer, and provider versus provider. In each case, he shows how the US system is different and why it matters.

THE UNIVERSALITY OF COLLECTIVE FINANCE

In all developed societies, the financing of health care is primarily a collective process. Pools of funds, described by White as "shared savings," are assembled through more or less compulsory levies on the general population, within or outside the formal tax system.[1] These funds are then transferred to the providers of care through institutional structures and processes that vary considerably from one country to another. But in no high-income country does direct payment by the user of services account for a major part of the total cost of health care.

Care is not, of course "free"; the residents of each country must bear, one way or another, the cost of that country's health care system. But the amount that each must contribute is largely unrelated to his/her own personal use of care. The political struggles over who pays, and who gets what, are played out through the collective funding processes specific to each country.

The results determine how much care is provided, of what types, and for whom. But they also determine who must pay—how the costs will be distributed over the population—as well as who will be paid, and how much, for providing care. This distribution of economic benefits and burdens, through the political process, is at least as contentious as the process of health care provision itself.

One might expect the United States, with its emphasis on "private" funding, to be an exception to this generalization. But it is not. Direct payments by users of care are projected to make up only 13.5% of total American health spending in 2005.[2] The rest flowed through various collective channels. One would have to go back to the end of the 1950s to find a time when out of pocket payment accounted for as much as half of the total; the collective share has been rising slowly but steadily for about half a century.[3]

What *is* unusual about the United States is the extent to which the assembly of these collective funds is carried out by private institutions. A substantial majority of Americans rely primarily on private insurance against health care costs. Holahan and Wang report that 65.1% of the non-elderly, non-institutionalized civilian population in 2002 had employer-paid coverage, while another 5.3% had private nong-roup coverage.[4] Assuming that the elderly, military, and institutionalized all relied primarily on some form of public insurance or support, this implies that about 60% of the American population depends primarily on private coverage, while many of the elderly also have supplementary "Medigap" coverage as a retirement benefit or individually purchased. Yet the proportion of total health *expenditures* covered by private insurance is much less, about one third (35.7% in 2005). Private insurers, perfectly understandably, prefer not to cover people in poor health or otherwise at high risk, and place a variety of limitations on the coverage they do offer. Any shortfalls in private coverage must be paid out of pocket by beneficiaries, or shifted to the public sector.

The public sector now accounts for about 46% of health care expenditures in the United States.[5] (Another 4.8% comes from other private sources.) This is still a remarkably low proportion, well below that in other developed countries. The average public share in the other high-income countries of the OECD is about three-quarters.

But the official figure is in fact a substantial understatement, because American governments also provide a large public subsidy for private health insurance, in the form of tax exemptions for coverage bought by employers for their employees.[6] This, in addition to several smaller subsidies, has been estimated at $209.9 billion in 2004, or roughly 11% of total health care expenditure.[7] If they were recorded on the federal government's books as expenditures, the public share of total health care costs would be over 55%; adding in other government contributions recorded as "private" brings the total public share to about 60%.[8] The contribution of private insurance (net of public subsidy) to financing American health care is only about 25%. In fact, total American *public sector* spending on health care now absorbs a larger share of national income—about 9%—than in any other country, and exceeds total spending in most. An extra 6% of private spending is added on top.

What is perhaps remarkable, then, is the predominant role that private insurers play both in Americans' (and others') perceptions of their health care system, and in the formulation of health care policy, despite raising a relatively small share of the money. This role sharply distinguishes the United States from all other developed countries. What are the implications of this role, in reality?

What it does *not* mean is that "private" insurance coverage in the United States is a commodity bought over the counter by individual consumers, along with boxes of soap flakes or cans of beans. Although it is often treated as a private consumption purchase in national statistics, and particularly in formal economic analyses, this is in fact misleading non-sense. The public subsidy to employment-based insurance, plus the problems of information flow in insurance markets—the well-known process of "adverse selection"—result in a minimal market for individual private coverage.[9] Most private health insurance in the United States is *de facto* compulsory, not "voluntary." It comes with the job—and leaves with it.[10]

Private health insurance is not only collectively purchased and heavily subsidized; it is also subject to considerable public regulation. In these respects it is similar to the social insurance systems in several of the European countries. There are, however, critical differences between private health insurance in the United States, and the various insurance organizations in each of the countries conforming to what White calls the "International Standard" (see Chapter 20). These latter have public roles and responsibilities that are quite foreign to American experience.

First, private insurers bear no collective responsibility for the population as a whole. Over 15% of Americans, about 45 million people in 2003, have no health coverage at any one time, and that number is estimated to rise to 56 million by 2013.[11] An estimated 16 million more, non-elderly and continually "insured" adults are in fact underinsured, exposed to serious financial burdens.[12] In total, then, about one-third of non-elderly American adults are un- or underinsured, and the proportion is likely to rise significantly over the next decade. In other developed countries the public requirement of universal, comprehensive coverage implies that all residents must have adequate coverage from *some* agency. Insurers collectively cannot simply wash their hands of a substantial part of the population as "not our problem." But for-profit firms, competing in private markets can, do, and indeed must. They cannot profitably take on such public functions, and the United States is correspondingly unique in the radical incompleteness of its coverage.

Second, private insurance premiums are explicitly risk-based. People and groups at higher risk pay more. If the resulting premiums are beyond their means, they must "go bare"—or try to find some form of public assistance specific to their circumstances. Social insurance premiums, by contrast, are largely or wholly unrelated to risk status. Moreover they typically bear some relation to wage or income level. Thus wealthier people pay a larger share of total health care costs, and sicker people pay less, than under private health insurance.

On the other hand, the premiums levied in social insurance systems are themselves less closely related to income than are the taxes in tax-financed systems. The latter thus distribute the overall burden of health care costs still more closely in accordance with ability to pay. But regardless of how, and

from whom, the "shared savings" are raised, public systems do not impose higher costs on individuals with higher risk of illness.[13] Private insurance does.

Third, private insurers cannot be involved in the management of the health care system itself.[14] In other countries, control of the payment process is a critical lever whereby governments try to influence the evolution of system capacity, costs, and coverage. Payments may come directly from governments, as in Canada, the United Kingdom, or Sweden, or flow through a large (Germany, Switzerland) or small (France, Belgium) number of health insurers that are non-profit and closely regulated. Such organizations occupy a middle ground between the strictly "private" (for-profit, commercial) and strictly "public" (line civil service) sectors. They are being subjected to increasing public regulation and accountability, largely in response to cost pressures. But a large and fluctuating group of private insurers, competing in a private marketplace, cannot be coordinated to manage the system as a whole.

The impossibility of global system management in the United States lies behind the increasing divergence between expenditure patterns in the United States, and in the rest of the OECD. Figure 21-1 shows comparative data, from the OECD Health Data File for 2005, on health expenditures relative to Gross Domestic Product (GDP) from 1960 to 2002. The average of this ratio (unweighted, for those twenty countries with continuous data available from 1960) is bracketed by the United States on the high side, and the United Kingdom on the low. (Canada is included because of its similarity in other respects to the United States.)

From 1960 until the mid-1970s, the OECD average ratio rose roughly in parallel with the United States, though about 1 to 1.5% below. These observations led several analysts in the mid-1970s to conclude that the factors driving health care costs were common to all countries, and essentially immune to public policy. The United States was more expensive only because it was somewhat farther advanced down the common trajectory.

After the mid-1970s, however, the general experience is of much slower escalation, more or less

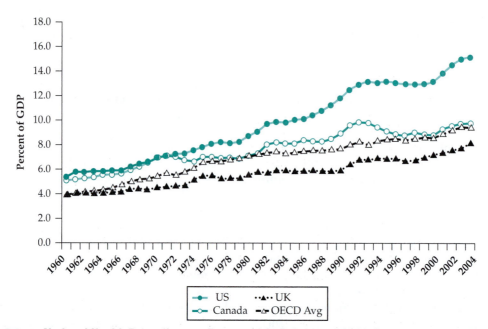

Figure 21-1 National Health Expenditure as Percent of GDP, Selected OECD Countries, 1960-2004

parallel to the United Kingdom. Between 1960 and 1977 the ratio of health expenditures to GDP rose at an average annual rate of 2.83% in the United States and slightly faster, 3.17% in this subset of OECD countries. But from 1977 to 2002 the average annual rate in the OECD countries fell markedly, to 1.26% while the rate in the United States has slowed only slightly, to 2.33%. Over this quarter century, these differential growth rates cumulate to 30%.

It was also during the mid- to late 1970s that governments in most European countries became concerned over the rate of escalation of health costs, and began developing mechanisms to control them.[15] It became obvious that health care cost trends were indeed controllable, though with considerable political difficulty, through the choice of institutions and policies. The cost problem never goes away, but there are more and less effective approaches to management.

Concerns over cost escalation were also being expressed in the United States as early as 1970, but they could not be translated into effective policy. It has become increasingly apparent that the United States is "not a country like the others," but is rather the "odd man out," as Abel-Smith pointed out twenty years ago. And the deviation in costs has risen, over the last quarter century, from 1.4% points of GDP to 5.4. This is a massive difference: had American health care costs simply risen (relative to national income) in line with the rest of the countries in Figure 21-1 they would now be lower by about $420 billion (or roughly 25%) a year. This is the price of "American exceptionalism," and it continues to grow.

The United States, like every other developed country, raises by far the bulk of the revenue for health care through collective institutions. Moreover, although the role of private funding is much greater in the United States than in other developed countries, private insurance (after accounting for the public tax expenditure subsidy) raises less than half as much money as the public sector. Yet this mix of financial sources has been sufficient to prevent the United States from developing public mechanisms for management and control similar to those that were worked out throughout the OECD during the 1970s, and have been progressively refined since.

The result has been a health care system that is, relative to the "international standard," inequitable, inefficient, unpopular, and spectacularly expensive— but also enormously profitable for some Americans. The latter feature is, of course, the key to its survival.

PLANES OF CLEAVAGE I: PROVIDERS VERSUS PAYERS

The revenues raised to pay for health care, whether through taxes or social insurance contributions, private insurance premiums, or out of pocket payments, make up one component of a fundamental three-part accounting identity that must always hold, by definition, over all systems of health care finance. The total revenues raised to pay for health care in any society must be equal to the expenditures on health care, and each in turn must exactly equal the total incomes earned from its provision:[16]

TOTAL REVENUE = TOTAL EXPENDITURE = TOTAL INCOME

These can then be factored as:

$$T + R + C = P \times Q = W \times Z$$

where T or taxes represents revenue raised through the public sector, R represents private insurance premiums, and C is direct charges to patients. Total expenditures, in turn, are the product of the quantities of health care services provided, Q, and their average prices, P, while total incomes earned can be factored into average rates of pay, W, and the total volumes of "factor inputs" used—person-hours, for example, or capital services—that we label Z.

The incomes earned from health care may be salaries or net incomes from professional practice; they also include interest on hospital bonds or dividends from private pharmaceutical or equipment companies. They are earned by doctors and nurses, dentists and pharmacists, but also by employees of firms selling health insurance or providing management consulting services to hospitals or ministries of health. The channels through which funds flow may be multiple and complex, but at the end of the day every dollar that someone has paid out must have been received by someone else. And if the goods or services which that dollar of expenditure bought were defined (albeit somewhat arbitrarily) as health care, then the corresponding dollar of income was by the same definition earned by providing health care. And someone, somehow, had to contribute an equal amount of revenue to pay for it.

This elementary accounting fact underlies the primary political conflict in every health care system— that between the payers for care and the providers of care.[17] There are also secondary conflicts on each side of this divide, among providers and among payers. But the most prominent division follows the income/expenditure distinction.

This political struggle is most evident in the universal discussions, even lamentations, over "cost explosions." In political rhetoric, health care cost trends are commonly presented as if they were some elemental force of nature, like tides or earthquakes, against which all those concerned with health policy struggle as best they can but with indifferent success. This image, assiduously promoted by providers— and some economists—is false and deceptive.[18] The *real* dynamic at work was expressed quite succinctly by Aaron Wildavsky as the Law of Medical Money: ". . . costs will increase to the level of available funds . . . that level must be limited to keep costs down."[19]

Those who *pay* for care are to a greater or lesser degree concerned to limit the escalation of costs. Those who *are paid* for care, however, are engaged in discouraging or avoiding any controls and in trying to keep the costs rising. For the sake of political credibility they may wish to be seen to share in the general hand-wringing about the relentless pressure of health care costs. But in actual fact, many if not most providers of health care believe that the adoption of appropriate priorities would lead to *more* spending, not less—at least on those services in which they have a professional interest and typically a commercial interest as well. This in turn would by definition increase the total of incomes earned from health care, making a larger total pie to share. When $P \times Q$ rises, so does $W \times Z$—that is what an identity means. Successful cost containment, on the other hand, means that someone in the system takes a wage or fee cut (W falls), or loses a job (Z falls). It cannot be otherwise.

Meeting Needs or Marketing Services: How Much Care Is Enough?

In making their case to the rest of society for more resources, and resisting pressures for cost containment, those who are paid for providing care focus primarily on the quantity of services. No matter what the current level of provision, there are always alleged to be unmet needs, and more money is needed to meet them. Furthermore these needs are constantly being increased by allegedly external forces of one sort or another—the aging of the population, the progress of technology, public expectations, AIDS, violence . . . .

Specific "explanations" of increased need may in principle be tested empirically. Some have been shown to be valid, others have been conclusively refuted. But general claims of increasing need survives any particular specific refutation, because they are in reality offered not as a testable account of causality, but as a form of product advertising. They are the classic "Your money or your life!" argument; if more resources are not forthcoming people will die, or at least suffer, unnecessarily. We *must* "meet the needs."

Such an argument is probably as old as medicine itself. At the individual level, it is the standard method whereby the therapist exerts power over the patient—which may well be in the patient's best interest. "Doctor's Orders" are most effective when combined with an explanation of the beneficial results of compliance—and the ill effects of noncompliance. The relationship has a fundamental political dimension—"orders" are the exercise of power backed up by the perception of superior knowledge, and thus the ability to make credible, if not always specific, threats. "Do this, or else." Again one must

emphasize that, in the individual clinical encounter, both the language and the intent may be entirely benevolent.

But since in developed societies the financing of health care is collectivized, providers must influence the controllers of those collective funds and induce them to spend more, on more different types of services. Political pressure is therefore brought to bear by convincing the relevant constituency (voters, employees, or premium-payers) of the adverse consequences of refusal. "Heartless" bureaucrats, politicians, employers, (even economists) are placing dollars above peoples' lives. Such claims, supported by human-interest anecdotes, are politically very powerful, and also sell newspapers.

Of course, as Williams has pointed out, if there is no natural limit to the scope of medicine, and if there is always *some* small benefit which might be gained, through sufficiently large expense, then logically it is impossible for *any* society to "meet all the needs" in a technical sense. Needs are infinite. It is then fundamentally a political question as to which needs—and whose—are "worth" meeting. Technical expertise may be necessary to determine what the payoffs to further expenditure in a particular situation might be, but the expert is no more qualified than any other citizen to state whether the benefits are worth paying for. In a democratic society everyone gets one vote.[20]

Providers accordingly seek to persuade their fellow citizens that the benefits of further expenditures are large, i.e., more "medical miracles." But they emphasize especially the catastrophic consequences, in health and human happiness, of any (successful) attempt to restrain the escalation of costs. In other fields of endeavor this activity would immediately be recognized as marketing.

In the United States in particular, the technique has been refined into the specter of "rationing." Ever-advancing technology is portrayed as constantly enhancing the ability to extend and improve the quality of life and maintain function, but at ever greater cost. Sooner or later, it is argued, we shall be forced to "ration"—deny people access to effective services, let them suffer or die—for sheer lack of the necessary resources.[21] But in the meantime, and to postpone the evil day—send more money![22]

Health care is valued by its users, not for itself but for its anticipated (positive) impact on health. Absent this payoff, most health care services are "bads," not "goods." No sane person knowingly undergoes health care that is ineffective or harmful. But ineffective or harmful services are just as effective as necessary care in generating employment and incomes, thus adding to total. Furthermore, both effective and ineffective care may be provided at different levels of technical efficiency. One country may spend more, not because it is getting more health benefits, or even more health care, but simply because its institutions for providing care are less efficient and more wasteful of human and physical resources.

Those who argue the inevitability of rationing must necessarily assume away the existence, on any significant scale, of either inefficient or ineffective care—and they do. They thus slide smoothly past a large and steadily growing body of contrary evidence—in effect ignoring what they cannot refute. But if the "rationing" story in health care is, at its core, not an intellectual investigation but rather part of a propaganda campaign to try to secure more resources and incomes for the health care sector, there is no reason to expect its advocates to take account of the now overwhelming (at least in the United States) contrary evidence.

"It is foolish to believe that increases in health care inputs and throughputs lead to increases in health status outcomes."[23] But it is not at all foolish to try to persuade others to this belief, if one can thereby enhance their willingness to pay for one's own services, and avoid awkward questions. The assumption that all care currently being provided is effective, and that any reductions must represent a threat to health, is not taken seriously by any student of health services in any country, least of all in the United States. But the specter of "rationing" plays the very important political role of diverting public attention from the question of whether the services *now* being provided, are effective and appropriate. Instead we are led back into the familiar bog: "How else will we meet the needs? We *must* have more money!"

The specter of "rationing" may possibly become reality at some time in the indefinite future. But it is not now, and may never be, in any of the wealthier industrialized countries. There is, at present, no direct linkage between levels of expenditure on health care, and the achievement of health outcomes, in any health care system in the industrialized world.[24] We are all a long way from the grim trade-off of "Your money or your life."

Paying for More Care, or Just Paying Higher Prices?

But a moment's reflection should also remind us that more money does not necessarily buy more services, effective or otherwise. It may, as Joseph White points out in Chapter 20, simply support higher prices. This point emerged very clearly from an analysis of OECD data by Gerdtham and Jönsson (1991b), in which they were able to identify the extent to which differences among countries in health care costs were a result, not of differences in levels of care, but simply of differences in the *relative* prices of health care services, from one country to another.

Gerdtham and Jönsson began by converting health care expenditures *per capita* in each of the OECD countries from domestic currency into US dollars. Typically this is done using purchasing power parities (PPPs) rather than exchange rates.[25] When PPPs are based on comparisons of the relative prices of all the commodities in the GDP, one finds very large differences between *per capita* spending in the United States, and in all other countries. Americans, at the time of this analysis, were spending about 50% more than the next two most expensive countries, Canada and Switzerland, 75% more than France and Germany, and more than twice as much as any of the rest.

But if instead one converts other countries' currency into US dollars using PPPs specific to the health care sector, Gerdtham and Jönsson found that much of this differential disappeared. In this alternative comparison, Canada spent as much *per capita* as the United States, Japan spent almost as much, and Sweden spent substantially more. Every country in the OECD moves up relative to the United States, some by a small amount and others by a great deal.

Other studies support this inference. Schieber et al. (1994) also show significantly higher rates of relative inflation of health sector prices in the United States than in other OECD countries. Several comparisons of the Canadian and American health care systems have shown rates of service use that are on average very similar, with Canadians receiving more of some forms of care, and less of others. Most recently Anderson et al. (2003, 2005) have reached the same conclusion from the OECD data.[26]

More narrowly focused, but with by far the best comparative data, is a recent study of costs of coronary artery bypass grafting in hospitals in Canada and in the United States that all employ a common accounting system.[27] Using chart review, the researchers were able to identify patient characteristics and outcomes, and to calculate within a similar accounting system the costs of comparable cases. Outcomes for comparable cases were the same on both sides of the border, but in-hospital costs per case in the United States were nearly twice those in Canada. Why do Americans spend so much more for health care? "It's the prices, stupid!"[28]

Why should care be so much more expensive in the United States? Apologists for the current system either avoid the question entirely, or try to argue that the quantity comparisons are invalid. Americans pay more because they get higher "quality." But this alleged higher quality is not reflected in better outcomes, or better population health status, or even greater public satisfaction. So what is it?

Apologists trained in economics may then shift into theological arguments that reduce in essence to such comments as: "The quality *must* be higher, or else rational patients making informed choices in free markets would not have paid for it. Objective data are irrelevant; it is [my] *theory* that must be decisive." And so it may be, in some world far from the one we actually live in. Those whose religious faith is weaker refer instead to the excellence of the care received and the outcomes achieved by *some* Americans—and nobody can deny that these are indeed excellent. But systems must be judged on their overall performance,

bad as well as good, and it is hard to find there any justification for higher prices in the United States. In any case Eisenberg et al. find no evidence of quality differentials between procedures in the United States and Canada, despite the dramatic difference in expenditures.

Bargaining Over Incomes—How Much Are Providers Worth?

High prices have two possible sources, high incomes and low efficiency. Comparative price data show the powerful effect of these factors taken together, but do not disentangle them.

Taking the first point first, much of health policy is taken up with, in Reinhardt's phrase, "the allocation of life-styles to providers."[29] How much shall providers earn, relative to the rest of the community, or more generally how shall this be decided? Although this is obviously a critical factor in determining the costs of health care, it is not one that health care providers typically wish to discuss explicitly— at least not the highest-earning ones. They would rather talk about unmet needs, and the escalating costs of providing quality care.

In a competitive marketplace, relative incomes are determined by "demand and supply" and are not amenable to political bargaining. In the real world of health care, however, the boundaries set by market forces tend to be broad and indistinct, and to leave a wide band of discretion. International comparisons of physicians' incomes, for example, show that their skills and long education periods lead to correspondingly high incomes everywhere, just as "demand and supply" would predict. But the *size* of their income advantage relative to the rest of the community is highly variable, both from country to country, and over time within countries. It is relatively low in the Nordic countries, and particularly high in the United States. Physicians were in the past very well off in both Germany and Canada, but have lost some ground (in Germany quite a lot) relative to the general income level.[30]

Much less attention has been given to international comparisons of incomes for other classes of health care personnel. Redelmeier and Fuchs (1993), however, found that overall, the average rates of income of hospital workers were very similar in Canada and in the United States—about 4% higher in the United States. But the wages of more highly skilled workers—head and general duty nurses—were about 20% higher in the United States, while wages of housekeepers and aides were about 20% lower. This may well reflect the greater role of unions in Canadian hospitals; if so European countries may show patterns more similar to that in Canada.

The point for our purposes, however, is simply to emphasize the variability in worker incomes in the health care sector, across countries and over time, relative to the rest of the community. They are not dictated by "the market"; institutional environments matter. Accordingly efforts by payers to control rates of pay—wages, salaries, fees, and prices—in the face of counter-pressures from providers, make up a large part of the process of cost containment in national health care systems. The political dimension of this process of bargaining over provider incomes is quite overt, in negotiations over the level of fees or salaries that will be paid by public or quasi-public insurers, and over the opportunities which physicians in particular will or will not have to increase their incomes by charging patients directly.

The process of bargaining over provider incomes varies with the structure of the delivery system in each country. In a number of countries physicians may be independent practitioners who are paid by fees for service. In Canada this is true of both generalists and specialists; in several of the European countries specialists may be hospital-based and on salary.[31] Most other health workers are salaried employees of hospitals or clinics that are themselves typically funded through some form of budgetary process. As a general observation, however, bargaining tends to evolve from specific items to more comprehensive budgets.

One may begin by negotiating fees with physicians. But payers rapidly discover that, depending upon the rules for payment, the total volume of billings per physician can be quite elastic. Hillman et al. (1990) provide a particularly dramatic example.[32] Which items are in the fee schedule—does it cover all diagnostic tests, for example?—and who can be reimbursed for particular services—all practitioners, or only selected ones?—may be as important for the evolution of total costs, as the actual level of fees.

The same problem emerges for pharmaceuticals, where again prescriptions are typically reimbursed on an item of service basis. The price of any given drug may be stable or falling over time, but the constant introduction of "new" drugs, real or apparent, keeps increasing both the number of prescriptions per capita and the average price per scrip.

Indeed the pharmaceutical industry provides the most naked examples of efforts by providers—the pharmaceutical manufacturing industry or "Big Pharma"—to manipulate the regulatory process in order to inflate costs, i.e., industry revenues. The strategy is two-pronged; the regulatory process is infiltrated and used to suppress competitive market forces and prevent the emergence of anything resembling price competition for prescription drugs, while at the same time undermining any efforts to regulate prices or industry incomes. It has been remarkably successful; pharmaceutical costs are the fastest growing component of health care costs in all developed countries despite growing evidence of inappropriate prescribing and excessive pricing.

Perhaps the most breathtaking example is that of (former) Representative Billy Tauzin, "a principal architect of the new Medicare drug law," who then resigned to "become president of the Pharmaceutical Research and Manufacturers of America, the chief lobby for brand-name drug companies" at a salary estimated at about $2 million a year.[33] Tauzin's services to the industry? "The law steers clear of price controls and price regulation . . . [and] forbids the government to negotiate with drug manufacturers to secure lower prices for Medicare beneficiaries."

Other countries have been somewhat more successful in imposing some institutional limits on the pharmaceutical industry's ambitions, but in the present era the industry has been using its extraordinary influence in Washington to undermine those efforts through bilateral trade agreements between the United States and other governments. The industry's agenda is front and centre, as it was in the case of the Medicare benefit law, with the United States government essentially acting as the industry's agent abroad as well as at home.

More generally, the attempt to control provider incomes leads payers through increasing restrictions on service volumes, towards some form of global budget within which the negotiation of prices for individual items of service may continue. Physicians— and drug companies—respond by trying to open up or expand access to the private funds of patients. In a number of the OECD countries they are employing the currently fashionable rhetoric of the marketplace. But that rhetoric—privatization, competition, efficiency, and so on—is simply window dressing behind which providers are still following Wildavsky's Law. They are trying to keep expenditures on health care expanding, in the face of relatively successful (outside the United States) cost control in the public sector, by seeking other sources of funds to absorb.

In terms of the balancing equation, they are trying to expand the revenue side by increasing direct charges (C) and then private insurance (R) to compensate for the restrictions on public funding through various forms of taxes (T). This would then permit continuing increases in either or both of average prices (P) and volumes of services (Q), and correspondingly increased provider incomes. Demands for extra-billing, and for expanded private "markets" more generally, in all public systems of health care finance, are thus quite understandable attempts to subvert cost *containment*, which threatens provider incomes, and replace it with cost *shifting*, which does not.

Apart from the pharmaceutical benefit debacle, the United States Medicare system has moved quite rapidly through the common stages of fee negotiation, establishing a Resource-Based Relative Value Scale (fee schedule), and introducing measures both to encourage "assignment" (discourage extra-billing) and to discourage multiplication of services—Volume Performance Standards.[34]

The result has been that over the long term, per enrollee cost has escalated less rapidly than in the private insurance sector.[35] Between 1970 and 2000 per enrollee costs for comparable services rose at an average rate of 9.6% for Medicare and 11.1% in the private insurance sector. This relatively small annual advantage, less than 1.4% per year, cumulates over thirty years to about 50%. If Medicare's control performance had been equivalent to that in the private sector, Medicare outlays per enrollee would have been 50% higher. Boccuti and Moon attribute the difference to "Medicare's ability to price aggressively." The pharmaceutical industry drew the same conclusions, and used its control of Congress to ensure that the drug benefit law, passed the next year, would forbid Medicare from using that ability.

But the principal difficulty for cost control is that American Medicare operates alongside a private insurance system that has no such controls, and much less potential for introducing them. This alternative, uncontrolled "market"—which is in reality quite unlike any normal market—weakens the bargaining power of the public program. Accordingly one finds that although Medicare pays lower fees than private insurers, it still pays very high fees by international standards. Thus the preservation of private insurance has been of vital importance to physicians in maintaining their fees and incomes, even though it pays only one third of total health care costs.

In contrast physician incomes, and where relevant, fees, have been more or less restrained— though often with bruising political struggles—in most of the other countries of the OECD. More detailed comparisons with Canada have shown quite clearly that the centralization of bargaining over physicians' fees resulted in a slowing in the escalation both of fees, and of overall outlays on physicians' services.[36] This slowing is observed relative to both previous patterns in Canada, prior to the establishment of the public universal insurance plans, and contemporaneous experience in the United States. The private insurance sector in the United State has thus played precisely the "safety valve" role that Canadian physicians have identified for it in Canada—a way of protecting their incomes in the public plan, and thus resisting cost containment.

"Interfering in the Practice of Medicine"

As noted above, health care—or anything else—can be expensive either because the people who produce it are paid a lot, or because they are not very productive. High levels of W (rates of payment), or of Z/Q (inputs per unit of output), are both reflected in higher prices P. The latter we may call technical inefficiency—more resources than necessary used up in production. Such inefficiency can show up either in the provision of health care *per se*, or in the operation of the payment system. This section focuses on health care; the organization of the payment process will be considered later.

Traditionally the payers for care, whether public or private, have avoided "interfering in the practice of medicine." They have not enquired into the details of servicing patterns, or how or why providers made their diagnostic and therapeutic decisions. Political and administrative negotiations or conflicts have focused on financial issues—fees, salaries, and budgets.

Payers in virtually every country have also tried to exert some control over the total capacity in the health care system, particularly hospital and major equipment capacity. There is general understanding that utilization of health care is predominantly capacity-driven, heavily influenced by the availability of facilities and personnel, independent of the "needs" (however defined) of the populations served.

Capacity control contributes to, but is not sufficient for, overall cost control, as American health planners have learned long ago. Culyer argues that Canada and the European countries have been more successful because they have also placed global restraints on total financing rather than relying only on controls of "demand," "supply," or capacity.[37]

Such global controls leave the maximum scope for provider autonomy within the overall physical and financial limits. The process of determining those limits, however, becomes rather arbitrary. Providers can always allege that the limits are too

tight, and that serious needs are going unmet—people dying on the waiting lists. Payers counter with the rhetoric of cost explosions—more than the country can afford. The general public, in its various roles as actual or potential patient, taxpayer, or voter, is unlikely to find the facts of the case significantly clarified by either side.

For decades, however, researchers have been observing that there are large and unexplained variations among patterns of practice and servicing rates—differences among countries, and among regions in the same country, and among individual practitioners—which seem to bear no identifiable relation to the needs of the populations served.[38] These variations show up in the fine structure of care—in particular procedures, not just aggregate utilization rates.[39]

At the same time, a considerable proportion of diagnostic and therapeutic interventions are carried on in the absence of any scientific evidence that they actually benefit patients, and in a non-trivial number of cases have been shown to do actual harm. A still more important problem, quantitatively, are those interventions which have been shown to benefit certain patients with particular conditions, but which are offered to a much wider range of patients for whom no such evidence is available.[40] This is a particularly serious problem with pharmaceuticals, since the typically very large margins between prices and costs of production create powerful incentives for maximum sales efforts, and generate the resources to support them.

The widely documented variations in patterns of health care, now stretching back over nearly 40 years, have for an equally long period been noted and then ignored. The typical response is some combination of undocumented claims that variations correspond to differences in patient needs, and when no such differences are found, some variant of "But who knows which rate is right?" Business continues as usual. But a group of researchers at Dartmouth College, under the leadership of John Wennberg, have been doggedly pursuing evidence on that question, and have begun to report findings that tie variations in health outcomes directly to variations in practice patterns.

In a series of related studies of particular procedures in the Medicare population, Fisher et al. have now shown not only that there is wide variation in patterns of utilization and cost per enrollee across hospital service areas in the United States, but that mortality is actually *higher* in the high service, high cost areas, while satisfaction levels are essentially similar. Regional populations are adjusted for age, sex, and (proxy) measures of health status. Higher rates of care use are in large part associated with higher levels of hospital and specialist availability, but the additional care does not simply add nothing to health, it is actually a threat to health. These findings have not been successfully challenged, but in the conventional rhetoric about rising needs and demands they are simply ignored.[41]

On the same theme, Baicker and Chandra report that when states are ranked on their scores on a widely accepted measure of the quality of medical care, there is a strong *negative* correlation between cost per Medicare enrollee, and also availability of specialists, and quality of care so measured. (The availability of general practitioners, however, is positively correlated with quality rankings).[42] The evidence is increasingly solid that higher costs, at least in the United States, are associated not with better quality of care, but with worse.

Such findings confirm long-standing suspicions that there is a huge potential, especially in the United States, for containing or reducing health care costs, with no harm or even benefit to patients. There is NO evidentiary basis for claims of the "Painful Prescription" variety, and much to show that the health care system of the United States is simply grossly over-funded for the work it does, and even more for what it should be doing. There is no need to "ration" access to effective care, and rationing of ineffective care is a solution, not a problem.

Realization of this potential depends, however, on improving the management of the health care system. More specifically, the system must be managed explicitly to achieve health outcomes, and to identify and eliminate ineffective and wasteful practices and procedures, rather than just to sustain traditional practices and to add whatever other new ideas attract the attention of clinicians.[43]

This realization had begun to sink in quite widely nearly twenty years ago and to emerge in serious political debate.[44] But the collapse of the Clinton national health insurance plan led to abdication by the federal government, and widespread embrace of the ideologically more comfortable faith that somehow the private business sector would be capable of managing health care for better outcomes and lower costs. The broad popularity of the idea of private "managed care" should have been a warning that it was unlikely to result in effective cost control.[45]

The principal reason for political reluctance, in virtually all countries, to tackle this issue, is that such management directly challenges the professional prerogatives of providers. Practitioners everywhere have always insisted that the "best" medicine was practiced by trained and experienced clinicians relying on their own individual clinical judgement. This is an article of faith, unshaken by observations of wide variations in clinical practice, or examples of clinical practices unsupported by and even in defiance of experimental evidence. The threat of accountability to others, who may draw on statistical and experimental evidence in evaluating and even directing their performance, strikes directly at professional autonomy. It is likely to excite even more severe political counterattacks than attempts at economic control, and may elicit substantially less support among the general public.

"Cost control" and fee/income bargaining seem to be viewed by the public, in most countries, as legitimate roles for payers. But it is not clear whether there would be political support for more detailed intrusion into the way care is provided. Even if there is widespread and very solid evidence—and there is—that a great deal of inappropriate and unnecessary care is being provided, members of the general public are not familiar with that evidence. As users of that care, they believe their needs are being met.

Thus it is probably not accidental that it is only in the United States that the political debate has most clearly turned to the evidence of specific inefficiencies in the provision of health care, and the need for detailed utilization review.[46] Other countries have managed to contain their overall costs at an acceptable level, without taking on the political dangers inherent in appearing to attack professional autonomy. But the United States has thus far completely failed to achieve such control, while simultaneously failing to provide adequate coverage for its population. There appears to be widespread and long-standing agreement among the American population that major reform is called for, but as President Clinton discovered, no agreement at all on what form it should take.[47]

Desperate times call for desperate measures. In these circumstances the United States has developed a high degree of sophistication in the technical aspects of health care management. The rapid spread of payer-enforced "guidelines" for patient treatment—*de facto* constraints—in the private sector amounts to precisely the direct "rationing" that Americans have been led to fear from state-financed systems. The ironic result has been that, in successfully fighting off "socialized medicine," American physicians have found themselves confronted with far more intrusion from payers than would be imaginable in any other country. And American patients find their choices of provider increasingly restricted, again in a way unlike any other national system.

This is not to say that providers are not restricted in other countries. Budgets are never large enough; there is never enough equipment, sufficiently up to date, or enough support staff, to do all the things physicians would like to do—especially if they are paid fees for their services. Canadian physicians feel particularly hard done by, as they compare themselves with their colleagues in the United States. But nowhere else do payers require physicians to justify and seek approval for their proposed care plans for individual patients, in order to ensure reimbursement. Payer-imposed guidelines constitute precisely the "cookbook medicine" that clinicians regard as unprofessional and dangerous for patients.

It is, of course, conceivable that if the guidelines were both valid and flexible, the care of patients could actually be improved. When there are wide variations in patterns of practice, it seems highly unlikely that *all* represent best practice—that "everything is optimal in its own way." But the private agencies that develop and enforce guidelines are trying to limit their own outlays, not to reform the practice of medicine. What they want are defensibly cheaper patterns of care; there is no reason why these should necessarily be better for patients.

It may be that the vigilance—and economic and professional interests—of providers, combined with the natural emotional bias against those who "sacrifice lives for dollars," will provide sufficient check on the stinginess of payers to prevent patients from being put at risk. But there is no guarantee of this. There may be a real need for "political entrepreneurship" to design institutions and assemble coalitions capable of offsetting payer interests, as the balance of power swings in their direction. But the present political climate is not propitious.

In any case, there is as yet no indication that the rationing of care by private payers has had more than a temporary impact on the global problems of the American health care system—uncontrolled costs, incomplete and inequitable coverage, and public dissatisfaction. There *have* been large changes in patterns of care, including major declines in the use of inpatient hospital care, over the last two decade. But any savings appear to have been absorbed in increased costs of management.

PLANES OF CLEAVAGE II: HOW DO WE SPLIT THE BILL?

Foreign experience indicates that these global problems can only be successfully addressed by coordinating the behaviour of payers, while making them politically accountable. Most other OECD countries have passed this stage, and have either a unitary payment system (the UK, Canada), or tight regulation and coordination of multiple payment agencies (Germany, France). That unity or coordination, however, is not a once-for-all achievement. It must be maintained in the face of continuing pressures from providers who recognize very clearly the connection between "sole source funding" and overall cost control—and who reject both. In the debates over "privatization" in Canada and Western Europe, providers have always been quite explicit in their attempts to expand the flow of resources to allegedly "underfunded" health care systems by diversifying the sources of funding.[48]

The assembly or maintenance of payer coalitions is made difficult not only by the efforts of providers, but also by the natural conflicts of interest among payers for and users of services. However a society determines the share of its economic resources to be given to the providers of care, it must still allocate that burden among its various members. At the same time, the terms and conditions of access to the health care goods and services provided, i.e., "Who gets what, when and how," will also depend on the structural and administrative framework.

As noted above, in a tax-financed system the distribution of economic burden is related to ability to pay, with the closeness of the relationship depending on the overall tax structure. Taxes on income tend to be roughly proportional to incomes, or even somewhat progressive, i.e., taking a larger share of income from those with higher incomes. Sales or consumption taxes are generally regressive, taking a larger share of the incomes of people with lower incomes and resting more lightly on the better off. Payroll taxes or "social insurance" premiums result in a more regressive distribution of burden, particularly if there is a ceiling for individual contributions. But in any case an individual's share of total health care costs does not depend on his/her health status.[49]

Private insurance systems, by contrast, set premiums on the basis of expected claims, as indicated by past experience. Elderly people or those with chronic illnesses will carry a larger share of health expenditures, in the form of significantly higher premiums for coverage. Competition among insurers dictates this result; a company that tried to cover all comers at the same premium ("community rating") would find that it attracted all the worst risks.[50] Direct charges to patients distribute costs according to actual illness/care experience, rather than prior expectation of expense. Which pattern of distribution is "fairer" is a political value judgment. As an empirical matter there does appear to be a broad consensus that people *should* contribute to the cost of

health care in proportion to their ability to pay, and should receive care according to their needs.[51]

Illness and income are everywhere negatively correlated, though the strength of the correlation varies across countries. A truly private financing system would thus assign the largest share of cost to those with the least resources as well as the greatest needs. But it is manifestly impossible to finance a modern health care system solely on the basis of such a distribution. The unhealthy and unwealthy would simply not get care at all. The use of health care is highly concentrated on a small proportion of the population, who are predominantly elderly and/or chronically ill.

Berk and Monheit, for example, found that among the non-institutionalized US population in 1987, the highest-using 1% accounted for 30% of all health expenditures, while the top 10% accounted for 72% of costs.[52] The lowest-using *half* of the population, on the other hand, accounted for only 3%. Forget et al. found very similar results ten years later for physician and hospital services used by the population of Manitoba population; over the period 1997–99. The highest-using 1% of the population accounted for 26% of expenditures, and the lowest half accounted for 4%. Analysis by age strata did not change this pattern.[53]

Hence the universal predominance of public payment, even in the United States. Unless a new political consensus emerges that would simply exclude a significant proportion of the population from access to health care, it is hard to see how that predominance could be challenged. On the other hand, the fact that *at any one point in time* a majority of the population is very little touched by health care costs, means that most people would not immediately be hurt by a reduction in public funding. Some would be hurt a great deal, but they are a minority.

Maintenance of the political consensus for public payment thus depends on a combination of a sense of solidarity with the less fortunate, and a prudential realization that most of us *will* become old, if we are not already, and many of us, or those close to us, will develop chronic illnesses. Only the very well off can be confident that they will never need some form of collective support, and that they can afford top priority in a private system. For them, shrinking the public sector is a rational agenda. But it follows that that political consensus is threatened by both increasing inequality of wealth and ever-escalating health costs—precisely the current trends in the United States.

In most countries, individual contributions to collective financing are simply detached from health status. The United States, however, provides public programs for those with the greatest needs and least resources (Medicare and Medicaid), and public subsidies (through income tax exemptions) for the private insurance system. The resulting distribution of burden is shown in Figure 21-2.[54] In total, health expenditures in the United States take a much smaller share of income from the highest income groups than from the lowest, even though higher income people contribute a substantially larger amount per capita.[55] The key observation, however, is that private insurance and self-payment have very

similar distributions of burden—highly regressive—while tax-financed health spending is actually mildly progressive.

This observation frames the debate over the appropriate roles of user charges and private insurance. Shifting costs from public to private budgets, implies shifting them down the income distribution, and conversely. How Joe White's shared savings (see Chapter 19) are assembled determines, to a considerable extent, what share each of us must contribute. Thus the endless debates, in every country, over the "public–private" mix of financing, are largely about how to shift the cost of care onto someone else. They never end, because they emerge from real conflicts of economic interest between the healthy and wealthy on the one hand, and the unhealthy and unwealthy on the other. Such conflicts cannot be resolved by "fact and argument."

But these struggles divert attention from the primary questions of how much to spend, and on what.

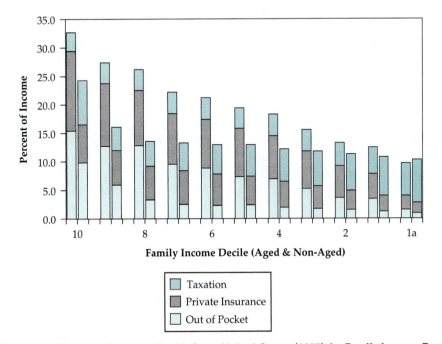

Figure 21-2 Share of Income Spent on Health Care, United States (1987), by Family Income Decile and Payment Form

It is as if a group of diners at a restaurant, greatly disturbed at the size of their total bill, and very suspicious about its contents, nevertheless spend all their energy debating who was to pay what share, rather than calling in the manager to demand an accounting for the overall cost.

Needless to say, the restaurant manager would prefer that the guests argue among themselves, rather than presenting him with a united front and demanding that he justify, and lower, his charges. The simplest summary explanation for the failure of cost control in the United States is that the institutional framework of health finance makes it easy and natural for the payers to try to pass the costs on to someone else, and very difficult for them to confront providers directly.

The intellectual framework provided by the rhetoric of the marketplace also tends to focus attention on the distribution among payers. The American economic literature perpetuates endless discussion of "deterrent charges," and the almost universal conviction that cost escalation results from low or zero "prices" to "consumers" at point of service, in spite of the obvious counter-examples in the rest of the world. Thus efforts by employers to shift the burden of health care costs to their workers—an understandable but unhelpful response to unchecked escalation—are applauded as "welfare-improving" despite their obvious lack of effect on overall costs.[56, 57]

Tax-financed systems, in which the principle of universal coverage has long been accepted, are less vulnerable to these diversions. They do, however, show increasing conflict over access to care. If the community as payer controls outlays by limiting its overall "willingness-to-pay," there will remain individuals who, perhaps encouraged by their physicians, want more. Or they may want care on more favorable terms, e.g., shorter waiting lists, more convenient bookings, nicer surroundings. Pressure from unsatisfied users generates cleavages of two kinds, between users and payers, and among users themselves.

The split between users and payers is quite straightforward. As noted above, payers are ultimately responsible to some user constituency, whether it be voters,

premium-payers, or employees. (In the final analysis, in a democratic society, they are always responsible to voters.) If the relevant constituency comes to believe that payers' efforts to contain cost escalation are threatening their own health, the controls will fail.

A delicate balance must thus be maintained between the voter-as-payer and the voter-as-(actual or potential) patient. Much of the political activity by both payers and providers is intended to elicit from voters the identification favorable to their cause. People who think of themselves as actual or potential patients are likely to support increased health care spending; people who think of themselves as taxpayers or premium-payers are more likely to support efforts to control costs. The pharmaceutical industry provides, as usual, the clearest example, spending billions on advertising and lobbying, and the subversion of individual physicians, researchers, politicians, and even economists to convince Americans, their physicians, and their political representatives that the extraordinarily high costs of drugs in the United States are justified by an ever-larger flow of health benefits.[58]

But the more contentious question concerns the treatment of those who want more services, even though there is a well-established political consensus for restraint. Should they be able to pay for more timely or perceived higher quality services, within or separately from the collective system? The affirmative argument is usually presented as an alleged "natural" right to spend ones own resources as one sees fit, spiced with anecdotes of patients dying for lack of care. But the issue is, in reality, rather different. Very few people are really willing or able to cover the full costs of medical care for serious illness out of their own pockets, so there is very little demand, in any country, for a truly private, parallel system of care in which neither providers nor patients receive any direct or indirect support from the public sector.

Rather, those who are relatively healthy and wealthy tend to favour "moderate" deterrent charges or copayments to restrict access by those with lower incomes, or the right to "go private"—in effect buying their way to the front of any queue by a relatively small extra payment.

Many providers, of course, would be only too pleased to enhance their incomes by charging additional amounts for preferential treatment, as has been the practice in the United Kingdom for years. Very few providers, if any, imagine that they could survive in a system where more than a small minority of users had to pay the full cost of their own care. But a "multi-class" system not only enables providers to charge extra for preferred access to care which is predominantly collectively financed, it also permits them to "whipsaw" payers and undermine global restraints by selectively withholding services from the patients of a particular payer, as American physicians do when they refuse to take Medicaid patients. Multiple income sources give one a stronger bargaining position. A perception that those who pay a bit extra are getting *therapeutically* superior care, i.e., better outcomes, not just better amenities, will in a democratic society eventually lead to extra payments for everybody.

All such discussion sidesteps the more fundamental issue of whether the services currently provided are medically necessary, or efficiently produced. As noted, there is substantial evidence that the short answer is "No," and that even the health care systems of Canada and Western Europe are in fact overfunded. In these circumstances, further expenditures whether individual or collective would seem ill-advised, to say the least.[59]

But the specter of "rationing," the threat that some will be denied "needed" services, is a very potent mechanism for undermining the unity of users. The least sick, and most well off, whether as voters or as patients, may be persuaded that they might fare better in a fragmented financing system with a greater element of user-pay.

And indeed some of them would. A shift from public to private funding definitely *will* move money, on average, from the less to the more wealthy as well as from the less to the more healthy—that is the message of Figure 21-2. The losers will be those, whether poor or moderately well off, who have the misfortune to become seriously ill. Providers who seek to

fragment the sources of funding, and to increase the overall flow of funds by drawing in more private money, thus have natural allies in those towards the top of the income distribution. The unique American outcome of uncontrolled overall costs and a highly regressive distribution of the burden of paying for those costs—plus much better access for the wealthy and unhealthy—reflects the success of this political coalition.

PLANES OF CLEAVAGE III: HOW MANY SPOONS IN THE DISH?

The fragmentation of financing systems, under various justifications, is accordingly a common objective of providers the world over. They look for greater ability to negotiate increased resources from the rest of society, and to protect their own autonomy from external accountability. From a professional perspective, a multiplicity of funders with deep pockets and few questions represents the ideal environment both for doing good and for doing well. But can such conditions last? Again the United States experience is critical, though the results are not all in yet. Certain generalizations, however, seem secure.

First, economic success brings competitors. Large and rapidly growing pies attract others who would like to share. The normal reaction of a competitive marketplace to a "growth industry" is that new suppliers offer the same or better products at lower prices. The customer benefits from improved quality and falling costs—consider, for example, the case of personal computers. But health care is not and never has been a competitive marketplace. The growth of the total revenues of the industry—health expenditures and incomes—has indeed drawn in new sharers, but the process and the results have been quite different from the predictions of hypothetical models of the competitive marketplace.

The first form of potential competition, starting in the 1960s, came from substitute personnel—nurse practitioners, midwives, dental therapists, chiropractors, denturists, etc. In some cases these practitioners could offer the same or better services at lower cost; in others the question of quality and servicing patterns was more open. But extensive research has left no room for doubt that, technically, such persons could significantly reduce the costs of health care services by substituting for the services of the higher-cost peak professionals, physicians and dentists.[60]

But they would in the process also reduce the income streams of such personnel—the expenditure–income identity again. Accordingly during the 1970s professionals in all countries, including the "highly competitive" United States, used their political control of the self-regulatory process to suppress the development and deployment of their potential competitors. New forms of practitioners *did* emerge, but only under the economic control of the established professions. A potentially significant form of inter-provider conflict was thus strangled at birth. The victory of the peak professionals was swift and complete.[61]

Learning from this experience, alternative practitioners have in subsequent years tried to present themselves as complementary to rather than substitutes for the established professions. They offer new and different product lines, thus trying to add to the total flow of income, and expenditures, rather than competing for a share of the existing flow. But it is pretty obvious to payers that adding still more income claimants—increasing the factor inputs (Z) in the balancing identity—is unlikely to mitigate cost pressures.

Lawyers, on the other hand, have in the United States been relatively successful in appropriating a share of the gross revenues of the health care system, through malpractice litigation.[62] In terms of the overall equation, the prices P of health services are increased to cover the costs of legal services—both plaintiffs and defendants—used up in association with health care delivery and paid for from health budgets. Lawyers have inserted themselves among the Z, raising the Z/Q ratio.

Physicians tend to be particularly bitter about this incursion, and commonly attribute rising health care costs to the pressures placed on them by the tort system.[63] The direct costs of the tort system, however, as reflected in malpractice judgments and settlements, are in fact a small and stable share of overall health care costs.[64] Lurid anecdotes about huge jury awards and the problems of particular specialties, regions, or individual practitioners grossly misrepresent the overall picture. The general rapid escalation of American health costs is drawing the cost of malpractice claims up with it. The claim that malpractice costs are responsible for that escalation is a myth.

Faced with such findings, clinicians often emphasize the addition to servicing made necessary by "defensive medicine," a cost allegedly several times greater than actual malpractice payments themselves. Such an argument implicitly concedes that a considerable proportion of servicing is "medically unnecessary," but shifts the blame from clinicians to lawyers. The solution to inappropriate care and escalating costs is . . . tort reform!

But do those who make this argument, really believe that in the absence of the malpractice threat, rates of servicing—and costs—would fall sharply? How then would provider incomes be maintained, if they were not providing, and being paid for, the additional services which make up "defensive medicine"? In reality, the lawyers provide a justification for the increase in servicing, even as they skim off a (relatively small) share of the gross revenue and subject physicians to the miseries of litigation. Blaming the lawyers is simply another diversionary tactic to shift attention away from providers themselves.

The really serious economic challenge to clinicians, however, has arisen not from lawyers but from managers and marketers. By the end of the 1980s, payment administrators and system managers had in the United States become established as the most potent new competitor for a share of health budgets.[65] They are impossible for providers to dislodge, because they have successfully integrated their services with the delivery and particularly the reimbursement of health care. Their relationship is not so much competitive as a complex combination of symbiosis and parasitism.

The fragmented funding system that prevents the containment of overall expenditures, also costs a great deal to administer. The difference between premium or tax payments *to* insurance agencies, public or private, and claims or benefits paid *by* such agencies, is an overhead cost of the payments system. It is the cost of marketing, premium setting and collection, and claims adjudication and payment, rather than of paying for services. Some such cost is unavoidable; complex institutions are not self-administering and would simply collapse without these services. But these costs are much larger in the United States than anywhere else for which data is available, and the difference adds literally tens of billions of dollars to American health care costs. Moreover they have risen dramatically over the last three decades.

Corresponding to these costs of insurance and prepayment are the large and increasing administrative costs within physicians' offices, hospitals and other care institutions made necessary by the process of complying with an increasingly complex payment system. These internal costs, which are recorded as part of the cost of providing care but again are simply "paper-pushing," add further tens of billions to expense without corresponding benefit to patients.

The team of David Himmelstein and Steffie Woolhandler, and their colleagues have been tracking these costs in a series of papers dating back over 20 years.[66] They estimate that by 1999, the *extra* administrative costs generated by the private insurance system—in both payment agencies and provider institutions—relative to the corresponding costs in a unitary, universal payment system (Canada) was $209 billion, or 17% of total US health care expenditures.[67] If this same ratio held in 2005, the excess cost—administrative waste—associated with the operations of the private health insurance system would be $330 billion.

No other country incurs administrative costs on this scale. Indeed according to the WHO (2004), no other country in the world spends as much on its entire health care system, as the United States spends to support the huge "private bureaucracy" required by its idiosyncratic system of health insurance.[68] These excess administrative costs, by themselves, account for about half the cost difference between the United States and the next most expensive countries in the world—Switzerland, Germany, Canada, France. But while they amount to pure waste motion in the financing of health care, they also account for $330 billion in incomes—wages and profits—in the insurance industry itself, in the non-clinical divisions of health care organizations, and in the benefits departments of private corporations. As President Clinton learned, those incomes are very powerfully defended.

Some may question the identification of these extraordinary administrative costs as pure waste, noting that they support a much more elaborate and sophisticated systems of management than are found in any other country. This is undoubtedly true, but rather misses the point. When more activity is paid for, more activity occurs. But this extra administrative activity yields no benefits, relative to the much simpler and less costly systems in place in other countries. The American health care system is not more efficient or less costly, indeed quite the contrary, and Americans are neither healthier not happier as a result of all this activity allegedly on their behalf. This is hardly surprising if, as noted above, the principal reason for America's much higher expenditure on health care is the much higher prices.

It is also important to be clear that "waste" is defined from the aggregate, system-wide perspective. For the individual insurance company, hospital, or physician's office, these expenditures are essential to continuing operations. But they are essential for each participant only in order to deal with the behaviour of other participants. They add nothing to, indeed detract from, the effectiveness of the system as a whole. In a more rational payment system, such as that in Canada, they vanish.

This massive bureaucracy has been built up over decades. "Between 1969 and 1999, the share of the US health care labor force accounted for by administrative workers grew from 18.2 percent to 27.3 percent. In Canada, it grew from 16.0 percent in 1971 to 19.1 percent in 1996."[69] And these data do not include insurance industry personnel. It is the product of a sort of "administrative arms race" between providers and payers in which insurers attempt to control their own liabilities by shifting costs onto others—by limiting what and whom they will reimburse. Providers, correspondingly, have had to add ever more layers of administration to get their bills paid.

In terms of the restaurant analogy, our embattled diners have each called in their own accountants and lawyers to help them minimize their share of the total bill. But the total cost of the meal is predictably escalating further, as it includes the payments to all these non-culinary personnel. The restaurant is becoming increasingly noisy and crowded, and the manager is becoming somewhat nervous. These new participants are disturbing the smooth functioning of the restaurant, and they do not order anything to eat! Furthermore, they are taking a share of his customers' money, threatening to reduce the amount available to pay his bill. So far, however, that does not seem to be happening, and he keeps on quietly padding the bill.

American providers have been caught in a dilemma. The financing system that by its diversity and complexity has protected them from external financial control is absorbing a larger and larger share of health system incomes just to keep it running. And to add insult to injury, pressures from payers have led to greatly increased attempts to influence the practice patterns of individual physicians. Physicians' autonomy is under threat from the payment system itself. Their former allies have become very expensive, and more aggressive in grabbing for the levers of power.[70] Machiavelli would have appreciated the irony of the situation.

CONFLICT MANAGEMENT? OR SAUVE QUI PEUT?

The planes of cleavage described above are universal. The management of these fundamental conflicts of interest—and particularly that between payers and providers—makes up a large part of the politics of health care finance in all developed countries. In no system can the conflict be avoided, but how it is managed makes a great deal of difference both to the balance of gains and losses, and to the amount of "collateral damage" generated in the process.

All other high income countries have created collective institutions—either public single-payer or publicly coordinated multiple-payer—for negotiating between payers and providers. The United States is unique in that the conflict remains largely decentralized even though the financing is largely collective. The results are much more advantageous to providers, at least in total, but there is a remarkably high level of collateral damage in the form of administrative waste motion as well as major financial damage to patients caught in no-man's-land. As the experience of US Medicare shows, Americans are perfectly capable of designing public payment systems that place some limits on cost escalation.[71] But as the fate of the Clinton plan and the career of the egregious Billy Tauzin demonstrate, providers are able to penetrate the political system and use the media to undermine this process or even foreclose the possibility.[72]

The most striking features of the American health care system all arise from this decentralization and fragmentation of the payment process. Most obvious is the extraordinary level and apparently uncontrollable escalation of expenditures. Present projections are that by 2014, health spending will pass 18.7% of GDP. Second is the extraordinary proportion of this expenditure absorbed in administrative waste motion. This is in turn a partial explanation of a third feature—the vastly higher American costs buy neither more care nor better health but merely support higher prices. And finally, a significant share of the non-elderly American population have grossly inadequate insurance coverage or simply none at all. This proportion, too, is projected to rise over the next few years.

The continuing cost escalation, however, will be the driver of future change. The majority of Americans can live with the problems of the uninsured, who are after all mostly other people. And those with insurance or private means appear to have been convinced that their extraordinary expenditures, while perhaps painful, are buying the "world's finest care"—technological miracles every day. The reality, that hundreds of billions are being siphoned off in useless administrative paper-pushing, has not penetrated.

Indeed one could perhaps argue that the American system, massively expensive as it is, does exactly what the dominant groups in American society *want* it to do. Bearing in mind Marmor's paraphrase of Hegel; "Nothing that is regular, is stupid," critics of that system may simply be applying inappropriate criteria. Perhaps those Americans who matter do not *want* an efficient, effective, or—heaven forbid!—equitably financed system.

Perhaps they want a system that imposes no effective limits on the business opportunities of providers of care or support services, individual or increasingly corporate. That is the other side of the expenditure coin. Accepting uncritically the marketing message that "More (and more expensive) is better," they want care unlimited in quantity or quality readily accessible at need—to those able to pay. But they refuse to be taxed to pay the corresponding costs of those less fortunate.

Such a system inevitably provides access to care that is steeply graded by social class.[73] Those at the top get the best care, easily accessible; those at the bottom are cared for, if at all, on terms that would be a political scandal in any other wealthy country. And the burden of payment will be distributed much more regressively than elsewhere—which is just fine, for those on top. If the result is greatly inflated costs and a grossly inefficient financing system, well, that is a price worth paying in order to avoid the more egalitarian outcomes of more efficient systems. Beyond rhetoric, America's current leaders have no detectable concern for improving the efficiency or effectiveness of their health care system, much less for the health of the American population. Reinhardt put it well:

That no one in the U.S. Congress shows much interest in the glaring inefficiencies that could easily be addressed within the current Medicare program speaks volumes about the true, but hidden, agenda that actually drives the quest for privatizing . . .
Crisply put, the objective is to shift responsibility for health spending on older persons from the general taxpayer onto the older people themselves . . .[74]

The various gimmicks being proposed for "reform" of America's version of Medicare illustrate Reinhardt's point. Medical Savings Accounts, Medicare + Choice, and the whole rhetoric of "consumer-directed health care," are all marketing terms for plain old-fashioned user-pay—rolling back or even eliminating Medicare, shifting costs from taxpayers to users—and thus shifting the burden of payment down the income distribution and further steepening the gradient in access. "Consumers" are people with money. Sick people are patients.

At the same time the coverage of the employment-based private insurance system has begun to erode under the pressure of ever-rising costs. General Motors provides a dramatic symbol, as the "legacy costs"—pensions and health benefits for retirees—threaten to bankrupt one of the world's greatest companies. Whether or not they do, post-retirement benefits are already being cut while current employees are facing an increasing share of health care costs. The relentless pressure of escalation leaves little choice.

The shifting of both public and private costs to users is encouraged by those American economists with the deeply held religious faith that insurance leads to "overuse."[75] Requiring users to pay more of the costs of their own care will somehow improve the efficiency of the health care system and in any case will lead to lower costs. This faith, rooted not in economic analysis but in personal ideology, has for a generation defied the American and international experience. It serves to clutter and confuse the American policy debates, but in the now relatively naked contest of class interests the economist advocates of user-pay appear to be essentially cheerleaders rather than players.

While cost-shifting strategies are a popular response to cost escalation, there is no reason to believe that, even if successful, they will halt that escalation. So what next?

National health insurance, universal and single-payer (or coordinated multiple payers) remains the only known way of containing costs, but it seems at least as remote as ever in the American political context. Perhaps a dramatic loss of coverage over the next decade will produce a political earthquake, but present signs are hard to find. "Managed care" mechanisms appeared to yield a certain amount of success in the mid-1990s; perhaps they can be revived and adapted to make these more acceptable and effective.[76] Perhaps.[77]

A very clear-eye view of the options emerges from a confidential memorandum drafted for the Board of Directors of Wal-Mart.[78] The memorandum considers both variants on the "managed care" strategies—steering employees ("associates" in Wal-Mart-speak) toward more conservative and less costly providers—and increases in deductibles and copayments. But it concludes that while both should be expanded, neither approach is likely to have significant impact.

The memorandum then notes that, as in all populations, a high proportion of health care costs are generated by a relatively small proportion of employees. If one could identify these employees and find ways to outplace them, or better still to avoid hiring them in the first place, that *could* have a significant impact on Wal-Mart's costs. Crudely put: "Dump the Dogs."

This could work. And it is highly doubtful that Wal-Mart is the only American company to have thought of it. Why not? Private employers, like private insurers, are not charities. Employment-based coverage already excludes those with the highest risks—the elderly, the unemployable, the poor—leaving them for the public sector to cover. It is a logical extension of the basic principles of private insurance. What happens to those higher-risk people? Well, that is not Wal-Mart's problem.[79]

Perhaps government will step in again? The Bush administration has been steadily weakening the fiscal position of the federal government—quite possibly deliberately—through tax cuts and military

spending. Large deficits have cumulated into a rising burden of public debt (relative to national income). Without tax increases there is little scope for increased public spending, even if the will were there.

If employers begin to follow the route suggested in the Wal-Mart memorandum, the high users may simply be pushed over to uninsured employment, or out of the workforce. The consequences are well-known—health care costs draining family savings, accumulating medical debt, and increasing difficulty of access to poorer quality care.[80] Solving the corporate cost problem by dumping the dogs will reduce access for precisely those who need care most, while transferring more of the financial burden onto the weaker shoulders (which may include state Medicaid programs). But at least it will finally moderate the cost escalation.

Or will it? No scenario is plausible that fails to consider the reaction of providers. [This has been the great, gaping flaw in discussions of the health care sector in the American economics literature.] If the Wal-Mart approach works, it will threaten the ever-growing revenues of the American health care industry. How will they react?

An emerging answer is suggested by "concierge" or "boutique" doctors, "who, in exchange for a yearly cash retainer, lavish time, phone calls and attention on patients, using the latest in electronic communications to streamline their care."[81] The yearly cash retainers are set high enough that they represent "a huge increase in per-patient reimbursement [that] allows the patient loads to be kept low." In short, concierge doctors—general practitioners and internists—make much more money while seeing far fewer patients, but caring for them much more intensively. And wealthy patients are in fact delighted to pay what is for them a relatively small annual retainer for highly personalized care, including hands-on guidance through the jungle of the American medical system.

The "value-added" services offered by concierge care include" same-day or next-day appointments and 24-hour telephone access to the doctor" and at the high end "home visits, deliver[ing] medications and accompany[ing] patients on visits to other doctors." These hardly seem like the most effective use of the physician's time, but wealthy patients are willing to pay. Unwealthy patients, who do not pay the retainer, are someone else's problem.

Without trying to speculate as to how large this particular market might become, one can easily see the general principle behind it—greatly enhanced revenue per patient. If insurance coverage shrinks, so does the revenue potential from those with lower incomes. In terms of the fundamental balancing equation above, if T and R begin to shrink, providers can maintain their incomes only by finding ways to increase C. And they will.

Those who can pay must be induced to pay more, by the offer of value-added services, where "value" is defined as anything they are willing to pay for. What forms these innovations will take is difficult to predict; markets are endlessly imaginative. (Regular and comprehensive diagnostic imaging as "preventive" screening—MRI for those willing to pay—appears to offer substantial opportunities.) But the combination of eroding insurance coverage—public and private—and continuing pressure to maintain provider revenues seem likely to drive an increasing separation between access and need.

As providers, like the famous bank robber Willie Sutton, "go where the money is," access to care will over time become increasingly determined by willingness/ability to pay, and less and less by actual need for care. This is, after all, the way normal markets work, and it is the pattern that many American economists have been advocating for a generation. It is not a healthy situation, certainly not for the unhealthy and unwealthy.

At least so go the current trends. The interesting question, however, is whether, as those in the middle income ranges become increasingly vulnerable while costs continue to escalate, an effective constituency finally emerges for major political change. But that is too far down the road to see at this point. For now, most Americans still seem willing to believe that they have the world's finest health care. As

James Thurber said: "You can fool too many of the people, too much of the time."

STUDY QUESTIONS

1. What proportion of American health care is purchased out-of-pocket? What are the other main payers in the American system?
2. What sets the purchase of health care apart from that of commodities in a market system?
3. How has the United States become the 'odd man out' in terms of international trends in health expenditure?
4. According to Evans' analysis, what broad factors contribute to cost escalation in American health care?
5. What are the main threats to the professional autonomy of providers in the contemporary American system?
6. What does the evidence suggest when it comes to the question of whether Americans receive 'enough' or 'superior' health care?
7. What are some ways providers can continue to increase health costs, even while fewer people can afford care?
8. What are the three broad planes of conflict that mark every system?
9. For each of the three broad planes of conflict, what is unique about the American system?

NOTES

1. Joe White, 1995.
2. Heffler et al., 2005.
3. Remarkably, however, out of pocket payments *as a share of GDP* have not changed much: 2.12% in 2005, down from 2.60% in 1960, and the ratio has fluctuated within a relatively narrow band. Meanwhile the share covered through collective mechanisms has gone up five times, from 2.7% to 13.5% of GDP.

4. Holahan and Wang, 2004.

5. Heffler et al., 2005.

6. The premiums are deductible from the employer's taxable income, but not taxed as income in the hands of the employee. This public subsidy provides the greatest benefits to people in the highest tax brackets; those with no taxable income receive no support from the general taxpayer. This "reverse Robin Hood," or "Sheriff of Nottingham" feature no doubt accounts for its political resilience.

7. Sheils and Haught, 2004. It is not obvious whether private health insurance could survive in the United States without this "life support" from the public treasury.

8. Woolhandler and Himmelstein, 2002.

9. There is a market for individual coverage, but in these contracts only about one dollar in two is actually paid out in benefits. Marketing expenses eat up much of the rest, since bad products take a lot of selling. Holahan and Wang (2004) find that private non-group insurance is the primary form of coverage for only 5.3% of their study population, which would amount to 4.5% of the total US population in 2002. There is, of course, an active individual market for "medigap" insurance to cover the holes in the public Medicare program for the elderly; but this is a low-risk product precisely because it is only supplementary.

10. Fein, 1986.

11. Gilmer and Kronick, 2005.

12. Schoen et al., 2005.

13. All generalizations are false. *Individuals* at higher risk do not make larger contributions. But in employment-based systems, of which Germany is a leading example, people (and their employers) do contribute a larger or smaller proportion of their earnings for coverage, depending upon the overall income and health status of the membership of the Sickness Fund to which they belong. Within each fund, however, the contribution percentage is the same for all, so higher income people pay more, and sicker people do not. But the range of variation among funds is limited by law, and there is enforced cross-subsidization. A portion of the contributions of members of "healthier" funds is transferred to "sicker" funds to reduce the burden on their membership. In particular, retired members are supported from a separate pool, drawn from the contributions of working members of all Sickness Funds. Such cross-subsidization is found in all systems of social insurance built up from separate funds.

14. They may become heavily involved, through setting criteria for reimbursement, in the standards of care for individual patients. But the implications, if any, for system-wide behaviour are far from clear.

15. Abel-Smith, 1992; Abel-Smith and Mossialos, 1994.

16. Strictly speaking, in an open economy the identity must be extended to account for external purchasers and suppliers of health care—exports and imports. It would also require an explicit inter-temporal structure to allow for changes in asset levels. But these additional complications are well known from national income accounting, and add no further enlightenment to compensate for the extra notation.

17. Not "buyers" and "sellers." The dominance of collective funding, combined with professional self-regulation and external public regulation, and rooted ultimately in the obvious fact that most users of health care are not able to define their own needs without professional help, implies that the images of the "free market," with voluntary exchange of goods/services for money, between fully informed, self-interested, autonomous and unconstrained transactors, exist only in the dreamworld of neoclassical economic theory.

18. Evans, 1985, 1986.

19. Wildavsky, 1977.

20. Williams, 1978. Some might wonder why the question of "What is worth paying for?" is treated as political rather than economic. For many commodities we appeal to the principle of Consumer Sovereignty, and rely on individuals to indicate, in the marketplace, what commodities each of them believes is worth paying for.

The choice process is decentralized. But the decision to leave that process to the free market—where among other things peoples' preferences are weighted by their wealth, not by their needs—is itself a political choice. For a variety of reasons, no country in the world has seen fit to do this for health care. In the United States, however, the very strong ideological commitment to free markets as ends in themselves is in continuous tension with powerful humanitarian values. These make citizens very uncomfortable with the results inevitably generated by markets in health care. The result has been a form of schizophrenia in health policy, and a lurching back and forth from one approach to another.

21. The "Painful Prescription" popularized by Aaron and Schwartz, 1984.

22. It may seem strange that we have grouped those who call for ever more money to "meet the needs," with those who argue that ultimately there will not *be* more money, because ever-growing demands will run into fundamental resource constraints. The critical linkage is that both assume that "more is better," and dismiss or more often simply ignore extensive evidence to the contrary. Thus in the near term, the "rationing" rhetoric serves to promote the further expansion of health care.

23. Maynard, 1981, p 145.

24. Mackenbach, 1991.

25. These are less volatile than exchange rates, not being sensitive to the effects of short-term capital movements. They attempt to compare the relative costs of similar baskets of commodities in each country.

26. Fuchs and Hahn, 1990; Nair et al., 1992; Redelmeier and Fuchs, 1993: Anderson et al., 2003, 2005.

27. Eisenberg et al., 2005.

28. Anderson et al., 2003. This finding implies that a large part of the differential is due to higher relative prices of health care in the United States, not to higher levels of services. It is not just that prices for health care goods and services were higher in the United States than elsewhere. They were; but the point is that the ratio of health care prices to the general price level was also much higher in the United States than in other countries. Americans received on average (at that time), no more care than Canadians, very little more than Japanese, and much less than Swedes. But they paid much more, relatively, for what they got. In terms of the equation above, P (the price) is higher in the United States than anywhere else.

29. Reinhardt, 1987.

30. OECD, 1987, p 76; Gerdtham and Jönsson, 1991a; Groenewegen et al., 1991; Fein, 1992.

31. But if salaried practitioners are also permitted to engage in some level of private fee practice, the level of effort (not) devoted to the salaried service and the steering of patients toward more remunerative private care become continuing problems that seem beyond the reach of negotiation or monitoring.

32. They found that, for patients with clinically equivalent problems, physicians who owned their own diagnostic radiology facilities took on average *four times* as many films, and charged 40% more, for a total cost over six times higher, than physicians who referred to arm's-length radiologists. Such observations rather undercut the claim that the volume of services provided is simply a response to patient needs—or for that matter, demands.

33. Pear, 2004.

34. There has always been a fee schedule for services paid by Medicaid, but this is generally viewed as "welfare medicine," outside the American mainstream. Not all practitioners accept Medicaid patients, because the fees are considerably lower than those of Medicare, let alone private insurance.

35. Boccuti and Moon, 2003.

36. Barer et al., 1988; Evans, 1987.

37. Culyer, 1988.

38. Lewis, 1969; Bunker, 1970; Vayda, 1973; McPherson et al., 1982; Roos et al., 1986; Chassin et al., 1986; Ham, 1988, and many more.

39. The distinction between inefficient production, and ineffective care, becomes fuzzy here. If a stay in hospital is unnecessarily prolonged, is this the

inefficient production of an episode of care, or the production of ineffective hospital days? At the most aggregated level, all ineffective care represents the inefficient production of health.

40. Banta et al., 1981; Feeny et al., 1986.
41. Fisher et al., 2003a, 2003b.
42. Baicker and Chandra, 2004.
43. Wennberg, 1984, 1988.
44. *The Economist*, 1988; Roper et al., 1988; Andersen and Mooney, 1989.
45. In fairness, the aggregate cost trends of the mid-1990s gave some reason to hope that this might happen, though many observers of the industry remained skeptical. Since then, their skepticism has been amply justified.
46. Roper et al., 1988.
47. Blendon, 1989.
48. Weller and Manga, 1983.
49. Of course total financial outlays are only one component of cost. Being ill or injured is a significant burden in itself; it may also result in loss of income and/or other additions to living expenses. The direct burden is inevitably borne by the patient; other economic losses are at best partially compensated.
50. The non-profit "Blue" plans in the United States began in the 1930s by community rating, with exactly this result. Competition from the for-profit sector forced a shift to experience rating, or charging different premiums to different groups on the basis of estimated risk (Fein, 1986).
51. van Doorslaer et al., 1993.
52. Berk and Monheit, 1992.
53. Forget et al. (2002). It is important to appreciate that this heavy concentration of costs does not represent a random distribution of misfortune. The heavy users are typically carrying a long-term burden of illness.
54. Figure II drawn from Rasell et al., 1993.
55. Families in the top 5% of the income distribution contributed $13,234 to health care in 1987, but this was only 10.2% of their incomes, while the $960 contributed by families in the lowest decile was 26.9% of their much smaller incomes. Taxation to support health care funded through the public sector accounted for most of the difference in dollar amounts. The top 5% contributed $9,650 in taxes or 7.3% of their incomes; the bottom 10% were taxed only $214 per family or 6.8% of income. But their average payment of $746 for insurance and direct charges was 20.2% of income, compared with the 3% ($3,584) paid out by the 5% of families at the top (Rasell et al., 1993, table 1).
56. There is also a very strong ideological component to the conflict among payers and users (Weller and Manga, *op. cit.*). Since illness is inversely correlated with social class, whether measured by income, or education, or looser measures of status, the detachment of economic burden from either actual or expected illness results in a corresponding redistribution of income from higher to lower levels in the social hierarchy. To some this egalitarian effect is offensive *per se*, even if it is associated with a lower overall burden of expenditures.
57. Manning et al., 1987.
58. Pear, 2003.
59. Rachlis and Kushner (1989) have written a comprehensive and very accessible survey of that evidence for the Canadian system. The western European systems show a similar pattern (Maynard, 1981; Enthoven, 1985, Culyer et al., 1988). Yet Canada and the major European nations spend between 8 and 10% of their national incomes on health care, while the United States spends over 15%, and still rising.
60. E.g., Record, 1981; Spitzer, 1984.
61. Spitzer, 1984.
62. The lawyer's fees are paid from the plaintiff's award, which is paid by the malpractice insurer, who in turn collects a share of the physician's gross receipts as malpractice premiums. The physician passes on this cost in higher fees, and/or increased rates of servicing, to the patient or the patient's insurer. The latter, government or employer, passes the cost to taxpayers or customers. At no point is there an agency

with the authority or the incentive to control the process.

63. Hence the bumper sticker: "Support a lawyer; send your child to medical school." Defenders of the tort system argue that the increase in legal inputs "buys" an improvement in the quality of output, keeping doctors on their toes in a way that regulation—especially self-regulation—never could. But this argument appears to be largely *a priori*, presented by interested parties operating in a data-free environment.

64. Chandra et al., 2005.

65. Lee and Etheredge, 1989.

66. Himmelstein and Woolhandler, 1986; Woolhandler and Himmelstein, 1991; Himmelstein *et al.*, 1996; Woolhandler *et al.*, 2003.

67. Woolhandler et al., 2003.

68. Woolhandler et al., 2003.

69. Woolhandler et al., 2003.

70. Webber and Goldbeck, 1984; Roper et al., *op. cit.*; Lee and Etheredge, *op. cit.*

71. Boccuti and Chandra, *op. cit.*

72. Pear, 2004.

73. E.g., Scott, 2005.

74. Reinhardt, 2001, p 201.

75. It is critical to understand that this economic concept of "overuse" bears absolutely no relation to patient needs or the effectiveness or appropriateness of care. It is defined solely in terms of "willingness"—i.e., typically ability—to pay, and is thus a purely ideological concept. Economists, however, all too rarely make this clear.

76. Schur et al., 2004.

77. In considering the relative long-term prospects for either single-payer or managed care, it may be relevant that the payment systems in place in other countries have only two roles for private insurance, (i) much reduced, or (ii) none. Managed care offers a continuing and even expanded role (and revenue) for private insurers as system managers. Against this enormous advantage, the fact that it may not work is a trivial objection.

78. Chambers, 2005; Greenhouse and Barbaro, 2005.

79. We may anticipate some accompanying rhetoric about high-risk people having deserved their fate—obesity, smoking, etc. There may also be quietly increased

80. Collins et al., 2004.

81. Zuger, 2005.

REFERENCES

Aaron, H.J., and W.B. Schwartz. 1984. *The Painful Prescription: Rationing in Health Care.* Washington DC, The Brookings Institution.

Abel-Smith, B. 1985. "Who is the odd man out: the experience of Western Europe in containing the costs of health care," *The Milbank Quarterly* 63 (1): 1–17.

Abel-Smith, B. 1992. "Cost Containment and New Priorities in the European Community," *The Milbank Quarterly* 70 (3): 393–416.

Abel-Smith, B., and E. Mossialos. 1994. "Cost containment and health care reform: A study of the European Union," *Health Policy* 28: 89–132.

Andersen, T.F., and G. Mooney, eds. 1990. *The Challenges of Medical Practice Variations.* London: MacMillan.

Andersen, G.F., et al. 2003. "It's the Prices, Stupid: Why the United States Is So Different from Other Countries," *Health Affairs* 23 (3): 89–105.

Anderson, G.F., P.S. Hussey, B.K. Frogner, et al. 2005. "Health Spending in the United States and the Rest of the Industrialized World," *Health Affairs* 24 (4): 903–14.

Baicker, K., and A. Chandra. 2004. "Medicare Spending, the Physician Workforce, and Beneficiaries' Quality of Care," *Health Affairs* Web Exclusive (April 7): 184–97.

Barer, M.L., R.G. Evans, and R.J. Labelle. 1988. "Fee Controls as Cost Control: Tales from the Frozen North," *The Milbank Quarterly* 66 (1): 1–64.

Banta, H.D., C. Behney, and J.S. Willems. 1981. Toward Rational Technology in Medicine: Considerations for Health Policy. New York: Springer.

Baumol, W.J. 1988. "Price Controls for Medical Services and the Medical Needs of the Nation's Elderly," Paper prepared with the financial support of the American Medical Association and presented before the Physician Payment Review Commission, Washington DC, February 11.

Berk, M.L., and A.C. Monheit. 1992. "The
Concentration of Health Expenditures: An Update,"
Health Affairs 11 (4): 145–9.

Boccuti, C., and M. Moon. 2003. "Comparing Medicare
and Private Insurers: Growth Rates in Spending
Over Three Decades," *Health Affairs* 22 (2):
230–7.

Blendon, R.J. 1989. "Three Systems: A Comparative
Survey," *Health Management Quarterly* 11 (1):
2–10.

Bunker, J.P. 1970. "Surgical Manpower. A Comparison
of Operations and Surgeons in the United States
and in England and Wales," *New England Journal of
Medicine* 282 (3 January 15): 135–44.

Chambers, S. 2005. Reviewing and Revising Wal-Mart's
Benefit Stratety. BOC Retreat FY06.

Chandra, A., S. Nundy, and S.A. Seaberg. 2005. "The
Growth of Physician Medical Malpractice Payments:
Evidence From the National Practitioner Data
Bank," *Health Affairs* 5 (May 31): 240–9.

Chassin, M.R., R.H. Brook, R.E. Park, et al. 1986.
"Variations in the Use of Medical and Surgical
Services by the Medicare Population," *New England
Journal of Medicine* 314 (5 January 30): 285–90.

Collins, S.R., M.M. Doty, K. Davis, et al. 2004. The
Affordability Crisis in U.S. Health Care: Findings
From the Commonwealth Fund Biennial Health
Insurance Survey. Commonwealth Fund publication
#723, New York (March).

Culyer, A.J. 1988. Health Expenditures in Canada:
Myth and Reality, Past and Future. Toronto:
Canadian Tax Foundation.

Culyer, A.J., J.E. Brazier, and O. O'Donnell. 1988.
*Organizing Health Service Provision: Drawing on
Experience*, working paper no. 2. Working Party on
Alternative Delivery and Funding of Health
Services, London: Institute of Health Services
Management.

The Economist. 1988. "Fallible Doctors. Patient's
Dilemma," 309 (7581 December 17): 19–21.

Eisenberg, M.J., K.B. Filion, A. Azoulay, et al. 2005.
"Outcomes and Cost of Coronary Artery Bypass
Graft Surgery in the United States and Canada,"
Archives of Internal Medicine 165: 1506–13.

Evans, R.G. 1985. "Illusions of Necessity; Evading
Responsibility for Choice in Health Care," *Journal
of Health Policy, Politics and Law* 10 (3): 439–67.

—— 1986. "Finding the Levers, Finding the Courage:
Lessons from Cost Containment in North America,"

Journal of Health Politics, Policy and Law 11 (4):
pp 585–616.

Evans, R.G., M.L. Barer, and G.L. Stoddart. 1994.
*Charging Peter to Pay Paul: Accounting for the
Financial Effects of User Charges.* Toronto: The
Premier's Council on Health, Well-being and Social
Justice, June.

Enthoven, A.C. 1985. *Reflections on the Management of
the National Health Service.* London: The Nuffield
Provincial Hospitals Trust (Occasional papers No. 5).

Feeny, D., G. Guyatt, and P. Tugwell. 1986. *Health Care
Technology: Effectiveness, Efficiency and Public
Policy*. Montreal: Institute for Research on Public
Policy.

Fein, R. 1986. Medical Care, Medical Costs: The Search
for a National Health Policy. Cambridge, MA:
Harvard University Press.

—— 1992. "Health Care Reform," *Scientific American*
267 (5): 46–53.

Fisher, E.S., H.G. Welch, and J.E. Wennberg. 1992.
"Prioritizing Oregon's Hospital Resources: An
Example Based on Variations in Discretionary
Medical Utilization," *Journal of the American
Medical Association* 267 (14): 1925–31.

Fisher, E.S., et al. 2003a. "The Implications of Regional
Variations in Medicare Spending: Part 1. The
Content, Quality and Accessibility of Care," *Annals
of Internal Medicine* 138 (4): 273–87.

Fisher, E.S., et al. "The Implications of Regional
Variations in Medicare Spending: Part 2. Health
Outcomes and Satisfaction with Care," *Annals of
Internal Medicine* 138 (4): 288–98.

Forget, E., R. Deber, and L.L. Roos. 2002. "Medical
Savings Accounts; Will They reduce Costs?"
Canadian Medical Association Journal 167 (2):
143–7.

Fuchs, V.R., and J.S. Hahn. 1990. "How Does Canada
Do It? A Comparison of Expenditures for
Physicians' Services in the United States and
Canada," *New England Journal of Medicine* 323
(13): 884–90.

Gerdtham, U.-G., and B. Jönsson. 1991a. "Health care
expenditure in Sweden—An international
comparison," *Health Policy* 19: 211–28.

—— 1991b. "Price and quantity in international
comparisons of health care expenditure," *Applied
Economics* 23: 1519–28.

Gilmer, T., and R. Kronick. 2005. "It's the Premiums,
Stupid: Projections of the Uninsured Through

2013," *Health Affairs* Web Exclusive (April 5) W5: 148.

Greenhouse, S., and M. Barbaro. 2005. "Wal-Mart Memo Suggests Ways to Cut Employee Benefit Costs," *New York Times* October 26.

Groenewegen, P.P., J. van der Zee, and R. van Haaften. 1991. *Remunerating General Practitioners in Western Europe*. Aldershot: Avebury, p 125.

Ham, C., ed. 1988. *Health Care Variations: Assessing the Evidence*. London: The King's Fund Institute (Research Report No. 2).

Heffler, S., S. Smith, S. Keehan, et al. 2005. "U.S. Health Spending Projections for 2004-2014," *Health Affairs* (February 23) W5: 74–85.

Hillman, B.J., et al. 1990. "Frequency and Costs of Diagnostic Imaging in Office Practice—A Comparison of Self-referring and Radiologist-Referring Physicians," *New England Journal of Medicine* 323 (23): 1604–8.

Himmelstein D.U., and S. Woolhandler. 1986. "Cost Without Benefit: Administrative Waste in U.S. Health Care," *New England Journal of Medicine* 314 (7): 441–5.

Himmelstein, D.U., J. Lewontin, and S. Woolhandler. 1996. "Who Administers Who Cares? Medical Administrative and Clinical Employment in the United States and Canada," *American Journal of Public Health* 86 (2): 172–8.

Holahan, J., and M. Wang. 2004. "Changes in Health Insurance Coverage During the Economic Downturn: 2000-2002," *Health Affairs* (January 28) W4: 31–42.

Lee, P.R., and L. Etheredge. 1989. "Clinical Freedom: Two Lessons for the UK from US experience with Privatisation of Health Care," *The Lancet* (February 4): 263–6.

Levit, K.R., et al. 1994. "National Health Spending Trends, 1960-1993," *Health Affairs* 13 (Winter 5): 124–36.

Mackenbach, J.P. 1991. "Health Care Expenditure and Mortality from Amenable Conditions in the European Community," *Health Policy* 19 (2+3): 245–55.

Marmor, T.R. 1983. *Political Analysis and American Medical Care: Essays*. Cambridge: Cambridge University Press.

Manning, W.G., J.P. Newhouse, N. Duan, et al. 1987. "Health Insurance and the Demand for Medical Care," *American Economic Review* 77 (3): 251–77.

Maynard, A. 1981. "The Inefficiency and Inequalities of the Health Care Systems of Western Europe," *Social Policy and Administration* 15 (2): 145–63.

McPherson, K., J.E. Wennberg, O.B. Hovind, and P. Clifford. 1982. "Small Area Variations in the Use of Common Surgical Procedures: An International Comparison of New England, England and Norway," *New England Journal of Medicine* 307 (21): 1310–4.

Nair, C., R. Karim, and C. Nyers. 1992. "Health Care and Health Status: A Canada-United States Statistical Comparison," *Health Reports* 4 (October 2) Ottawa: Statistics Canada (cat. no. 82-003), pp 175–83.

OECD. 1987. Financing and Delivering Health Care: A Comparative Analysis of OECD Countries. Social Policy Studies No. 4, Paris: OECD.

—— 1994. The Reform of Health Care Systems: A Review of Seventeen OECD Countries. Health Policy Studies No. 5, Paris: OECD.

Pear, R. 2003. "Drug Companies Increase Spending to Lobby Congress and Governments," *New York Times* May 31.

—— 2004. "House's Author of Drug Benefit Joins Lobbyists," *New York Times* December 15.

Rachlis, M., and C. Kushner. 1989. Second Opinion: What's Wrong With Canada's Health-Care System and How to Fix It. Toronto: Collins.

Rasell, M.E., J. Bernstein, and K. Tang. 1993. "The Impact of Health Care Financing on Family Budgets," Economic Policy Institute Briefing Paper (April). Washington DC: Economic Policy Institute.

Record, J.C., ed. 1981. Staffing Primary Care in 1990: Physician Replacement and Cost Savings. New York: Springer.

Redelmeier, D.A., and V.R. Fuchs. 1993. "Hospital Expenditures in the United Staes and Canada," *New England Journal of Medicine* 328(11 March 18): 772–8.

Reinhardt, U.E. 1987. "Resource Allocation in Health Care: The Allocation of Lifestyles to Providers," *The Milbank Quarterly* 65 (2): 153–76.

—— 1988. "On The B-Factor in American health care," *Washington Post* August 9, p 20.

—— 2001. "Commentary: On the Apocalypse of the Retiring Baby Boom" in "Northern Lights: Perspectives on Canadian Gerontological Research", Special Supplement *Canadian Journal of Aging* 20 (supp1, Summer): 192–204.

Roos, N.P., G. Flowerdew, A. Wajda, and R.B. Tate. 1986. "Variations in Physicians' Hospitalization Practices: A Population-Based Study in Manitoba, Canada," *American Journal of Public Health* 76 (1): 45–51.

Roper, W.L., W. Winkenwerder, G.M. Hackbarth, and H. Krakauer. 1988. "Effectiveness in Health Care: An Initiative to Evaluate and Improve Medical Practice," *New England Journal of Medicine* 319 (18 November 3): 1197–202.

Schieber, G.J., J.-P. Poullier, and L.M. Greenwald. 1994. "Health System Performance in OECD Countries, 1980-1992," *Health Affairs* 13 (3): 100–12.

Schoen, C., M.M. Doty, S.R. Collins, and A.L. Jolmgren. 2005. "Insured but not Protected: How Many Adults Are Underinsured?," *Health Affairs* (June 14) W5: 289–302.

Schur, C.L., M.L. Berk, and J.M. Yegian. 2004. "Public Perceptions of Cost Containment Strategies: Mixed Signals for Managed Care," *Health Affairs* (November 10) W4: 516–25.

Scott, J. 2005. "Life at the Top in America Isn't Just Better, It's Longer," *New York Times* May 16.

Sheils, J., and R. Haught. 2004. "The Cost of Tax-Exempt Health Benefits in 2004," *Health Affairs* (February 25) W4: 106–12.

Spitzer, W.O. 1984. "The Nurse Practitioner Revisited: Slow Death of a Good Idea," *New England Journal of Medicine* 310 (16 April 19): 1049–51.

van Doorslaer, E., A. Wagstaff, and Frans Rutten, eds. 1993. *Equity in the Finance and Delivery of Health Care: An International Perspective.* Oxford: Oxford University Press.

Vayda, E. 1973. "A Comparison of Surgical Rates in Canada and in England and Wales," *New England Journal of Medicine* 289 (23 December 6): 1224–9.

Webber, A., and W.B. Goldbeck. 1984. "Utilization Review," in P.D. Fox, W.B. Goldbeck, and J.J. Spies, eds. *Health Care Cost Management: Private Sector Initiatives.* Ann Arbor: Health Administration Press, pp 69–90.

Weller, G.R., and P. Manga. 1983. "The Push for Reprivatization of Health Care Services in Canada, Britain and the United States," *Journal of Health Politics, Policy and Law* 8 (3): 495–518.

Wennberg, J.E. 1984. "Dealing With Medical Practice Variations: A Proposal for Action" *Health Affairs* 3 (2): 6–32.

—— 1988. "Practice Variations and the Need for Outcomes Research," in C. Ham, ed. *Health Care Variations: Assessing the Evidence.* London: The King's Fund Institute (Research Report No. 2), pp 32–5.

White, J. 1995. Competing Solutions: American Health Care Proposals and International Experience. Washington DC: The Brookings Institution.

Wildavsky, A. 1977. "Doing Better and Feeling Worse: The Political Pathology of Health Policy," *Daedalus* 106 (1): 105–24.

Williams, A. 1978. "Need: An Economic Exegesis," in *Economic Aspects of Health Services*, A.J. Culyer and K.G. Wright, eds. London: Martin Robertson, pp 32–45.

Woolhandler, S., and D.U. Himmelstein. 1991. "The Deteriorating Administrative Efficiency of the U.S. Health Care System," *New England Journal of Medicine* 324 (18): 1253–8.

—— 2002. "Paying for National Health Insurance—and Not Getting It," *Health Affairs* 21 (4 July-August): 88–98.

Woolhandler, S., T. Campbell, and D.U. Himmelstein. 2003. "Costs of Health Care Administration in the United States and Canada," *New England Journal of Medicine* 349 (8 August 21): 768–75.

World Health Organization. 2004. *World Health Report 2004—changing history.* (Annex tables 5 and 6). Geneva: WHO.

Zuger, A. 2005. "For a Retainer, Lavish Care by 'Boutique Doctors'," *New York Times* October 30.

Ted Marmor, Richard Freeman, and Kieke Okma

The following Consider This… concludes the section on international politics by explaining how to compare systems and how to learn about health care from other nations. Looking at other nations can be a marvelous way to stretch the mind and expand our knowledge of what is possible. On the other hand, the authors warn against treating comparative studies like a sports tournament (which system wins?) or a shopping trip (can we pick up these policy items and use them back home?).

We are constantly bombarded by health care information from other countries.[1] Yet, despite the volume and velocity of the information flows, it is not easy to learn useful lessons from foreign experience. A large gap falls between promise and performance in comparative health policy studies.[2] Misdescription and superficiality are common.

Unwarranted inferences, rhetorical distortion, and caricatures all regularly show up in both scholarship and policy debates. In this chapter, we suggest how to avoid the common pitfalls and learn useful lessons from other nations.

THE POLITICAL CONTEXT: WELFARE STATE DEBATES AND HEALTH REFORMS 1970–2000

Health policy is prominently on the public agenda of most if not all of the industrial democracies. Canada's universal health insurance is a model of achievement for many observers, the subject of considerable intellectual scrutiny, and the destination of many policy travelers searching for illumination. Yet both the national government and a majority of its provinces have felt sufficiently concerned about the condition of Canadian Medicare to set up advisory commissions and chart adjustments.

The United States has been even more obvious about its medical care worries, with crisis commentary a fixture for decades on the national agenda. Fretting about medical care costs, quality, and access is not limited to North America. Disputes about reforming Dutch medical care have been going for decades. Any review of the European experience would discover persistent policy controversies in Germany (burdened by the fiscal pressures of unification), in Great Britain (with recurrent debates about the National Health Service), and in Italy and Sweden (both facing fiscal and unemployment pressures).

The puzzle is not why there is such widespread interest in health policy, but why now. Why does international evidence (arguments, claims, caricatures) seem so much more prominent at the turn of the 21st century than, say, during the fiscal strains of the mid-1970s or early 1980s? What can be usefully said not only about the substance of the experience of different nations, but about the political processes of introducing and acting upon policy change in a national context?

There is a simple answer to these questions. Medical care policy came to the forefront of public agendas for the following reasons. First, the financing of personal medical care everywhere became a major financial component of the budgets of mature welfare states. When fiscal strain arises, policy scrutiny is the predictable result. Second, mature welfare states have less capacity for bold fiscal expansion in new areas. This means that managing existing programs assumes a more prominent place on the public agenda.[3] Thirdly, the post war consensus about the welfare state is wearing out (perhaps wearing down). We see the effects of more than two decades of fretfulness about the affordability, desirability, and governability of the welfare state.

The reexaminations of health care arrangements began in earnest when the 1973–74 oil shock exacerbated high levels of unemployment and persistent stagflation. Critics became bolder, bolstered by the electoral victories of conservative parties opposed to welfare state expansion. Mass publics increasingly heard challenges to programs that had for decades seemed sacrosanct. From Mulroney (Canada) to Thatcher (Britain), from New Zealand to the Netherlands—the message of serious problems requiring major change gained support. Accordingly, when economic strain reappears, the inner rim of programmatic protection—not just interest group commitment, but social faith—weakens, and the incentives to explore transformative but not fiscally burdensome options become relatively stronger. Those factors help to explain the pattern of welfare state review—including health policy—over the past three decades across the industrialized world. But there still remains the question of why these pressures gave rise to increased attention to other national experiences.

Pressures for policy change increase the demand for new ideas—or at least new means to old ends. Rudolf Klein once argued "no one wants to be caught wearing yesterday's ideas."[4] Everywhere, policy makers and analysts looked across the border to search for the latest policy fashion. Just as American reformers turned to Canada, many Canadian, German, Dutch, and other intellectual entrepreneurs reviewed recent American, Swiss, and Swedish experience. In the 1990s, many conferences followed this pattern. International conferees were interested in getting better policy answers to the problems they faced at home. Many were explicit about cross-border learning: how to find a balance between "solidarity and subsidiary?" How to maintain a "high quality health system in times of economic stress?" Even the optimistic search for "optimum relations between patients, insurers, providers, and the government?"

Understood as simply wanting to stretch ones mind—to explore what is possible conceptually, or what others have managed to achieve—these questions are useful. This is the kind of learning anthropologists have long extolled—understanding the range of possible options and seeing one's own circumstances more clearly by contrast. But as a simple search for the best model—like shopping abroad for the best answer to problems back home—this is wishful thinking.

What about drawing policy lessons from international experience? What are the rules of cross-national learning? The truth is that, whatever the appearances, most policy debates in most countries are (and will remain) parochial affairs. They address national problems, they emphasize national developments in the particular domain (pensions, medical finance, transportation), and embody conflicting visions of what policies the particular country should adopt. Only occasionally are the experiences of other nations—and the lessons they embody—seriously examined. When cross-national experiences are employed in such parochial struggles, their use is typically that of policy warfare, not policy understanding and careful lesson-drawing. And, one must add, there are few knowledgeable critics at home of ideas about "solutions" abroad.

In the world of American medical debate, the misuse of British and Canadian experience surely illustrates this point. The National Health Service was from the late 1940s the specter of what "government medicine" or "socialized medicine" and "rationing" could mean. In recent years, mythmaking about Canada has dominated the distortion league in North America. The reasons are obvious. Policy makers are busy with day-to-day pressures. Practical concerns incline them, if they take the time for comparative inquiry, to pay more attention to what appears to work, not academic reasons for what is and is not transferable and why. Policy debaters— whether politicians, policy analysts or interest group figures—are in struggles, not seminars. Like lawyers, they seek victory, not illumination. For that purpose, compelling stories, whether well-substantiated or not, are more useful than careful conclusions. Interest groups, as their label suggests, have material and symbolic stakes in policy outcomes, not reputations for intellectual precision to protect.

Once generated and communicated, however, health policy ideas are adopted more readily in some contexts than in others. These patterns of adoption and adaptation have to do with the machinery of government, as well as with local cultural understandings. The autonomy and authority of government in parliament in the United Kingdom, for example, as well as its position at the apex of a nationalized health service, means that, "ideas can make a difference more quickly in Britain than in America."[5] It may be, too, that policy ideas transfer more easily between similar types of health systems. Institutional similarity—facilitated the spread of managed competition among the national health services of northern and southern Europe.[6]

However, lessons from abroad often meet strong local cultural resistance. Globalization may be putting economic pressure on social programs, as Giaimo and Manow observe, but even a quick look at the political response makes it clear that "the national markets for ideas" have yet to be fully liberalized.[7] Morone similarly remarks of Canada's experience with universal health insurance:

It is difficult to imagine a lesson that is more foreign to the American experience. Instead of hard conscious choices, we have sought painless automatic solutions. Rather than explicit programmatic decisions Americans prefer hidden, implicit policies. Rather than centralize control in governmental hands, we would scatter it across many players. In short the Canadian lessons . . . are not just different— they challenge the central features of American political culture, at least as they have manifested themselves in health care policy.[8]

It is not clear, then, whether what matters most is administrative infrastructure or national values and assumptions. Different systems operate with different organizational rules. And perhaps more important, different national policy communities—however well networked internationally—simply see problems differently.[9]

PURPOSE, PROMISE, AND PERILS OF COMPARATIVE INQUIRY IN HEALTH POLICY

Comparative analysis in health policy can serve various purposes: learning about national health arrangements and how they operate, learning why they take the forms they do, and learning policy lessons from those analyses. Much of the comparative commentary on health care neither clarifies the different modes of comparison nor addresses the difficulties of drawing policy lessons from the experience of other countries.

First, there is the goal of learning about health policy abroad. Comparative work of this sort can illuminate and clarify national arrangements without addressing causal explanation or seeking policy transplantation. Its comparative element remains for the most part implicit: in reading (or writing) about them, we make sense of other systems by contrasting them with our own. The process of learning entails, a deeper appreciation of something familiar by contrasting it what it is like or unlike. This is the gift of perspective.

The second purpose served by comparison is to generate causal explanations without necessarily seeking policy transplantation: that is, learning why policies develop as they do. Many of the historical and developmental studies of health care fall into this category. This approach uses cross-national inquiry to check on the adequacy of nation-specific accounts. Let us call that a defense against explanatory provincialism. Many different things may seem decisive in explaining why country A adopted a policy. How do we know if a feature is truly decisive as opposed to simply present? One answer is to look for similar outcomes elsewhere. Do the same factors seem to drive country B to the same policy? Or are those apparently "decisive" factors in country A missing or configured differently in country B?

An example from North American health policy provides a good illustration of how and how not to proceed. Some policy makers and academics in North America regard universal health insurance as incompatible with American values. They rest their case in part on the belief that Canada enacted health insurance and the United States has not because North American values are sharply different. In short, they attribute a different outcome to a different political culture in the United States. In fact, the values of Canada and the United States, while not identical, are actually quite similar.[10] Like siblings, differences are there, sure, but Canada's distribution of values is closer to that of the United States than any other modern, rich democracy. In fact, the value similarities between Western regions like British Columbia and Washington State are greater than

those between either of those jurisdictions and, say, New Brunswick or New Hampshire along the east coast. Similar values are compatible with different outcomes, which in turn draw ones attention to other institutional and strategic factors that distinguish Canadian from American experience with financing health care.[11] The important point is simply that comparing the United States and Canada give us explanatory checks that are unavailable by simply looking at one nation's history alone. Why doesn't the United States have national health insurance. The comparison with Canada is what tells us that culture alone is inadequate—we have to find other explanations.

The third category of work explicitly draws lessons from the policy experience of other nations. The international organizations which support policy work have this as part of their rationale. The World Health Organization, for example, is firmly in the business of selling "best practices." The OECD regularly produces extensive, expensive, hard to gather, statistical portraits of programs as diverse as disability and pensions, trade flows and the movement of professionals, education, and health care. No one can avoid using these studies, if only because the task of collecting data and discovering "the facts" in a number of countries is so daunting. But the portraiture that emerges requires its own very careful review. Even data as simple as "*health spending*" is full of hidden questions. What Germany spends on spas may count as public health expenditure; in the United States it would, of course, fall under an entirely different category. Often the same words do not mean the same things. And different words may denote similar phenomena.

For now, it is enough to restate that looking carefully at the experience of other nations is a precondition for understanding why change takes place in one's own country. International experience can stretch the mind and offer us perspective on our own experience. It can help identify (or refute) causal explanations. And it can help generate policy lessons; this last category, however, must be approached carefully, with close attention to the many factors that shape the politics, the institutions, the culture, and even the definitions in another nation.

CONCLUSIONS

The last decades have seen a growing body of comparative study in health policy, but this growth was not matched by a growing understanding of the processes of policy learning from the experience of other countries. There is, in fact, little attention to methodological questions about this learning process.

The confluence of economic, demographic, and ideological factors that led to extensive debate about the future of the welfare state also created pressure to reform health care systems. Fiscal strains and declining political support for an active role of the state undermined support for welfare state expansion and that strain also affected health policy. There was, indeed, growing pressure to seek out new policy solutions abroad. That pressure also gave rise to a new body of research within national communities as well as international agencies like the World Bank, OECD, World Health Organization, and the European Union. However, to date most of that research consists of merely descriptive studies of health care systems and policy measures within national boundaries. The studies pay little attention to the question of what experience can be applied in another country under what circumstances. Institutional and cultural factors are important elements in the policy context as determinants of successful reception and implementation of ideas.

In practice, there is much mislearning and misrepresentation by omission. Policy makers and politicians feel pressured to change, but have little or no time (or willingness) to critically assess claims about policy experience across the border. Potentially, comparison can bring learning opportunities as other countries can serve as natural experiments, in particular when the policy contexts are similar. Some lessons apply across many different countries. Similar pressure can create opportunities for learning, and international organizations serve as platforms for debate and potential sources for comparative studies. Existing research largely ignores the important difference between the process of learning about other countries' experience, learning why certain change takes place, and drawing lessons from that experience. But the basic ingredients for improved policy learning are there: the statistical database, the first generation of descriptive country studies and the experience of academics and international organizations.

NOTES

1. For a longer, more fully annotated version of this article, see *Journal of Comparative Policy Analysis* 7 (4): 331–48, December 2005. ISSN 1387-6988 Print/1572-5448 Online/05/040331-18 ª2005, Taylor & Francis.
2. Klein, 1997.
3. Klein, 1988, pp 219–24.
4. Klein, 1996.
5. Marmor and Plowden, 1991, p 810.
6. Freeman, 1998.
7. Giaimo and Manow, 1997, p 197.
8. Morone, 1990.
9. Freeman, 1999.
10. Lipset, 1990.
11. White, 1995; Maioni, 1998.

REFERENCES

Freeman, R. 1998. "Competition in context: the politics of health care reform in Europe, International," *Journal for Quality in Health Care* 10 (5): 395–401.

—— 1999. "Policy transfer in the health sector." European Forum conference paper WS/35, Florence: European University Institute.

—— 2000. *The Politics of Health in Europe.* Manchester: Manchester University Press.

Giaimo, S., and P. Manow. 1997. "Institutions and ideas into politics: health care reform in Britain and Germany," C. Altenstetter and J.W. Bjorkman, Eds., *Health Policy Reform, National Variations and Globalization.* Basingstoke: Macmillan.

Klein, R. 1997. "Learning from others: shall the last be the first?," *Journal of Health Politics, Policy and Law* 22 (5): 1267–78.

—— 1996. Commentary at Second Annual Meeting of the Four Country Conference on Health Policy, Montebello, Canada.

Klein, R., and M. O'Higgins. 1988. "Defusing the crisis of the welfare state: a new interpretation," T.R. Marmor and J. Mashaw, Eds., *Social Security: Beyond the Rhetoric of Crisis.* Princeton, NJ: Princeton University Press.

Lipset, S.M. 1990. *Continental Divide: The Values and Institutions of the United States and Canada.* New York: Routledge.

Maioni, A. 1998. *Parting at the Crossroads: The Emergence of Health Insurance in the United States and Canada.* Princeton, NJ: Princeton University Press.

Marmor, T.R. 1994. "Patterns of fact and fiction in the use of the Canadian experience; and Implementation: making reform work," in *Understanding Health Care Reform.* New Haven, CT: Yale University Press, pp 179–94.

Marmor, T.R. 1993. "Understanding the welfare states: crisis, critics, and countercritics," *Critical Review* 7 (4): 461–77.

Marmor, T.R., and K.G.H. Okma. 2003. "Review essay: health care systems in transition," *Journal of Health Politics, Policy and Law* 28 (4): 747–55.

Marmor, T.R., and W. Plowden. 1991. "Rhetoric and reality in the international jet stream: the export to Britain from America of questionable ideas," *Journal of Health Politics, Policy and Law* 16 (4): 807–12.

Morone, J.A. 1990. "American political culture and the search for lessons from abroad," *Journal of Health Politics, Policy and Law* 15 (1): 129–43.

Report Four Country Conference. 1995. "Health care reforms and health care policies in the United States, Canada, Germany and the Netherlands," Amsterdam, February 23–25, The Hague: Ministry of Health, Welfare and Sports.

White, J. 1995. *Competing Solutions: American Health Care Proposals and International Experiences.* Washington DC: Brookings Institution.

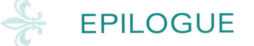

Health Politics and Policy: Issues and Challenges for the 21st Century

Leonard S. Robins

Health politics and policy for the last twenty years have been dominated by two major issues: trying to control constantly increasing health care costs, and reversing the trend in the ever growing number of persons without health insurance. Each of these has been extensively addressed in this volume and some final thoughts on them will be presented in the context of the discussion of national health insurance, which concludes the epilogue. First, however, let me reflect on some issues that health specialists often overlook.

Abortion and the right to die are also high on the nation's political agenda. Although their politics are more similar to "social" issues (like gay rights) rather than health issues, they deserve comment here. The politics of abortion has been a highly contentious national social issue since the *Roe v. Wade* decision in 1973. Although there is little likelihood of *Roe* being totally overturned, the bitter divisions it has

produced clearly remain—if anything, they have grown with time.

The issue of "death and dying" is likely to become an increasingly major political and policy issue as the percentage of elderly in the population increases. While seemingly identical to the abortion issue (except that it occurs at the other end of life) the politics of death and dying is in fact, somewhat different.

THE POLITICS OF ABORTION

Having an abortion requires, at a minimum, that a woman consider the following issues:

- whether or not she wants to have a baby
- the relative safety of having a baby as opposed to the risks of having an abortion

- the relative cost of having a baby as opposed to that of having an abortion
- possible legal penalties associated with having an abortion as opposed to those associated with having a baby

In China, the government encourages women in a variety of official and unofficial ways to have abortions if they have had one child and that child is still alive. The government of the United States has never encouraged abortion: Between the 1870s (before that date, abortions were common in the United States) and 1973, most of the states—the level of government that had primary policy responsibility for this issue—made abortions illegal except under certain limited (usually very limited) circumstances.

In 1973, the U.S. Supreme Court radically changed this in *Roe v. Wade*. It made all abortions legal in the first trimester of pregnancy, severely limited the right of the states to restrict abortions in the second trimester, and granted considerable discretion to states only in the last trimester. Since the vast majority of abortions occur in the first trimester, the Supreme Court essentially created a full right to an abortion.

Whether *Roe* was a wise legal decision is a matter of great dispute among scholars of constitutional law. There is more agreement, however, that since *Roe* has been the law of the land for over thirty years, the Supreme Court—even a more conservative Supreme Court —is unlikely to overturn *Roe* unless there is a massive shift in public opinion against abortion rights.

As a consequence of the *Roe* decision, those opposed to abortion rights have had to limit themselves to actions designed to "induce" women not to have an abortion and to incrementally "chip away" at *Roe*. These actions go far beyond mere persuasion. If, for example, physicians and hospitals are successfully pressured to not perform abortions, then a woman desiring to have one might reconsider because she feared the health consequences of a poorly performed abortion. Similarly, while abortions are much cheaper than pregnancies, Medicaid's refusal to pay for them means they are

more expensive to the woman and she may, therefore, decide to have a baby.

The political strength of the "pro-life" and "pro-choice" movements has varied over time. At least since the 1980s, however, there have been two constants. First, while opinion polls give a somewhat varying picture of public opinion, depending on how and when the questions are asked, the majority of the public has at times wanted to keep abortions legal in most of the circumstances under which they occur. However, the key to the strength of the pro-life movement is the greater intensity of feeling on the subject by pro-life supporters in contrast to those who are pro-choice. Second, while initial polls showed more Republican than Democratic support for *Roe*, the national Republican Party has been solidly against *Roe* since 1980 and the national Democratic Party has been solidly for abortion rights.

Given these political facts, there have been two basic strategies in the political struggle over abortion rights. First, pro-life activists have worked to elect pro-life candidates (usually Republican) and pro-choice activists have worked to elect pro-choice candidates (usually Democrats). Second, each side tends to emphasize those aspects of the issue where public opinion is most supportive of its position. Thus, pro-lifers stress such things as the need for parental notification and approval before an abortion is performed and opposition to "partial birth" abortions. Pro-choice activists, by contrast, are, for example, increasingly stressing the importance of birth control as a useful alternative to abortion, both because they believe this and because they know it splits the pro-life coalition, some of which opposes contraception as well as abortion.

The politics of abortion is also shaped, as are many other aspects of health politics and policy, by changes in science and technology. Pro-lifers will benefit from the fact that fetal viability will occur at an earlier and earlier period. Pro-choicers will benefit from developments like the "morning-after" pill and RU-486.

A current fascinating development is the extension of the abortion debate into the issue of stem cell research. Perhaps the pro-lifers will be lucky and ways will be found to obtain the hoped-for benefits of stem cell research in treating diabetes and other diseases through the use of adult stem cells. If not, they are likely to lose to those willing to trade the death of viable embryos for the potential health of a friend or loved one. The political fallout against the pro-life movement will become especially strong if it embraces the views of some of its activists in opposition to *in vitro* fertilization itself.

Republicans have dominated recent American politics—at least between 1994 and 2006, arguably since Ronald Reagan's election in 1980. Perhaps as a result, the pro-life movement has been politically stronger than the pro-choice movement. Conversely, perhaps the limited progress—even in some ways, retrogression—of the pro-life agenda during conservative and Republican domination suggests that, in the long run, it is doomed to fail.

THE POLITICS OF DEATH AND DYING

There are at least three different and, despite superficial similarities, quite distinct subjects that fall within the death and dying rubric: medical care at the end of life, physician-assisted suicide, and euthanasia.

Euthanasia will not be adopted anywhere in the United States in the near future. While many opponents of physician-assisted suicide argue that it will inevitably lead to euthanasia, and they may be right, the fact that euthanasia is so often and so successfully used as the ultimate pejorative suggests that it is politically untenable for the foreseeable future.

The reverse is true regarding medical care at the end of life. There is now overwhelming support for giving patients the right to refuse medical treatment. The most dramatic manifestation of our changed attitudes regarding end-of-life medical care is the evolution of public policy regarding living wills. Up until the mid-1980s, living wills were explicitly and consciously ignored by health providers

in the vast majority of states where they were not legally recognized. Today, by contrast, they are, for all practical purposes, legal and universally encouraged everywhere in the United States.

The controversy surrounding the death of Terri Schiavo, in 2005, illustrates this shift in attitudes. Those opposed to removing Ms. Schiavo's life support did not argue against following her wish to die, but rather contended that *they were doing what Terri wanted* in striving to keep her alive. The overwhelming reaction against Congressional intervention and the urgent effort of hundreds of thousands of people to obtain or clarify their living wills provide further testament to the growing consensus supporting the right to refuse treatment.

What accounts for this change in public policy? The growing longevity of our population coupled with the increased sophistication of end-of-life medical care provide the structured basis for everyone now being able to foresee friends, loved ones, or themselves facing these conditions. In my view, it is the desire of patients and their families to control end-of-life medical care decisions that is the driving force behind the movement giving patients and their surrogates the right to deny care that in fact often delays death more than prolong life.

While many physicians support a health care approach that emphasizes pain alleviation and patient autonomy rather than delaying death, many others view their primary imperative as saving life and consider a patient's death as a "defeat." Trends in medical education coupled with growth in the hospice movement are likely to result, however, in growing acceptance of patient choice in end-of-life decision-making and, when the choice is necessary, to favor pain alleviation rather than death delay.

Many of the groups supporting patient autonomy in end-of-life decisions do not, however, support physician-assisted suicide. To my knowledge, all or nearly all major religions in the Untied States oppose physician-assisted suicide. The hospice movement opposes physician-assisted suicide in the belief that effective hospice care, stressing effective pain control and bonding with patients, eliminates all the reasons for suicide, except for depression, which itself is a clinically treatable condition. Finally, the American Medical Association and the vast majority of physicians in the United States officially and publicly oppose physician-assisted suicide.

At the time of this writing, physician-assisted suicide is only legal in one state (Oregon) and is being challenged in the Supreme Court for violating federal law opposing physician-assisted suicide.

While the outcome of the case is unknowable at this time, it really is just another illustration that as individuals and as a society, we are conflicted in our attitudes toward physician-assisted suicide. To the extent that physician-assisted suicide appears to be equivalent to euthanasia, we oppose it. Conversely, when it appears similar to patient choice in end-of-life treatment, we support it.

What will happen in the future? In the short run, the most probable outcome is a continuation of current trends. Specifically, physician-assisted suicide is likely to remain illegal, but will also be performed more frequently, though still rarely, on a de facto basis without punishment.

A long-range prediction is, of course, highly speculative. Nonetheless, to this author it seems on balance likely that physician-assisted suicide will become much more acceptable over time. The main reason is that the argument that "big government" should not be allowed to interfere with the doctor-patient relationship is likely to provide ultimately persuasive in the most libertarian country in the world.

THE POLITICS OF NATIONAL HEALTH INSURANCE

When I first began to study health politics and policy in 1969, national health insurance appeared to be an idea whose time had come and its enactment seemed almost inevitable by the mid 1970s. Today, the reasons for it are even more compelling but its enactment seems further away than ever.

This book has presented overwhelming evidence that costs have and will continue to escalate and the number of uninsured and underinsured has and will continue to grow under the current structure of our health care system. Therefore, rather than once again making the case for why national health insurance could and probably would lower overall (public and private) health care costs while obviously increasing access to health care, my focus here will be first, on understanding why it has been so hard to enact national health insurance and second, offering some thoughts—a complete strategy is beyond the scope of our epilogue and the capacity of the author—for overcoming the opposition to national health insurance.

First, those interest groups currently opposed to national health insurance are much stronger than those supporting it. Organized labor is the primary interest group supporting national health insurance. While some argue that unions whose members have particularly good health coverage have been lukewarm in their support, the more important problem for supporters of national health insurance is that the union movement—sadly, in the author's view—is weaker today than at any time since before the presidency of Franklin Delano Roosevelt.

The American Medical Association (the nation's largest physician organization) and the Health Insurance Association of America (representing small health insurers) have and will continue to oppose national health insurance. It is important to always remember that, as Chapter 22 put it, one person's cost containment is another person's income reduction. Therefore, while medical care cost increases elicit growing concern among policy experts and fear and anger among the public, they also paradoxically increase the stake of vested interests in the preservation of the status quo and their willingness to go to great lengths to defend it. Thus, while former President Clinton devoted great time and energy to promoting his national health insurance plan, his efforts were dwarfed by the resources devoted by the Health Insurance Association of America and the National Federation of Independent Businesses (small businesses, often and increasing typically not providing health insurance) to opposing it.

It might, at first glance, seem that businesses not providing insurance to their employees would especially benefit from national health insurance, but this is incorrect. Not providing health insurance gives them a cost advantage over their big business competitors—who are increasingly weighed down by costs. Moreover, when a small business's employees receive uncompensated care from health providers, it is actually paid out of higher billings to those who are insured, i.e., their big business competitors!

Surely, one would think, big business can easily be persuaded to support national health insurance. Going beyond the labor-liberal base and achieving business support was the control political strategy of the Clinton administration in its efforts to achieve national health insurance. Unfortunately, as discussed in Chapter 13, this effort was poorly managed and probably fundamentally flawed.

The understandable anti-government ideology of business and its fear of setting a precedent by supporting government control and regulations is likely to mean that the neutrality of business is the best national health insurance advocates can hope for.

A more likely ally would be the provider community. For decades, health professionals fought the idea of losing power to government only to see control over medicine transferred to the market. It is not at all clear that either health professionals' interests or their ideology make market power preferable to government power—on the contrary, they fought long and hard against one perceived threat (government) only to lose power and autonomy to an entirely unexpected party (the market—corporations, payers, and managed care).

It must be admitted that the provider community (medical students and nurses being an exception) has shown little interest in supporting any national health insurance program that has effective cost-containment provisions. Whether they would be willing to accept compromise national health insurance proposals from a labor-liberal coalition seeking a true alliance is unknown. Unfortunately, however, it

has not been tried since each party has viewed the other as its primary enemy in medical care politics and policy. This may have been true in the past, but it is surely no longer true today.

The second major obstacle to national health insurance is public opinion. In Chapter 11, Brodie and Blendon demonstrate that when public opinion is carefully analyzed, it is much less supportive of major change than many politicians and policy experts realize. In earlier pieces, Robert Blendon has shown that when publics evaluate their medical systems, the United States ranks highest on dissatisfaction. On the surface, this would seem to be an argument for change. However, for purposes of political change, comparative dissatisfaction is irrelevant. The big issue is whether the public in any given country is relatively satisfied or dissatisfied with their medical care system. Moreover, those who are relatively satisfied tend to have higher social status and income and thus greater political influence than those who are relatively dissatisfied.

Two things will be necessary to overcome the public's fears concerning national health insurance. First, any proposal should be designed as simply as possible and analogized to popular programs with which the public is familiar. Thus, if one advocates a single-payer system, it should be described as "Medicare for all Americans" (or, simply, "Medicare for all") rather than the "Canadian system."

Second, it should be recognized that any new proposal will need considerable time to "sink in" with the public and become increasingly acceptable to it. It took Medicare eight years to move from introduction to passage and any specific national health insurance proposal is likely to take as long.

Unfortunately, supporters of national health insurance bitterly fight over their respective versions of national health insurance; they also constantly tinker and revise their plans in the mistaken belief that "one more technical improvement is the key to victory." How supporters can be united around one basic approach—and stick to it— is not clear to me. But it is one key to political success. Enacting a plan and then, if necessary, modifying it is far preferable to the continual struggles over comparative plan strengths and weaknesses. That leads, inevitably, to nothing ever getting done.

One final point. As we saw in Chapters 5 and 14, the key to winning Medicare was the election of an overwhelmingly Democratic (and liberal) congress and president. The issue of Medicare helped get them elected, but it was not the main reason for their election. It was *after* the passage of Medicare, as Brandon and Alt note in Chapter 18, that the elderly became a more conscious and cohesive interest group. Perhaps national health insurance will also have to wait for a political climate conducive to major health reform, but it will powerfully redound to the political benefit of those who are responsible for its enactment.

INDEX